COGNITIVE-BEHAVIORAL INTERVENTIONS IN EDUCATIONAL SETTINGS

A Handbook for Practice

3rd Edition

Edited by
Ray W. Christner, Psy.D., NCSP, ABPP and
Rosemary B. Mennuti

Routledge
Taylor & Francis Group
NEW YORK AND LONDON

Designed cover image: ©Getty

Third edition published 2025
by Routledge
605 Third Avenue, New York, NY 10158

and by Routledge
4 Park Square, Milton Park, Abingdon, Oxon, OX14 4RN

Routledge is an imprint of the Taylor & Francis Group, an informa business

Second edition published by Routledge 2012

Library of Congress Cataloging-in-Publication Data
Names: Christner, Ray W., 1972– editor. | Mennuti, Rosemary B., 1947– editor.
Title: Cognitive-behavioral interventions in educational settings : a handbook for practice / Edited by Ray W. Christner, Psy.D., NCSP, ABPP, Rosemary B. Mennuti.
Identifiers: LCCN 2024027248 (print) | LCCN 2024027249 (ebook) | ISBN 9781032491677 (hardback) | ISBN 9781032491660 (paperback) | ISBN 9781003392439 (ebook)
Subjects: LCSH: School psychology—Handbooks, manuals, etc. | Cognitive therapy for children—Handbooks, manuals, etc. | Behavior modification—Handbooks, manuals, etc.
Classification: LCC LB1027.55 .C63 2025 (print) | LCC LB1027.55 (ebook) | DDC 370.15/28—dc23/eng/20240626
LC record available at https://lccn.loc.gov/2024027248
LC ebook record available at https://lccn.loc.gov/2024027249

ISBN: 978-1-032-49167-7 (hbk)
ISBN: 978-1-032-49166-0 (pbk)
ISBN: 978-1-003-39243-9 (ebk)

DOI: 10.4324/9781003392439

Typeset in Times New Roman
by codeMantra

Access Support Material: http://www.routledge.com/9781032491677

COGNITIVE-BEHAVIORAL INTERVENTIONS IN EDUCATIONAL SETTINGS

The thoroughly updated third edition of *Cognitive-Behavioral Interventions in Educational Settings* offers readers a way to think strategically about individual students and plan for effective interventions based on the student's age, developmental level, and presenting problem.

Written in a forward-thinking manner, this volume presents evidence-based interventions and offers both innovative and well-established approaches to working with children and adolescents in a school setting. This book begins by establishing foundational skills that provide updated information on cognitive behavior therapy (CBT) and a framework for working with youth and addresses timely issues such as schoolwide approaches to intervention, brief care models, ethnicity and race, and wellness programs. The second part of this volume uses CBT to explore strategies for building relationships, assessment, intervention, progress monitoring, and more. Case studies and specific techniques are provided throughout each chapter.

Cognitive-Behavioral Interventions in Educational Settings provides a complete overview for effective practice using CBT in schools.

Ray W. Christner, PsyD, NCSP, ABPP, is a licensed psychologist in Pennsylvania, a nationally certified school psychologist, and a nationally registered health service psychologist. He is board certified in behavioral and cognitive psychology.

Rosemary B. Mennuti, EdD, NCSP, is a professor emerita and former director of School Psychology Programs in the Department of Psychology at the Philadelphia College of Osteopathic Medicine.

We dedicate this book to Dr. Arthur Freeman, whose guidance and belief in us resulted in the early editions of this work. His mentorship is not only reflected in these pages, but in our continued growth and collaboration on many projects. Though Dr. Freeman's voice has fallen silent, his influence continues in our work. This revised edition is not only a tribute to the knowledge he has imparted but also a testament to the enduring legacy of his mentorship.

– Ray W. Christner and Rosemary B. Mennuti

CONTENTS

CONTRIBUTORS

Kathryn Arcari, PsyD, is a licensed psychologist and clinical neuropsychologist in New Jersey with over 18 years of experience working with children and adolescents in various settings.

Justin Ayoub, PsyD, is a licensed psychologist and certified school psychologist. He works as a school psychologist, has a part-time private practice, and is an adjunct instructor at Adelphi University.

Samantha Baker is a clinical psychology doctoral student at the Philadelphia College of Osteopathic Medicine and a clinician at the Temple University Child and Adolescent Anxiety Clinic.

Jacqueline Blass, PhD, is a research fellow at the University of Massachusetts, Amherst.

Jessica Bolton Petronis, PsyD, NCSP, is a school psychologist and licensed psychologist in Pennsylvania. She serves students in the Cumberland Valley School District.

Caroline L. Boxmeyer, PhD, is Associate Dean for Academic and Faculty Affairs in the College of Community Health Sciences at The University of Alabama and Professor in the Department of Psychiatry and Behavioral Medicine.

Hannah Brimkov, MEd, is a doctoral candidate in the PhD Program in School Psychology of Indiana University of Pennsylvania.

Ray W. Christner, PsyD, NCSP, ABPP, is a licensed psychologist, a certified school psychologist, and an elected fellow of the Association of Behavioral Cognitive Therapies (ABCT). He is the president of Cognitive Health Solutions in Pennsylvania.

Celenia L. DeLapp, PhD, received her doctorate from The Catholic University of America. She is a clinical psychology intern at Montefiore Medical Center.

Ryan C. T. DeLapp, PhD, is a child and adolescent psychologist who treats anxiety, depression, and cultural stress in children, adolescents, and young adults. He is the director of The REACH Program at The Ross Center.

Diana M. Diaków, PhD, NCSP, is a multilingual psychologist, psychotraumatologist, and trauma therapist, renowned for her research focused on trauma, resilience, and culturally responsive mental health.

Randolph Dupont, PhD, is a doctoral student at the University of Nevada, Las Vegas.

Chuck Emig, EdS, NCSP, is a school psychologist in the Cumberland Valley School District (PA) serving students in elementary and high school.

Sarah Fefer, PhD, is a professor and Associate Director of the Center for Youth Engagement and Associate Dean for Research and Faculty Development at the University of Massachusetts, Amherst.

Eva L. Feindler, PhD, is Co-Director of Clinical Training and Professor of Psychology at Long Island University Post. She specializes in cognitive-behavioral interventions with children and adolescents, anger management, and clinical supervision/mentorship.

Michael Fensken, M.A., is a doctoral student in the clinical psychology program at the University of Nevada, Las Vegas.

Amanda Guld Fisher, PhD, BCBA-D, is a certified behavior analyst (doctoral level) and is currently an associate professor in the School of Professional and Applied Psychology at the Philadelphia College of Osteopathic Medicine.

Emily S. Fisher, PhD, is a professor in the Department of Specialized Programs in Professional Psychology at Loyola Marymount University in Los Angeles, CA. Dr. Fisher has published extensively on school-based supports for LGBTQ youth.

Elizabeth A. Gosch, PhD, ABPP, is a professor of Psychology at the Philadelphia College of Osteopathic Medicine and Lead Clinical Supervisor at the Temple University Child and Adolescent Anxiety Clinic. Her research and publications focus on anxiety in youth.

Barbara Katic, PhD, is an assistant professor at Loyola Marymount University. She earned her PhD in school psychology from the University of California Riverside, Riverside, CA.

Christopher A. Kearney, PhD, is Distinguished Professor and Chair of Psychology at the University of Nevada, Las Vegas. He is also the director of the UNLV Child School Refusal and Anxiety Disorders Clinic.

Jessica Glass Kendorski, PhD, NCSP, BCBA-D, is a licensed psychologist in Pennsylvania, and maintains certifications as a board certified behavior analyst (BCBA). She is Depart Chair and Director of the MS and Certificate Programs.

Courtney L. Leone, PhD, NCSP, is a professor in the Psychology Department at Indiana University of PA. She directs the PhD Program in School Psychology.

Sarah Liberti, BA, is pursuing her doctorate in school psychology at Adelphi University.

John E. Lochman, PhD, ABPP, is the Saxon professor emeritus of Psychology at The University of Alabama and a senior fellow in the Alabama Life Research Institute. He is the recipient of numerous awards for his work.

Kristen E. Mahony, PhD, is a postdoctoral scholar at the University of South Florida College of Education.

James J. Mazza, PhD, is a professor in the School Psychology Program at the University of Washington. His current research focus is centered around the implementation of a universal emotion regulation SEL curriculum *DBT STEPS-A*.

Rosemary B. Mennuti, EdD, NCSP, is a professor emerita and former director and founder of School Psychology Programs at the Philadelphia College of Osteopathic Medicine. She has presented nationally and written numerous books and articles on the use of CBT.

Dana Milakovic, PsyD, is a mental wellness and trauma specialist at the Pennsylvania Department of Education. She is certified as a cognitive behavioral therapist and school psychologist.

David N. Miller, PhD, is a professor in the School Psychology Program at the University at Albany (SUNY). He is Past President of the American Association of Suicidology and the author of numerous publications.

Laura W. Monahon, PsyD, is a licensed psychologist in New Jersey and a certified school psychologist. She specializes in using CBT to treat a variety of emotional and psychological concerns across the lifespan.

Christy A. Mulligan, PsyD, is an assistant professor in School Psychology in the Derner School of Psychology at Adelphi University. She also serves as Assistant Editor for the New York Association of School Psychologists (NYASP) newsletter.

Julia Ney is a doctoral student in clinical psychology at Temple University and a clinician at the Temple University Child and Adolescent Anxiety Disorders Clinic.

Nicole P. Powell, PhD, MPH, is a research psychologist at the University of Alabama's Center for Youth Development and Intervention. She has played influential roles in conceptualizing and conducting intervention research, including with the Coping Power Program.

Kristina Puzino Lenker, PhD, is an assistant professor in the Department of Psychiatry & Behavioral Health of Penn State College of Medicine as well as a clinical psychologist specializing in Behavioral Sleep Medicine at Penn State Health Sleep Research & Treatment Center.

Dawn M. Richards, PhD, is a Clinical Assistant Professor, Fieldwork Coordinator, School Psychology Program in the Department of Specialized Programs in Professional Psychology at Loyola Marymount University in Los Angeles, CA.

Meghann Sallee, PhD, is a staff psychologist in the Couples and Family Clinic in the Orlando VA health system and Clinical Assistant Professor in the Psychiatry Department at Nova Southeastern University's Dr. Kiran C. Patel College of Osteopathic Medicine.

Salma Siddiqui, PhD, is Dean of the School of Social Sciences and Humanities at the National University of Sciences & Technology, Islamabad, Pakistan and professor and the founding chair of the Department of Behavioral Sciences.

Jessica L. Stewart, PsyD, is a clinical psychologist in Providence, Rhode Island, who specializes in working with adolescents, adults, and families.

Sara L. Stromeyer, PhD, is a licensed clinical psychologist who specializes in treatment of children and adolescents. Dr. Stromeyer is primarily focused on clinical practice with The Birmingham Psychology Group and teaches and collaborates on research projects.

Dr. Shannon M. Suldo, PhD, is a professor of School Psychology and a licensed psychologist at the University of South Florida. Her research interests are in positive psychology and how they relate to children and adolescents.

Katy Tresco, PhD, is an associate professor and director of the PsyD Program in School Psychology at the Philadelphia College of Osteopathic Medicine (PCOM).

Hilary B. Vidair, PhD, is the program director and an associate professor in the Clinical Psychology Doctoral Program at LIU Post. She is specialized in CBT for children and adolescents, behavioral parent training, and dialectical behavior therapy (DBT).

Sally M. Weinstein, PhD, is Associate Professor of Clinical Psychology in the Department of Psychiatry at the University of Illinois at Chicago, with a specialization in pediatric mood disorders.

Amy E. West, PhD, is Professor of Clinical Pediatrics, Psychology, and Psychiatry & the Behavioral Sciences and Director of the Child Clinical and Pediatric Psychology Internship at Children's Hospital Los Angeles/Keck School of Medicine at the University of Southern California.

PART I

Building Foundations

1

BUILDING A FOUNDATIONAL FRAMEWORK OF COGNITIVE-BEHAVIOR THERAPY (CBT) IN SCHOOLS

Ray W. Christner and Rosemary B. Mennuti

In today's society, we are currently facing a mental health crisis, and we hear about the challenges people experience on a daily basis (The White House, 2023). Since the first edition of this book, there have been many changes in the field of school-based mental health—both positive and concerning. On a positive note, research and social movements have increased the acceptance of mental health treatment, offered new and innovative ideas to help marginalized groups, and expanded the training in and dissemination of evidence-based interventions. However, the rate of mental health concerns surrounding youth has continued to rise and intensify over the years (Phillips & Yu, 2021). In addition, societal complexities, such as the COVID-19 pandemic, school shootings, social media and excessive device use, the political divide in America, and the continued stressors on families and schools, have resulted in disconnection and increased isolation. This change in connection, which is a basic human need, has manifested in increased rates of anxiety, depression, suicide, anger, aggression, functional changes, and, at times, even further isolation. Subsequently, the prevalence of mental health concerns has accelerated at alarming rates (Bell et al., 2023).

Along with these difficulties remains the longstanding challenge of accessing appropriate mental health treatment for youth (Kuehn, 2022; Shidhaye, 2023). This has placed even a larger emphasis on the need for school-based mental health. Schools remain a promising setting to provide efficient, connecting, and evidence-based care that overcomes other barriers that prevent intervention. When we wrote the first edition of this book, there were few resources available on applying cognitive-behavior therapy (CBT) in schools. However, because of the need and effectiveness of CBT in schools, there have been a number of excellent resources developed (see Creed et al., 2011; Joyce-Beaulieu & Sulkowski, 2015; Joyce-Beaulieu & Zaboski, 2021; Mendez, 2016).

This has prompted us also to rethink our approach and revise *Cognitive-Behavioral Interventions in Educational Settings: A Handbook for Practice*. This revision has been an exciting process for us, as we have drawn upon our experiences over the years working with children, training professionals, offering supervision, and collaborating with others. In this edition, we continue to highlight the growing body of research and literature on the effectiveness of CBT with children and adolescents. However, it was important for us to take this book further and increase school-based clinicians' awareness of integrating CBT with relational-cultural theory (see Miller & Stiver, 1997). The idea of ensuring that we remain focused on students within the context of connection and providing the skill-building

 DOI: 10.4324/9781003392439-2

interventions of CBT is the driving force behind this book. In other chapters, you will find information on working with specific populations and issues, including examples of evidence-based practices and programs. Still, here, we will present our approach to benefit the well-being of children and adolescents with a relational CBT approach.

Evidence-Based Practice of CBT

Those working in mental health and education continue to hear about the need to provide "evidence-based" interventions and services. Within mental health literature, CBT is one approach that has continually proven to be effective and efficacious for a variety of mental health concerns with children and adolescents (Chorpita & Wisz, 2009; Weisz & Kazdin, 2010). The efficacy of CBT in treating a range of psychological disorders in children and adolescents is well-documented. Meta-analytic studies demonstrate that CBT is effective for conditions such as anxiety disorders, depression, and externalizing problems, among others. For instance, James et al. (2020) found that CBT significantly reduced symptoms of anxiety and depression in adolescents when compared to control groups. Similarly, research by Riise and colleagues (2021) underscored the effectiveness of CBT in addressing externalizing problems in children, noting significant improvements in behavior and social functioning.

Although much of the research on CBT with youth has been in clinical settings, we are now seeing a growing body of literature regarding its application and effectiveness in schools (Chui et al., 2013; Werner-Seidler et al., 2021). This research has been promising, supporting the use of CBT in the increasing school-based mental health movement. Moreover, because of its time-limited and skill-based approach, CBT is a natural fit within schools, resulting in it being more accepted by other educational professionals. Because of its natural fit within the educational model, research has found that school professionals, even with minimal training, can effectively identify students appropriate for CBT interventions (Choi et al., 2022).

Manual vs. Transdiagnostic Approaches

When implementing CBT with children and adolescents, therapists may choose between manualized interventions and transdiagnostic interventions. Manualized interventions involve structured, session-by-session guidelines, clearly defined procedures, and specific activities that are often disorder-specific. Many of these programs are highlighted throughout chapters within this book, including *Coping Cat* (Kendall & Hedtke, 2006), *Coping Power* (Lochman, et al., 2008), and *Adolescent Coping with Depression Course* (Clarke et al., 1999), to name a few. These are designed to ensure fidelity to the treatment model and are highly effective in research settings where control over variables is essential. However, in clinical practice, such rigidity can be limited, as young clients often present with comorbid conditions or unique circumstances that may not fit neatly into a single diagnostic category. Because of this, there has been a greater shift and emphasis on using flexibility and building connections with individuals while still delivering the interventions with fidelity. For an excellent reference, see Phillip Kendall's (2021) book, *Flexibility within Fidelity: Breathing Life into a Psychological Treatment Manual.*

In contrast, transdiagnostic interventions represent a more flexible approach. These interventions target common underlying processes across different disorders, such as emotion regulation or cognitive distortions, rather than focusing on disorder-specific symptoms. This approach is gaining popularity due to its flexibility, efficiency, and potential for broader applicability, including its use in schools. As with manualized programs, transdiagnostic approaches share strong support for their effectiveness (Qanbari Alaee et al., 2022). However, the use of transdiagnostic approaches has a targeted focus on the higher rate of occurrence of different disorders, such as anxiety and depression (Brown & Barlow, 2009). Within transdiagnostic approaches, two sub-approaches should be discussed—unified and modular.

Unified Approach

The unified approach, such as the *Unified Protocol for the Treatment of Emotional Disorders in Children and Adolescents* (Ehrenreich-May & Kennedy, 2021), is a single, comprehensive treatment designed to address multiple disorders simultaneously. It is based on the premise that various psychological disorders share common underlying factors. While the strategies used still have the structure and step-by-step processes seen with manual intervention, there is greater flexibility in how the interventions are applied to an individual. By focusing on these shared elements, the unified approach aims to treat the underlying processes common in coexisting disorders in a cohesive, streamlined manner. Research has shown that unified approaches can be particularly beneficial for clients with multiple comorbid conditions (van Doorn et al., 2023; Schniering & Rapee, 2020).

Modular Approach

On the other hand, modular approaches, such as the *Modular Approach to Therapy for Children with Anxiety, Depression, Trauma, or Conduct Problems* (MATCH-ADTC; Chorpita & Wisz, 2009), consist of various modules, each targeting specific symptoms or processes. Therapists can tailor the intervention by selecting relevant modules based on the individual needs of the child or adolescent. This approach offers high flexibility, allowing therapists to adapt the treatment to the client's unique profile of symptoms and changing needs throughout therapy. It is important with modular approaches that clinicians select interventions based on a solid case conceptualization. Studies have found modular approaches to be highly effective, including in community settings where client presentations are diverse (Harmon et al., 2021; Weisz et al., 2020).

The choice between manualized and transdiagnostic interventions (whether unified or modular) should be guided by the individual needs of the child or adolescent, the clinician's expertise, and the intervention setting. Each of these approaches can have value within the school setting to meet the needs of students. While manualized interventions offer the benefit of a structured, evidence-based framework, transdiagnostic approaches, both unified and modular, provide the flexibility needed to address the diverse and often complex presentations seen in practice. As research progresses, these interventions will likely become increasingly nuanced, enhancing the ability of therapists to provide effective, personalized treatment to this population.

Multidirectional Approach to CBT Formulation

In working with individuals using a multidirectional approach, it is understood that emotions and behaviors are influenced by a combination of reasons that interface and form a dynamic of their own. CBT formulation is often described as "activating event/situation," "belief/thought," and "consequence/behavior." While this view can be helpful, our experiences have been that, in most cases, the process is not linear, following a simple cause-and-effect pattern. We see the theoretical formulation as more of a dynamic process including four interacting elements—social, cognitive, affective/physiological, and behavioral, which are illustrated in Figure 1.1. Our approach brings to life the theoretical formulation, using knowledge of CBT research and the individual to serve as a lens through which the child's areas of concern are fully understood. Each of these elements interacts in a complex, multidirectional way to create a unique picture of the child's experience.

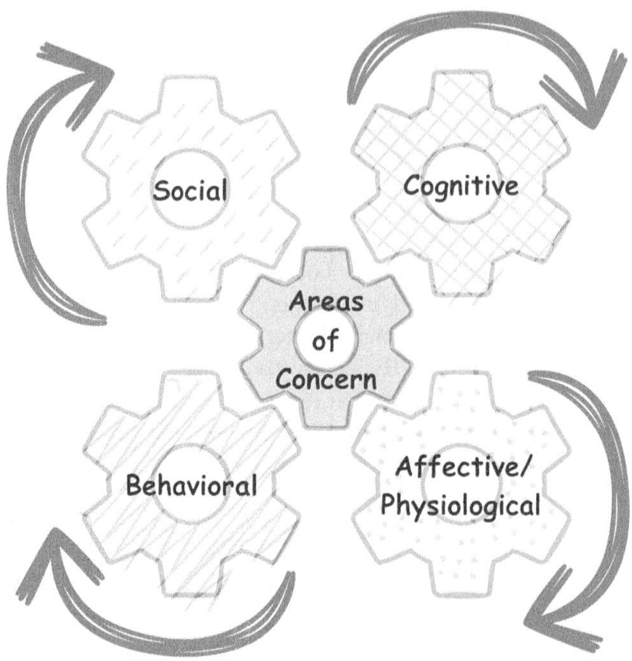

Figure 1.1 Multidirectional Interaction of Factors in CBT

In practice, we may see two children with the same presenting concerns, yet their stories and the underlying factors driving their experience will be very different. It is through this multidirectional lens that we can develop an individualized and effective approach to treatment. Each of these four elements discussed can be an entryway to start the treatment process. For some children, we might need to rely more heavily on behavioral interventions at first, whereas for others, our initial focus might be on social or cognitive factors. By examining each of these, we open a door for numerous possibilities to select interventions or components of practice tailored to the individual child. As we discuss each of these elements in detail, specific case examples will be provided.

Social Factors

In CBT, social factors are critical as they play a significant role in shaping an individual's cognitive processes and behaviors. This begins at an early age with initial attachment and develops through the lifespan. Very young children might focus on the relationship and connection with their parents; as they mature, the desire and need for peer interaction are more pronounced. The lack of meaningful connection can lead to a negative cognitive bias and create feelings of social isolation and loneliness. It is essential to remember that social isolation and loneliness are not merely emotional states but are deeply interconnected with cognitive patterns and well-being. Being isolated can lead to a host of negative health outcomes, which could present as somatic complaints, stomachaches, headaches, nausea, and heart racing. Research has shown that if this continues into adulthood, major health issues can then arise, such as cardiovascular conditions. In addition, isolation and loneliness can exacerbate mental health issues, hopelessness, antisocial behaviors, and impaired executive functioning. These then can lead to increased addictive behaviors, destructive behaviors, depression, anxiety, and risk of suicide and violence.

Conversely, positive social interactions can serve as a buffer against these adverse effects. This can build a sense of self-worth and a desire for more relationships. Not all individuals will need or want the same level of social interaction. For some, maybe they feel best with only a few close friends, whereas other individuals have a desire for many acquaintances and frequent interactions. As clinicians, we must not assume that a child is lonely because they have only a few friends; this might be "right" for them. In addition, not every child will want to be in a social activity every night; some may be content and happy with a mix of time alone and time with others. Our role as clinicians is to try to find the relational harmony that is best for each individual without imposing our or the parents' expectations on the child.

To highlight this, we use the term "connectedness prescription," which includes several dimensions: the personal nature of good interactions (where can they be themselves and feel comfortable), the frequency and intensity of connections (how often), the time spent in each interaction (how long), and the type of activities shared (what are they comfortable doing). Using this, you can work with individuals to determine the social needs most fitting for them.

Consider the case of Zareea, who is a 12-year-old girl attending a public school. She has a history of moving frequently, as her parents both work for the military. Although she possesses good social skills, making deeper connections is hard for her. She has attended her current middle school for about a year and has yet to develop a peer group. She has tried to enter different groups by changing her interests or engaging in behaviors that she thought would make her more popular. However, she continues to feel like an "outsider." Currently, she attempts to connect with others by "pushing herself" into conversations, resulting in her peers blatantly ignoring her and pushing her away. She becomes increasingly isolated and depressed, feeling she is inadequate. In our time with Zareea, we must understand and validate her, avoiding the risk of reinforcing her feelings of disconnection. If we start with teaching her "social skills" or "behavioral strategies" before understanding how her isolation is currently serving a protective role, she could see this as discounting her feelings and further increasing her isolation and feeling misunderstood. By taking time to understand her loneliness, we have an opportunity to tactfully see her contributions to her social difficulties and collaborate to develop a plan. This is not going to be moving straight to "having a best friend," but instead, it will involve a gradual movement toward improved interactions.

Cognitive

Cognitive factors play a pivotal role in CBT, influencing how individuals perceive and react to the world around them. CBT posits that an individual's thoughts can affect their feelings and behaviors, and by examining and modifying these thoughts, they can change how they feel and act. At the heart of these cognitive processes are automatic thoughts, intermediate beliefs, core beliefs, cognitive distortions, and cognitive deficiencies. Figure 1.2 illustrates the hierarchy and interactions of these different levels of cognition.

Automatic thoughts are the involuntary thoughts and images that immediately pop into one's mind in response to a situation. These thoughts are often habitual and reflexive, occurring without deliberate consideration or conscious awareness. These can be both positive and negative. In treatment, we often refer to positive and productive thoughts as "positive encouraging thoughts" (PETs) and negative thoughts as "automatic negative thoughts" (ANTs) or "junk thoughts." For instance, a student might automatically think, "I'm going to fail," when handed a test, reflecting a pattern of negative thinking without evidence.

Intermediate beliefs include the attitudes, rules, and assumptions those hold that influence how they interpret life's challenges and stressors. These beliefs are the "if-then," "must," and "should" statements we carry within us, such as, "I must be perfect, or then I'm a failure." These beliefs can shape our responses to difficult situations, often in ways that are not helpful.

Core beliefs are the deeply held beliefs people have about themselves, others, and the world. They are fundamental and generalized, often inflexible, and form the foundation upon which we interpret

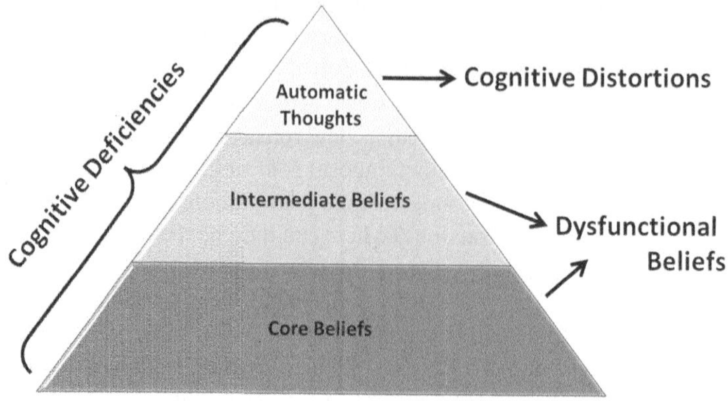

Figure 1.2 Levels of Cognition

Table 1.1 Examples of Cognitive Distortions

Dichotomous thinking—This is when an individual perceives situations in extremes without recognizing any middle ground or spectrum of possibilities. For example, a student might think, "If I'm not the best in my class, then I must be the worst."

Overgeneralization—This involves drawing broad, generalized conclusions from a single event. A new example could be, "I stumbled during my presentation, so I'm always going to be terrible at presenting in the classroom."

Mind reading—This is when an individual assumes they know what others are thinking without any concrete evidence. For example, "Everyone in this room must think I'm boring."

Emotional reasoning—Here, an individual lets their feelings dictate their perception of reality. For instance, "I feel nervous, so this must be an impossible test to pass."

Disqualifying the positive—This occurs when someone ignores or dismisses positive experiences or aspects, focusing only on the negative. For example, "I only got a compliment on my work because they were being polite, not because it was actually good."

Catastrophizing—This is when an individual anticipates the worst possible outcome and reacts to it as if it were a certainty. For example, "Alice did not say hello today; she truly doesn't like me."

Personalization—This involves attributing personal responsibility, including the blame for events outside the individual's control. For example, "My friend is upset today; it must be because of something I did."

Should/must statements—Rigid thinking patterns characterize this, using "should," "must," or "ought" to impose unrealistic expectations on oneself or others. For instance, "I should never feel tired or take breaks if I want to be the best."

Comparing—This involves measuring personal worth or abilities against others, often feeling inferior. For example, "Everyone else seems to manage their time better than me; I'm just not as smart."

Selective abstraction—This is focusing exclusively on a single negative detail and ignoring the broader context. An example could be, "I got one question wrong in the quiz; I must be really bad at this subject."

Labeling—This is when an individual assigns a global, negative label to themselves based on specific actions or events. For example, "I forgot to submit my homework; I'm such a disaster."

our experiences. For example, a core belief might be, "People can trust me" or "People cannot be trusted." These beliefs are formed and reinforced throughout life and, once engrained, can be difficult to change.

Cognitive distortions are inaccurate or irrational ways in which people process information, leading to misinterpretations of a situation or event. There are numerous cognitive distortions, and we provide examples of the more common ones seen in children and adolescents in Table 1.1.

Cognitive deficiencies refer to weaknesses in cognitive processing skills, such as problem-solving or impulse control. A student with cognitive deficiencies may act impulsively or struggle to focus attention, often leading to difficulties in both academic and social situations. There are times in which we might see a child have both cognitive distortions and deficiencies. For instance, a child who struggles to manage anger might be in a situation where they see other students laughing, and they have the automatic thought, "They're making fun of me." And, due to a lack of behavior inhibition skills, they react to this thought by punching one of the children in the group.

Dysfunctional beliefs act like negative filters, coloring the way an individual perceives and interprets their experiences. These are the beliefs that guide attention in a biased way, often leading to negative interpretations and emotions like anxiety and depression. These are seen when at the immediate and core belief level and are more deeply rooted negative thought patterns that are not just a reaction to a single situation. Often, these dysfunctional beliefs can be the driving force that leads to more frequent ANTs.

In the context of CBT, especially within schools, clinicians need to help children recognize and address these cognitive factors. By doing so, they can guide students toward acquiring improved cognitive and behavioral skills. This includes teaching strategies to challenge and modify unhelpful thoughts and beliefs, thus facilitating a change in cognitive processes and thinking patterns. Through CBT, children can learn to view situations more accurately, respond to challenges with more adaptive thought processes, and ultimately develop healthier patterns of behavior.

Affective/Physiological

When working with individuals, multiple factors interface that we must consider in how they respond. It is common for clinicians to discuss concepts related to "fight and flight" or "physiological arousal" when someone is upset. Often, this leads to interventions such as "take a deep breath" or "count from one to 10." However, the affective and physiological aspects related to well-being go beyond these simple concepts.

Damasio (2000) discusses the concept of *embodied cognition*, which posits that there is an inextricable link between one's rational thought processes and the emotions that manifest within the body. This theory suggests that emotional experiences are not just abstract concepts but are rooted in bodily sensations that influence cognitive processing. The body's responses to various stimuli are thus integral to understanding how individuals perceive and interact with the world. In CBT, this emphasizes the importance of acknowledging the individual's physical experiences as part of the cognitive framework, allowing for a more holistic approach to therapy that addresses both the mind and the body. When working with a student who is feeling depressed, we might work with them to position their body differently to see if it impacts their mood and cognitive response. Often, we employ the *Wonder Woman Pose*, discussed by Amy Cuddy (2016), as an example.

Equally important is the idea of *interoception*, a term detailed by Khalsa et al. (2018), which refers to the process by which the nervous system senses, interprets, and integrates signals from within the body, offering a continuous mapping of the body's internal landscape. This mapping occurs at both conscious and unconscious levels, affecting emotional regulation and perception. Clinicians using CBT can use the concept of interoception to help individuals become more attuned to their bodily sensations as they relate to their emotions, facilitating a greater understanding of their internal states. This awareness is crucial in helping individuals learn to manage and respond to their feelings more adaptively. For an individual who is processing through trauma, we work with them to understand the link and cognitive chain that is triggered by specific sensory experiences. For instance, how certain sounds that occur might result in them anticipating a series of negative events.

Table 1.2 Affective Primes in User-Friendly Language

Affective Primes	*Alternate Wording*
Rage (Anger)	Angry, Pissed Off, Frustrated, Explosive, and Rage
Panic/Grief (Sadness)	Sad, Depressed, Down, Blue, Lonely, and Grief
Fear (Anxiety)	Anxious, Nervous, Tense, Scared, Worried, and On Edge
Play (Social Joy)	Connected, Happy, Joyful, Fun, and Engaged
Seeking (Expectancy/Enthusiasm)	Excited, Enthusiastic, Hopeful, and Zestful
Lust (Sex)	Attracted, Desire, Wanting, and Longing For
Care (Nurturing/Loving)	Care, Love, Warm, Adoring, Concerned, and Affectionate

A theory that has been written about extensively, especially when working with trauma, is the *polyvagal theory* (Porges, 2009). This theory further expands the understanding of how the autonomic nervous system governs the body's response to stress and safety. It outlines a hierarchy within the autonomic nervous system that dictates our physiological state and, consequently, our behavioral responses. Clinicians may incorporate principles from polyvagal theory to help individuals recognize and shift their physiological states, which can lead to changes in their emotional and cognitive experiences. By doing so, individuals can develop strategies to engage their social engagement system and manage their fight, flight, or freeze responses more effectively. For example, for a student who struggles to manage anger and a "fight" response, we work with them to use diaphragmatic breathing to help decrease arousal.

Another area of important work when exploring affective and physiological factors is *affective primes* (Panksepp, 2004; Panksepp & Biven, 2012). Panksepp's work identifies core emotional feelings such as rage, panic/grief, fear, play, seeking, lust, and care as intrinsic values that guide individuals in their survival. These affective states are not merely emotions but are primal forces that drive behavior. In CBT, understanding these affective primes can be instrumental in addressing the root causes of maladaptive behaviors and cognitive patterns. When working with children, we might need to redefine or re-term these states. In Table 1.2, we provide the terms we might use with youth. By exploring these fundamental emotional drives, we can help individuals develop more constructive ways of responding to their emotional states and the challenges they face in their environment. There are a lot of labels to describe emotions, and we can find resources that present "101 Emotions." Rather than expanding these visceral emotional responses to vague terms, we encourage clinicians to help individuals obtain a deeper understanding of these core emotions. For example, when a student comes to our office, rather than having them select their "feeling for the day" from a chart of many emotions, we have them focus on an understanding and reaction related to the seven emotional primes.

Behavioral

Behavioral components with children and adolescents can be influenced by environmental factors or be a result of skill deficits. By combining the understanding of environmental factors, classical and operant conditioning principles, self-reinforcement strategies, and motivation enhancement, CBT provides a robust framework for facilitating positive behavioral change in students.

When examining the impact of environmental influences, clinicians may evaluate classroom management practices, school climate, teaching and parenting styles, or past traumatic experiences. This understanding helps in conceptualizing the concerns faced by children and adolescents across their functional environments (e.g., school, home, community, recreational, and so on). Sometimes, the most effective intervention is to modify the environment itself, which can be achieved through positive behavioral supports, creating token economies, or other similar strategies. Such interventions aim to alter the external factors that may be contributing to the areas of concern.

Behavioral skill deficits, such as poor self-regulation or underdeveloped social skills, are another significant area of focus in CBT. This might include teaching or coaching students in skills such as self-awareness, communication, self-regulation, self-monitoring, and so on. Often, these involve collaborating with the child to identify the skills needed and then providing direct instruction, modeling, role-playing, and later involving exposure activities to practice and reinforce the skills. The goal is to encourage the development of improved and more adaptive behaviors or to minimize the impact of less desirable behaviors. When working with students, we need to view this process in stages involving skill acquisition, skill implementation, and skills maintenance. Thus, for each skill, we teach or coach, practice, and build a plan for continued use.

Self-reinforcement is a crucial aspect of behavioral change. It involves individuals learning to reward themselves and seeing the benefit of making progress and change. This is particularly important when addressing escape/avoidance behaviors, where a student may try to avoid a situation that they find unpleasant or challenging. By recognizing their progress and rewarding themselves for facing difficult situations, students can gradually overcome avoidance behaviors. While there can be some controversy around people needing rewards to complete tasks, there are longstanding psychological theories to support its use, such as the Premack Principle (following a less desirable task with a more desirable task). However, we must focus on how we word these approaches, and rather than saying, "If you do your homework, you can play 30 minutes on your iPhone," we should rephrase to say, "When you complete your homework, you can play 30 minutes on your iPhone." The reward is not to "bribe" them to complete an activity but to engage in self-care and celebrate the successes experienced.

CBT in Schools

CBT is increasingly recognized as a versatile and effective approach for addressing mental health issues within school settings. Its compatibility with educational cultures stems from its structured, goal-oriented nature, mirroring the systematic approach of educational services. The congruence between CBT and the educational framework paves the way for its integration into school-based mental health services, making it an acceptable approach in school-based mental health (Mennuti & Christner, 2005; Mennuti et al., 2012).

Multi-Tiered System of Supports

CBT's practicality for school implementation lies in its time-limited, present-focused, and solution-oriented methodology, as noted by Reinecke and others (2003). This approach aligns seamlessly with the educational model, emphasizing immediate, actionable strategies. The adaptability allows it to fit within the already existing multi-tiered system of supports (MTSS) structure of schools, offering services at varying levels of specificity, complexity, and intensity. This continuum ranges from universal prevention programs to targeted interventions for students with identified needs. Within the MTSS framework, mental health services are often categorized into three tiers: universal, selected, and targeted interventions, which are described in Table 1.3.

Integration of CBT in Educational Settings

The structure of CBT, which focuses on psychoeducation, skill building, between-session work (i.e., homework), agenda setting, and progress monitoring, is congruent with most activities that already

Table 1.3 MTSS Levels of Services in School-Based Mental Health

Universal interventions: These are preventive measures applied school-wide, aiming to foster a healthy psychological environment for all students. CBT principles can be incorporated into classroom teachings, focusing on general emotional well-being, stress management, and resilience building.
Selected interventions: Targeting groups of students who are at risk or showing early signs of mental health concerns, selected interventions offer more focused CBT strategies. These might include group sessions that address common issues like mild anxiety or social skills deficits.
Targeted interventions: For students with more pronounced or specific psychological needs, targeted interventions provide intensive, individualized CBT. These could include one-on-one sessions addressing complex issues like severe anxiety, depression, or behavioral problems.

exist in today's school settings. Thus, although these components assist in providing intervention services, they also strengthen the link between psychological counseling and other services provided in schools. CBT's emphasis on practical, present-focused solutions aligns with the resource-limited reality of schools, where time and support are often scarce. Rather than dwelling on diagnosing specific pathologies, CBT in schools focuses on addressing students' immediate issues, enhancing their coping skills in the context of their educational and social environments.

Proving CBT in schools lends itself to being a natural laboratory for which students can learn new skills and immediately applied in real-time, everyday situations. For example, Katie is a third-grade student who is shy and experiences high levels of social anxiety. Although she attends school daily, she often finds participating in class discussions and socializing with others difficult. Within her counseling session, she has started learning relaxation and self-talk strategies to increase Katie's comfort with herself and enhance her relational experiences with others. Katie and the clinician practice in session (e.g., role-play), but these interventions come to life when the "experiments" can expand activities, such as taking a note from the clinician to a teacher Katie does not know or saying "good morning" to the custodian who is working in the hallway. These small real-time exposure opportunities can build her confidence and be used in ways that she and her clinician can process immediately after they occur. The ability to provide these in close proximity to learning and working on skills is invaluable.

Conclusion

Given the need for short-term, flexible mental health services within school settings, the CBT model is ideal. The structure and framework of CBT parallel the existing organization of school systems while allowing for interventions that focus on social, cognitive, affective/physiological, and behavioral elements inherent in many difficulties seen in youth. CBT has much promise to build healthy relationships at a time when our youth are feeling more isolated and disconnected. It also can be used to enhance and modify existing programs delivered in schools and has the potential to go beyond providing interventions to individual students. School-based clinicians must use their knowledge of CBT, as well as their understanding of youth in general, to develop effective and efficient treatment or intervention planning.

Furthermore, notwithstanding the need for school-based mental health programs, there is a question of whether school-based clinicians are sufficiently trained to provide CBT interventions. This is a challenge facing university training facilities, as well as those organizations providing continuing professional development for school-based clinicians. Finally, using CBT as a means of addressing students' problems will require a paradigm shift for many educators. While many services provided for emotional and behavioral issues in schools have focused on behavioral interventions, current trends are moving to a more integrative approach. This involves not only the combined use of cognitive and behavioral intervention but also taking into consideration the social and relational dynamics and the personal stories students share. It is this comprehensive understanding that will help children and adolescents grow toward greater well-being.

Reflection Questions

1. What is your current theoretical approach to psychotherapy? How might you incorporate CBT into your practice and move toward a CBT orientation?
2. When working with a student, how might you use the multidirectional formulation approach to determine an entry point to begin intervention?
3. What barriers might you face when implementing CBT in schools, and how might you overcome these?

Professional Resources

Association of Behavioral and Cognitive Therapies (ABCT). www.abct.org.
Academy of Cognitive Therapy (ACT). www.academyofct.org.

References

Bell, I. H., Nicholas, J., Broomhall, A., Bailey, E., Bendall, S., Boland, A., Robinson, J., Adams, S., McGorry, P., & Thompson, A. (2023). The impact of COVID-19 on youth mental health: A mixed methods survey. *Psychiatry Research, 321*, 115082. https://doi.org/10.1016/j.psychres.2023.115082

Brown, T. A., & Barlow, D. H. (2009). A proposal for a dimensional classification system based on the shared features of the DSM-IV anxiety and mood disorders: Implications for assessment and treatment. *Psychological Assessment, 21*, 256–271. https://doi.org/10.1037/a0016608

Choi, S. Y., Rusch, A., Koschmann, E., Bilek, E. L., Lane, A., Abelson, J. L., Eisenberg, D., Himle, J. A., Fitzgerald, K. D., Liebrecht, C., Kilbourne, A. M., & Smith, S. N. (2022). How effective are school professionals at identifying students who might benefit from cognitive behavioral therapy? Baseline data from the adaptive school-based implementation of cognitive behavioral therapy trial. *Frontiers in Education, 7*, 814157. https://doi.org/10.3389/feduc.2022.814157

Chorpita, B. F., & Wisz, J. R. (2009). *MATCH-ADTC: Modular approach to therapy for children with anxiety, depression, trauma, or conduct problems.* Satellite Beach, FL: PracticeWise, LLC.

Chui, A. W., Langer, D. A., McLeod, B. D., Har, K., Drahota, A., Galla, B. M., Jacobs, J., Ifekwunigwe, M., & Woods, J. J. (2013). Effectiveness of modular CBT for child anxiety in elementary schools. *School Psychology Quarterly, 28*, 141–153. https://doi.org/10/f43nx9.

Clarke, G., Lewinsohn, P. M., & Hops, H. (1999). *The adolescent coping with stress class: Leader's guide.* Portland, OR: Kaiser Permanente Center for Health Research.

Creed, T. A., Reisweber, J., & Beck, A. T. (2011). *Cognitive therapy for adolescents in school settings.* New York: Guilford Press.

Cuddy, A. (2016). *Presence: Bringing your boldest self to your biggest challenges.* Boston, MA: Little, Brown & Company.

Damasio, A. R. (2000). A second chance for emotion. In R. D. Lane & L. Nadel (Eds.), *Cognitive neuroscience of emotion* (pp. 12–23). New York: Oxford University Press.

Ehrenreich-May, J., & Kennedy, S. M. (eds.) (2021). *Applications of the unified protocols for transdiagnostic treatment of emotional disorders in children and adolescents.* New York: Oxford University Press.

Harmon, S. L., Price, M. A., Corteselli, K. A., Lee, E. H., Metz, K., Bonadio, F. T., Hersh, J., Marchette, L., Rodriguez, G., Raftery-Helmer, J., Thomassin, K., Bearman, S., Jensen-Doss, A., Evans, S., & Weisz, J. R. (2021). Evaluating a modular approach to therapy for children with anxiety, depression, trauma, or conduct problems (MATCH) in school-based mental health care: Study protocol for a randomized controlled trial. *Frontiers in Psychology, 12*, 639493. https://doi.org/10.3389/fpsyg.2021.639493

James, A. C., Reardon, T., Soler, A., James, G., & Creswell, C. (2020). Cognitive behavioural therapy for anxiety disorders in children and adolescents. *The Cochrane Database of Systematic Reviews*, *11*(11), CD013162. https://doi.org/10.1002/14651858.CD013162.pub2

Joyce-Beaulieu, D., & Sulkowski, M. L. (2015). *Cognitive-behavioral therapy in K-12 school settings: A practitioner's toolkit.* New York: Springer Publishing Company.

Joyce-Beaulieu, D., & Zaboski, B. A. (2021). *Applied cognitive behavioral therapy in schools.* New York: Oxford University Press.

Kendall, P. C. (2021). *Flexibility within fidelity: Breathing life into a psychological treatment manual.* New York: Oxford University Press.

Kendall, P. C., & Hedtke, K. A. (2006). *Coping cat workbook* (2nd ed.). Ardmore, PA: Workbook Publishing.

Khalsa, S. S., Adolphs, R., Cameron, O. G., Critchley, H. D., Davenport, P. W., Feinstein, J. S., Feusner, J. D., Garfinkel, S. N., Lane, R. D., Mehling, W. E., Meuret, A. E., Nemeroff, C. B., Oppenheimer, S., Petzschner, F. H., Pollatos, O., Rhudy, J. L., Schramm, L. P., Simmons, W. K., Stein, M. B., Stephan, K. E., … & Interoception Summit 2016 Participants (2018). Interoception and mental health: A roadmap. *Biological psychiatry. Cognitive Neuroscience and Neuroimaging*, *3*(6), 501–513. https://doi.org/10.1016/j.bpsc.2017.12.004

Kuehn, B. M. (2022). Clinician shortage exacerbates pandemic-fueled "mental health crisis." *JAMA, 327*, 2179–2181. https://doi.org/10.1001/jama.2022.8661

Lochman, J., Wells, K., & Lenhart, L. (2008). *Coping power: Child group facilitators guide.* New York: Oxford Press.

Mendez, L. R. (2016). *Cognitive behavioral therapy in schools: A tiered approach to youth mental health services.* New York: Routledge.

Mennuti, R., & Christner, R. W. (2005). School-based cognitive-behavioral therapy (CBT). In A. Freeman (Ed.), *International encyclopedia of cognitive behavior therapy* (pp. 343–347). New York: Kluwer.

Mennuti, R. B., Freeman, A., & Christner, R. W. (2012). *Cognitive-behavioral interventions for educational settings: A handbook for practice* (2nd ed.). New York: Routledge.

Miller, J. B, & Stiver, I. P. (1997). *The healing connection: How women form relationships in therapy and life.* Boston, MA: Beacon Press.

Panksepp, J. (2004). *Affective neuroscience: The foundations of human and animal emotions.* New York: Oxford University Press.

Panksepp, J., & Biven, L. (2012). *The archaeology of mind: Neuroevolutionary origins of human emotion.* New York: W. W. Norton & Company.

Phillips, S. P., & Yu, J. (2021). Is anxiety/depression increasing among 5–25 year olds? A cross-sectional prevalence study in Ontario, Canada, 1997–2017. *Journal of Affective Disorders, 282*, 141–146. https://doi.org/10.1016/j.jad.2020.12.178

Porges, S. W. (2009). The polyvagal theory: New insights into adaptive reactions of the autonomic nervous system. *Cleveland Clinic Journal of Medicine*, *76*(Suppl 2), S86–S90. https://doi.org/10.3949/ccjm.76.s2.17

Qanbari Alaee, E., Saed, O., Khakpoor, S., Ahmadi, R., Ali Mohammadi, M., Yoosefi Afrashteh, M., & Morovati, Z. (2022). The efficacy of transdiagnostic cognitive behavioural therapy on reducing negative affect, anxiety sensitivity and improving perceived control in children with emotional disorders – A randomized controlled trial. *Research in Psychotherapy*, *25*, 588. https://doi.org/10.4081/ripppo.2022.588

Reinecke, M. A., Dattilio, F. M., & Freeman, A. (Eds.). (2003). *Cognitive therapy with children and adolescents: A casebook for clinical practice* (2nd ed.). New York: The Guilford Press.

Riise, E. N., Wergeland, J. H., Njardvik, U., & Ost, L. (2021). Cognitive behavior therapy for externalizing disorders in children and adolescents in routine clinical care: A systematic review and meta-analysis. *Clinical Psychology Review, 83*, 1–15. https://doi.org/10.1016/j.cpr.2020.101954

Schniering, C. A., & Rapee, R. M. (2020). Evaluation of a transdiagnostic treatment for adolescents with comorbid anxiety and depression. *Journal of Affective Disorders Reports*, *2*, 1–8. https://doi.org/10.1016/j.jadr.2020.100026.

Shidhaye, R. (2023). Global priorities for improving access to mental health services for adolescents in the post-pandemic world. *Current Opinion in Psychology, 53*, 101661. https://doi.org/10.1016/j.copsyc.2023.101661.

The White House. (2023). White house report on mental health research priorities. Washington, DC: Author.

van Doorn, M., Monsanto, A., Wang, C. L., Verfaillie, S. C. J., van Amelsvoort, T. A. M. J., Popma, A., Jaspers, M. W. M., Öry, F., Alvarez-Jimenez, M., Gleeson, J. F., & Nieman, D. H. (2023). The effects of a digital, transdiagnostic, clinically and peer-moderated treatment platform for young people with emerging mental health complaints: Repeated measures within-subjects study. *JMIR mHealth and uHealth*, *11*, e50636. https://doi.org/10.2196/50636.

Weisz, J. R., Bearman, S. K., Ugueto, A. M., Herren, J. A., Evans, S. C., Cheron, D. M., Alleyne, A. R., Weissman, A. S., Tweed, J. L., Pollack, A. A., Langer, D. A., Southam-Gerow, M. A., Wells, K. C., & Jensen-Doss, A. (2020). Testing robustness of Child STEPs effects with children and adolescents: A randomized controlled effectiveness trial. *Journal of Clinical Child & Adolescent Psychology, 49*, 883–896. https://doi.org/10.1080/15374416.2019.1655757

Weisz, J. R., & Kazdin, A. (2010). *Evidence-based psychotherapies for children and adolescents* (2nd ed.). New York: Guilford.

Werner-Seidler, A., Spanos, S., Calear, A. L., Perry, Y., Torok, M., O'Dea, B., Christensen, H., & Newby, J. M. (2021). School-based depression and anxiety prevention programs: An updated systematic review and meta-analysis. *Clinical Psychology Review, 89*, 102079. https://doi.org/1016/j.cpr.2021.102079

2

REVOLUTIONIZING COGNITIVE-BEHAVIOR THERAPY (CBT) WITH CHILDREN AND ADOLESCENTS

An Integrative-Relational Model of CBT

Rosemary B. Mennuti and Ray W. Christner

Being an effective therapist involves an evolution over time consisting of increased knowledge of the literature, a better understanding of the processing, and increased comfort in our professional identity and authentic self. However, we both can remember the days of floundering over learning new techniques and skills and figuring out "when to use what strategy with whom and how." In those early years, we sometimes complicate what is needed to impact the children and adolescents we work with. It is exciting to see and follow the ever-changing world of psychotherapy, especially cognitive-behavior therapy (CBT) and its use with youth. However, with this growth, there are also times of confusion as we have an expanding "psychotherapy alphabet soup." This can make determining what to do even more challenging for clinicians. We are not only choosing from many available strategies but also the multitude of psychotherapy approaches, such as those in the 3rd wave of CBT (e.g., dialectical behavior therapy, acceptance and commitment therapy, etc.). While we respect and have been trained in many of these newer approaches, in our clinical and scholarly work, we have avoided establishing another "new approach to psychotherapy." Instead, we have followed suit with the psychotherapy integration movement, focusing on the critical aspects of all psychotherapy approaches.

This has led to the model we present here, constructed from distilled information from our clinical practices and the empirical literature on what factors enhance the psychotherapy experience and allow for movement through the change process. We refer to this model as an Integrative-Relational Model of Psychotherapy (see Figure 2.1). While this can be used no matter your approach to psychotherapy, we focus on using it from a traditional CBT theoretical orientation. The Integrative-Relational Model of CBT is organized around psychotherapy constructs intertwined within a relational framework and our general understanding of the change process. At the root of our model, the individual and the therapist come together in a real way with a common goal leading to well-being. The relational framework is embraced as a key component of this model. The work in psychotherapy is held together by the relationship formed, nurtured, and developed throughout the treatment. The connection is characterized by mutual empowerment and awareness where both individuals are fully present, responsive, and able to reconnect when a disconnect occurs. While this dynamic is imperative in psychotherapy,

DOI: 10.4324/9781003392439-3

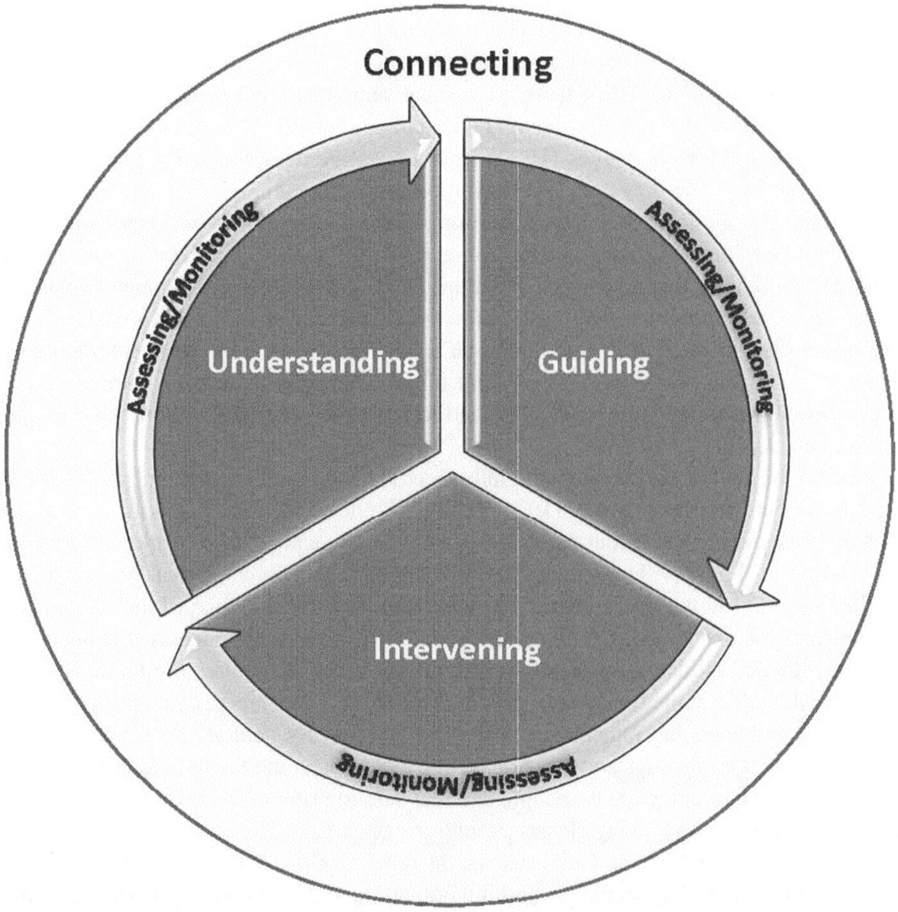

Figure 2.1 Integrative-Relational Approach to CBT

it alone is insufficient for change to occur, thus requiring us to also focus on other aspects of the psychotherapy process.

The relational framework (connecting) is embedded and valued in all three main areas of psychotherapy, including case conceptualization (understanding), session structure (guiding), and intervention modules (intervening). You will notice in Figure 2.1 and in the previous sentence that we refer to the areas of psychotherapy by the function each aims to achieve. As a reader and clinician, we want you to be able to avoid the jargon of what we do in psychotherapy and keep in mind the "why" of each of those parts of therapy. As practitioners, this model is to help empower you and the individual to determine the treatment process and interventions to address the presenting problem within the context of an authentic connection.

Relational Consideration in Treatment (Connecting)

The centerpiece of psychotherapy with children and adolescents is the evolution of the relationship. Research has continually shown that the relationship between therapist and individual is an essential aspect of the treatment outcome (see Norcross & Lambert, 2019; Norcross & Wampold, 2019). Interestingly, an often-stated criticism of CBT is that it is manualized and that it ignores the relevance of the "therapeutic relationship." Those trained in CBT and effectively practicing inherently know that this claim is far from accurate. While there are manual approaches that exist, the way in which those interventions are delivered still hinges on the underlying interaction between therapist and child.

Aaron T. Beck and his colleagues (1979) emphasized the need for active interaction between therapist and "patient," and they note that "slighting the therapeutic relationship" (p. 27) is a common error in the therapy process. This interaction should be empathetic and empowering to allow the individual to explore and give voice to their genuine thoughts, feelings, and true needs in such a way that allows for insight and change in action. Positive movement and change happen through the awareness of self and others while in connection. The impact we have on each other in connection, rather than in separation, modifies one's relational view and future interactions, which impact identity development, self-concept, and individual wellness. Clinicians must incorporate the specific strategies and techniques of CBT and Relational Theory throughout the conceptualization and treatment.

A pioneer in the field of psychology who influenced much of our thoughts and practices regarding relational factors is Jean Baker Miller (1976, 1987), who developed the Relational-Cultural Theory (RCT). Her work established a foundation for how we view and use the relational components of therapy, leading to the individual's relational development and psychological health. In RCT, the relationship is central to the psychotherapy process and the understanding of the factors contributing to problem areas and subsequent treatment goals. It focuses on the increased connection that is mutually empathetic, validating, and empowering. This practice requires the therapist to be fully present and real. Unlike some thoughts in psychotherapy, RCT encourages therapists to be emotionally responsive and engaging rather than remaining emotionally neutral. Therefore, it is okay for therapists to reveal their feelings and reactions while always keeping the individual's interests at the forefront. In a setting of authenticity, people can feel safe to bring more of themselves into the session, thereby exploring and looking closely at their experiences.

When working with children and adolescents, the relationship is one of connection and collaboration. It is a combination of spontaneous and intentional interactions that occur between two people over time. In this approach, we get a sense of how each other feels and thinks, and we come to know each other and ourselves. This way of relating is mutually empowering and growth-producing for both parties. It provides new experiences and perceptions in relating that combine with prior information and memories, forming healthy relational images. Miller and Stiver (1997) describe the five good things of healthy relationships as signs of (1) zest, (2) action, (3) clarity, (4) a sense of increased worth, and (5) the desire for more connection. In therapy, there is an emphasis on the importance of relationships and their impact on each of us. When the connection between therapist and individual is a positive, authentic relationship, it facilitates growth and well-being. By modeling good relationships, we aim to help individuals generalize these relational dynamics to life and promote further connection.

On the other hand, it is imperative to recognize that the relational dynamic includes a deep sense of connection and moments or periods of disconnection. Just as we recognize and promote good connections, we must also not ignore the rough spots, rifts, and ruptures that are experienced along the journey. If left unattended, these conflicts lead to the opposite of the five good things—less energy, isolation, lack of trust, and movement toward decreased self-worth and understanding. These patterns lead to lowered self-esteem, shame, isolation, anger, and depression. This spiral often results in a greater sense of disconnection, which underlies mental health issues (e.g., anxiety, stress, depression, etc.), health concerns (e.g., sleep problems, cardiovascular concerns, etc.), addiction, suicide, and other detrimental behaviors (see Novotney, 2019).

It is important to recognize that there are times of disconnection or rupture in all relationships, whether in therapy or daily life. Some of these are minor conflicts (little c's) that can be easily overlooked. At other times, the disruptions can be major conflicts (big C's) that require resolution and repair. Whether little c's or big C's, all conflict needs attention so that reconnection can occur. Unresolved issues, no matter how big or small, cause a break in the relationship. The resulting distance can cause isolation and distress and impede growth. Mending the disconnection is vital and includes listening compassionately to each other's point of view or even spontaneous humor to move toward greater understanding. The completed cycle of connection, disconnection, and reconnection leaves people feeling cared about, safe, and valued, improving the quality and strength of their relational abilities.

Conversely, if the resolution is done incorrectly, further distance can be created. For instance, if one person feels unable to use their voice or be heard, this causes a power-over dynamic—one person becomes dominant, and the other is silenced and relinquishes part of themselves. In an attempt to stay in the connection or to "fit in," authenticity is lost in this situation. Losing "who you are" interferes with development, and the power of relationships in therapy helps individuals reclaim their authentic selves while in connection, which is vital to well-being.

Taking this knowledge of RCT and relationships, we must remember that a collaborative, working relationship between a clinician and an individual is beyond "getting along" or having a friendship. A positive healing relationship is a complex dynamic in which a bond exists that promotes a connection and trust between two people. Once a sense of safety and trust is established, children can risk being open about who they are and what they believe and are willing to share sensitive information. Thus, attention to relationships in their world and therapy is acknowledged and examined. We believe that it is the relationship that runs through the therapy process that becomes the foundation of understanding, guiding, and intervening. It is what helps the strategies and techniques come alive and thrive. Although collaboration generally suggests an "equal" or 50/50 involvement between the clinician and individual, this is not always the case in actual treatment. In fact, a clinician needs to meet the child at their level (based on age, motivation, etc.) while holding a place for dignity and respect (Mennuti & Christner, 2005). Initially, until the individual matures in the therapy process, the ratio of clinician-to-individual work may be 30/70 or 40/60. As the process unfolds, children experience increased inclusion, respect, concern, and a deeper sense of self in connection.

A number of basic resources are available to help clinicians facilitate an authentic relationship. For instance, frequent and brief summations throughout the session will likely assist in keeping focus and demonstrating involvement within the session while further establishing and maintaining the relationship. These summations convey that the clinician is emotionally available and understands what is being said and felt. In addition, it is useful to acquire feedback that will help clarify information or misunderstandings. Providing time for relational practice in real time through role-playing is often an effective approach. Creating an atmosphere of empowerment and freedom to question further facilitates sharing and learning together. Finally, the permission and expectation of individuals to question, examine, and explore is often uncharacteristic of most interactions experienced by children yet lies at the heart of growth and change for children.

Responsive Evaluation of the Person (Assessing/Monitoring)

The idea of assessment begins with the initial moment that a clinician and individual meet or even make eye contact. When working with a student, we will begin with simple observations and casual discussion, which leads to more intentional conversation. While we advocate for the use of a semi-structured interview approach, for some individuals and clinicians, a more structured approach might be a better fit. However, with either, keeping the relationship and connection at the forefront is important. To do this, our use of questions and dialogue should remain conversational to avoid the perception of being interrogated. Clinicians must have the knowledge and automaticity to be able to ask the questions and listen while also formulating follow-up questions to obtain an even deeper understanding of the individual and their strengths and problems. This is a fluid discussion that results in obtaining data and an understanding of the individual. We obtain necessary data to help with the formulation of the case while further enhancing the relationship through the use of active listening, clarification of key concerns, and validation. By doing this, we can follow a structured approach to interviewing with fidelity while also exploring the individual's personal experience interactively, allowing us to integrate the individual's personal story with clinical information into a meaningful case conceptualization to help drive treatment. This same approach is used throughout the therapy process to monitor progress.

When conducting a semi-structured interview, the clinician must be familiar with the model and the specific questions they will be asking. In doing this, clinicians will create an environment that allows the interview to flow as a natural conversation, which will provide the opportunity for the

Table 2.1 Guiding Questions When Conducting Individual Interviews

Getting to know you
- Tell me some things about you.
- How do you describe yourself?
- What is something important about yourself you'd be willing to share?

Knowing the authentic self
- How would you describe yourself to yourself?
- What would you say about you?
- Tell me some things that are true for you.
- How do you describe yourself to other people? (e.g., friends, family, school)

[a]*Recovery questions*
- Tell me about your favorite place to be in your house.
- What's in there?
- What do you like to do in there?
- What is safe about that space for you?

Understanding the dynamics of relationships (e.g., power over, mutuality, acceptance, self-worth within the relationship)
- How do others describe you? (e.g., friends, family, school)
- Describe your relationship with other important people in your life. (e.g., friends, family, school)
- Tell me some people you can count on (e.g., adults and peers). Follow-up: What about them makes you feel that way?

[a]*Recovery questions*
- Who do you enjoy being around?
- What do you like doing together?

Closing comments
- Anything else I should know about you or the other people in your life?
- Is there anything else I didn't ask that you want to tell me?
- Before we wrap up, are there any questions you might have for me?
- I appreciate you sharing this with me. Thank you.
- Provide reassurance and remind them of confidentiality.

[a] Given that the previous questions could be emotionally charged for some, the use of recovery questions creates a lighter discussion to help recenter the individual before transitioning to the next part of the interview.

connection to deepen or be enhanced. In this approach, all of the needed questions will be addressed to gather comprehensive information, yet they will not follow a specific order, and the information will be obtained through a natural ebb and flow of conversation. Knowing the questions, clinicians will avoid repeating questions at a later time and will let you spontaneously probe further to obtain deeper information and clarification. This creates the opening for you to pick up on their thinking and expressions and allows them to guide you and share their story while remaining within the bounds of clinical structure. It is essential to listen for keywords or phrases that the child uses, which often offers insight into areas that need further clarification. For example, let's say you are interviewing a student who is talking about school and states, "I'm the worst kid in school." This statement gives several areas that require additional exploration, including their self-perception as "the worst kid" and the connection of that perception to school. You might say, "You said 'worst kid,' what does that mean for you?" This could be followed further by questioning them about school, "Could you give me an example of what happens at school?" Their responses provide you not only with the perceived school stressors but also a description of their relational images within the school environment. There are many phrases and questions you might use to engage the individual in providing additional information and expanding their comments. Some examples include:

- "Tell me more about..."
- "What did you mean by..."
- "Can you give me an example of..."
- "Help me understand what that is like for you."

There are a number of structured and semi-structured interview formats that are available to help guide you through the process of conducting an assessment interview with a child or adolescent. In the Appendix of this book, we provide the *Clinical Psychological Evaluation Interview Guide* that can be used to provide a format to help gather information in a number of important areas. In addition, Table 2.1 offers suggestions of specific questions you should make part of your interview question bank to help understand relational aspects, build a further connection with the student, and give data for a more robust case conceptualization and treatment planning.

Collateral Data

Beyond the interview that allows the student to guide us in their story, additional data from multiple sources helps us understand the student's experience and the perception of others within the context of the home, school, and social environments. All of the collateral data is gathered in anticipation of developing a case conceptualization to understand the individual and frame their difficulties in a manner that leads to enhanced collaboration and effective treatment. Thus, information should be gathered with this purpose in mind. It is easy to become overwhelmed with too much information that is not relevant and does not lead to interventions or outcomes. Therefore, clinicians should be thoughtful in what information they gather and how it is relevant to this case. Although this is not an exhaustive list of options, we encourage clinicians to consider completing record reviews, interviewing other important people in the student's life, and obtaining objective symptom-related data from rating scales. While collateral information is often used at the initial phase of treatment, additional information may be needed and incorporated as the treatments unfold. Moreover, clinicians can use this information to help with determining progress in treatment. For instance, the number of office discipline referrals collected prior to therapy can serve as a baseline, and frequency can be monitored over time.

Interviews with Others

When initiating treatment with a student, we focus on giving them the opportunity to tell their story, no matter their age. However, it is also important to gather the perceptions of others to understand problem areas and the relational dynamics in various contexts. As with the student interview above, we encourage clinicians not to simply ask questions about problem areas but to use this time with others to obtain further understanding of who the student is. When working in schools, collateral interviews are most common with parents and teachers. Yet, the school environment creates opportunities for observations and to explore further relationships, such as with coaches, classroom aides, or others with a personal connection to the child. Some of the most valuable information might come from those who have a relationship with the student where the student's problem areas are less prominent, and we will learn about the student's strengths and assets. It lets us see what relationships create a positive opportunity for the child, which is information that might be vital in creating interventions for this student. Table 2.2 provides samples of guiding questions to use when conducting collateral interviews with others. This does not take the place of a clinical interview but is a way to enhance the interview. Also, these are starting questions, and we encourage you to obtain additional detailed information by asking, "Tell me more" or "Help me understand what you mean."

Observations

One advantage of providing services within a school setting is the opportunity to have observations in a natural setting. Not only do we have a chance to see behaviors in real time, but we also can witness interactions and relationships with others. Conducting classroom observations is a common component of psychoeducational evaluations. However, for therapeutic interventions, we suggest that observations go beyond the classroom setting. This information adds a personal component to the assessment that serves as a helpful adjunct to interviews, checklists, and other measures. This lets us see the student's spontaneous behaviors and reactions within the classroom, on the playground, in the

Table 2.2 Guiding Questions When Conducting Collateral Interviews

Getting to know your perceptions of the child

- Tell me some things about your time with [the student].
- How would you describe them?
- What do you like about [the student]?

Knowing the student's relationships

- How would you describe your relationship with them?
- How do they relate or get along with others? (e.g., friends, family, school)
- Who does [the student] connect best with? What makes that a good relationship?
- Who does [this student] count on?

Understanding the student

- Do you have any concerns with [the student]?
- What do you see as their assets or strengths?
- What changes could help [this student] be successful at [home, school, etc.]?
- What has worked best with [this student]?

Closing comments

- Is there anything else I didn't ask that you want to tell me?
- Before we wrap up, are there any questions you have for me?
- I appreciate you sharing this with me. Thank you.
- Provide reassurance and remind them of confidentiality.

cafeteria, at home, or even in a counseling session. The educational setting is a "natural laboratory" for school-based clinicians to observe interpersonal dynamics and to gather data about the problems facing students, including antecedents, consequences, and general level of functioning (Christner et al., 2007; Mennuti & Christner, 2005; Mennuti et al., 2012). The information from the observations is qualitative data that can be collected in a narrative that can be easily interwoven into the case conceptualization. In addition, we can use our observations to prompt discussion and examples with the student. For instance, in a session when a student is responding impulsively, the clinician can use the observation to increase self-awareness (e.g., "I notice when we were talking, you sometimes answered the question before hearing the whole thing. Do you know that happens?"), discuss the student's perception and insight (e.g., "What do you think is going on when that happens?"), and provide direction or intervention (e.g., "Let's think of some strategies to help with this.").

Rating Scales

Several rating scales and behavioral inventories exist for use with children and adolescents. These instruments often provide comparative data to same-age peers, which can assist in examining the severity of behaviors in relation to others. These tools can be classified into two areas—(1) broadband instruments and (2) narrowband instruments. Broadband instruments look at a variety of symptoms and adaptive skills and are often useful in the initial treatment phase. Narrowband instruments are more symptom-focused and can provide information to look more deeply at a specific area of concern. Narrowband instruments are also useful as progress monitoring tools. Discussing all available instruments is beyond the scope of this chapter or book. However, we recommend readers to *Clinical Assessment of Child and Adolescent Behavior and Personality, Fourth Edition* (Frick et al., 2020) for a review of available rating scales. In addition, throughout the chapters of this book, the authors offer specific assessment tools to use with each specific area.

Case Conceptualization (Understanding)

Case conceptualization in CBT is a cornerstone in the effective application of this therapeutic approach, serving as a roadmap for both the clinician and the individual, patient, or student. It is our way as clinicians to "understand" the person. As we do our work in therapy or counseling, our mutual growth and understanding expand, and the shared experiences are real and need validation. This comprehensive understanding of the individual's presenting issues, background, and psychological patterns contributes to our relationship with the person and becomes a guide that informs the therapy process. This systematic approach allows the clinician to tailor interventions that are specific to the individual's needs, thereby enhancing the effectiveness of therapy. The process of case conceptualization in CBT is not static. This is the dynamic and ongoing part of the therapeutic journey, requiring continuous refinement as both the clinician and the individual gain more understanding. While this understanding is often thought to be about the individual or student, we as clinicians further develop an understanding of ourselves and how we respond and intervene with the person. The framework of case conceptualization is crucial in identifying and challenging unproductive thinking, unhealthy reactions, or relational concerns, which are central to CBT's effectiveness in helping others reach their goals.

For a more in-depth exploration of this topic, Chapter 3 of this book delves into the nuances of case conceptualization in CBT with youth. We offer a detailed discussion on each component to consider, providing practical examples and guidelines that are essential for both new and experienced clinicians. The chapter emphasizes the importance of a collaborative relationship between the clinician and the individual in developing a shared understanding of what is needed to increase well-being.

This collaboration is vital in ensuring our energy is focused on the individual in the room and the desired goals, fostering a sense of empowerment and engagement. By understanding the principles and framework outlined in Chapter 3, clinicians can enhance their skills in creating effective, personalized treatment plans that are at the heart of successful CBT interventions.

Session Structure (Guiding)

This section of the model sets the structure for carrying out the actual therapeutic sessions. This helps provide consistency in sessions that will help the child or adolescent be able to predict what will occur in sessions. This predictability and structure can lessen their anxiety about "what will happen in each session." This is not to say that we can identify everything that will occur in a session, but instead, we can provide a guide that will be used to organize the flow when working with the individual. The session length must be appropriate for the specific child, often influenced by age and developmental level. The structure of the session is somewhat flexible depending on the child's needs and the therapist's clinical judgment. Table 2.3 offers a sample session structure for consideration, and we describe each below.

Checking in Relationally

Each session begins with the opportunity to connect with the individual in front of us, showing the child that we genuinely are interested and care about them. It is the lead-in to help a child open and be spontaneous in their time with us. While this often begins with simple statements, such as "How has your week been," "Tell me how you've been," or "How are you doing," it is our response that shows the child our authentic curiosity and true interest in them and their lives. This time helps the child transition from either home or the classroom to relate to themselves and to be present in the session. The connection goes both ways so that the child and therapist reunite for a mutual flow of thinking and feeling for each session.

For most children, this relational check-in is easy and a natural part of the therapeutic relationship. However, for some, this might present as difficult. Some might struggle to initiate this connection and respond in a short and vague manner, such as "Good," "Fine," or "Okay." In these cases, we as clinicians need to explore this further with curiosity and zest. We may encourage further responses through comments, such as "Awesome! Tell me about it" or "Great, I would love to hear more." If they still struggle, we might need to help this evolve by being more specific, such as, "Great, can you tell me one thing that made it good?" On the other hand, we might have a child who provides an extensive response and a minute-by-minute script of what has happened since we saw them last. In

Table 2.3 Sample Session Structure

- Checking in relationally (e.g., "Tell me about your week.")
- Setting the agenda
- Soliciting feedback about the previous session
- Reviewing the current status and events since the last session
- Reviewing homework from the previous session
- Focusing on specific skills and interventions for that session
- Developing new between-session actions
- Reflecting on session and connection (e.g., "Tell me how you think today's session went" or "On a scale of 0 (not well) to 10 (awesome), how did you think today's session went and why?")

these cases, our response needs to be one of helping the child in give and take and to regulate their response. This can be done by providing a higher level of structure, such as using a timer and saying, "Let's take 5 minutes for you to tell me about the week." Or, we might structure through reframing the question to something like, "Tell me one thing new that happened this week." In all cases, it is focused on the needs of the child and how we build connections together while also making good use of therapy time.

Setting the Agenda

The use of an agenda is common practice in CBT. It is the means by which the actual session is structured, and it is done in a way that provides a consistent approach and predictability to each meeting. Each of the areas we are addressing here is part of that agenda. We encourage clinicians to write out the agenda on a whiteboard or piece of paper and provide the child with opportunities to contribute. Once the agenda is written, simply asking, "Is there anything we are missing or that you would like to add today?" can be a way to increase collaboration and respect for the child's voice. At times, this might be information directly related to the interventions (e.g., "I want to talk about getting in trouble at school"), but other times, it might be more relational (e.g., "I want to tell you about my new dog"). Both can be valuable in the session and can be put into the agenda.

Soliciting Feedback about the Previous Session

Before moving into new content, it is vital to take a moment and review the last meeting. This provides a chance for the child to discuss their experience in the last session and any concerns or things that went well but also gives a chance to clarify any misunderstandings. This is done by asking, "In thinking about our last meeting, is there any part of the last session we should talk about further?" and "Since you've been able to think about the session, did it bring up any emotions?" Also, it is our time to provide feedback to the child. This can be in the form of praise (e.g., "I was really impressed with how you were willing to role play with me."), though it can also be in a way to provide helpful feedback (e.g., "Last session when I asked about your homework, you seemed angry. When that happened, it made me feel I did something wrong and think you might not want to be here. Can we talk through the situation to find out what happened and what we each could have done differently?").

This part of the agenda is about making sure we are allowing space for authenticity about the thoughts and feelings that occurred since the last session. This is the part of the therapy process that can help the therapeutic relationship occur.

Reviewing the Current Status and Events Since the Last Session

Once we solicit feedback and empower the student to share their thoughts, we transition to obtaining information about their current status and any new information that might have occurred since we last met. When discussing current status with individuals, a common mistake is to simply ask about specific symptoms and to ignore the relational aspects this might have on them. To highlight this, let's use an example of a ten-year-old girl who presents with test/performance anxiety. While we might first ask about the presentation of symptoms (e.g., "I know you had a spelling test this week, how did it go?"), we also need to explore the functional or relational aspects of the experience. In this case, we might follow up by asking, "What were you saying to yourself at that time?" or "What was going through your mind?" In this example, maybe the child reveals that she and her mother "studied for hours," and her mother told her, "You got this." However, when experiencing difficulty during the test it brought up thoughts, "I'm letting my mother down" or "I'm not as smart as my mother thought." This line of questioning helps go beyond "How high was your anxiety?". It lets us then explore underlying factors contributing to her concerns with performance and its impact on herself and others. We can then use this information when working on specific interventions with the child to find ways to avoid thinking traps and develop more non-negative thinking.

Reviewing Between-Session Work from the Previous Session

As will be discussed below, we encourage clinicians to work with individuals on between-session work or "homework" to help reinforce skills. If we are asking students to complete tasks between sessions, we must dedicate time to discuss how it went. The focus is to ask about how it went, what difficulties might have occurred, and how it might have helped. Let's take an example of a 12-year-old boy who has social anxiety. Maybe the between-session work involved him introducing himself to two people over the past week. We might ask, "Let's talk about the between-session experiment from the last session—you were to introduce yourself to two people. How'd it go? How did you feel? What went through your head during and after?" We will likely have cases where, despite collaborating on what the child will practice, they will come in and not have completed the task. This, too, can be useful and is worth exploring with them. We would respectfully say, "It's okay that you were unable to practice. Let's talk about it. What happened that made that difficult for you?" We can also follow up by stating, "It is important that you practice, so what might we do to make this easier?" It is essential to convey a sense of understanding and support of their experience and focus on self-worth and the importance of their ownership in this process.

Focusing on Specific Skills and Interventions for That Session

This part of the session focuses on building or practicing new skills with the individual. We might choose to focus on these interventions that become needed based on earlier parts of the agenda. Let's take the student we discussed above with test anxiety. During our discussion of her experience since the last session, she disclosed to us thoughts that she has about letting her mother down. We would be remiss to ignore issues specific to her experience and not make them part of the process for the current session. So, even if something else might have been planned, this is an opportune time to work on thought restructuring or addressing thinking traps. For others, there might not be specific issues brought up, and we might follow through with a planned course of treatment, such as working on problem-solving or relaxation during the session. Clinicians must be flexible and be sure to take advantage of topics important to reaching treatment goals that naturally present themselves. This not only makes progress toward treatment goals but also shows the student we are listening to their experiences and addressing issues that are specific to them and how they respond.

Developing New Between-Session Actions

The use of "homework" or between-session work is common in CBT, and it has been shown to improve long-term outcomes (Helbig-Lang et al., 2013; Kazantzis et al., 2000). Beyond the outcomes, this use of between-session work is about bridging what is taught in the therapy room to real-life scenarios. This provides needed practice but also offers practice at a time when the child can return to the therapy session to discuss what they may face when implementing inventions in the real world. Children return after this situation with vulnerability, and because of the therapeutic relationship, this discussion will be one of validation and support. This support will encourage them to take additional risks to practice and build their skills without fear of being judged if the practice does not go as planned. If we do not validate them and the difficulties, the child becomes less likely to share out of fear of "not being good enough." They will present in session based on what they "think we expect" in order to preserve the relationship and connection.

When developing between-session work, the focus needs to be on the skill or intervention introduced in the session. This should be developed in conjunction with the student or others collaboratively and relate specifically to the individual child. It needs to be linked to the child, their thinking, and their experiences in the world. It is important that when developing this in collaboration, the between-session work be challenging enough to further their skill development but manageable enough not to overwhelm them. This could include simple exposure tasks (e.g., introducing yourself to two people, singing in front of someone, playing a frustrating game, role-playing with a parent), activity scheduling (e.g., doing one thing each day that you enjoy), thought records, journaling, or other tasks that reinforce skills and bringing them into the real world. Novice clinicians might rely more heavily upon specific manuals, books, programs, and virtual resources for which there are many suggestions to come up with these tasks (see Friedberg & McClure, 2015; Kendall, 2021; McClure et al., 2019). In addition, many activities will be discussed in chapters throughout this book. However, those clinicians who are more seasoned and have more resources available in their "toolbox" might be able to be more creative and take risks in developing between-session activities with the child based on solid theoretical underpinnings.

Reflecting on Session and Connection

As we wrap up our time with the child, the goal is to complete the cycle and bring closure to the work that was done in session. This begins with a relational check-in at the start to build skills and practice skills and then return to the connection. At this time, we reflect together what happened today, obtain the child's reactions to the session, and again check in on the relationship. Although many sessions are likely to go well and smoothly, in this process there will inevitably be ruptures or disconnects that happen. Maybe the child was not heard, or maybe we pushed "too far." In any case, it is a time to have the child express their concerns so that they can be collaboratively discussed to facilitate new and stronger reconnection.

Components of Practice (Intervening)

In Chapter 1, we explored the differences between manualized and transdiagnostic approaches, including differentiating between unified and modular approaches. When selecting interventions to use with children and adolescents, it is important that clinicians also consider their comfort level to implement these interventions. So, for beginning clinicians, using a predetermined treatment protocol or an already-developed therapeutic game is a great option. This helps build skills and an understanding of the underlying theoretical framework of CBT and its application. Throughout Part III of this book, a number of programs will be offered. As clinicians become more seasoned and comfortable, they will be better able to use their case conceptualization knowledge and skills to use a tailored approach, individualizing the treatment while still adhering to the fundamental evidence-based principles. This personalization and adaptation of strategies is built upon the collaboration, relationship, and understanding of the individual.

When discussing a modular approach to intervening, we use the term *components of practice* to refer to the different modules that can be used to create an intervention plan for an individual. The modules are the specific areas we are going to focus on with an individual to help them meet their goals. They serve as the scaffolding for crafting and personalizing effective intervention strategies that are attuned to the distinctive psychological landscape of a child or adolescent. Within each module, we may utilize any number of interventions or strategies to increase the skill and application

Table 2.4 Examples of CBT Modules

Module	*Description*	*Example*
Setting goals (goal setting)	Aims to empower children and adolescents to set and achieve goals through structured and realistic planning. Emphasizes the importance of flexibility in adjusting goals as needed and recognizing and celebrating achievements.	Emma, a 15-year-old, feeling overwhelmed by her desire to improve her grades across all subjects, defined specific, achievable goals for each subject.
Staying motivated (maintaining motivation)	Focuses on strategies to keep children and adolescents motivated toward their goals, including setting achievable targets and recognizing accomplishments.	Mark, a 15-year-old, lost interest in his goal to improve his grades. By setting smaller weekly study targets and rewarding himself for each achievement, Mark's motivation and grades improved.
Understanding emotions (emotional awareness)	Helps children and adolescents recognize and understand their emotions, teaching them to identify emotional triggers and differentiate between various feelings.	Riley, a ten-year-old, often felt overwhelmed but couldn't articulate her emotions. Through activities like emotion mapping and storytelling, she learned to identify and label her feelings as anxiety, frustration, or sadness, leading to better emotional communication with her parents and teachers.
Decreasing physical sensations (confrontation of physical sensations)	Aims to desensitize individuals to physical sensations associated with anxiety, such as a racing heart or dizziness, through gradual, controlled exposure.	Alex, a 14-year-old, experienced panic attacks characterized by intense physical sensations. Through controlled breathing exercises and gradual exposure to exercise-induced heart rate increases, Alex learned to manage his fear of these sensations, reducing the frequency of his panic attacks.
Facing body sensations (interoceptive exposure)	Targets the fear of bodily sensations by safely exposing individuals to these sensations in a controlled manner, teaching them that these sensations are not dangerous.	Lily, a seven-year-old with severe anxiety about fainting, engaged in interoceptive exposure exercises like spinning in a chair to induce dizziness. Over time, Lily's anxiety diminished as she realized she could manage and tolerate these sensations.
Building communication (communication skills)	Enhances effective communication by teaching listening skills, assertiveness, and how to express needs and feelings appropriately.	Josh, a six-year-old, struggled with making friends due to poor communication skills. Through role-playing exercises and feedback, he learned how to initiate conversations, listen actively, and express his thoughts and feelings more clearly, leading to improved peer relationships.

(*Continued*)

Table 2.4 (Continued)

Module	*Description*	*Example*
Learning from others (modeling)	Uses role models to demonstrate positive behaviors and coping strategies, encouraging children and adolescents to emulate these behaviors.	Sara, a 13-year-old, observed her mentor calmly handling criticism and resolving conflict. By modeling this behavior, Sara learned to approach disagreements with peers more constructively.
Maintaining progress (maintenance)	Teaches strategies to sustain progress made in therapy, including identifying potential triggers and developing a plan for dealing with setbacks.	After making significant progress in managing her social anxiety, 17-year-old Zoe worked with her therapist to create a maintenance plan that included joining a social skills group to continue practicing her new skills.
Regulating emotions (emotional regulation)	Focuses on teaching children and adolescents how to identify, understand, and manage their emotions. Techniques include mindfulness practices, cognitive reframing, and the use of emotional thermometers to gauge the intensity of feelings.	Jamie, a 14-year-old, struggled with anger management issues at school, often resulting in conflicts with peers. Through the emotion regulation module, Jamie learned to recognize the early signs of anger and applied mindfulness techniques to calm down before reacting. Over time, Jamie's ability to manage anger improved, leading to fewer conflicts and better relationships with classmates.
Challenging our thoughts (cognitive restructuring/ reframing)	Helps individuals identify and challenge negative, irrational thoughts and beliefs, replacing them with more positive, realistic ones. Techniques include the identification of cognitive distortions, thought records, and the evidence-based challenge of negative thoughts.	Sandy, a 12-year-old, often felt overwhelmed by academic pressures, leading to thoughts like "I'm not smart enough." Through cognitive restructuring, Sandy learned to identify and challenge these thoughts, replacing them with "I can improve with effort and help." Her academic confidence and performance gradually improved.
Solving problems (problem solving)	Teaches children and adolescents systematic steps to solve problems, including identifying the problem, generating possible solutions, evaluating and selecting solutions, and implementing the chosen solution.	Mark, a ten-year-old, faced difficulty completing group projects, often feeling left out. Through the problem-solving module, Mark learned to express his feelings to his group and brainstorm solutions, such as assigning clear roles. This led to better group integration and project outcomes.
Engaging in activation (behavioral activation)	Focuses on increasing engagement in positively reinforcing activities to improve mood and reduce avoidance behaviors. Techniques include activity scheduling and participation in social, physical, or creative activities.	Emily, a 13-year-old, experienced social withdrawal and loss of interest in activities she once enjoyed. Through behavioral activation, Emily identified and engaged in activities like joining a school art club, which helped improve her mood and social connections.

(Continued)

Table 2.4 (Continued)

Module	*Description*	*Example*
Facing uncomfortable situations (exposure)	Aims at reducing fear and avoidance behaviors through gradual, systematic exposure to feared stimuli or situations, combined with coping strategies to manage anxiety.	Alex, a 15-year-old, had a severe fear of public speaking, impacting his school presentations. Through gradual exposure exercises, starting with speaking in front of a mirror, progressing to small groups, and finally, larger audiences, Alex's anxiety significantly decreased.
Refining social skills (social skills)	Enhances interpersonal effectiveness through teaching communication skills, assertiveness, and empathy. Techniques include role-playing, feedback, and practice in real-life situations.	Lisa, an 11-year-old, struggled with making friends due to shyness. The social skills training module helped Lisa learn and practice initiating conversations and joining group activities, leading to the development of new friendships.
Pausing on purpose (mindfulness/ relaxation)	Teaches techniques to focus on the present moment and reduce stress through practices like deep breathing, progressive muscle relaxation, and guided imagery.	Kevin, a nine-year-old, experienced high levels of anxiety, especially during tests. Mindfulness and relaxation techniques taught Kevin how to calm himself before and during tests, improving his performance and reducing anxiety.
Monitoring emotions (emotional self-monitoring)	Empowers children and adolescents to enhance self-awareness by tracking their emotional states, triggers, and patterns over time. It utilizes techniques such as maintaining an emotion diary, rating emotion intensity, and reflecting on the causes and effects of emotional responses to foster an understanding of the link between thoughts, feelings, and behaviors.	Bella, a nine-year-old, often experienced sudden outbursts of frustration during homework time, leading to tears and refusal to complete assignments. She started keeping a simple diary to track her emotions, noting what was happening before, during, and after her frustration spikes.
Monitoring behaviors (behavioral self-monitoring)	Enhance self-awareness by teaching children and adolescents how to observe and record their behaviors, thoughts, and feelings in real time. Techniques include the use of diaries or digital apps for tracking behaviors, thought logs to capture cognitive patterns, and mood charts to document emotional fluctuations.	Nina, a 16-year-old, struggled with procrastination, affecting her homework and project deadlines. Through self-monitoring, Nina identified patterns in her procrastination and set realistic goals for completing tasks, leading to improved time management and academic performance.
Managing stress (stress management)	Teaches strategies for identifying sources of stress and implementing effective coping mechanisms, such as time management skills, setting priorities, and using relaxation techniques to manage stress.	Tom, a 17-year-old facing college application deadlines on top of his regular schoolwork, learned to manage his stress by breaking down tasks into manageable steps, setting realistic deadlines, and using deep breathing techniques when overwhelmed.

(*Continued*)

Table 2.4 (Continued)

Module	*Description*	*Example*
Managing attention (attention regulation)	Designed to improve focus and attention control through exercises that enhance sustained attention, selective attention, and attention-switching capabilities.	Derek, an eight-year-old with ADHD, struggled with paying attention in class. Attention regulation exercises, combined with teacher collaboration to provide structured learning activities, helped improve Derek's focus and academic performance.
Being assertive (assertiveness)	Focuses on developing the ability to express thoughts, feelings, and needs in a direct, honest, and appropriate way. It includes learning the difference between passive, aggressive, and assertive communication styles.	Anna, a 13-year-old, often felt bullied into doing things she didn't want to do by her peers. Assertiveness training helped Anna learn to say no respectfully and express her own needs, improving her self-esteem and peer relationships.
Focusing on gratitude (gratitude)	Encourages the identification and appreciation of positive aspects of life, fostering a sense of gratitude. Techniques include gratitude journaling and engaging in acts of kindness.	Chloe, a 15-year-old, felt depressed and disconnected from her school community. By participating in gratitude exercises and focusing on positive interactions, Chloe's mood improved, and she felt more connected to her peers and teachers.
Resolving conflict (conflict resolution)	Teaches strategies for constructively resolving interpersonal conflicts. This includes understanding others' perspectives, communicating effectively, and finding mutually beneficial solutions.	Ethan, a 12-year-old, frequently got into arguments with classmates. The conflict resolution module helped Ethan develop skills to understand his classmates' points of view and to resolve disputes calmly and fairly.
Building resiliency (resilience building)	Aims at strengthening the ability to cope with adversity, bounce back from failures, and adapt to change. Techniques include fostering a growth mindset, setting realistic goals, and building a support network.	Sophia, a 14-year-old, faced significant anxiety after failing a math test. The resilience module helped her understand failure as a learning opportunity, leading to improved academic resilience and performance.
Celebrating successes (self-reward/praise)	Encourages the use of positive reinforcement to motivate behavior change, teaching individuals to reward themselves for achieving personal milestones.	Danny, a seven-year-old, struggled with completing homework on time. He implemented a self-reward system, where he enjoyed extra video game time for each week he completed all his assignments, leading to consistent homework completion.
Creating a support network (parents, teachers, and others) (parent, teacher, and other psychoeducation)	Offers education and resources to parents, teachers, and others to support the child's or adolescent's mental health, covering topics such as effective communication, behavior reinforcement, and stress management.	The parents of eight-year-old Mia attended a series of workshops on supporting children with ADHD. They learned strategies for providing structure, encouraging positive behaviors, and managing their stress, which in turn improved Mia's behavior and family dynamics.

in that area. For instance, for relaxation (what we refer to as "Pausing on Purpose"), clinicians might choose to use diaphragmatic breathing, progressive muscle relaxation, guided imagery, or other mindfulness-based interventions. This nuanced approach to CBT emphasizes the importance of selecting and applying specific CBT modules and strategies based on the individual rather than applying a one-size-fits-all strategy. The flexibility and adaptability allow school-based clinicians to address a broad spectrum of emotional and behavioral challenges, making it an invaluable approach for school-based clinicians.

It is beyond the scope of this chapter to cover the full range of strategies that could be at a clinician's disposal. In Table 2.4, we offer the modules that we focus on with youth, including the wording we use to frame each module as actions to be reached, a description of each, and case examples. We also encourage clinicians to explore the many excellent resources available that offer extensive practical tools for working with youth, including *Clinical Practice of Cognitive Therapy with Children and Adolescents: The Nuts and Bolts* (Friedberg & McClure, 2015), *Cognitive Therapy Techniques for Children and Adolescents: Tools for Enhancing Practice* (Friedberg et al., 2009), and *CBT Express: Effective 15-Minute Techniques for Treating Children and Adolescents* (McClure et al., 2019). These resources are invaluable for clinicians seeking to refine their approach and enhance the effectiveness of their interventions.

CBT has developed to be the "go-to" or "gold standard" treatment for many areas of concern that children and adolescents face, including anxiety, depression, anger, adjustment, trauma, stress, and so on. The evidence for CBT is robust and ongoing. Because of its strong theoretical framework and the research to support its use, CBT affords clinicians the opportunity to be creative and personalize interventions even further while in connection with the individual. The foundation of CBT provides a platform from which originality can be used to enhance already developed practices and procedures (Rozmid & Friedberg, 2022). This can be done through using metaphors, games, pop culture, superheroes, play, humor, and improv. While beginning clinicians might not pursue this initially, as their clinical skills increase and their understanding of the theoretical underpinnings becomes more secure, they will be more comfortable and confident. This will allow them to focus on being present and connected to the child or adolescent with them, resulting in greater creativity and authenticity within the therapy sessions.

There are many ways to personalize and make CBT fun for children and adolescents. Clinicians might use readily available games as a way to enhance treatment, such as playing *Jenga* to improve self-regulation or using *Perfection* to help expose a student to being startled. As exposure to being embarrassed, the clinician and child might engage in karaoke, improv acting, or stand-up comedy in session. Cognitive restructuring could be discussed as *Jedi Thinking* to connect to a specific child or lyrics from a song might be used for self-talk, like "Shake it Off" (by Taylor Swift). Again, the options are endless to be creative while still adhering to the theoretical underpinnings of CBT.

Conclusion

In conclusion, it is essential to highlight the profound journey that both clinicians and individuals embark upon in the realm of psychotherapy. The intricate dance of forming authentic connections, understanding deeply, guiding effectively, and intervening strategically underscores the transformative power of the Integrative-Relational Model of CBT. Our approach, rooted in the principles of CBT and enhanced by the richness of Relational Theory, serves not only as a framework for therapeutic intervention but also as an example for navigating the complex, ever-evolving landscape of mental health care. By embracing the relational dynamics at the heart of therapy, clinicians are equipped to forge meaningful, empowering connections with their individuals, fostering an environment where genuine growth and healing can occur. The emphasis on relational considerations, combined with a commitment to responsive evaluation and tailored intervention, underscores the pivotal role of the therapist-individual relationship in facilitating positive change. This approach not only aligns with the current evidence base but also resonates with the core human need for connection, validation, and understanding.

As we reflect on our time with individuals throughout our career in psychotherapy, the path to effectiveness is multifaceted, requiring a thoughtful balance of knowledge, skill, and empathy. The journey from novice to expert therapist is marked by continuous learning, self-reflection, and adaptation. However, the essence of therapeutic success lies in the ability to remain present, authentic, and responsive to the unique needs of each child and adolescent. By integrating the critical elements of various psychotherapeutic approaches within a relational framework, we offer an approach that transcends traditional boundaries, advocating for a holistic, personalized, and caring approach to treatment. This model not only champions the significance of the therapeutic relationship but also highlights the clinician's role in facilitating a time of discovery, empowerment, and transformation. In doing so, we pave the way for a future where psychotherapy continues to evolve, informed by both science and the profound human capacity for connection and change.

Reflection Questions

1 How might you weave the relational framework into your practice? Think of one of your current cases.
2 How might you approach the case differently using modular-based interventions?
3 How do you handle conflicts and heal ruptures in relationships both in your personal life and when interacting in therapy, whether it be with the child, their parents, or school personnel?

References

Beck, A. T., Rush, A. J., Shaw, B. F., & Emery, G. (1979). *Cognitive therapy for depression.* New York: Guilford Press.

Christner, R. W., Forrest, E., Morley, J., & Weinstein, E. (2007). Taking cognitive-behavior therapy to school: A school-based mental health approach. *Journal of Contemporary Psychotherapy, 37*, 175–183. https://doi.org/10.1007/s10879-007-9052-2

Frick, P. J., Barry, C. T., & Kamphaus, R. W. (2020). *Clinical assessment of children and adolescent personality and behavior* (4th ed.). New York: Springer.

Friedberg, R. D., & McClure, J. M. (2015). *Clinical practice of cognitive therapy with children and adolescents: The nuts and bolts* (2nd ed.). New York: Guilford Press.

Friedberg, R. F., McClure, J. L., & Garcia, J. H. (2009). *Cognitive therapy techniques for children and adolescents: Tools for enhancing practice*. New York: Guilford.

Helbig-Lang, S., Lang, T., Gloster, A. T., Fehm, L., Gerlach, A. L., Strohle, A., Deckert, J., Kircher, T., Hamm, A. O., Alpers, G. W., Arolt, V., & Wittchen, H. U. (2013). Specificity of homework compliance effects on treatment outcome in CBT: Evidence from a controlled trial on panic disorder and agoraphobia. *Journal of Clinical Psychology, 69*, 616–629. https://doi.org/10.1002/jclp.21975

Kazantzis, N., Deane, F. P., & Ronan, K. R. (2000). Homework assignments in cognitive and behavioral therapy: A meta-analysis. *Clinical Psychology: Science and Practice, 7*(2), 189–202. https://doi.org/10.1093/clipsy.7.2.189

Kendall, P. C. (2021). *Flexibility within fidelity: Breathing life into a psychological treatment manual.* New York: Oxford University Press.

McClure, J. M., Friedberg, R. D., Thordarson, M. A., & Keller, M. (2019). *CBT express: Effective 15-minute techniques for treating children and adolescents.* New York: Guilford.

Mennuti, R., & Christner, R. W. (2005). School-based cognitive-behavioral therapy (CBT). In A. Freeman (Ed.), *International encyclopedia of cognitive behavior therapy* (pp. 343–347). New York: Kluwer.

Mennuti, R. B., Freeman, A., & Christner, R. W. (2012). *Cognitive-behavioral interventions for educational settings: A handbook for practice* (2nd ed.). New York: Routledge.

Miller, J. B. (1976). *Toward a new psychology of women*. Boston, MA: Beacon Press.
Miller, J. B. (1987). *Toward a new psychology of women* (2nd ed.). Boston, MA: Beacon Press.
Miller, J. B., & Stiver, I. P. (1997) *The healing connection: How women form relationships in therapy and life*. Boston, MA: Beacon Press.
Norcross, J. C., & Lambert, M. J. (eds.) (2019). *Psychotherapy relationships that work: Evidence-based therapist contributions*, Volume 1 (3rd ed.). New York: Oxford University Press.
Norcross, J. C., & Wampold, B. E. (eds.) (2019). *Psychotherapy relationships that work: Evidence-based therapist responsiveness*, Volume 2 (3rd ed.). New York: Oxford University Press.
Novotney, A. (2019). The risk of social isolation: Psychologists are studying how to combat loneliness in those most at risk, such as older adults. *Monitor on Psychology, 50*, 32–37.
Rozmid, E. V., & Friedberg, R. D. (2022). Incorporating humor, superheroes, and improvisational theatre exercises into CBT with Youth: "Just because something works, it doesn't mean it can't be improved". In R. D. Friedberg & E. V. Rozmid (Eds.), *Creative CBT with youth: Clinical applications using humor, play, superheroes, and improvisation* (pp. 1–8). Cham: Springer Nature.

3

ENHANCING CASE CONCEPTUALIZATION

Integrating CBT and Relational Perspectives

Ray W. Christner and Rosemary B. Mennuti

When providing psychological counseling to youth, it involves more than just knowing a variety of techniques. Clinicians need to understand when and how to apply these techniques effectively with specific clients. Gordon Paul (1967, 1969) posed what he referred to as the ultimate question—"What treatment, by whom, is most effective for this individual, with that specific problem, under which set of circumstances, and how does it come about?" While at first glance, this question might appear to be complex, it is actually quite simple and elegant. It takes our focus away from a problem focus and moves it to individual focus. That is, it is more important to understand the individual who has the problem rather than trying to understand the problem that an individual has. Taking this point of view is key when working from an integrative relational model of CBT where both the student and the therapist are fully engaged and present throughout treatment.

Before discussing our approach to case conceptualization and each of its components, let's start with a working definition of case conceptualization. Christner (2022) provides the following:

> A clinical strategy and process by which a clinician obtains and organizes information about a patient/student to understand a patient's/student's situation and current problems, to inform and guide treatment and interventions, to anticipate challenges, and to determine outcomes in the change process.

This definition highlights several key aspects, including data collection, organization and understanding, and informed decisions about treatment strategies and progress monitoring. Clinicians using CBT are not just randomly selecting interventions to see "what works;" they are making thoughtful decisions about the child and their knowledge of evidence-based inventions to provide targeted interventions. They are conducting a functional assessment of the child to make informed treatment decisions. Through a process of predetermined progress monitoring, the clinician is able to adjust as needed to help the individual progress toward goals and appropriate outcomes. School-based providers are likely familiar with this model through work on prereferral teams (e.g., MTSS or child study teams) or the completion of functional behavioral assessments (FBAs). Each of these has a similar framework when developing strategic interventions, though what we propose when working with mental health provides a more comprehensive approach.

There are a number of models of case conceptualization, though many of these are designed with adults in mind (see Needleman, 1999; Persons & Davidson, 2010; Sperry & Sperry, 2020). Murphy

DOI: 10.4324/9781003392439-4

and Christner (2006, 2012) proposed a case conceptualization model that integrated information from existing models while keeping in mind unique aspects specific to children and adolescents. Our current model is an extension of this work, and it has been refined over 15 years based on our work with clinical and school cases. The goal of our case conceptualization model is to move from a "one-size-fits-all" approach to treatment toward one that is "what-size-fits-you." This highlights the need to be focused on the specific child or adolescent in front of us and to tailor our interventions and time with them. So, we are moving past the days of understanding the child's problems, and we are now appreciating the child to help them with their problems and move toward healthy relationships and well-being.

Using this dynamic and relational model, clinicians can develop individualized treatment plans and adapt their approach and interventions as new information becomes available during treatment, ensuring interventions remain relevant and effective for the individual. This suggests that our interventions are always a work in progress, and there are usually times that, with more information, we will need to change paths more than once. Thus, the case conceptualization process is continuous throughout the treatment process. An example to illustrate this is Cole—a 14-year-old boy who was referred for school-based counseling due to disruptive behaviors and anger outbursts in class. Upon the initial case conceptualization, Cole's problems presented as issues with anger and emotional control, and treatment proceeded in that direction. However, although initial progress was limited, the connection with Cole grew, which resulted in him being more open about his experiences and what led to his outbursts. Rather than it being simple as an anger issue, Cole began discussing feelings of embarrassment and anxiety in class, which resulted in behaviors that provided a mechanism for him to escape. With this new information, a change in treatment occurred, with the focus being on addressing thought traps leading to embarrassment and then behavioral addressing issues of avoidance and escape. The new information brought forth through the working relationship with Cole became vital and resulted in him making notable progress in the next six sessions.

Relational CBT Case Conceptualization Model

In our clinical work, we have combined the use of CBT and relational theories as described in Chapter 2. Our case conceptualization model has grown from this approach and offers a comprehensive, dynamic approach to understanding and intervening with various concerns experienced by children and adolescents. Our goal is to balance the uniqueness of each individual with the need for evidence-based treatments and interventions. We describe each of the components that we believe are necessary to have an integrative understanding of the individual and can be used to develop an effective approach to supporting and helping those with whom we work. Table 3.1 provides a list of each element that we will describe below, and in the Appendix of this book, we share our *Cognitive-Behavior Case Conceptualization Worksheet*.

Identifying Data/Personal Information

The initial information gathered on the student can often be from the chart or history forms used. Here, we want to gather identifying information such as their preferred name or nickname, age, ethnoracial information, preferred pronouns, and basic family information. Although this information seems basic, asking about and using the individual's preferred name or pronouns can be an initial signal to the individual about the clinician's approach. Although much of this information will be listed on paperwork completed before the session, clinicians should take a moment and "double-check" with the individual.

Table 3.1 Components of CBT Case Conceptualization

Components of an Interactive-Relational CBT Case Conceptualization
Self-view—This should include information from the individual on how they describe themselves and include information on interests that might be able to be tied to treatment.
Relational view—This should include how the individual describes themselves within relationships.
Reported concerns—This should be a comprehensive list of areas of concern across settings—home, school, social, and community.
Antecedents/triggers—This should include events that activate thoughts, feelings, actions, and reactions.
Developmental considerations—This should include developmental variables that are important in understanding the individual and might be important to modify interventions (e.g., language delays, cognitive level, or motor difficulties).
Ethnoracial/cultural considerations—This should include information related to racial, ethnic, and cultural experience. This might include preferences, socioeconomic issues, discrimination experienced, perception of mental health and trust in providers, and beliefs about treatment.
Wellness and resiliency factors—This should include individual, family, peer, education, and community variables that provide support and help promote positive well-being.
Roadblocks and barriers to progress—This should include individual, family, systemic, and teacher/classroom factors that might be sustaining the difficulties or create challenges to successful treatment.
Readiness to change—This should include determining where the individual is in the change process for the approach to be adjusted to "where they are" in the change process.
Relevant assessment data—This should include a summary of standardized assessment data from rating scales and self-ratings of thoughts and behaviors to understand the level or severity of difficulties.
Working hypothesis(es)—This should include information to summarize how triggers, social experiences, thoughts, feelings, physical reactions, and behavioral reactions lead to short-term (what problems now) and long-term (what problems could get worse) outcomes.
Diagnostic impressions/educational classification—This should include specific clinical diagnoses or educational classifications, if any.
Goal setting—This should include clearly articulated and measurable goals that can be included in an intervention or treatment plan.
Levels of care—This should include the identification of the care level that might be most appropriate for the individual—this could include more than one service or a determination for other referrals.
Frequency of services—This should include how often an individual will be seen for intervention.
Comments/notes—This should include any other information that could be relevant when planning and moving through the intervention/treatment process with the individual.

Self-View

When working with youth clients, many people often provide information about them and inform the clinician "who they are." We find it vital to obtain information from the individual about how they view and describe themselves. This might be hard for some children and adolescents in the first session, but this might unfold with time. In the Assessing section of Chapter 2, we provide guiding questions for clinicians to use as a starting point. Sometimes, it is easier for children and adolescents to identify personal information about themselves—what they are into, what they like/dislike, hobbies, etc. This information can be very useful when connecting with the student, planning inventions, or developing metaphors to use in treatment. For instance, maybe a child with anger issues has a strong interest in Marvel movies. With this information, we might use it to start conversations and build common dialog. We might use this information to personalize strategies, such as making the *Subjective Units of Insights, Thoughts, and Experiences* (SUITE) scales or *Subjective Units of Distress Scale* (SUDS) from Bruce Banner to the Incredible Hulk rather than simple numbers from 0 to 10. This simple adaptation can sometimes build interest and buy-in from the individual.

Relational View

Beyond having a child or adolescent provide information on self-view, we also want to obtain how they view themselves in relationships and their relational experience. What is their role, how do they connect, disconnect, and heal ruptures, and where do they fit in within the scope of family, friends, and general social relationships? Again, in Chapter 2, we provide questions in the Assessing section to help guide inquiry about these factors. Going back to the social factors of the multidirectional model, understanding the individual's relational view can help us understand connections, isolation, and social vulnerability that can be used as a resource (e.g., building on existing connections) and as a treatment need (e.g., decreasing isolation and lack of connectedness). We can also use this to aid in developing supplemental interventions or building further connections. For instance, we might help identify a supportive adult in school with whom a student can interact or connect.

Reported Concerns

There is also a need to understand the problems or challenges that individuals are facing. This list is often started through the referral process, as the referral source provides areas of concern or problem areas. For case conceptualization, clinicians need to articulate these challenges in clear, behavioral language. It is not enough to say a child is "depressed." What does that look like for the specific child in front of you, and how do we move them toward less suffering and a more fulfilling life experience? It is also important to understand problems in different settings, including school, home/family, social, and community. Historically, a number of CBT experts have underscored the importance of an exhaustive problem list (Nezu & Nezu, 1993; Persons & Davidson, 2010), which will become more refined as the case conceptualization comes together. A comprehensive list from various domains helps to spot patterns that emerge in the child's behavior and to ensure no critical aspect is overlooked. This is essential for comprehending the root causes of the child's issues. Also, being thorough at this phase of the treatment process minimizes the introduction of new problems mid-treatment by the child, parents, or teachers.

Persons and Tompkins (2007) proposed that formulation occurs at several levels—symptom, disorder or problem, and case. We advocate for rethinking this and conceptualizing the child and how the problems, symptoms, and possible disorders manifest for the individual and affect their functioning. A comprehensive problem list serves as a means for the clinician to collaborate with the child and key adults in their life to dissect and understand the diverse and sometimes conflicting issues they face, paving the way to uncover the core reasons behind the reported concerns and help them develop new ways of enjoying a healthy life. We recommend describing these problems in specific, measurable, and observable terms—for example, rather than stating a child "is anxious," describing exact moments when a child experiences anxiety (and when they don't). For instance, "Maya experiences anxiety in the cafeteria every day, including sweaty palms, heart racing, and worry about getting sick, and she rates it as a 7 out of 10 on a SUITE scale."

We understand that creating a comprehensive list can be challenging, especially when behaviors overlap or are ambiguous. To manage this, clinicians should use various assessment tools, such as rating scales, and conduct in-depth interviews with the child, parents, and teachers.

Antecedents/Triggers

Consistent with functional behavior assessments (FBAs) commonly used in school settings, it is important also to identify the triggers or precursors that activate specific behavioral patterns. These antecedents or precipitating factors act as catalysts for the student's thoughts, feelings, and behaviors, and understanding them can help inform interventions. Antecedents or triggers can either directly influence the individual or create a context in which behaviors are more likely to occur (Chu & Pimentel, 2023; Friedberg & McClure, 2015; McClure et al., 2019). It is important to keep in mind that triggering events can be an external situation (e.g., being in crowds or taking a test). Still, there are times when individuals are triggered by their internal thought processes (e.g., telling themselves they will never have friends).

For instance, consider Shayzear's case, which illustrates a direct link between an antecedent and behavior. While playing soccer with others at recess, other students would competitively take the ball from him, which resulted in him stating that they were "bullying" him and would result in him crying. So, competitive games, even when age-appropriate, resulted in negative thoughts and behaviors for Shayzear. On the other hand, the relationship between triggers and actions can be less direct, as seen in Andrea's case. Andrea often became tearful and reported others were picking on her, though others did not observe this. However, through gathering data, the clinician identified that these tearful days often occurred when she transitioned from one parent's home to the other's, which was part of a change in custody arrangements.

Developmental Considerations

While some professionals unfamiliar with CBT may criticize it as a rigid, manual-driven approach, experienced CBT practitioners understand this is a misconception. In practice, CBT is a dynamic process where clinicians use data from assessments and case conceptualizations to tailor strategies to the individual's age, developmental stage, specific problem areas, individual interests, and relational awareness and capabilities. A critical aspect of working with school-aged children is a deep understanding of child and adolescent development. Clinicians with a solid grounding in developmental principles are more likely to select and adapt interventions that align with a child's functional level, avoiding a trial-and-error approach. Since CBT strategies often require a child's ability to focus, understand language, use working memory, employ executive functions, and communicate verbally, practitioners need to evaluate and consider these factors when creating interventions for each student. The balance of cognitive and behavioral techniques must be carefully adjusted according to the student's developmental needs. For example, students with limited cognitive and language skills or those with severe behaviors are likely to benefit more when interventions emphasize behavioral elements at first. While this does not mean cognitive techniques are unsuitable for younger children or those with severe behavioral issues, it does highlight that the balance of cognitive to behavioral interventions may lean more toward behavioral-based approaches. When thinking about development, clinicians must keep in mind that a child's developmental level may not always align with their chronological age. As such, clinicians will look at cognitive levels (think Piaget), social skills and maturity, language skills, attention skills, self-insight, and self-regulation when considering developmental levels.

Ethnoracial/Cultural Considerations

When understanding a child and adolescent, we must do so within the context of one's sociocultural experience. This includes processing information regarding race, ethnicity, gender and sex, socioeconomic status, and cultural beliefs, values, and experiences. It also involves embracing diversity and understanding the role discrimination plays in the individual's experiences and perceptions. These factors can have an impact in various ways, including problem recognition, the decision to seek help, selecting services, and patterns related to service utilization (e.g., treatment adherence, service providers, etc.). Eiraldi and colleagues (2006) discuss these patterns within the context of service delivery for ADHD, though we believe it is vital to consider these across the mental health spectrum.

Understanding racial, ethnic, and cultural components in case conceptualization and treatment is beyond what we can cover appropriately here. However, we dedicated a full chapter to this book, and we encourage readers to read the comprehensive review and suggestions provided by DeLapp and DeLapp in Chapter 6.

Wellness and Resiliency Factors

Research in developmental psychopathology, particularly concerning risk, protective, and resiliency factors, has been present for over 25 years (see Coie et al., 1993; Doll & Lyon, 1998). This research has contributed valuable insights for those working with young people. Risk factors are generally organized into five areas—individual (e.g., predisposition, attitudes, skills, etc.), social (e.g., activities, norms, connection), family (e.g., conflict, parenting, relationship, abuse), education (e.g., connection, climate, performance), and community (e.g., norms, resources, poverty, etc.). When thinking of risk factors, it is important not to focus on any one event or issue, as risk tends to be more of a cumulative effect—that is, the more risk factors, the higher the probability of mental health issues. It is also noteworthy to mention that for some youth, there might not be any apparent risk factors, yet mental health concerns arise. It is equally important to recognize that not every child with risk factors will face poor outcomes.

While it is important to understand factors that contribute to risk for mental health concerns, it is more important in treatment to draw from the impact of those factors to build wellness and resiliency. Protective factors are thought to serve as a buffer that can reduce the negative effect of adversity on child outcomes. According to Coie et al. (1993), protective factors can (1) directly reduce risk, (2) act as buffers interacting with risk factors, (3) interrupt the progression from risk factors to disorders, and (4) prevent the initial occurrence of risk factors. When thinking about protective factors, we recommend organizing thoughts into the same five areas of risk noted above, with the focus being on how to build or enhance positive aspects within each. A description and examples of each are provided in Table 3.2.

Clinicians can use their understanding of these risks and protective factors to modify interventions for students, aiming to mitigate risks while enhancing strengths and building competency. Early interventions might focus on skill-building through psychoeducation, transforming maladaptive behaviors, and enhancing protective factors such as peer relationships, self-monitoring skills, parent-child interactions, therapist interactions, and academic success.

Roadblocks and Barriers to Progress

In addressing the challenges faced by children and adolescents, clinicians must consider various factors that might sustain a student's difficulties or impede their progress. It is a common oversight for clinicians to attribute an individual's lack of progress solely to the student's shortcomings. While personal responsibility and individual issues are factors, there are other critical elements that clinicians should explore to understand the individual fully and to be prepared to use problem-solving to work around these barriers. According to Christner (2004), clinicians should evaluate four key areas when looking at what maintains these challenges or hinders progress:

> **Individual Factors.** These are specific to the individual and can include a lack of readiness or motivation for change, pervasive negative thoughts or feelings, deficiencies in essential skills (e.g., problem-solving), difficulty developing healthy connections, or lack of personal responsibility.
>
> **Family Factors.** These pertain to the individual's home environment and can include the dynamics of home-school collaboration. Clinicians should consider the level of caregiver

Table 3.2 Protective Factor Descriptions and Examples

Descriptions	*Examples*
Individual—focuses on personal characteristics that mitigate risk and engagement in negative emotions and behavior.	• High expectations • Positive temperament • Social competencies • Problem-solving skills • Self-efficacy • Healthy beliefs • Spirituality
Family—focuses on the family structure, support, culture, and functioning that affect positive and negative outcomes.	• Positive parenting • Family stability • Relationship with parents/siblings • Extended family relationships
Peer—focuses on peer norms, connection, socialization, and interaction processes that can build resilience and promote healing.	• Peer connection and support • Embrace and work through healthy conflict • Appropriate involvement in extracurricular activities • Positive peer role models
Education—focuses on attention, effort, performance, and relationships within the school environment that build a sense of connection, purpose, and involvement.	• High expectations and achievement • High-quality schools • Clear standards for appropriate behavior • Involvement in class activities • A feeling of school connectedness • Positive staff/faculty role model
Community—focuses on the general physical environment, availability of opportunities (e.g., recreational), and existing social supports that promote the individual's growth.	• Safe and supportive neighborhood • Involvement within community • Connection to caring/supporting adults • Prosocial opportunities (e.g., recreational activities) • Community service or volunteer opportunities

involvement and cooperation, the family's views on education and mental health services, the effectiveness of collaboration with the school, and any family-related stressors or conflicts, such as mental health issues.

Systemic Factors. These relate to the school environment itself and how it might be impacting the student. Factors in this category can range from ineffective school disciplinary practices (e.g., suspensions), stringent policies (e.g., zero-tolerance rules), overall school climate, and safety concerns (e.g., bullying). A lack of evidence-based educational programs or services to meet the child's needs also falls under this category.

Teacher/Classroom Factors. This area focuses on the characteristics or actions of teachers and classroom procedures that might be limiting the individual's progress. It includes issues such as ineffective behavior management, poor planning, lack of teacher training, and negative perceptions or attitudes of the teacher towards the student or their own professional role. This is not to blame the teacher, but instead, it is a way to identify a need beyond the child, which can promote better consultation with the teacher.

Finally, while the factors above highlight the barrier clinicians should consider when working with children in schools, it is also essential for clinicians to look inward at "clinician factors." Sometimes, the barriers to change can also lie with us, which are often easy to miss. Being reflective about our time and approach to youth can often reveal factors that might be limiting progress. From a more evidence-based approach, clinicians should ensure they are delivering interventions and strategies with fidelity. We encourage readers to explore Dr. Phillip Kendall's book (2021), *Flexibility within Fidelity: Breathing Life into a Psychological Treatment Manual*, as a resource that discusses essential components of empirically supported treatments and how to maintain fidelity while meeting an individual's specific needs. However, sometimes, the clinician factors are beyond issues of treatment fidelity and are related more to relational factors.

The therapeutic relationship is not about being nice or having the child see you as a friend. Instead, it is about how we develop healthy connections with appropriate boundaries and be present with the truth of their stories. This does not mean that there should not be a friendly and inviting relationship. However, there is a boundary set that the clinician is someone who is there to help and can provide an opportunity and safety for the child to share in an open and real manner. We encourage building a connection that can be, at times, fun and engaging, yet it is also a relationship that, at other times, involves intense discussions and content. Clinicians must be aware of the connection with the child while also being aware of times of disconnection and ruptures and use those to navigate conflict and promote growth in a healthy manner on both sides of the relationship. This ultimately can help make the therapeutic relationship stronger, as it demonstrates to the child that conflict is not only common but can be growth fostering. Often, with difficult cases, the stories shared might be difficult and involve vulnerability in both the child and therapist. When clinicians see a stall or lack of progress in treatment, we encourage clinicians to first look toward the therapeutic relationship as a variable.

Readiness to Change

An area that school-based clinicians might not commonly consider is the concept of readiness to change and the child's understanding of the therapy process. When working in schools, because others working with children are "ready for the child to change," that does not suggest that the child is equally ready. However, in reality, while the adults in the child's life want "action" to happen, the child may not be at that point. Being aware of these factors is pivotal not only for establishing a collaborative relationship but also for the respect and understanding of the journey, which guides the effectiveness of interventions and their outcomes.

The readiness to change model developed by Prochaska and DiClemente (1982) and Prochaska et al. (1992) is widely referenced in the mental health literature, detailing six stages of change: Precontemplation, Contemplation, Preparation for Action, Action, Maintenance, and Relapse. A more recent revision by Freeman and Dolan (2001) expands his model to outline ten stages in the change process: (1) Noncontemplation, (2) Anticontemplation, (3) Precontemplation, (4) Contemplation, (5) Action Planning, (6) Action, (7) Prelapse, (8) Lapse, (9) Relapse, and (10) Maintenance. While there is less research on the Freeman and Dolan model, we have found using this breakdown in clinical practice with youth more useful as it provides different and realistic entry points for working with youth. In Table 3.3, we provide definitions and examples of each of these stages.

In the early phases of interventions, clinicians might be most focused on obtaining buy-in from the child. Consider an adolescent referred for being disruptive and rude in class. A direct approach (e.g., why the student should not disrupt the class) may face resistance from the student and prove ineffective. Instead, a skilled clinician might leverage the student's motivation, such as using a shared goal of reducing the teacher's "being on their back" to enhance adherence to the intervention and strengthen the partnership with the student. While this initial buy-in is important, we believe the role of the relationship is vital throughout the change process and can be a catalyst for readiness to change.

Throughout therapy, the clinician and child move through the dynamic process of stages of change together. This progression through this process and the growth of the relationship are interwoven,

Table 3.3 Stages of Change with Youth

Readiness to Change Stages	*Examples*
Noncontemplation—the student is not aware that change is necessary or possible.	Jerry is frequently having meltdowns in class and other students start avoiding him. He is unaware of how his actions in class are affecting others wanting to play with him.
Anticontemplation—the student actively (or reactively) opposes the need for change.	Margie is failing several of her classes for not completing work. When this is discussed, she becomes upset and states, "The teachers expect too much. No one can pass these classes."
Precontemplation—the student becomes aware of the purpose and possible benefits of change.	Cesear has struggled with social interactions. In therapy, he begins discussing how "kids don't ever pick" him to be a partner in activities. In discussion, he sees he might need to change what he does in interactions to change the actions of others.
Contemplation—the student is directly and actively considering change, though they are unsure what to do.	Emma is an 11th-grade student who is not doing well academically. She recognizes that she needs to change how she studies and prepares for classes but does not know where to begin.
Action planning—the student is collaboratively thinking about what they can do to take action.	Donnie has been spending time alone, not interacting with others, and not eating. These things have increased his feelings of being depressed and isolated. He and his counselor begin brainstorming action steps that he can take to increase interactions with others.
Action—the student is ready to take steps and engage or experiment in activities to help reach their goals.	Jaynaya has anxiety when talking with new people or being in social situations. After learning several strategies, she begins "behavioral experiments" to try to engage with three new people the next week.
Prelapse—the student has overwhelming thoughts related to the new ideas and plans and is thinking about returning to previous reactions and behaviors.	Simon has been doing well with managing his anger at school but begins having thoughts that "others think I'm a wimp" and "this isn't working." While he has not had old behaviors, he questions if doing the work is worth it.
Lapse—the student begins ignoring the skills and strategies from therapy that have been helping, and they start returning to previous behaviors.	Alina is working on school attendance and has been following through on a number of interventions (e.g., setting an alarm, texting mom when she leaves the house, etc.). She began being inconsistent with the strategies, and over the past two weeks, her attendance has become inconsistent.
Relapse—the student returns to previously maladaptive behaviors or reactions that caused the original referral.	With Alina, although she and the counselor collaborated to avoid a backslide to past behaviors, she did not make the needed adjustments, resulting in her absenteeism returning to previous rates.
Maintenance—the student has made changes and consistently adjusts strategies to maintain successful behaviors and avoid slipping back.	John has been in an emotional support program throughout his education and has shown consistently positive behaviors. After a successful trial in a general education program with limited support, he has proven he can manage setbacks, uses strategies he has learned, and knows how to reach out for support when needed. John, his parents, and the school team agree that he no longer needs special education services.

resulting in each affecting the other—that is, the growth of the relationship facilitates movement through the stages and movement through the stages deepens the relationship. This is not to say the process is smooth. There will likely be ruptures in the relationship to some extent that need to be addressed (e.g., the child gets upset with the clinician or expresses frustration) along with times when treatment is not successful (e.g., a behavioral experiment did not go well or the skill was not accessible for use and they defaulted to past behaviors). When the relationship allows for the vulnerability of both parties and offers a space for the individual to be open and honest about the difficulties, it provides an opening for the student to discuss the "barriers" or "rough spots" that occur in both treatment and everyday life without having a fear of judgment. We can use this process to reengage in "action," using new skills or reusing previously ineffective skills to continue moving toward the individual achieving their goals. Doing this process together with the student will help facilitate self-regulation for later use of this process independently in the future.

We can illustrate the common experience of making changes in behavior (stages of change) with the case of Henry, a 12-year-old student struggling with work completion. The classroom teacher has tried many interventions without success, and she referred him for services so they could join together to work through this issue. At this point, the school-based clinician is brought in as an additional team member to take a "deeper dive" into the situation. Both Henry and his teacher are at the *contemplation stage* at the onset of intervention, as both are aware of the concerns and are thinking about what they can do but are unsure of how or what to try. At this stage, the school-based clinicians provide psychoeducation about the change process. Change is not linear but a progression that has an ebb and flow and requires simple modifications or the development of new ideas when interventions are not working. This includes providing real-life examples (including those provided by the teacher or Henry) to show how setbacks occur and can be overcome to reach goals.

One of the past strategies tried was a "homework book," though this did not help, as Henry either would forget to write down the assignments each day, would forget the book at school, or would not reference the book once he was home, all of which resulted in work not getting done. Although the homework book was unsuccessful, the school-based clinician decided to revisit this and discuss what barriers occurred that made it unsuccessful to brainstorm ways around them and create new actions using the same intervention. When discussing the barrier of forgetting to write down assignments, Henry states, "I wanted to write them; I just forgot." This led to a discussion between Henry and his teacher on what each of them could do differently (*action planning*) and move to new ways of thinking and a new plan. Through this, Henry and his teacher decided on new *actions* that included his teacher taking a few minutes each day to make sure all of the assignments were in his book and the book was placed in his book bag. Henry's new behavior was to set the alarm on his cellphone, "alerting him" at 5 PM each day to check his assignment book and begin his work (***Note:*** Henry chose this time as the best time to get work done.).

These changes in behaviors resulted in Henry improving his work completion to 90%, and this lasted over three weeks. Henry began thinking he did not "need" the support anymore, and he did not want to continue checking in with the teacher at the end of the day (*prelapse*). This led to Henry returning to past behaviors, and the work did not get done. At the next meeting, the school-based clinician pointed this out, but not in a punitive way—"Henry, you've been awesome with getting things done. I noticed there were a few days that did not go as well lately. What got in the way?" It is important to note here that prior to the group meeting, the school-based clinician spoke with the teacher as well to approach this interaction in a problem-solving manner rather than "pointing out" what Henry did "wrong." In the meeting, Henry states, "I'm the only one that needs the teacher to check me at the end of the day. I want to do it on my own." This is a good time to return the discussion to the change process and how it is okay to want to be independent, but creating new habits takes time. The clinician can refer to this as a "setback" rather than a relapse and collaborate with Henry and his teacher on a timeline to move toward *maintenance*. This can involve starting to fade out interventions, monitoring their success (or not), and adjusting the maintenance process as needed.

Relevant Assessment Data

In Chapter 2, we discussed assessment in detail from initial interviews to gain the individual's personal story, observations, and the use of rating scales from both the individual and collateral informants. All of that information is part of the initial case conceptualization, though we encourage providers to obtain ongoing assessment data to help refine the conceptualization, treatment, and relationship. This can be ongoing interview data and the unfolding narrative presented during sessions. However, it can also be more formal to include the use of narrow-band rating scales (e.g., PHQ-9, SCARED, and CES-D). One of the best measures, in our view, is simply using Subjective Units of Distress (SUDs). However, as noted above, we recommend a revised approach titled *Subjective Units of Insights, Thoughts, and Experiences* (SUITE) scales, as the data that is important does not always have to be distressing.

We might ask a student to focus on the success they had with a between-session activity and relational experiences rather than solely focusing on the distressing aspects (e.g., "On a scale of 1 to 10 (10 being great), how well did you do getting along with others this week?"). This could focus on interactions with others, such as acts of kindness, helping others, obtaining support, or the receipt of positive feedback. There are times when obtaining symptom information will also be essential, and a clinician might ask, "On a scale of 1 to 10 (10 being the worst), how high has your anxiety been?" This is useful progress monitoring data regarding symptom relief or exacerbation that can help look at outcomes. Finally, the use of SUTEs can also be used to look at the relational dynamics between the clinician and student to take the pulse of the therapeutic connection. For instance, at the end of the session, the clinician could ask, "On a scale of 1 to 5 (5 being the strongest), how well do you feel we connected today?" or "On a scale of 1 to 10 (10 being best), how did you feel today's session went?" This empowers the student to have a voice in the session, develop relational insight, and provide feedback to continue the work being done together.

Working Hypothesis(es)

The working hypothesis represents the clinician's tailored application of cognitive-behavioral theory to an individual client, bridging general cognitive and behavioral theories to create a personalized formulation. This is instrumental in understanding the child and the dynamics around them and dissecting areas of concern to facilitate a relational and strategic approach to intervention. Echoing the approach of Jacqueline Persons and colleagues (2013), we emphasize the importance of examining historical situations that reveal how individuals developed specific thoughts and behaviors. Good working hypotheses integrate these historical factors with schema development, levels of functioning, behavioral actions, and the current strengths and needs presented by the individual in front of us. Clinicians use this hypothesis statement as a way to collaboratively determine goals and select strategies to help the student reach their goals.

For example, let's consider different hypotheses that might help us understand three different students presenting with test anxiety—Hector, Anna, and Jossie. All three manifest the same presentation of symptoms, including anxiety prior to tests, poor test performance despite studying, and worry about tests several days before they occur. However, the reasons that lead to their anxiety are very different. Hector has thoughts of, "If I don't get straight A's, I'm a failure, will let my parents down, and never get into law school." The hypothesis for Hector could be *Hector's test anxiety is triggered by negative thoughts about success and his concern about others being critical of him if he does not show perfection in his performance*. In Anna's case, she describes thoughts of "If I don't do well, I'm not smart or good enough to hang out with the 'popular' kids." The hypothesis for her might be *Anna's test anxiety is due to a fear of 'not being good enough' and not fitting in*. Jossie is a very confident student, yet her commitments outside of school as a competitive horseback rider result in limited time for test preparation. Thus, the working hypothesis for her is that *Jossie's test anxiety is triggered by being overwhelmed with commitments and having difficulty managing and organizing her time to be prepared*. For each of these, while the reason for the referral is the same, understanding their unique and personal stories helps us target interventions to meet their needs.

In the *Cognitive-Behavior Case Conceptualization Worksheet*, which is Form 2 in the Appendix of this book, we provide a visual diagram to organize a clinician's analysis of an individual's situation. This focuses on summarizing triggers and how they affect the interactive aspects of social, cognitive, affective/physiological, and behavioral factors. With this, we then look at both the short-term and long-term outcomes of the individual's situation. Short-term outcomes might include outcomes such as avoiding a social situation to reduce feelings of anxiety. However, the long-term outcomes for this example might be increasing isolation and losing friendships.

Diagnostic Impressions/Educational Classifications

In education contexts, the role of diagnosis remains a topic of debate. While many professionals advocate for its utility, others view it as a potentially harmful label that can follow students throughout their educational journey and life, skewing their self-view and the view of others. Despite imperfections in the diagnostic process, we see it as a valuable tool in individual case conceptualization and intervention planning. There are clear drawbacks to relying solely on diagnosis. Most profoundly, diagnosis tells us little about the child in front of us. This is why we advocate the need for a more comprehensive case conceptualization process. However, that does not mean there is no benefit to understanding diagnosis. Most of the evidence-based treatments and programs showing efficacy and effectiveness are based on an understanding of specific diagnoses or clusters of diagnoses. We believe clinicians need to understand and use diagnosis in that manner—a guide to help look at what evidence-based treatments and interventions might be useful for a specific problem. But, our job does not stop there; we must use this knowledge within the context of understanding the individual and tailoring our approach to use empirically supported treatments that are personalized to engage and build resilience in the person.

Levels of Care

When providing mental health services to children in schools, it is essential to realize that services may be delivered at different levels. The idea of different levels of intervention is common in school, with most MTSS programs looking at interventions provided on universal, selected, and targeted levels. However, when we are working with individual students for case conceptualization, we must also consider the specific level of care that will best meet their needs. We understand that not all schools or school-based clinicians will be able to offer all levels that we offer below. However, ensuring that there are different options available to reach the best outcome is needed. In Table 3.4, we provide a brief description of the different levels of care we use and consider when working with students. While for some students, only one service might be needed, other students might need a combination of these services. For instance, when working with an autistic child, we might decide to provide brief services on a weekly basis to help teach self-regulation skills; however, it is also necessary to provide parent and teacher consultation to bridge the skills building to everyday situations and system consultation to address issues in the environment that are contributing the student's needs (e.g., sensory

Table 3.4 Levels of Service and Care

Levels of Service/Care	*Description*
Supportive care	A brief interaction with the child to check in and provide individual acknowledgment and support as needed.
Ultra brief care	Individual skill-building services that involve up to six sessions, each session lasting 15–20 minutes.
Brief care	Individual skill-building services that involve up to 12 sessions, each session lasting 20–30 minutes.
Standard care	Individual services that involve a combination of interpersonal, solution-focused, and skill-building interactions up to 25 sessions, each session lasting approximately 45 minutes.
Extended care	Individual services that involve a combination of interpersonal, solution-focused, and skill-building interactions *that reach a deeper understanding* of the individual and require over 25 sessions and/or fewer sessions requiring up to 60 minutes.
Group intervention	Group intervention that is addressing and skill-building around specific targeted areas (e.g., anger, anxiety, depression, etc.)
Teacher/parent consultation	A varying number of sessions with the clinicians meeting with teachers/ parents to involve them as positive resources and to support them in carrying out interventions outside of the session.
Systematic consultation	A varying number of sessions with school administration to help address larger changes that will help promote the mental health and well-being of not only the individual child but also the greater population.

issues in the cafeteria). On the other hand, for an adolescent dealing with depression, we might decide that a more traditional, standard care approach with weekly, 45-minute sessions will be the best and most appropriate option. Understanding these levels of care and what services we can provide within our setting also offers clearer guidance and when we need to refer to services outside of the school setting.

Goal Setting

The use of goals in treatment is common for those who have worked with a CBT or behavioral therapy approach. Goal setting in these approaches is necessary, given they are both goal-driven and time-limited. We advocate fully for setting goals when providing services to students. However, when setting goals in relational CBT, we draw upon both the underpinnings of cognitive and behavioral approaches to treatment, as well as relational theory. While we will have those goals that are traditional to CBT (e.g., "Anna will reduce her anxiety in social situations, rating herself below a 4 out of 10 on a SUTES rating"), we also need to ensure that embedded in the goal setting are the goals to help the individual when dealing with themselves and others (e.g., "Anna will collaboratively problem solve and engage in discussion regarding her expectations about social relationships with peers.").

When we consider goals in therapy, the goals must address two factors—the wording needs to meet regulations or professional standards and the wording that is personal and motivating to the child. In some cases, a single goal might meet both of these expectations, while other times, we might have goals that are for the "treatment plan" and then goals that are written in a way that the student understands and has the motivation to accomplish. This simple change in semantics during the session can increase buy-in by working collaboratively with her. The measurable goals that we need to monitor progress are not often interesting to students and, in some cases, might be met with resistance. However, when we take the child's interest and desire and work collaboratively and respectfully, we can increase interest in the process of therapy.

For instance, Lucy is a 16-year-old student with depression that affects her motivation to complete tasks. Her depression manifests as sadness but also involves behaviors that reinforce her depression, such as spending excessive time on social media (e.g., making social comparisons) and not wanting to get out of bed, resulting in her having a lack of involvement and not completing needed tasks. For her intervention plan, the goal might be written as "Lucy will improve her activity level to include spending at least 30 minutes a day involved in one activity after school." The others in her life initially want this to involve activities that are important to them, such as joining a club, getting a job, etc. However, these activities are met with resistance from Lucy, as she views them as having no value, boring, and being "just more work." When exploring with Lucy, we began getting insight into what is important to her. She revealed that her "real goal" is to be able to obtain her learner's permit so she can get her driver's license and hang out with friends. Although this is something that she is passionate about, she feels "stuck." This is an example of collaboratively creating actions by listening to the student, validating what she desires, and ultimately helping her find new ways to reach the goal. Although the goal is the same (e.g., increase activity), how we get there has to be collaborative and be worded differently. It is important to recognize that this approach not only helps reach the current goal but also serves as a springboard to later exploration of the interpersonal experiences and connection with others, further reducing her isolation.

Conclusion

Our goal of this chapter is to emphasize the complexity and individualized nature of providing CBT interventions for youth, especially when also considering the relational dynamics and needs at play when providing counseling or therapy services. The approach provided is to encourage clinicians to go beyond a one-size-fits-all approach and to focus on understanding the unique aspects of each child or adolescent rather than just the problems they present with. Case conceptualization is a key strategy for the work we do as clinicians, and it provides us with an understanding of the person and serves as a guide to positive outcomes. Our goal is to collect and analyze data to inform decision-making about treatment strategies, considering the individual's personal story, developmental stages, cultural background, and various other individual factors. By using a thoughtful and strategic approach that is personalized for the individual, we increase our chances of both buy-in and positive outcomes from interventions.

Reflection Questions

1 In thinking about a recent case, how might you find the child's self-view of value for use in the conceptualization and treatment process?
2 Take a moment to reflect on yourself as a clinician; what lies within you that could be a roadblock when working with a child?
3 After reading this chapter, how would you use any new information to inform your work with a child?

References

Christner, R. W. (2004). The development and validation of the Impediments to Change Scale—Educational Version: A study of children and adolescents with emotional disturbance. Unpublished doctoral dissertation, Philadelphia College of Osteopathic Medicine, Pennsylvania.

Christner, R. W. (2022, October). *Beyond diagnosis: Using test data for case conceptualization.* Presented for the PARtalks series for Psychological Assessment Resources (PAR) [Virtual].

Chu, B. C., & Pimentel, S. S. (2023). *CBT treatment plans and interventions for depression and anxiety disorders in youth.* New York: Guilford.

Coie, J. D., Watt, J. F., West, S. G., Hawkins, J. D., Asarnow, J. R., Markman, H. J., Ramey, S. L., Shure, M. B., & Long, B. (1993). The science of prevention: A conceptual framework and some direction for a national research program. *American Psychologist, 48*, 1013–1022.

Doll, B., & Lyon, M. A. (1998). Risk and resilience: Implications for the delivery of educational and mental health services in the schools. *School Psychology Review, 27*, 348–363.

Eiraldi, R. B., Mazzuca, L. B., Clarke, A. T., & Power, T. J. (2006). Service Utilization among ethnic minority children with ADHD: A model of help-seeking behavior. *Administration and Policy in Mental Health, 33*(5), 607–622. https://doi.org/10.1007/s10488-006-0063-1

Freeman, A., & Dolan, M. (2001). Revisiting Prochaska and DiClemente's stages of change theory: An expansion and specification to aid in treatment planning and outcome evaluation. *Cognitive and Behavioral Practice, 8*, 224–234.

Friedberg, R. D., & McClure, J. M. (2015). *Clinical practice of cognitive therapy with children and adolescents: The nuts and bolts* (2nd ed.). New York: Guilford Press.

Kendall, P. C. (2021). *Flexibility within fidelity: Breathing life into a psychological treatment manual.* New York: Oxford University Press.

McClure, J. M., Friedberg, R. D., Thordarson, M. A., & Keller, M. (2019). *CBT express: Effective 15-minute techniques for treating children and adolescents.* New York: Guilford.

Murphy, V. B., & Christner, R. W. (2006). A cognitive-behavioral case conceptualization approach for working with children and adolescents. In R. B. Mennuti, A. Freeman, & R. W. Christner (Eds.), *Cognitive-behavioral interventions in educational settings: A handbook for practice* (pp. 37–62). New York: Routledge.

Murphy, V. B., & Christner, R. W. (2012). A cognitive-behavioral case conceptualization for children and adolescents. In R. B. Mennuti, R. W. Christner, & A. Freeman (Eds.), *Cognitive-behavioral interventions in educational settings: A handbook for practice* (2nd ed.) (pp. 81–114). New York: Routledge.

Needleman, L. D. (1999). *Cognitive case conceptualization: A guidebook for practitioners.* Mahwah, NJ: Lawrence Erlbaum.

Nezu, A. M., & Nezu, C. M. (1993). Identifying and selecting target problems for clinical interventions: A problem-solving model. *Psychological Assessment, 5*, 254–263.

Paul, G. L. (1967). The strategy of outcome research in psychotherapy. *Journal of Consulting Psychology, 31*, 109–118.

Paul, G. L. (1969). Behavior modification research: Design and tactics. In C. M. Franks (Ed.), *Behavior therapy: Appraisal and status* (pp. 29–62). New York: McGraw-Hill.

Persons, J. B., Beckner, V. L., & Tompkins, M. A. (2013). Testing case formulation hypotheses in psychotherapy: Two case examples. *Cognitive and Behavioral Practice, 20*, 399–409.

Persons, J. B., & Davidson, J. (2010). Cognitive-behavioral case formulation. In K. S. Dobson (Ed.), *Handbook of cognitive-behavioral therapies* (pp. 172–195). New York: Guilford Press.

Persons, J. N., & Tompkins, M. A. (2007). Cognitive-behavioral case formulation. In T. D. Eells (Ed.), *Handbook of psychotherapy case formulation* (pp. 290–316). New York: Guilford.

Prochaska, J. O., & DiClemente, C. C. (1982). Transtheoretical therapy: Toward a more integrative model of change. *Psychotherapy: Theory, Research and Practice, 19*, 276–288.

Prochaska, J. O., DiClemente, C. C., & Norcross, J. C. (1992). In search of how people change: Applications to addictive behaviors. *American Psychologist, 47*, 1102–1114.

Sperry, L., & Sperry, J. (2020). *Case conceptualization. Mastering this competency with ease and confidence.* New York: Routledge.

4

TRANSDIAGNOSTIC TREATMENT IN SCHOOLS

Eva L. Feindler and Hilary B. Vidair

Child and adolescent mental health problems are associated with impaired functioning in school, such as problems with academic performance, school attendance, and degree attainment (Agnafors et al., 2021; Esch et al., 2014; Lereya et al., 2019). During the COVID-19 pandemic, child and adolescent emotional and behavioral problems increased (Meherali et al., 2021). Ideally schools are equipped to address these problems, as children spend the majority of their time each day at school. In fact, schools are one of the most common settings for children to receive mental health services (Duong et al., 2021).

School-based mental health (SBMH) services can be universal, such as prevention programs involving all students, selective, such as identifying students at risk for mental health issues or targeted toward children who are already experiencing mental health problems (McKenzie et al., 2017). Unlike in clinical settings, however, SBMH personnel often work with children who have received a classification through the special education system rather than DSM-5 diagnoses (Shaw & Edwards, 2019). In addition, children often present with multiple problems and need help with different issues throughout treatment (Weisz et al., 2015). This can make it difficult for SBMH clinicians to identify appropriate evidence-based treatment (EBT) manuals, which are typically focused on specific disorders. Furthermore, school stakeholders are likely most interested in mental health treatment when programs can positively impact academic outcomes, yet many SBMH programs have not included this dual focus (Vidair et al., 2013).

There are additional barriers to implementing EBTs in schools. For example, training staff in a number of EBTs for a variety of problems is often not feasible, as this requires a variety of implementation facilitators, such as stakeholder buy-in, experts to provide training and ongoing supervision or consultation on specific EBTs, and time and incentives for SBMH professionals to participate in each training (e.g., Forman et al., 2009; Vidair et al., 2013). It would be more efficient to train SBMH clinicians in treatments that can be used across different types of childhood internalizing and externalizing problems, preventatively or for children with subthreshold diagnoses, a particular diagnosis, or comorbid problems. Programs that address multiple childhood problems would also have the best chance of being sustained in schools over time.

The Development of Transdiagnostic Interventions for Children and Adolescents

The comorbidity of psychological symptomatology for children and adolescents has long been known (Angold et al., 1999; Merikangas et al., 2010). In fact, for youth, comorbidity is more the rule than

DOI: 10.4324/9781003392439-5

the exception, and many note the pervasiveness and regularity of comorbidity (Weersing et al., 2012). Transdiagnostic interventions are designed to use therapeutic techniques that address the mechanisms of problems across a variety of diagnoses (e.g., Chu, 2012; Marchette & Weisz, 2017). These interventions are theorized to reach more youth because clinicians can be trained to use one protocol to address a variety of child and adolescent problems.

Effective CBT interventions for children and adolescents have a long history and much research evidence to support the effectiveness of interventions for a host of childhood disorders (Weisz et al., 2005). Interestingly, there are some historical underpinnings for interventions with a transdiagnostic focus as well. In the early development of CBT therapeutic interventions, children were often grouped into diagnostic categories of externalizing and internalizing symptomatology. Early treatment strategies were based on effectiveness across diagnostic categories. For example, treatment approaches for externalizing disorders (including ADHD, oppositional defiant disorder, and conduct disorder) had common elements such as impulse control, problem-solving, self-regulation, and social skills training (Chase & Eyberg, 2008; Lochman et al., 2011). The same research support has been reported for internalizing disorders, including anxiety, depression, obsessive-compulsive disorder, and post-traumatic stress disorder in children and adolescents (Wergeland et al., 2021).

Additionally, there has been success in delivering group CBT in school settings for both internalizing and externalizing problems (Eiraldi et al., 2016). Finally, a recent systematic review and meta-analysis of 3rd-wave CBT interventions for youth indicated significant outcomes for emotional/internalizing problems (Perkins et al., 2023). These interventions include acceptance and commitment therapy, mindfulness-based cognitive therapy, compassion-focused therapy, and metacognitive therapy. These 3rd-wave approaches are transdiagnostically focused on common psychological processes rather than diagnostic categories.

Another set of effective interventions for youth has been parent training programs, as either standalone treatments for internalizing or externalizing problems or as an adjunct to child treatment. There is evidence that parent training programs developed for the treatment of childhood disruptive disorders have a positive impact on comorbid internalizing symptoms (Zarakoviti et al., 2021). There is also a strong research base for a transactional model in children's development. Both parent pathology and parental stress influence child development and children's presenting symptoms and vice versa. So, independent of the child's actual diagnosis, most clinicians accept the parents' role in perhaps the onset of symptomatology and certainly the maintenance of behavior disorders. Most parent training programs can be applied transdiagnostically and seem critical for positive child outcomes. However, Scott and Dadds (2009) indicate that despite the solid research support for behavioral parent training programs, a quarter to a 3rd of children and families do not benefit. In response to that, current parent training researchers have focused on other aspects of the parent-child relationship that contribute to children's disorders. A recent meta-analysis of attachment- and emotion-focused parenting programs for internalizing and externalizing youth disorders indicated that these programs effectively help parents to understand and respond to their child's emotional needs (Jugovac et al., 2022). The focus on attachment security and caregiver sensitivity is related to emotional co-regulation in the parent-child interaction and represents a transdiagnostic approach to parent training.

Over the last couple of decades, many CBT treatment developers have turned to a transdiagnostic approach to helping youth with both internalizing and externalizing problems. Since these approaches target common mechanisms related to emotion regulation and cognitive processing, they would be advantageous for addressing problems with comorbidity (Bullis et al., 2019). Rather than specific CBT interventions for broad categories of dysfunction in children, clinical researchers have looked toward developing effective interventions that can be applied across diagnostic categories and problems. For example, the *Unified Protocol for Adult Disorders* developed by Barlow (Barlow et al., 2010) was extended downward into the *Unified Protocol for Children* (UP-C) and the

Unified Protocol for Adolescents (UP-A) (Ehrenreich-May & Kennedy, 2021). These protocols are emotion-focused, evidence-based treatments for youth with emotional disorders between the ages of six and twelve for UP-C and 12–18 year olds for UP-A. In addition, Chorpita and Weisz (2009) developed the MATCH (Modular Approach to Therapy for Children with Anxiety, Depression, Trauma, or Conduct Problems) approach. This approach was developed as a distillation and matching model with key "practice elements" (Chorpita et al., 2005). According to Chorpita and colleagues, many of the manual-based diagnostic-specific protocols can be distilled into their common elements. Subsequently, practitioners can then select specific practice elements that would be effective given particular child characteristics (Chorpita et al., 2007). Practice elements include psychoeducation, cognitive coping, problem-solving, activity scheduling, and social and communication skills (see Chorpita et al., 2007 for a more detailed listing). These protocols address the lack of feasibility and acceptability for manualized treatments expressed by practitioners in the field and circumvent the need for specialized training in specific diagnostic-based protocols.

Overall, many transdiagnostic programs have been developed and tend to focus on core cognitive dysfunction, emotion regulation, and behavioral difficulties that are common in childhood disorders. The following section reviews the major transdiagnostic intervention programs for youth that have been implemented in school settings, highlighting treatment components and research support. Then, there is a brief review of some universal CBT prevention programs with school applications that can be considered as transdiagnostic programs. Table 4.1 presents a brief overview of these programs, including the following: population focus, problem or content focus, delivery format, number of sessions, available languages, factors the researchers discuss related to their implementation in schools, the most rigorous research method used in schools, and websites for further information.

Major Transdiagnostic Intervention Programs in School Settings

Unified Protocols for Adolescents (UP-A) and Children (UP-C)

Both the UP-A and the UP-C are focused on the following three main targets: altering antecedent cognitive appraisal, the prevention of emotional avoidance, and the modification of behavioral action tendencies (Ehrenreich-May & Kennedy, 2021). The foundational aspects of this transdiagnostic approach are emotion education, cognitive flexibility, and opposite action during intense emotions. Specific treatment strategies seek to teach youth more adaptive coping skills to emotional reactions.

The UP-A protocol includes eight modules for the adolescent plus several parenting sessions focused on parenting the emotional adolescent (García-Escalera et al., 2020). Designed for ages 12–18 as a downward adaptation of the adult protocol, the UP-A was developed for individual treatment and varies in length from 12 to 16 sessions. Treatment strategies target underlying dysfunctions such as engagement in maladaptive action tendencies, such as cognitive or behavioral avoidance, distress intolerance, and aversive reactions to emotion. Some of the intervention components are motivational enhancement, emotion-focused behavioral experiments (i.e., behavioral activation and exposure), antecedent cognitive reappraisal, problem-solving strategies, and awareness and mindfulness strategies (see Gruen & Braun, 2021 for a complete overview). The parenting module includes one to three sessions designed to target ineffective emotional parenting responses of over-control, inconsistent discipline, criticism and having the parent model healthy emotion regulation strategies. Recently, Vivas-Fernandez and colleagues (2023) have reported on a group-based abbreviated version of the UP-A, which is delivered online using a Google Meet platform. Two trained therapists offered eight sessions and a follow-up booster session to groups of six to eight adolescents. There were also add-on modules available for higher risk adolescents that targeted specific risk factors: social rejection and peer victimization, stress-related in relation to COVID-19 and healthy habits.

Table 4.1 Overview of Universal CBT Prevention Programs

Program Name	*Population Focus*	*Problem or Content Focus*	*Format*	*Number of Sessions*	*Languages Beyond English*	*Implementation Factors*	*Most Rigorous Research Method in Schools*	*Website for Further Information*
UP-C	Elementary school students	–	Child group, caregiver sessions, joint child and caregiver sessions; also integrated into regular classes	15	Spanish	Includes caregiver and parent/child sessions	Not yet conducted	unifiedprotocolkids.com
UP-A	Middle and high school students	–	Individual adolescent sessions, parent sessions	12–16	Spanish	Individual and a shortened group format	RCT	unifiedprotocolkids.com
MATCH	Ages 6–15	Elevated symptoms of anxiety, depression, trauma, and conduct problems	Individual sessions, caregiver sessions	No set #	–	–	RCT	www.practicewise.com/portals/0/MATCH_public/index.html
EMOTION	Elementary school students and parents	–	Group plus eight parent sessions	20	Norwegian	–	Cluster RCT	www.cebc4cw.org/program/emotion-coping-kids-managing-anxiety-and-depression
SUPERSKILLS	Elementary school students	–	Group	8	Spanish	–	Cluster RCT	www.superskillsforlife.com
UP2-D2	Ages 8–15	Broadband prevention	Group implemented by teachers	12	Japanese	Implemented by teachers in the classroom	Open trial	–
DBT STEPS-A	Middle and high school students	Universal skills-based curriculum	Integrated into regular classes	30	–	–	Quasi-experimental	www.dbtinschools.com

(*Continued*)

Table 4.1 (Continued)

Program Name	*Population Focus*	*Problem or Content Focus*	*Format*	*Number of Sessions*	*Languages Beyond English*	*Implementation Factors*	*Most Rigorous Research Method in Schools*	*Website for Further Information*
CSB-DBT	Elementary, middle, and high school students	–	Individual, group, and caregiver sessions	No set #	–	Components include individual, group, in-school coaching, and therapist consultation team	Open trial	www.cbc-psychology.com
BRISC	School-based mental health practitioners	Program for practitioners working with students experiencing mental health stressors	Individual	4	–	–	Cluster RCT	smartcenter.uw.edu/programs-services/brisc/
L2B	High school students	Universal mindfulness curriculum	Integrated into regular classes	10	Chinese	–	Pilot RCT	learning2breathe.org
.b	Ages 11–18	Universal mindfulness curriculum	Integrated into regular classes	6–9	Multiple languages	Brief motivational booster session	Cluster RCT	mindfulnessinschools.org
RULER	Pre-K through high school	Universal social-emotional learning program	Integrated into regular classes	N/A	–	–	Cluster RCT	www.rulerapproach.org

UP-C brings together cognitive-behavioral and mindfulness-based techniques in a single group treatment package flexible enough to address multiple symptom pictures (Gruen & Braun, 2021). This protocol includes 15 90-minute group sessions for children between 6 and 12 years old. Further, there are caregiver sessions and parent-child sessions. Caregivers are much more involved in the UP-C as compared to the UP-A. Children are trained to become Emotion Detectives and learn each of the CLUES skills: Consider how I feel, Look at my thoughts, Use detective thinking and problem-solving, Experience my emotions, and Stay healthy and happy. Grossman and Ehrenreich-May (2020) provide implementation details in a case study for an eight-year-old girl presenting with irritability and anxiety related to sleeping alone and separating from her mother.

In a study of an earlier version of the UP-C at a summer camp setting, Ehrenreich-May and Bilek (2011) describe developmental adaptations to include many interactive activities and iterative practice through behavioral experiments, all designed to keep school-aged children engaged. Further, there has been an examination of a stepped-care UP-C approach (Kennedy et al., 2020) delivered via a telehealth platform.

Therapist manuals for both UP-C and UP-A are presented as two halves of a joint therapist guide (Ehrenreich-May et al., 2018). In a 2021 book, Gruen and Braun compare and contrast the two protocols in terms of the core components and treatment objectives and give a recommended session range. Another chapter in that same book details the evidence base for the two protocols (Tonarely & Phillips, 2021). Research using both open trials and randomized control trials indicates improvements in emotional disorder symptoms and negative affect from pre- to post-treatment. Both UP-A and UP-C protocols have shown good feasibility and acceptability with youth, parents, and clinicians as well. Program developers indicate that the UP-A can be used with groups, and the UP-C can be implemented in individual treatment. Training for the UP-A clinicians includes a 12-hour workshop focused on didactics, skill demonstrations, and role-plays, followed by ongoing weekly one-hour consultation calls.

In all of the recent studies of the UP-A, the protocol was adapted as a universal preventive program because there was a strong evidence base with at-risk populations, a manualized program with clearly defined modules/sessions and the need for flexible for group interventions, in schools (García-Escalera et al., 2020). Further, the emphasis on adaptive emotion regulation seemed well-suited for the prevention of clinical symptomatology. García and colleagues (2019, 2020) examined an adapted Spanish version of the UP-C in high schools in Spain. The 1st study (García-Escalera et al., 2019) was an uncontrolled trial for 28 9th-grade students (*M* age = 14.7 years). The UP-A protocol was altered to provide nine weekly 55-minute sessions for two groups using multiple outcome measures. There were significant decreases in anxiety symptomatology (specifically social phobia and GAD) assessed by the RCADS-30 scale but no significant differences in reported depressive symptoms. Acceptability and satisfaction ratings were moderate to high for both the participating adolescents and their parents. The authors suggest that there may need to be an increased emphasis on the usual CBT strategies for depression reduction (cognitive restructuring and behavioral activation) in this group treatment protocol.

In the next study reported by García-Escalara et al. (2020), the same nine-session universal prevention program adapted from the UP-A and translated into Spanish was examined in a randomized waitlist control trial with clusters of particular classes assigned randomly to either UP-A or waitlist control. A number of assessments were given pre-post as well as at a three-month follow-up for 151 9th and 10th-grade students. The parent module was not included. Unfortunately, there was a decline in both anxiety and depressive symptoms in both groups. The researchers offer some interpretations of their data and indicate that the size of the groups (usually 30) probably diluted the impact of the CBT-based protocol. Clearly, further research is needed.

Most recently, there is a report of another Spanish-based examination of the UP-A in school setting by Fonseca-Pedrero and colleagues (2023). This randomized controlled trial (RCT) included a ten-session adaptation of the UP-A protocol and an active control group receiving progressive muscle relaxation. A computerized screening questionnaire was administered to over 1,000 students between 12 and 18 years of age. Then, adolescents at risk of emotional disorders with a moderate score on both the PHQ-9 and GAD-7 were offered the treatment program as part of a nation-wide project entitled PSICE (Evidence-based Psychology in Educational Contexts). In preparation for this large program implementation, 10–20 school psychologists with at least two years of experience will be trained in the modified UP-A. The results of this large investigation have not yet been reported.

Although research has not yet been conducted on the use of the UP-C in school settings, there was a report on an earlier version of UP-C called Emotion Detectives used as a Prevention Program (EDPP) at a recreational summer camp (Ehrenreich-May & Bilek, 2011). The EDPP was originally a 15-session program developed as a downward extension of the Unified Protocol for adults. Later revised as the UP-C, this earlier version focused on psychoeducation and experiential activities designed to train adaptive coping skills applicable across a range of all emotional experiences. This prevention approach was presented to participants in a transdiagnostic manner that easily allowed for discussion of emotions of varying intensity. The EDPP was an optional program available to children ages 7–10 attending summer camp. Pre-post research was conducted in an open trial format in a non-randomized approach so that all campers whose parents provided consent were able to receive four large group sessions. Results from the sample of 40 children were mixed. Although there was evidence for self-reported decreases in anxiety symptoms, parent reports were not significant for change. Further, there were no differences in measures of depression or emotions regulation. There were reports of high acceptability and program satisfaction from both the child and parent participants. The researchers cite some situational barriers to conducting their research in the camp environment and note the dilution of the program into only four large group meetings may have impacted the results obtained.

Modular Approach to Therapy for Children

MATCH is considered a modular treatment developed to address comorbid problems in children ages 6–15 using a protocol where clinicians can flexibly select interventions based on an individual child's needs over time (Chorpita & Weisz, 2009). The protocol was designed to include the most common practice elements that have demonstrated research support for each disorder. Specifically, the MATCH protocol includes a variety of EBT strategies for treating children with anxiety, depression, trauma, and conduct problems, such as exposures, behavioral activation, trauma narrative, and reward systems, respectively (Marchette & Weisz, 2017). There is no set number of sessions for this treatment; rather, the clinician decides how long to focus on a specific intervention strategy and the order of strategies used based on a child's presenting problem and treatment response. The protocol includes an overall flowchart to help clinicians decide which intervention strategy to use and in what order, as well as flowcharts for each of the four problem areas. This approach utilizes the evidence base while also allowing the practitioner to use their clinical judgment when developing an individualized treatment plan. Training in the MATCH protocol typically involves six full days, followed by weekly consultation sessions with experts.

MATCH has been evaluated in a SBMH setting. Specifically, MATCH was examined in an effectiveness RCT for children ages 7–13, where it was compared to EBT manuals for singular disorders (e.g., CBT for anxiety, depression, and trauma, behavioral parent training for behavioral issues) as well as treatment as usual (TAU) in both SBMH and community clinic settings (Weisz et al., 2012). The study included 174 children who had been referred to treatment in these local settings. Community-based clinicians were randomly assigned to provide one of the three treatments. Clinicians in both the modular and the standard condition received six days of training on three protocols focused on treating anxiety, depression, and child behavior. These clinicians received weekly consultations from supervisors involved with the project, while those in TAU received supervision as usual. The average duration of treatment in the modular and singular treatment conditions was 16.17 sessions, and 41% of the sessions included a child and at least one family member. MATCH was found to be significantly more effective than both singular EBTs and TAU for a variety of child's internalizing and externalizing problems. Children who had participated in MATCH continued to show significant improvements over those in TAU at a two-year follow-up (Chorpita et al., 2013).

An innovative MATCH effectiveness RCT is now being conducted exclusively in schools with students in kindergarten through 8th grade who are actually referred for SBMH services rather than recruited for a research study (Harmon et al., 2021). Both clinical and academic outcomes are being examined for the 1st time, the latter of which includes attendance, grades, academic and behavioral competence as assessed by teachers, and cognitive, behavioral, and emotional engagement in school. In this trial, MATCH is being compared to TAU. Participants are being recruited across 27 schools in five Boston school districts, which ensures ethnic diversity. To the authors' knowledge, the results of this RCT have yet to be published. The researchers emphasized that the sustainability of MATCH in these schools will depend on the mitigation of typical implementation barriers, such as demands on school counselors to engage in other activities, large caseload size, and time allotted for therapy sessions.

EMOTION: Coping Kids Managing Anxiety and Depression

Originally designed as a group intervention protocol for children ages 8–13 who are experiencing anxiety and depression (Kendall et al., 2013), EMOTION: Coping Kids Managing Anxiety and Depression is considered transdiagnostic, but the focus is on internalizing symptoms and the underlying mechanism of emotion regulation. Children exhibiting symptoms related to anxiety and depression meet twice a week for 20 group sessions with no more than six participants. In addition, each child meets individually with the group leaders, who are school psychologists, for two individual sessions. For depressive symptoms, EMOTION emphasizes (a) building a positive self-schema and (b) behavioral activation. For anxiety problems, EMOTION emphasizes graduated exposure to feared situations, using the Brave Practice plan. In exposure tasks, the child will experience some anxious distress and is prevented from escaping or avoiding: the child confronts and faces increasingly challenging situations. Playful and experiential activities (e.g., the Solution Round Robin activity) are used to generate multiple ideas for handling certain situations. (See Martinsen et al. [2016] for a detailed description of the session content.) Further, the EMOTION program includes eight parent sessions that occur alongside the group sessions for children and can occur with children as well.

The EMOTION program was initially evaluated with 5th graders in a rural school in Norway (Martinsen et al., 2016). Martinsen et al. detail the objectives and activities for each of the group sessions. Psychoeducation about symptoms, problem-solving, cognitive restructuring, and emotion regulation skills were taught in creative ways to engage children and provide practice of new skills.

Twenty-two children signed up for this program evaluation and completed both an anxiety and depression self-report measure, while parents completed the Child Behavior Checklist pre- and post-intervention. A ten-question consumer satisfaction survey was completed by children, parents, and group leaders to determine the satisfaction, usefulness, and feasibility of the EMOTION program. Results revealed that children reported increased emotion-coping abilities and reductions in internalizing symptomatology (Martinsen et al., 2016).

In a subsequent larger investigation in Norway, Martinsen et al. (2019) used a clustered randomized design with 36 schools as the unit of randomization. Psychologists and school health nurses provided the EMOTION intervention after a three-day training, and CBT supervisors gave weekly supervision to EMOTION group leaders as they implemented the 20-session program to

8- to 12-year-olds ($n = 591$: 272 in the EMOTION program and 319 in the control condition) identified as at risk for emotional and behavioral difficulties. Seven sessions for parents were also included, and pre-post scores on self-report and parent report measures were compared to children in the control schools. Both parents and children reported significant reductions in depressive symptomatology as compared to the control group, while only the children reported significant decreases in anxiety symptoms. A further study in Norway used the same data set but specifically assessed changes in emotion regulation using the 23-item caregiver Emotion Regulation Checklist, which measures both positive and negative emotion regulation skills (Loevaas et al., 2019). Results indicated significant improvements in emotion regulation for children receiving the EMOTION program as compared to the control condition. These studies provide an evidence base for this school-implemented program, but there was also a substantial parent component, which may not be feasible in US school settings.

Super Skills for Life

The Super Skills for Life (SSL) protocol includes eight weekly group sessions focused on emotion education, problem-solving and social skills training, self-monitoring, and cognitive reappraisal for children from six to ten years of age (Fernández-Martínez et al., 2019). The group intervention protocol was based on a number of CBT elements, such as social skills training, problem-solving skills training, cognitive reappraisal, and behavioral activation (Essau et al., 2014). The authors indicated that the treatment components targeted typical risk factors for children, such as low self-esteem, deficits in social skills, and biases in social information processing. This SSL protocol also included video feedback to enhance children's self-appraisal of their skill development. In addition, this allowed researchers to code the two-minute speech videos made by the children in sessions 1 and 8. The protocol was designed for a school setting and facilitators who were not specialist psychologists but were social workers and school counselors with diverse experiences working with children (Essau et al., 2019).

The SSL transdiagnostic protocol was originally evaluated in an open clinical trial for 61 children ages 8–10 years whom their teachers referred to as having significant anxiety problems (Fernández-Martínez et al., 2019). Results indicated significant reductions in anxiety symptoms, as well as in other forms of difficulties such as hyperactivity, conduct, and peer problems at post-assessment and the six-month follow-up. In another study by Essau and colleagues (2019), the SSL was adapted into a transdiagnostic prevention program for children with both emotional and behavioral problems. This was another open clinical trial with 205 children between the ages of 8 and 12 years. Data from three assessment points (pre-post and at six-month follow-up) indicated significant reductions in total anxiety reported by children (using the SCARED measure) and reductions in emotional symptomatology on the Strengths and Difficulties Questionnaire completed by teachers and parents. Analyses of the speech videos also indicated reductions in indicators of social anxiety (changes in the length of gaze, vocal quality, length of speech, and conversational flow).

The SSL protocol was later translated into Spanish, and a larger school-based cluster-RCT for 123 young children between the ages of 6 and 8 years was reported (Fernández-Martínez, 2019). In this study, children whose parents indicated they had some emotional difficulties were recruited from ten schools and were randomly assigned to either the SSL intervention or the waiting list control group. Parents completed four assessment measures before and after the eight-week small group intervention. When compared to the control group, the children receiving the SSL program showed significant reductions in symptoms of depression, anxiety, social anxiety, physical injury fears, and emotional problems (i.e., both anxiety and depression). Data from a 12-month follow-up study with these same children and their parents were reported by 107 parents (Fernández-Martínez et al., 2020). Results indicated that reduction of anxiety and depressive symptoms was maintained at this follow-up, although effect sizes were lower.

Universal Unified Protocol for Diverse Disorders

The Universal Unified Protocol for Diverse Disorders (UP2-D2) program was developed as a broadband transdiagnostic prevention program for students ages 8–15, originally designed for use in grades 4–6 (Hida et al., 2020). It is a 12-session program that integrates many of the core CBT elements, including emotion education, behavioral activation, social skills training, and cognitive restructuring. The unique part of this program is that it was designed to be implemented in school settings and by teachers in the classroom environment. Ishikawa and colleagues (2019) described the development of the program, which is structured with specific lesson plans for each session, combined into an overall teaching plan to enhance effective implementation in the schools. Overall, the program has a positive orientation focused on strengths and resilience, along with a multi-element cartoon developed to have a storyline in which the four defined characters experience distress in common situations at school and learn how to cope with them. The authors believe that this creative element increases engagement, learning, and retention of protocol components. (See Ishikawa et al. [2019] for a detailed description of the treatment objectives and strategies taught in each of the 12 sessions. The cartoon elements are also described.) The protocol received high ratings from a sample of 213 children between 9 and 12 years of age for both acceptability and satisfaction.

Hida et al. (2020) reported outcome studies of the impact of UP2-D2 implementation in two different elementary schools in Japan. In the 1st school, 58 children participated in the UP2-D2 training twice a month for six months. For Study 1, two participating teachers received 1.5 hours of on-site training for learning rationales for interventions and how to run the program and then received ongoing supervision by professionals with mental health expertise. Results indicated some reductions for both internalizing and externalizing behavioral problems on a general measure but no significant changes on more specific measures of anger, anxiety, and depression. In Study 2, with 73 slightly older elementary students, three teachers implemented the program with the same frequency; however, their training was different. Specifically, the teachers were given self-learning DVD materials (lasting about 1.5 hours) to learn the rationale and management of the program, but they did not receive on-site teacher training and ongoing supervision. The outcomes for this school were negligible, allowing the researchers to emphasize the importance of the training conducted in the 1st school. Neither sample was compared to a control group, and all of the measures were self-report by the children. Kishida and colleagues (2023) suggest that additional more methodologically rigorous research is needed.

Kishida and colleagues (2023) conducted a very similar evaluation of the UP2-D2 program in a junior high school sample. However, this time, the program was implemented immediately after pandemic-related school closures had ended in Japan. One hundred and twenty students ages 12–13 from three classes at a public high school completed the UP2-D2 program as well as multiple self-report assessments pre-post and at a two-month and six-month follow-up. In this study, teachers received two hours of on-site training and three hours of supervision across time. Results indicated that anxiety for the whole sample decreased and was maintained for at least six months, but no significant improvement was observed for other mental health problems, such as depression and anger. Examining a subset of data ($n = 20$) for those students who started the program with clinically elevated anxiety, results showed greater reductions in self-reported anxiety as well as for general difficulties, emotional symptoms, conduct problems, and depression. This would support the notion that UP2-D2 might have the greatest impact on clinical or subclinical populations in the school setting.

DBT in Schools

Dialectical Behavior Therapy (DBT) is an evidence-based multicomponent treatment that blends standard CBT techniques with some Eastern meditation practices based on a dialectical worldview (e.g., Rathus & Miller, 2015). There has been a tremendous amount of research to date on the effectiveness of DBT intervention programs for the most difficult of populations. Dialectical behavior therapy for adolescents (DBT-A) teaches mindfulness, emotion regulation, distress tolerance, and interpersonal effectiveness. It includes walking the middle path, an added skill set related to adolescent-family challenges. This additional component can also include adolescents' interactions with other adults in school or community settings. Although originally developed for multiproblem, suicidal adolescents, in recent years, DBT-A has emerged as a transdiagnostic program for adolescents presenting with a wide variety of emotional and behavioral problems. This approach to reducing emotionally dysregulated behavior, especially non-suicidal self-injury and suicidal thoughts and behaviors in adolescents, is well-researched.

DBT STEPS-A (Dialectical Behavior Therapy Skills Training for Emotional Problem Solving for Adolescents) is a universal social-emotional curriculum for middle school and high school students based on DBT (Mazza et al., 2016). This curriculum includes 30 lessons designed for 50-minute class periods in school. The lessons are skills-based and include the same skills found in DBT: mindfulness, emotion regulation, distress tolerance, and interpersonal effectiveness. The premise for teaching these skill sets universally was that all adolescents can benefit from learning how to manage confusion about their identity, emotions, impulsive urges, and interpersonal interactions. The curriculum is intended to be administered by teachers or SBMH personnel.

Given the school setting is the most common place to encounter emotionally dysregulated students, DBT developers then designed CSB-DBT (Comprehensive School-Based DBT) (Miller et al., 2023). CSB-DBT involves a broad approach for students and school staff to learn a set of foundational skills. Further, the program aims to shift school culture from a reactive one to a proactive one, helping to reduce emotional distress and conflict in the school setting. Designed initially for middle to high school-level students, it has since been examined for use with elementary school students. CSB-DBT has four components: individual counseling, group skills training, coaching in school, and a consultation team (Miller et al., 2023). A 5th component, caregiver involvement, is recommended when feasible.

All CSB-DBT components are designed to achieve the following main aspects of the DBT approach: (1) the acquisition of new behavioral and emotion regulation skills, (2) an increase in students' motivation for change, (3) generating ways for skills to generalize to all facets of the students' environments (classroom, lunchroom, home, peers), (4) methods to increase motivation and skill development of DBT providers in the school setting, and (5) orchestrating change (such as regular times) so that the student can receive comprehensive DBT within the school (Miller et al., 2023). The 1st component of individual counseling is implemented by trained SBMH staff, and the frequency of sessions depends on an assessment of the emotional and behavioral difficulties of the individual student. Using a weekly diary card, treatment targets center around reducing life-threatening, quality of life-threatening, and therapy-interfering behaviors while increasing the various positive skills taught in the skills group. There are five modules in the skills group: emotion regulation, interpersonal effectiveness, distress tolerance, walking the middle path, and core mindfulness. See Miller et al. (2023) for a more thorough discussion of characteristics of dysregulation (emotional, behavioral, cognitive, interpersonal and self) and the associated DBT skills leading to better outcomes. In-school coaching is used to help generalize skills learned in groups to in-vivo occurrences of dysregulation. Students are encouraged to reach out to staff for in-vivo coaching when in distress. These contacts are brief (three to five minutes) and help both to prompt DBT skills application to natural triggers and to reduce distress in a preventative fashion. Either the individual student's clinician or other staff members trained in DBT can serve as a coach. Finally, of utmost importance is the weekly meeting of the CSB-DBT consultation team made up of staff members who have been trained and work directly with students in some CSB-DBT modality. This facilitates support and discussion for staff in a non-judgmental way so as to further staff skill development and reduce burnout/stress.

Research support for DBT STEPS-A has been accumulating during the past few years, with a number of studies completed in European countries (Chugani et al., 2022). In 2022, Chugani and colleagues examined the acceptability, appropriateness, and feasibility of implementation of DBT STEPS-A in a low-income high school setting. A school staff population of 29 general education and special education teachers, school counselors, and administrators were trained and assigned to co-teach two DBT classes per week during the high school health class. The program was delivered in a modified 19-lesson curriculum; however, no student outcomes were assessed. Staff who were trained found the program to be quite appropriate, although many times, modifications were required to adapt to the way a high school day runs. There was a desire for additional training and coaching support.

Martinez and colleagues (2022) examined the STEPS-A integrated into a classroom health and physical education curriculum with pretest and posttest nonequivalent groups quasi-experimental research design. Delivered by school counselors to 9th-grade classes in a rural area (two intervention and two regular curriculum classes), 42 co-ed students with a mean age of about 15 years completed pre-post measures of social-emotional competency and emotion regulation. Modified into a 20-module format, counselors delivered the program over 12 weeks and received DBT coaching/support from the researchers. Results indicated that students who received the STEPS-A classes reported significant improvements in social resiliency, emotion regulation, and acceptance/understanding of DBT skills. An exploratory analysis of the perceived self-efficacy of DBT skills, however, did not show a treatment effect, and the authors call for an examination of the importance of adapting the program to be more culturally sensitive when implemented with diverse student populations.

Unfortunately, to date, there have been no RCTs demonstrating the effectiveness of the CSB-DBT comprehensive program (Miller et al., 2023). Miller et al. describe the few small open trials and a comprehensive case study of CSB-DBT implementation in a large public school district of approximately 5,000 students, grade levels K-12. Their detailed, step-by-step implementation guide, as well as the "Do's and Don'ts" list, will help school personnel anticipate the complex process required to consider incorporating CSB-DBT.

BRISC: Brief Intervention for School Clinicians

Based upon the common elements approach to intervention for youth, this SBMH intervention approach (Brief Intervention for School Clinicians [BRISC]) for high schools is a stepped-care model designed to assess and triage students with emotional and behavioral issues (Lyon et al., 2015). Lyon and colleagues (2014, 2015) described several qualitative research projects conducted to guide the development of the BRISC approach such that it would align with the identified needs of the students and the SBMH providers and integrate service delivery into the school setting. The five primary elements of the BRISC protocol include a problem-solving approach to identify intervention targets and possible interventions, a common elements foundation to providing specific EBT modules to match the students' presenting problems, a stepped care/tiered structure, culturally sensitive student engagement and motivation strategies, and systematic data collection and outcomes evaluation (Lyon et al., 2014). Qualitative data from structured interviews with SBMH providers revealed three important themes: alignment with the school setting, a need for flexible and responsive treatment implementation, and effective use of data already available in the school context.

In 2015, Lyon et al. examined the acceptability, feasibility, and appropriateness for 11 high school students who received the BRISC intervention as part of a standard school-based health center appointment. The BRISC protocol outlined four sessions (each lasting between 30 and 60 minutes), based on the following treatment elements shared across effective interventions for internalizing and externalizing problems in adolescents: (1) assessments and problem identification,

(2) psychoeducation and problem-solving with a selection of a solution and the development of a behavioral experiment for that solution, (3) select and implement modules including cognitive restructuring, emotion regulation, motivation enhancement, and interpersonal communication, and (4) readminister assessment, identify progress, and troubleshoot. The 4th session included options for post-BRISC triage/planning should there be further need for service. Using a combination of qualitative and quantitative data, researchers determined that clinicians were able to deliver the intervention within the recommended time (four 30–60 minute sessions) and that 9 of 11 students attended all four sessions, indicating feasibility and acceptability. Further, students had significant improvements in coping and planful problem-solving skills on standardized measures. The authors note that BRISC appears useful for increasing student engagement and targeting individualized student needs.

In 2022, Crooks and colleagues reported on a five-year retrospective qualitative study on the implementation success and challenges using the BRISC intervention model. Participants in this study included 13 female school mental health clinicians responsible for supervising the use of BRISC in their respective schools. Coding of interview data revealed a number of themes supporting BRISC as an efficient and effective intervention and emphasizing the integrated data-informed decision-making process. Further, the importance of high-quality training/supervision and the attitudes and self-efficacy of clinicians were critical to successful implementation.

Most recently, Bruns and colleagues (2023) conducted a large RCT across three states, 49 schools and 457 high school students. The BRISC intervention was implemented by licensed mental health clinicians already conducting SBMH counseling in partnership with 15 school districts. The schools were randomly assigned to the BRISC condition (n = 259 students) or the service as usual (SAU) condition (n = 198). The SBMH practitioners received a day and a half of in-person training followed by biweekly phone consultations with the trainers. Students and SBMH practitioners completed a number of standardized self-report measures, fidelity checks, and survey assessments at baseline, two and six months post-intervention. Although fidelity measures showed excellent adherence and exit surveys supported the feasibility and acceptability of BRISC, student outcome data indicated few differences between the treatment and SAU students. There was a significant decrease in youth-reported top problems (YTPA) for the BRISC students, while both groups showed improvement for the other measures of anxiety, externalizing and internalizing problems, and impairment. Essentially, adolescent symptom and functioning measures showed significant improvement, but these changes did not differ by condition. This is unfortunate for such a well-designed and comprehensive study of the impacts of BRISC. However, further research will surely be ongoing as SBMH practitioners had such a positive evaluation of this brief intervention approach.

Other Prevention-Based CBT Programs in Schools

The promotion of mental well-being has been supported by the implementation of social-emotional learning (SEL) platforms. System-wide SEL approaches have been foundational in the development of CASEL: *Collaborative for Academic, Social, and Emotional learning* (see www.pg.casel.org). With a long history of successful school-wide implementation, SEL is a skills-based approach for helping students achieve the following competencies: self-awareness, self-management, social awareness, relationship skills, and responsible decision-making. Successful implementation usually involves SBMH staff, teachers, and administrators. The Program Guide for CASEL has a database that includes 85 programs and shows the types of outcomes these programs have been effective for, as well as some implementation facilitators of each program. Below, we review three of these programs that appear closely aligned with transdiagnostic and CBT approaches.

L2B: Learning to Breathe Program

Learning to Breathe (L2B) is designed as a universal school-based prevention program for adolescents (Eva & Thayer, 2017). This mindfulness curriculum for adolescents has a strong foundation in adolescent developmental processes and is designed to be implemented in a classroom setting. The overall goal is to cultivate emotional balance through the practice of mindfulness. Although there are similarities in CBT approaches to emotion regulation, there are also some important differences in the theoretical base. Both approaches view thoughts as connected to feelings and behaviors and help to build skills to be less reactive to emotional experiences. However, the mindfulness approach to emotion regulation does not involve restructuring cognitions related to the content of specific experiences. Rather, mindfulness approaches advocate for changing the nature of one's relationship to that emotional experience. According to Metz et al. (2013),

> Rather than directing attention to changing beliefs, mindfulness builds attentional capacity to become aware of and less reactive toward the whole range of pleasant, unpleasant, or neutral experience. Uncomfortable thoughts and feelings are viewed as temporary mental events that are allowed to exist without the need to challenge, change, or be captured by them.
>
> *(p. 254)*

Letting go of maladaptive thoughts and increasing self-compassion will result in greater distress tolerance and reduced experiential avoidance. (See the chapter by Broderick and Frank, 2014 for an expanded discussion of the rationale and foundations for teaching mindfulness to adolescents.)

Based on this approach, the L2B curriculum is designed around six core themes: body awareness, understanding and working with feelings and with thoughts, integrating awareness of body sensations, thoughts and feelings, reducing negative self-judgments, and integrating mindful awareness into everyday life (Broderick & Metz, 2009). These core themes line up with the acronym BREATHE: Body, Reflection/Thought, Emotions, Attention, Tenderness, Habits for a healthy mind, and Empowerment.

In some reports, the L2B curriculum was integrated into high school health classes as 45-minute sessions offered twice per week over five weeks (Broderick & Metz, 2009), while in others, shorter lessons (15–25 minutes) were integrated into elective choir classes for 18 sessions over four months (Metz et al., 2013). Class sizes were those of normal high school classes between 25 and 32 students. Each of the six themes is manualized, and the program includes workbooks and CDs/DVDs for in-home practice of mindfulness strategies. Regular classroom teachers volunteer for MBSR (Mindfulness-Based Stress Reduction) training over eight weeks and then receive a two-day in-service by program developers. The various versions of L2B are adjusted in terms of the number of sessions and the length of time from start to finish based on particular school needs and populations served.

There have been a number of evaluations of treatment outcomes for the L2B program, all in middle and high school settings (Broderick & Frank, 2014). The 1st pilot program evaluation (Broderick & Metz, 2009) was in an all-girls private high school where the program was linked to the school's health classes and implemented by the program developers. Outcome results on multiple measures for the 105 seniors indicated a significant decrease in negative affect, increases in emotion regulation, and increases in feelings of calm, relaxed, and self-accepting when compared to a sample of 30 juniors in a control group. Further, two-thirds of the target sample indicated the use of mindfulness practices outside of the classroom. Next, Metz and colleagues (2013) examined an altered version of L2B with public high school students from grades 10 to 12. The mindfulness-based curriculum was blended into mixed-gender elective choir classes and delivered in 18 shortened sessions over 16 weeks by the explicitly trained choir teacher. Class sizes were large for the 129 students receiving the program as well as for the 87 who just received regular choir instruction. Multiple self-report assessments from pre to post indicated significant gains in emotion regulation, decreases in psychosomatic symptoms and perceived stress, and increases in overall self-regulation efficacy.

Bluth et al. (2016) conducted a randomized pilot study on an alternative high school for ethnically diverse Hispanic youth. The L2B program was implemented by an experienced teacher and mindfulness practitioner across 11 sessions and was compared to an active control group of a usual, evidence-based substance abuse class. Comparisons of the youth receiving L2B (n = 14) to the active control group (n = 13) on multiple symptom, mindfulness, and self-compassion measures revealed significant reductions in only anxiety and depression for the treatment group. Qualitative data on variables related to program satisfaction indicated that students appreciated most the safe space created for the program, the flexibility of the curriculum to adapt to students' needs, and inviting students to participate and not judging students who opted out. Further, the data indicated that since an outside person did the program implementation, students appreciated having an in-house staff member as a program assistant.

Also, conducting a small pilot study, a staff educational psychologist at an alternative high school for youth at risk of school failure conducted the L2B program over six weeks for 23 youth ages 17–20 (Eva & Thayer, 2017). Post-intervention, students' scores on self-esteem and perceived stress scales improved; however, there were no significant gains on the Mindful Attention Awareness Scale, thus compromising the outcomes. Interestingly, eight students elected to participate in a post-intervention focus group, yielding qualitative outcomes. Coding data from the focus group, the following themes emerged as skills enhanced: self-regulation, attention awareness, and positive thinking.

Conducted in a boarding school for at-risk female adolescents, Rawlett et al. (2019) compared L2B to an attention intervention implemented by nurse practitioners in another pilot RCT. Both groups of ethnically diverse 6th graders met weekly for 1–1½ hours over six weeks. They completed the following standardized assessment before and after the interventions: *Response to Stress Scale, Positive and Negative Affect Scale for Children*, and the *Mindful Attention and Awareness Scale*. Although the intervention was deemed feasible as there was good attendance and engagement, there were no significant improvements on any of the three scales. Strengths of this study were the focus on the urban minority participants, the use of standardized outcomes assessment measures, and implementation by school health care providers. The small sample size (only 11–12 girls in each condition) and the possible intermixing of the interventions due to girls all living together during the week may have compromised the outcome results.

Finally, Lucas-Thompson and colleagues (2020) report on an enhanced curriculum, namely, L2B Plus, in order to support the practice of mindfulness in everyday life and during times of greater stress. This was accomplished by creating an on-demand library full of additional resources about mindfulness education and developing a cache of messages that functioned as reminders to engage in mindful practice, motivational messages to encourage mindful practice and positive self-efficacy messages. This focus on enhancing mindfulness practice at home is supported by previous research: children who reported more frequent use of the mindfulness practices had higher well-being scores at post-intervention and follow-up, lower depression scores at post-intervention, and lower stress scores at follow-up in a study reported by Kuyken et al. (2013) across a number of British schools. Further, another element of L2B Plus is ecological momentary assessments (EMA) that are used throughout the day to ask participants to report on their levels of stress/mindfulness so that intervention content can be delivered "*just-in-time*" (JIT) to real-time data from participants. See Lucas-Thompson et al. (2020) for examples of each of these messages. Adding this more technological aspect will likely appeal to adolescents; however, there is no data yet to support this enhancement.

.b: Mindfulness in Schools

Huppert and Johnson (2010) designed the .b program as an adaption of the mindfulness programs based on Kabat-Zinn's work. Mindfulness approaches target improvements in emotion awareness, sustained attention, and the regulation of both attention and emotions. Initially, this was a four session once per week program designed to offer the principles and practices of mindfulness. The session focused on the concepts of awareness and acceptance, practices of bodily awareness of contact points, mindfulness of breathing and finding an anchor point, awareness of sounds, understanding the transient nature of thoughts, and finally, walking meditation. Huppert and Johnston compared intervention and control groups on cognitive and affective mindfulness, resiliency, and overall well-being. Participants from the UK were 153 adolescent boys (ages 14–15 years) recruited from religious education classes. In six classes, the .b program was implemented by longstanding mindfulness practitioners, and five classes served as the usual curriculum control. Results showed that although there was no overall group difference between the groups, a multiple regression analysis revealed that significant changes in mindfulness and well-being were related to the frequency of between-session practice. The authors indicate that four 40-minute sessions were not sufficient and that 43% of the students wanted the .b program to be longer.

Volanen and colleagues (2016, 2020) expanded the .b curriculum to nine 45-minute sessions across nine weeks in their evaluation of a large non-clinical sample of 12- to 15-year-olds from 56 schools in Finland. Their cluster randomized control trial compared three groups: .b program, a standard relaxation program as an active control condition, and a non-treatment group. Classes were randomly assigned to these groups, and the program was implemented by 14 educated facilitators (teachers, school psychologists, and other health professionals). Students, teachers, and parents completed assessments of depressive symptoms, resilience, and strengths and difficulties at pre and post-treatment, as well as at 6 and 12-month follow-up. Complete data analyses were available for 970 students in the .b group, 1,034 in the relax group, and 308 in the non-treatment group. Modest improvements in resilience and social-emotional functioning were reported for the .b group, and reductions in depressive symptoms showed a decrease for girls. Further, those who completed the suggested independent mindfulness practice had greater increases in resiliency. The rigorous nature of this research and the use of an active control group in this relatively short school-based mindfulness intervention provide evidence for the effectiveness of .b (Volanen et al., 2020).

An associated research project (with the above data set) reported by Beattie and colleagues (2019) sought to identify predictors/determinants of sustained mindfulness practice after this .b program and to develop and test a booster intervention to increase independent mindfulness practice between sessions. Analyses of predictors of mindfulness practice from an early batch of .b program completers ($n = 177$) allowed for the creation of a brief motivational booster session to be added to a later batch received .b+ booster ($n = 152$). Students responded to questions about their expectations of mindfulness practice, their self-efficacy for doing it, their intentions to practice, their reason not to practice, and their perceptions about peers who practice mindfulness. Results indicated that the top reason for not engaging in mindfulness practice was that students did not find it helpful, and the strongest predictor of practice was the perception that peers were practicing. These two factors were then integrated into booster session activities (slideshow presentation of peer practice, a video about peers' experience with practice, and a group activity for identifying personal motives). Unfortunately, there was no significant impact for those students receiving the .b+ booster intervention, and researchers concluded that a higher "dose" of booster materials would be important to consider (Beattie et al., 2019). What is most commendable is the use of research data to develop the relevant content of booster sessions.

RULER

RULER is a program designed to enhance SEL for children from pre-K through high school (www.rulerapproach.org). The acronym represents five components of emotional intelligence: recognizing emotions, understanding their causes and consequences, labeling emotions with the right choice of words, expressing emotions as appropriate for societal or cultural norms, and regulating emotions (Brackett et al., 2012). This school-based curriculum is integrated into classroom lesson plans, typically in English and history courses, in developmentally appropriate ways across multiple years. Students are taught to identify feelings and connect them to personal experiences, identify them in the news and books they are reading, discuss them in class and with family members, and draw or write about them. Each feeling unit lasts approximately two weeks, with each curriculum designed to cover one academic year.

One quasi-experimental study assessed the effects of RULER on social and emotional competence as well as academic performance (Brackett et al., 2012). Specifically, the study included 273 5th and 6th graders from 15 classrooms across three schools. Schools were randomly assigned to implement RULER in either their 5th or 6th-grade classes. They then conducted school as usual in the remaining participating classes. All teachers received three hours of emotional literacy training, regardless of study condition. Those teaching RULER obtained an additional nine hours of training in the curriculum. To assess program adherence, researchers visited teachers four times during the year to address questions and review student work. In addition, the principal of each school reviewed lesson plans to check if RULER material was being adequately covered. Students' social and emotional competence was assessed via teacher's reports of student behavior, while academic performance was evaluated via report cards. Results indicated students in RULER classrooms had significantly higher social and emotional competence (e.g., social skills, leadership), fewer problems, and higher end-of-the-year grades in English language arts (ELA) and work habits/social development than students serving as controls. This study provided preliminary support for RULER's impact on student SEL and academic outcomes.

RULER's theoretical model suggests that implementation of the RULER curriculum facilitates classroom-level changes, including emotional support and literacy, which then lead to improvements in instructional support and classroom organization (Hagelskamp et al., 2013). These classroom-level changes are then theorized to lead to individual student improvements in SEL and academic outcomes. A cluster RCT was used to examine if RULER does, in fact, facilitate classroom-level changes in the order hypothesized. Sixty-two Catholic schools in the New York City area were randomly assigned to either teach RULER as part of their ELA classes or teach their classes as usual. Across schools, 164 5th and 6th students and 90 teachers participated. Schools offering RULER provided teachers with nine hours of training, as well as at least five coaching sessions across each year of the study. Teachers were also offered the training again at the start of the 2nd year. Teachers implemented the RULER lesson plans during their ELA classes, introducing a new feeling word unit every two to three weeks. Teachers reported completing an average of approximately seven units per year. Outcomes were tested at the classroom level via systematic observation of classroom quality (i.e., emotional support, organization, and instructional support). As hypothesized, at the end of two years, results indicated RULER classrooms demonstrated significantly more emotional and instructional support, as well as better organization. Instructional support and organization after year two were both partially explained by the amount of emotional support in year 1. This study provided support for the theory behind RULER and emphasized the importance of teaching SEL in schools.

Transdiagnostic Intervention Implementation Recommendations for SBMH Clinicians

The transdiagnostic interventions outlined in this chapter have all been found to have some empirical support in schools. These types of interventions are likely more amenable and useful to school settings than treatments focused on specific disorders due to their common practice elements and flexible protocols. At the same time, it is challenging to implement interventions conducted as part of research studies, even effectiveness studies conducted in real-world settings, on the ground in SBMH settings, outside of the context of research. Doing so requires a variety of implementation facilitators, including the following: key stakeholder buy-in (e.g., SBMH staff, teachers, administrators), funding, an intervention's fit with student needs, inclusion of SBMH staff, time to train and consult, ample time for SBMH personnel to conduct therapy, experts to provide training and consultation, parental/caregiver consent, time for students to attend therapy sessions, parent engagement, assessment of intervention adherence, and student, parent, and school staff satisfaction (e.g., Forman et al., 2009; Vidair et al., 2013).

Based on the aforementioned implementation facilitators and descriptions of transdiagnostic intervention research studies in schools to date, we provide several recommendations for SBMH clinicians interested in helping to implement transdiagnostic interventions in their schools.

Recommendations

1. Become well-versed in the rationale for transdiagnostic interventions and what makes them feasible to implement in schools, such as their common practice elements that reduce the need for training in multiple protocols and their ability to be used flexibly for individual student needs, as well as what can practically be done at school (e.g., number of sessions).
2. Identify the types of student problems most commonly found in your SBMH caseload and determine how they could be addressed through the use of any of the transdiagnostic protocols. Consider students who might benefit from universal, selective, and/or targeted approaches. For feasibility, consider students who are already slated to receive SBMH services.
3. Present the rationale for implementing transdiagnostic interventions to key school stakeholders, such as school administrators, other SBMH professionals, teachers, and parents. Advocate for the use of these protocols by highlighting how improvement in mental health can positively impact academic outcomes, such as school attendance, grades, and standardized test scores. Present these big ideas and also accept starting with partial implementation.
4. Identify interested SBMH clinicians and teachers who want to join your transdiagnostic intervention implementation efforts and in what capacity (e.g., recruit, advocate, treat students).
5. Determine if there are school funds that can be used to hire a transdiagnostic intervention expert for training and consultation. Even a small amount of funding/expert time is a useful start!
6. Identify times SBMH clinicians and teachers can use to attend transdiagnostic training, participate in consultation meetings, and treat students. Approach school administrators about protecting this time.
7. Consider ways to implement parts of a transdiagnostic intervention over time. Figure out what will likely be most feasible and start small!
8. Identify feasible ways to involve parents in transdiagnostic interventions (e.g., via telehealth, in various languages, providing child care, food, and transportation for in-person sessions, offering sessions after school hours and finding ways to compensate SBMH staff for this time).
9. Once you begin a transdiagnostic intervention, systematically track recruitment and participant data, including how students, parents, and school staff are approached to participate, who agrees to do so, the types of problems addressed in therapy, treatment attendance, and completion.
10. Systematically track which components of a transdiagnostic intervention each student received, as well as the school staff's experience implementing it.
11. Systematically evaluate a mix of student's clinical and academic outcomes prior to and after they receive the transdiagnostic intervention.

12 Once you implement a transdiagnostic intervention, assess student, parent, and school staff satisfaction with their experience and, when possible, make adjustments to how it is implemented based on their feedback.
13 Help set up methods for assessing school staff's adherence to the transdiagnostic intervention and work to improve adherence over time.

Please keep in mind we are not suggesting one SBMH clinician should be able to implement all of these recommendations at once or on their own. Even taking some or part of the steps listed can be a step toward making a school-based transdiagnostic intervention possible!

Conclusions

In this chapter, we review the critical intersection of mental health and education, particularly highlighting the escalation of child and adolescent mental health issues amidst the COVID-19 pandemic. We underscore the significant impact of mental health problems on school performance, attendance, and overall academic success. This highlights the importance of SBMH services as a primary avenue for intervention, given the substantial portion of time children spend in educational settings. There are challenges to adapting EBTs for educational contexts, including coexisting conditions among students and the need for SBMH professionals to be versatile in their approach due to the broad range of student needs. We propose transdiagnostic interventions as a more practical and effective strategy for tackling the diverse mental health issues present in schools. These interventions, by focusing on common underlying factors across disorders, offer a streamlined and adaptable approach to mental health care in educational settings.

Reflection Questions

1 What are the advantages of incorporating a transdiagnostic approach in a school setting?
2 What can you see as barriers to the implementation of transdiagnostic interventions for the mental health needs of youth in school settings?
3 What are some ways school-based practitioners can facilitate the implementation of transdiagnostic interventions in school settings?

References

Agnafors, S., Barmark, M., & Sydsjö, G. (2021). Mental health and academic performance: A study on selection and causation effects from childhood to early adulthood. *Social Psychiatry and Psychiatric Epidemiology, 56*(5), 857–866. https://doi.org/10.1007/s00127-020-01934-5

Angold, A., Costello, J., & Erkanli, A. (1999). Comorbidity. *Journal of Child Psychiatry and Psychology, 40*, 57–87. https://doi.org/10.1111/1469-7610.00424

Barlow, D. H., Ellard, K. K., & Fairholme, C. P. (2010). *Unified protocol for transdiagnostic treatment of emotional disorders: Workbook*. Oxford: Oxford University Press.

Beattie, M., Hankonen, N., Salo, G., Knittle, K., & Volanen, S.-M. (2019). Applying behavioral theory to increase mindfulness practice among adolescents: An exploratory intervention study using a within-trial RCT design. *Mindfulness, 10*(2), 312–324. https://doi.org/10.1007/s12671-018-0976-2

Bluth, K., Campo, R. A., Pruteanu-Malinici, S., Reams, A., Mullarkey, M., & Broderick, P. C. (2016). A school-based mindfulness pilot study for ethnically diverse at-risk adolescents. *Mindfulness, 7*, 90–104. https://doi.org/10.1007/s12671-014-0376-1

Brackett, M. A., Rivers, S. E., Reyes, M. R., & Salovey, P. (2012). Enhancing academic performance and social and emotional competence with the RULER Feeling Words Curriculum. *Learning and Individual Differences, 22*(2), 218–224. https://doi.org/10.1016/j.lindif.2010.10.002

Broderick, P. C., & Frank, J. L. (2014). Learning to BREATHE: An intervention to foster mindfulness in adolescence. *New Directions for Youth Development, 2014* (142), 31–44. https://doi.org/10.1002/yd.20095

Broderick, P. C., & Metz, S. (2009). Learning to BREATHE: A pilot trial of a mindfulness curriculum for adolescents. *Advances in School Mental Health Promotion, 2*(1), 35–46. https://doi.org/10.1080/1754730X.2009.9715696

Bruns, E. J., Lee, K., Davis, C., Pullmann, M. D., Ludwig, K., Sander, M., Holm-Hansen, C., Hoover, S., & McCauley, E. M. (2023). Effectiveness of a brief engagement, problem-solving, and triage strategy for high school students: Results of a randomized study. *Prevention Science, 24*(4), 701–714. https://doi.org/10.1007/s11121-022-01463-4

Bullis, J. R., Boettcher, H., Sauer-Zavala, S., Farchione, T. J., & Barlow, D. H. (2019). What is an emotional disorder? A transdiagnostic mechanistic definition with implications for assessment, treatment, and prevention. *Clinical Psychology: Science and Practice, 26*(2), Article e12278. https://doi.org/10.1037/h0101755

Chase, R. M., & Eyberg, S. M. (2008). Clinical presentation and treatment outcome for children with comorbid externalizing and internalizing symptoms. *Journal of Anxiety Disorders, 22*(2), 273–282. https://doi.org/10.1016/j.janxdis.2007.03.006

Chorpita, B. F., Becker, K. D., & Daleiden, E. L. (2007). Understanding the common elements of evidence-based practice: Misconceptions and clinical examples. *Journal of the American Academy of Child and Adolescent Psychiatry, 46*(5), 647–652. https://doi.org/10.1097/chi.0b013e318033ff71

Chorpita, B. F., Daleiden, E. L., & Weisz, J. R. (2005). Identifying and selecting the common elements of evidence-based interventions: A distillation and matching model. *Mental Health Services Research, 7*(1), 5–20. https://doi.org/10.1007/s11020-005-1962-6

Chorpita, B. F., & Weisz, J. R. (2009). Modular approach to therapy for children with anxiety, depression, trauma, or conduct problems (MATCH-ADTC). *Proprietary material*. Retrieved from http://www.practicewise.com/portals/0/MATCH_public/index.html.

Chorpita, B. F., Weisz, J. R., Daleiden, E. L., Schoenwald, S. K., Palinkas, L. A., Miranda, J., Higa-McMillan, C. K., Nakamura, B. J., Austin, A. A., Borntrager, C. F., Ward, A., Wells, K. C., Gibbons, R. D., & Research Network on Youth Mental Health (2013). Long-term outcomes for the Child STEPs randomized effectiveness trial: A comparison of modular and standard treatment designs with usual care. *Journal of Consulting and Clinical Psychology, 81*(6), 999. https://doi.org/10.1037/a0034200

Chu, B. C. (Ed.) (2012). Translating transdiagnostic approaches to children and adolescents. *Cognitive and Behavioral Practice, 19*(1), 1–4. https://doi.org/10.1016/j.cbpra.2011.06.003

Chugani, C. D., Murphy, C. E., Talis, J., Miller, E., McAneny, C., Condosta, D., Kamnikar, J., Wehrer, E., & Mazza, J. J. (2022). Implementing dialectical behavior therapy skills training for emotional problem solving for adolescents (DBT STEPS-A) in a low-income school. *School Mental Health*, 1–11. https://doi.org/10.1007/s12310-021-09472-4

Crooks, C., Fortier, A., Graham, R., Hernandez, M., Chapnik, E., Cadieux, C., & Ludwig, K. (2022). Implementing a brief evidence-based tier 2 school mental health intervention: The enablers and barriers as seen through a clinical team supervisor lens. *Canadian Journal of Community Mental Health, 41*(3), 139–156. https://doi.org/10.7870/cjcmh-2022-017

Duong, M. T., Bruns, E. J., Lee, K., Cox, S., Coifman, J., Mayworm, A., & Lyon, A. R. (2021). Rates of mental health service utilization by children and adolescents in schools and other common service settings: A systematic review and meta-analysis. *Administration and Policy in Mental Health, 48*(3), 420–439. https://doi.org/10.1007/s10488-020-01080-9

Ehrenreich-May, J., & Bilek, E. L. (2011). Universal prevention of anxiety and depression in a recreational camp setting: An initial open trial. *Child & Youth Care Forum, 40*, 435–455. https://doi.org/10.1007/s10566-011-9148-4

Ehrenreich-May, J., & Kennedy, S. M. (Eds.) (2021). *Applications of the unified protocols for transdiagnostic treatment of emotional disorders in children and adolescents*, ABCT Clinical Practice Series. Oxford: Oxford University Press. https://doi.org/10.1093/med-psych/9780197527931.001.0001

Ehrenreich-May, J., Kennedy, S. M., Sherman, J. A., Bilek, E. L., Buzzella, B. A., Bennett, S. M., & Barlow, D. H. (2018). *Unified protocols for transdiagnostic treatment of emotional disorders in children and adolescents: Therapist guide*. Oxford: Oxford University Press.

Eiraldi, R., Power, T. J., Schwartz, B. S., Keiffer, J. N., McCurdy, B. L., Mathen, M., & Jawad, A. F. (2016). Examining effectiveness of group cognitive-behavioral therapy for externalizing and internalizing disorders in urban schools. *Behavior Modification, 40*(4), 611–639. https://doi.org/10.1177/0145445516631093

Esch, P., Bocquet, V., Pull, C., Couffignal, S., Lehnert, T., Graas, M., Fond-Harmant, L., & Ansseau, M. (2014). The downward spiral of mental disorders and educational attainment: A systematic review on early school leaving. *BMC Psychiatry, 14*, 237. https://doi.org/10.1186/s12888-014-0237-4

Essau, C. A., Olaya, B., Sasagawa, S., Pithia, J., Bray, D., & Ollendick, T. H. (2014). Integrating video-feedback and cognitive preparation, social skills training and behavioural activation in a cognitive behavioural therapy in the treatment of childhood anxiety. *Journal of Affective Disorders, 167*, 261–267. https://doi.org/10.1016/j.jad.2014.05.056

Essau, C. A., Sasagawa, S., Jones, G., Fernandes, B., & Ollendick, T. H. (2019). Evaluating the real-world effectiveness of a cognitive behavior therapy-based transdiagnostic program for emotional problems in children in a regular school setting. *Journal of Affective Disorders, 253*, 357–365. https://doi.org/10.1016/j.jad.2019.04.036

Eva, A. L., & Thayer, N. M. (2017). Learning to BREATHE: A pilot study of a mindfulness-based intervention to support marginalized youth. *Journal of Evidence-Based Complementary & Alternative Medicine, 22*(4), 580–591. https://doi.org/10.1177/2156587217696928

Fernández-Martínez, I., Morales Sabuco, A., Espada Sánchez, J. P., Orgilés Amorós, M., & Essau, C. A. (2019). Effectiveness of the program Super Skills for life in reducing symptoms of anxiety and depression in young Spanish children. *Psicothema, 31*, 298–304. https://doi.org/10.7334/psicothema2018.336

Fernández-Martínez, I., Orgilés, M., Morales, A., Espada, J. P., & Essau, C. A. (2020). One-year follow-up effects of a cognitive behavior therapy-based transdiagnostic program for emotional problems in young children: A school-based cluster-randomized controlled trial. *Journal of Affective Disorders, 262*, 258–266. https://doi.org/10.1016/j.jad.2019.11.002

Fonseca-Pedrero, E., Pérez-Albéniz, A., Al-Halabí, S., Lucas-Molina, B., Ortuño-Sierra, J., Díez-Gómez, A., Perez-Saenz, J., Inchausti, F., Garcia, A. V., Garcia, A. G., Solana, R., Rodenas-Perea, G., Clemente, M., Lopez, A., & Debbane, M. (2023). PSICE project protocol: Evaluation of the unified protocol for transdiagnostic treatment for adolescents with emotional symptoms in school settings. *Clinical and Health, 34*(1), 15–22. https://doi.org/10.5093/clysa2023a3

Forman, S. G., Olin, S. S., Hoagwood, K. E., Crowe, M., & Saka, N. (2009). Evidence-based interventions in schools: Developers' views of implementation barriers and facilitators. *School Mental Health, 1*(1), 26–36. https://doi.org/10.1007/s12310-008-9002-5

García-Escalera, J., Chorot, P., Sandín, B., Ehrenreich-May, J., Prieto, A., & Valiente, R. M. (2019, February). An open trial applying the unified protocol for transdiagnostic treatment of emotional disorders in adolescents (UP-A) adapted as a school-based prevention program. *Child & Youth Care Forum, 48*, 29–53, Springer US. https://doi.org/10.1007/s10566-018-9471-0

García-Escalera, J., Valiente, R. M., Sandín, B., Ehrenreich-May, J., Prieto, A., & Chorot, P. (2020). The unified protocol for transdiagnostic treatment of emotional disorders in adolescents (UP-A) adapted as a school-based anxiety and depression prevention program: An initial cluster randomized wait-list-controlled trial. *Behavior Therapy, 51*(3), 461–473. https://doi.org/10.1016/j.beth.2019.08.003

Grossman, R. A., & Ehrenreich-May, J. (2020). Using the unified protocol for transdiagnostic treatment of emotional disorders with youth exhibiting anger and irritability. *Cognitive and Behavioral Practice,* 27(2), 184–201.

Gruen, R., & Braun, D. (2021). Delivery of standard UP-C and UP-A treatment for youth. In J. Ehrenreich-May & S. M. Kennedy (Eds.), *Applications of the unified protocols for transdiagnostic treatment of emotional disorders in children and adolescents*, ABCT Clinical Practice Series (pp. 17–30). Oxford: Oxford University Press. https://doi.org/10.1093/med-psych/9780197527931.003.0002

Hagelskamp, C., Brackett, M. A., Rivers, S. E., & Salovey, P. (2013). Improving classroom quality with the RULER approach to social and emotional learning: Proximal and distal outcomes. *American Journal of Community Psychology, 51*(3–4), 530–543. https://doi.org/10.1007/s10464-013-9570-x

Harmon, S. L., Price, M. A., Corteselli, K. A., Lee, E. H., Metz, K., Bonadio, F. T., Hersh, J., Marchette, L., Rodriguez, G., Raftery-Helmer, J., Thomassin, K., Bearman, S., Jensen-Doss, A., Evans, S., & Weisz, J. R. (2021). Evaluating a modular approach to therapy for children with anxiety, depression, trauma, or conduct problems (MATCH) in school-based mental health care: Study protocol for a randomized controlled trial. *Frontiers in Psychology, 12*, 639493. https://doi.org/10.3389/fpsyg.2021.639493

Hida, N., Ishikawa, S., Murasawa, T., & Oguni, M. (2020). Effect of universal unified prevention program for diverse disorders for junior high school students. *Doshisha Clinical Psychology: Therapy and Research, 10*, 3–13. https://doi.org/10.14988/00027868

Huppert, F. A., & Johnson, D. M. (2010). A controlled trial of mindfulness training in schools: The importance of practice for an impact on well-being. *The Journal of Positive Psychology, 5*(4), 264–274. https://doi.org/10.1080/17439761003794148

Ishikawa, S. I., Kishida, K., Oka, T., Saito, A., Shimotsu, S., Watanabe, N., Sasamori, H., & Kamio, Y. (2019). Developing the universal unified prevention program for diverse disorders for school-aged children. *Child and Adolescent Psychiatry and Mental Health, 13*(1), 1–15. https://doi.org/10.1186/s13034-019-0303-2

Jugovac, S., O'Kearney, R., Hawes, D. J., & Pasalich, D. S. (2022). Attachment- and emotion-focused parenting interventions for child and adolescent externalizing and internalizing behaviors: A meta-analysis. *Clinical Child and Family Psychology Review, 25*(4), 754–773. https://doi.org/10.1007/s10567-022-00401-8

Kendall, P. C., Stark, K. D., Martinsen, K., O'Neil, K. A., & Arora, P. (2013). *EMOTION: "Coping kids" managing anxiety and depression; group leaders manual.* Ardmore, OK: Workbook Publishing.

Kennedy, S. M., Lanier, H., Salloum, A., Ehrenreich-May, J., & Storch, E. A. (2020). Development and implementation of a transdiagnostic, stepped-care approach to treating emotional disorders in children via Telehealth. *Cognitive and Behavioral Practice, 28*(3), 350–363. https://doi.org/10.1016/j.cbpra.2020.06.001

Kishida, K., Hida, N., Matsubara, K., Oguni, M., & Ishikawa, S. I. (2023). Implementation of a transdiagnostic universal prevention program on anxiety in junior high school students after school closure during the COVID-19 pandemic. *Journal of Prevention, 44*(1), 69–84. https://doi.org/10.1007/s10935-022-00709-9

Kuyken, W., Weare, K., Ukoumunne, O. C., Vicary, R., Motton, N., Burnett, R., Cullen, C., Hennelly, S., & Huppert, F. (2013). Effectiveness of the mindfulness in schools programme: Non-randomised controlled feasibility study. *The British Journal of Psychiatry: The Journal of Mental Science, 203*(2), 126–131. https://doi.org/10.1192/bjp.bp.113.126649

Lereya, S. T., Patel, M., Dos Santos, J. P. G. A., & Deighton, J. (2019). Mental health difficulties, attainment and attendance: A cross-sectional study. *European Child & Adolescent Psychiatry, 28*(8), 1147–1152. https://doi.org/10.1007/s00787-018-01273-6

Lochman, J. E., Powell, N. P., Boxmeyer, C. L., & Jimenez-Camargo, L. (2011). Cognitive-behavioral therapy for externalizing disorders in children and adolescents. *Child and Adolescent Psychiatric Clinics of North America, 20*(2), 305–318. https://doi.org/10.1016/j.chc.2011.01.005

Loevaas, M. E. S., Sund, A. M., Lydersen, S., Neumer, S. P., Martinsen, K., Holen, S., Patras, J., Adolfsen, F., & Reinfjell, T. (2019). Does the transdiagnostic EMOTION intervention improve emotion regulation skills in children? *Journal of Child and Family Studies, 28*(3), 805–813. https://doi.org/10.1007/s10826-018-01324-1

Lucas-Thompson, R. G., Rayburn, S., Seiter, N. S., Broderick, P. C., Smyth, J. M., Coatsworth, J. D., & Henry, K. L. (2020). Learning to BREATHE "Plus": A multi-modal adaptive supplement to an evidence-based mindfulness intervention for adolescents. *Frontiers in Public Health, 8.* https://doi.org/10.3389/fpubh.2020.579556

Lyon, A. R., Bruns, E. J., Ludwig, K., Stoep, A. V., Pullmann, M. D., Dorsey, S., Eaton, J., Hendrix, E., & McCauley, E. (2015). The Brief Intervention for School Clinicians (BRISC): A mixed-methods evaluation of feasibility, acceptability, and contextual appropriateness. *School Mental Health, 7*(4), 273–286. https://doi.org/10.1007/s12310-015-9153-0

Lyon, A. R., Bruns, E. J., Weathers, E. S., Canavas, N., Ludwig, K., Vander Stoep, A., Cheney, D., & McCauley, E. (2014). Taking evidence-based practices to school: Using expert opinion to develop a brief, evidence-informed school-based mental health intervention. *Advances in School Mental Health Promotion, 7*(1), 42–61. https://doi.org/10.1080/1754730X.2013.857903

Marchette, L. K., & Weisz, J. R. (2017). Practitioner review: Empirical evolution of youth psychotherapy toward transdiagnostic approaches. *Journal of Child Psychology and Psychiatry, 58*(9), 970–984. https://doi.org/10.1111/jcpp.12747

Martinez Jr, R. R., Marraccini, M. E., Knotek, S. E., Neshkes, R. A., & Vanderburg, J. (2022). Effects of dialectical behavioral therapy skills training for emotional problem solving for adolescents (DBT STEPS-A) program of rural ninth-grade students. *School Mental Health, 14*(1), 165–178. https://doi.org/10.1007/s12310-021-09463-5

Martinsen, K. D., Kendall, P. C., Stark, K., & Neumer, S. P. (2016). Prevention of anxiety and depression in children: Acceptability and feasibility of the transdiagnostic EMOTION program. *Cognitive and Behavioral Practice, 23*(1), 1–13.

Martinsen, K. D., Rasmussen, L. M. P., Wentzel-Larsen, T., Holen, S., Sund, A. M., Løvaas, M. E. S., Patras, J., Kendall, P. C., Waaktaar, T., & Neumer, S. P. (2019). Prevention of anxiety and depression in school children: Effectiveness of the transdiagnostic EMOTION program. *Journal of Consulting and Clinical Psychology, 87*(2), 212–219. https://doi.org/10.1037/ccp0000360

Mazza, J. J., Dexter-Mazza, E. T., Miller, A. L., Rathus, J. H., & Murphy, H. E. (2016). *DBT Skills in schools: Skills training for emotional problem solving for adolescents (DBT STEPS-A).* New York: Guilford Press.

McKenzie, V., Vidair. H. B., Sauro, D., & Eacott, C. (2017). School mental health and psychological intervention in a school setting. In M. Thielking & M. D. Terjesen (Eds.), *Handbook of Australian school psychology, international research, practice and policy* (pp. 235–239). New York: Springer.

Meherali, S., Punjani, N., Louie-Poon, S., Abdul Rahim, K., Das, J. K., Salam, R. A., & Lassi, Z. S. (2021). Mental health of children and adolescents amidst COVID-19 and past pandemics: A rapid systematic review. *International Journal of Environmental Research and Public Health, 18*(7), 3432. https://doi.org/10.3390/ijerph18073432

Merikangas, K. R., He, J., Burstein, M., Swanson, S. A., Avenevoli, S., Cui, L., Benjet, C., Georgiades, K., & Swendsen, J. (2010). Lifetime prevalence of mental disorders in US adolescents: Results from the national comorbidity study-adolescent supplement. *Journal of the American Academy of Child and Adolescent Psychiatry, 49*, 980–989. https://doi.org/10.1016/j.jaac.2010.05.017

Metz, S. M., Frank, J. L., Reibel, D., Cantrell, T., Sanders, R., & Broderick, P. C. (2013). The effectiveness of the learning to BREATHE program on adolescent emotion regulation. *Research in Human Development, 10*(3), 252–272. https://doi.org/10.1080/15427609.2013.818488

Miller, A. L., Gerardi, N., Mazza, J. J., Dexter-Mazza, E., Graling, K., & Rathus, J. H. (2023). Delivering comprehensive school-based dialectical behavior therapy (CSB-DBT). *Psychology in the Schools, 60*, 2762–2781. https://doi.org/10.1002/pits.22887

Perkins, A. M., Meiser-Stedman, R., Spaul, S. W., Bowers, G., Perkins, A. G., & Pass, L. (2023). The effectiveness of third wave cognitive behavioural therapies for children and adolescents: A systematic review and meta-analysis. *The British Journal of Clinical Psychology, 62*(1), 209–227. https://doi.org/10.1111/bjc.12404

Rathus, J. H., & Miller, A. L. (2015). *DBT skills manual for adolescents*. New York: The Guilford Press.

Rawlett, K. E., Friedmann, E., & Thomas, S. A. (2019). Mindfulness based intervention with an attentional comparison group in at risk young adolescents: A pilot randomized controlled trial. *Integrative Medicine Research, 8*(2), 101–106. https://doi.org/10.1016/j.imr.2019.04.002

Scott, S., & Dadds, M. R. (2009). Practitioner review: When parent training doesn't work: Theory-driven clinical strategies. *Journal of Child Psychology and Psychiatry, 50*(12), 1441–1450. https://doi.org/10.1111/j.1469-7610.2009.02161.x

Shaw, S. R., & Edwards, M.-D. (2019). Integrating diagnostic systems in school psychology: DSM-5, ICD-11, and IDEA. In M. K. Burns (Ed.), *Introduction to school psychology: Controversies and current practice* (pp. 274–292). Oxford: Oxford University Press.

Tonarely, N., & D. Phillips (2021). Current evidence base for the UP-C and UP-A. In J. Ehrenreich-May & S. M Kennedy (Eds.), *Applications of the unified protocols for transdiagnostic treatment of emotional disorders in children and adolescents*, ABCT Clinical Practice Series (pp. 31–38). Oxford: Oxford University Press. https://doi.org/10.1093/med-psych/9780197527931.003.0003

Vidair, H. B., Sauro, D., Blocher, J. B., Scudellari, L. A., & Hoagwood, K. (2013). Empirically supported school-based mental health programs targeting academic and mental health functioning: An update. In H. M. Walker & F. M. Gresham (Eds.), *Handbook of evidence-based practices for students having emotional and behavioral disorders* (pp. 15–53). New York: Guilford Press.

Vivas-Fernandez, M., Garcia-Lopez, L. J., Piqueras, J. A., Muela-Martinez, J., Canals-Sans, J., Espinosa-Fernandez, L., Jimenez-Vasquez, D., del Mar Diaz-Castela, M., Morales-Hidalgo, P., & Ehrenreich-May, J. (2023). Retracted article: Randomized controlled trial for selective preventive transdiagnostic intervention for adolescents at risk for emotional disorders. *Child Adolescent Psychiatry Mental Health, 17*, 7. https://doi.org/10.1186/s13034-022-00550-2

Volanen, S. M., Lassander, M., Hankonen, N., Santalahti, P., Hintsanen, M., Simonsen, N., Raevuori, A., Mullola, S., Vahlberg, T., But, A., & Suominen, S. (2016). Healthy learning mind – A school-based mindfulness and relaxation program: A study protocol for a cluster randomized controlled trial. *BMC Psychology, 4*(1), 35. https://doi.org/10.1186/s40359-016-0142-3

Volanen, S. M., Lassander, M., Hankonen, N., Santalahti, P., Hintsanen, M., Simonsen, N., Raevuori, A., Mullola, S., Vahlberg, T., But, A., & Suominen, S. (2020). Healthy learning mind – Effectiveness of a mindfulness program on mental health compared to a relaxation program and teaching as usual in schools: A cluster-randomised controlled trial. *Journal of Affective Disorders, 260*, 660–669. https://doi.org/10.1016/j.jad.2019.08.087

Weersing, V. R., Rozenman, M. R., Maher-Bridge, M., & Campo, J. V. (2012). Anxiety, depression, and somatic distress: Developing a transdiagnostic internalizing toolbox for pediatric practice. *Cognitive and Behavioral Practice, 19*, 68–82. https://doi.org/10.1016/j.cbpra.2011.06.002

Weisz, J. R., Chorpita, B. F., Palinkas, L. A., Schoenwald, S. K., Miranda, J., Bearman, S. K., Daleiden, E. L., Ugueto, A. M., Ho, A., Martin, J., Gray, J., Alleyne, A., Langer, D. A., Southam-Gerow, M. A., Gibbons, R. D., & Research Network on Youth Mental Health. (2012). Testing standard and modular designs for psychotherapy treating depression, anxiety, and conduct problems in youth: A randomized effectiveness trial. *Archives of General Psychiatry, 69*(3), 274–282. https://doi.org/10.1001/archgenpsychiatry.2011.14

Weisz, J. R., Jensen Doss, A., & Hawley, K. M. (2005). Youth psychotherapy outcome research: A review and critique of the literature. *Annual Review of Psychology, 56*, 337–363. https://doi.org/10.1146/annurev.psych.55.090902.141449

Weisz, J. R., Krumholz, L. S., Santucci, L., Thomassin, K., & Ng, M. Y. (2015). Shrinking the gap between research and practice: Tailoring and testing youth psychotherapies in clinical care contexts. *Annual Review of Clinical Psychology, 11*, 139–163. https://doi.org/10.1146/annurev-clinpsy-032814-112820

Wergeland, G. J. H., Riise, E. N., & Öst, L. G. (2021). Cognitive behavior therapy for internalizing disorders in children and adolescents in routine clinical care: A systematic review and meta-analysis. *Clinical Psychology Review, 83*, 101918. https://doi.org/10.1016/j.cpr.2020.101918

Zarakoviti, E., Shafran, R., Papadimitriou, D., & Bennett, S. D. (2021). The efficacy of parent training Interventions for disruptive behavior disorders in treating untargeted comorbid internalizing symptoms in children and adolescents: A systematic review. *Clinical Child and Family Psychology Review, 24*(3), 542–552. https://doi.org/10.1007/s10567-021-00349-1

PART II

Embracing Inclusivity, Well-Being, and Diverse Services

5

CBT FOR PROMOTING WELL-BEING OF CHILDREN AND ADOLESCENTS

Shannon M. Suldo, Sarah Fefer, Kristen E. Mahony and Jacqueline Blass

Introduction and Overview of CBT to Fostering Well-Being

Best practices in school mental health care entail assessment and intervention practices to increase positive aspects of well-being alongside services to prevent and decrease symptoms of mental illness (Lazarus et al., 2021). Such comprehensive services are aligned with a dual-factor model of mental health, which recognizes that wellness and illness are related, separable, and both of importance. Indeed, the World Health Organization (WHO) affirms,

> Mental health exists on a complex continuum, with experiences ranging from an optimal state of well-being to debilitating states of great suffering and emotional pain. People with mental health conditions are more likely to experience lower levels of mental well-being, but this is not always or necessarily the case.
>
> *(WHO, 2022, p. xiv)*

Despite such clear calls to intentionally foster well-being in and of itself, substantially more research and practice has focused on cognitive-behavioral interventions intended to treat mental illness as compared to interventions intended to foster well-being. Advances in recent decades of clinical practice have yielded guidance for how to balance clinical interventions to both downregulate negative feelings and upregulate positive feelings and how to cultivate an optimal state of well-being in all individuals—not just those already suffering—through positive activities commonly drawn from the positive psychology literature. This chapter conceptualizes well-being in accordance with the wellness factor in a dual-factor model of mental health, describes corresponding assessment strategies, overviews relevant cognitive-behavioral interventions to address subjective well-being, and illustrates through case studies of applications of such interventions in school-based mental health care.

Understanding the Specific Issue—Subjective Well-Being

To properly conceptualize wellness, we begin by considering the arguably better understood illness factor (i.e., psychopathology). In cognitive-behavioral treatment of youth mental illness, practitioners seek to address multiple areas of potential vulnerability (e.g., cognitive, behavioral, affective) to reduce symptoms of psychopathology (Benjamin et al., 2011) in consideration of the behavioral,

DOI: 10.4324/9781003392439-7

biological, environmental, cognitive, social, and societal factors that may contribute to the maintenance of the presenting problem (Kuyken et al., 2009). Psychotherapeutic treatment of mental illness has heavily emphasized fixing and repairing weaknesses, like a remedial discipline (Rashid & Seligman, 2018). A narrow focus on listing, fixing, and monitoring problems assumes (incorrectly) that the absence of mental illness will translate to the presence of wellness. This can be a demoralizing experience for the client particularly when contrasted with strength-based approaches that intentionally evoke positive feelings (Geschwind et al., 2020; Suldo & Doll, 2021). The high prevalence of internalizing and externalizing forms of mental illness in children and adolescents—and the adverse outcomes associated with unmanaged mental illness—certainly justify the need for efficacious treatments, including evidence-based cognitive-behavioral interventions for various disorders, as described in other chapters of this book. However, the mere absence of clinical levels of internalizing and externalizing problems does not reflect an optimal state of well-being as reflected in the presence of healthy social-emotional experiences tied to positive outcomes.

Research within positive psychology has conceptualized optimal functioning as personal happiness (i.e., feeling good about life [hedonic tradition]) and/or striving for excellence and functioning well in life (i.e., eudaimonic tradition), and determined a biopsychosocial etiology of emotional and psychological well-being involving genetic predispositions, circumstantial variables, behavioral patterns, and relational components (Sheldon & Lyubomirsky, 2021). Personal happiness has been commonly operationalized as subjective well-being, which has cognitive and affective components (Diener et al., 2009). The cognitive component involves life satisfaction appraisals, in other words one's perceived quality of life as determined by personal standards for global/overall life or in specific domains of life (e.g., satisfaction with friends, family, school, self). The affective component involves the frequency of experiences of positive emotions (e.g., interest, joy, enthusiasm, pride, cheer) on a regular basis and in relation to the frequency of negative emotions (e.g., guilt, envy, sadness, worry) in the same time frame. Level of subjective well-being spans the full range from being acutely dissatisfied with life and experiencing a preponderance of negative emotions to judging one's life in neutral or mildly satisfactory terms, to being very satisfied with one's life and experiencing a preponderance of positive emotions.

Research with children and adolescents indicates positive, significant associations between subjective well-being and a host of positive outcomes, including concurrent and later academic achievement (Bucker et al., 2018; DiLeo et al., 2022). Moreover, numerous studies that have applied a dual-factor model of mental health in research with students in elementary, middle, high school, and college have illustrated that youth who experience a combination of high subjective well-being and few symptoms of psychopathology have superior academic, social, and physical health outcomes in comparison to peers whose absence of psychopathology co-exists with low subjective well-being (Suldo & Doll, 2021). Such findings support the importance of assessing and promoting subjective well-being among all youth, including those with and without symptoms of mental illness. Promising cognitive-behavioral interventions address the pathways to flourishing mental health, specifically activities that evoke **P**ositive emotions, increase **E**ngagement, strengthen **R**elationships, cultivate a sense of **M**eaning and purpose, and lead to **A**ccomplishments and achievements (PERMA; Seligman, 2011). Interventions that foster growth in subjective well-being alter behavioral, cognitive, and social patterns in a manner intended to mimic the practices of naturally happy people (Lyubomirsky & Layous, 2013). Collectively, these activities are often referred to as positive psychology interventions (PPIs) in recognition of the emphasis on fostering well-being through applications of the science of happiness.

Empirical Support of Interventions that Foster Subjective Well-Being

There is considerable theoretical and practical overlap between the bases of therapeutic activities intended to reduce symptoms or illness (i.e., traditional cognitive-behavioral therapy [CBT]), cultivate positive thoughts, behaviors, and feelings that underlie wellness (i.e., PPIs), and achieve both (e.g., positive psychotherapy; Rashid & Seligman, 2018). The interventions generally involve affect education to identify and understand emotions that are either distressing (i.e., negative affect) or uplifting (i.e., positive affect); examination, cultivation, or interruption of thoughts that sustain a given type of emotion; and initiation of behavioral practices that evoke positive feelings or reduce negative feelings. van Agteren and colleagues (2021) reviewed the effects of psychological interventions that have been examined in randomized controlled trials in clinical and non-clinical (i.e., general) samples in relation to change in indicators of subjective well-being (hedonic approach) or psychological well-being (eudaimonic approach). In this meta-analysis, the researchers classified interventions based on CBT as those that "target maladaptive thinking patterns, developing coping skills, emotional regulation and cognitive reappraisal," mindfulness interventions as those "solely focused on mindfulness or meditation… include diaphragmatic breathing, mind–body scan and mindful imagery," and PPIs as "activities or exercises stemming from positive psychology or interventions that focus only on building [a] positive construct" (van Agteren et al., 2021, p. 634). Further, they distinguished singular from multicomponent PPIs, with the former involving a single exercise such as Three Good Things (identify three good things that happened today and why those things occurred), Best Possible Self (visualize an ideal future life), or activities that cultivate gratitude (e.g., keep a gratitude journal, make a gratitude visit), use of character strengths, and savoring. Multicomponent PPIs include a combination of different positive psychology exercises often bundled into a lengthier program. Among samples from the general population, the meta-analysis found mindfulness-based interventions led to statistically significant small to moderate improvements, and singular and multicomponent PPIs yielded significant but small effects on well-being, but no effect of CBT on well-being. Among samples that had mental illness, mindfulness-based interventions had a moderate to large effect on well-being, followed by CBT with a small to moderate effect and multicomponent PPIs which were associated with a significant but small effect. The researchers concluded that well-being can be reliably improved using a variety of psychological approaches and that multicomponent PPIs and mindfulness-based interventions are two types associated with gains in well-being across sample types (general population vs. people identified with various forms of mental or physical illness). Whereas the van Agteren et al. (2021) study included all available evidence from experiments with youth and adults, in any setting, Tejada-Gallardo et al. (2020) conducted a meta-analysis that limited focus to outcomes from nine studies of multicomponent PPIs implemented in schools. This study found school-based multicomponent PPIs caused statistically significant, small effects on improving wellness (indicators of subjective well-being and psychological well-being) as well as on decreasing illness (indicators of depressive symptoms).

Taken together, a growing literature demonstrates that well-being can be reliably increased using programs and practices that cultivate positive interpretations of the past through activities that target gratitude, forgiveness, or visualization of positive experiences; positive behaviors in the present through activities that target kindness, use of character strengths, savoring, and relationship-enhancement; and positive thoughts about the future through activities that target hope and optimism. Positive results on well-being have been seen among general samples, supporting efforts to aim for flourishing among anyone seeking enhanced wellness, as well as among clinical samples, showing the applicability of PPIs to individuals experiencing mental illness. With the utility of PPIs being relatively established, current and future research entails integrating PPIs with mindfulness and other approaches to mental health treatment such as traditional CBT (e.g., positive psychotherapy; Rashid & Seligman, 2018), CBT and solution-focused brief therapy (e.g., positive CBT; Bannink & Geschwind, 2021) and Acceptance Commitment Therapy (e.g., Strong Minds; Burckhardt et al., 2016) and examining the impact of balanced approaches on wellness and illness outcomes.

Relational Consideration in Fostering Subjective Well-Being (Connecting)

As aforementioned, the PERMA model includes "strengthen relationships" as a central pathway to flourishing mental health (Seligman, 2011). Thus, relational considerations are particularly central to maximizing treatment outcomes within interventions that involve applications of positive psychology. Clinicians should attend to and prioritize the therapeutic relationship between themselves and the client throughout their work together, especially considering the positive impact that therapeutic alliance has on outcomes of CBT for youth (Bose et al., 2023). This alliance goes beyond client perceptions of the relationship and includes their willingness to collaborate with the clinician to work on intervention tasks and toward desired treatment outcomes. To foster a positive alliance, clinicians may consider incorporating intentional rapport building exercises or "icebreaker" activities in early sessions, demonstrate a willingness to share examples from their own lives while incorporating students' unique life experiences, consider feasibility and fit in selection of positive activities, and ensure consistency in warm interactions and predictable routines to encourage trust throughout all sessions. A focus on student strengths may also serve to build and strengthen relationships within and across sessions. For example, building rapport is an essential first step when using a specific therapeutic approach called positive CBT (Bannink & Geschwind, 2021). This starts with asking the youth questions about their daily life or interests which can function as icebreakers, allowing the clinician to unravel strengths and solutions that are already present within the youth's life. For example, questions such as "What grade are you in?", with follow-up questions such as, "What hobbies do you have?" or "What are you good at?", can be used to set a positive tone for the session, in a light-hearted manner, and inform case conceptualization and planning for future sessions.

Beyond the therapeutic alliance, clinicians should also encourage students to foster positive and supportive relationships with peers, teachers, and family members through their use of positive activities and by shifting their attention to strengths within these existing relationships. A small-group intervention modality lends itself particularly well to fostering peer relationships through practicing positive activities and strength-spotting in sessions to build peer-to-peer relationships. Activities like carrying out gratitude visits or performing acts of kindness lend themselves well to relationship building in daily life, and existing relationships across domains (e.g., school, home, extracurriculars) should be incorporated into our treatment planning as relationship building is a central strategy for improving well-being. Planning for positive activity use within existing relationships increases the likelihood that students will receive natural reinforcement to increase their motivation to use these activities in the future and provides opportunities for students to increase their access to social supports. It is important to note that some students may not have access to positive existing relationships and benefit from additional opportunities for practice and problem-solving to increase the likelihood of positive responses and/or to plan for potentially negative responses.

Interviewing and Assessing Subjective Well-Being (Assessing)

Assessing Wellness before and Throughout Interventions

Because mental wellness and illness are related yet separable constructs, practitioners are encouraged to supplement traditional approaches to clinical assessment that track symptoms of emotional and behavioral distress with measures that assess dimensions of emotional, social, and psychological flourishing. Such a comprehensive approach to measuring indicators of illness and wellness simultaneously permits clinicians to examine outcomes of their treatment with regard to decreasing distress and increasing positive mental health (Trompetter et al., 2017) and makes possible an understanding of clients' full range of recovery from mental illness, from less symptomatic to flourishing as indicated by high levels of positive emotional, social, and psychological outcomes (Rottenberg & Kashdan, 2022).

Assessment of subjective well-being entails use of self-report measure of life satisfaction and/or affect that have strong support for reliability and validity among the age range of relevance. Well-established measures of youth life satisfaction require children and adolescents to rate satisfaction with their life as a whole (i.e., global life satisfaction) or satisfaction with domain-specific areas of life that are considered central to overall appraisals of wellness (i.e., school, family, friends, self, living environment). Among youth in grades 3–12, the seven-item Students' Life Satisfaction Scale (SLSS; Huebner, 1991) and the 40-item Multidimensional Students' Life Satisfaction Scale (MSLSS; Huebner, 1994) are commonly used to assess global and multidimensional life satisfaction, respectively. Such measures can be interpreted in an ipsative manner (e.g., a child's satisfaction is lowest in this area and highest in this area) and provide a baseline level of wellness at the outset of any intervention. The six-item Brief Multidimensional Students' Life Satisfaction Scale (BMSLSS; Seligson et al., 2003), which estimates satisfaction in each of the five domains of life as well as globally, may be most useful in large-scale surveillance efforts as well as incorporated in universal screening to identify students with low life satisfaction. Whereas life satisfaction ratings are considered relatively stable and reflective of the conditions of one's life, measures of affect are more influenced by recent events as they inquire about a respondent's mood in the moment, or how often—from *not at all* to *frequently*—they have felt various positive emotions (e.g., interested, delighted) and negative emotions (e.g., lonely, mad) during a specified period of time (e.g., the past day or few weeks). The most commonly used self-report measures of affect validated for use with children and adolescents are the 10- or 27-item versions of the Positive and Negative Affect Schedule for Children (PANAS-C; Laurent et al., 1999), which assess frequency of positive and negative emotional experiences over the past few weeks.

The aforementioned measures of subjective well-being focus on the hedonic tradition of well-being which emphasizes *emotional* wellness. Seligman's (2011) PERMA model redirects attention to the salience of additional aspects of wellness aligned with the eudaimonic tradition—social and psychological strengths that reflect positive functioning. Measures of PERMA developed specifically for use with youth include the 20-item EPOCH Measure of Adolescent Well-Being (Kern et al., 2016). The EPOCH assesses Engagement, Perseverance, Optimism, Connectedness, and Happiness, characteristics in youth hypothesized to influence the PERMA domains later in life. The Social Emotional Health Survey (SEHS) developed by Furlong and colleagues is another comprehensive measure that assesses the promotive factors that underly emotional well-being. The 20-item SEHS-Primary (Furlong et al., 2013) assesses elementary school students' psychological strengths (i.e., gratitude, zest, optimism, and persistence) which collectively indicate *covitality*. The 36-item secondary version (SEHS-S; Furlong et al., 2014) yields 12 subscales that tap four expanded areas: engaged living (gratitude, zest, optimism), emotional competence (empathy, self-control, and emotion regulation), belief in self (persistence, self-efficacy, self-awareness), and belief in others (school support, family support, friend support). The EPOCH and SEHS can be included in a comprehensive assessment of assets and promotive factors that contribute to subjective well-being as indexed by the aforementioned narrowband outcome measures of life satisfaction and affect.

Interviewing for Strengths and Resources

A comprehensive clinical intake process involves formal assessment of emotional well-being using some of the aforementioned tools and identification of strengths and resources using measures of assets (e.g., SEHS; EPOCH) and/or intentional survey and interview questions about personal and social strengths. Direct inquiry about positive features of the student's self and environment conveys respect for the uniqueness of the student, uncovers assets for use in later intervention planning, and facilitates rapport.

Identification of the youth's strengths and resources, goals, motivation to change, and current experiences of hope and optimism are all foundational in the assessment process from a dual-factor model of mental health to gather sufficient information to develop a case conceptualization and intervention plan that both builds resilience and alleviates distress (Kuyken et al., 2009). Youth are not often aware of the coping strategies and strengths they use on a daily basis to be resilient; thus, a strengths-based approach offers the advantages of embedding their individual strengths in the change process to promote positive outcomes. Identifying youth's signature character strengths can help draw attention to the positive features of themselves, which they can lean into to improve their overall life functioning. Some youth—particularly those experiencing distress—may have difficulty recognizing any personal assets and strengths. In such cases, an objective assessment of one's top strengths may be useful. The VIA classification of character strengths advances 24 individual positive traits (e.g., kindness, curiosity, zest, bravery) within six virtue categories (Peterson & Seligman, 2004). The website viacharacter.org presents a description of each of the character strengths within the VIA framework and houses a free survey of these character strengths for either youth or adults to complete. The survey yields an ipsative identification of one's top strengths, referred to as "signature character strengths." After completion of the VIA Youth survey, students can record or print a screenshot of their signature character strengths and respond to questions that lead them to reflect on how they demonstrate these strengths in their daily life. Directly assessing student strengths through interviews or surveys allows for goal setting related to increased use of signature strengths, which emphasizes the possibility of change and allows the youth to focus on future possibilities (hope) rather than on problems.

Case Conceptualization (Understanding)

Understanding why a given person may present with a relatively low or high level of wellness requires appreciation for the range of biological, circumstantial and social, and behavioral factors that influence subjective well-being (Sheldon & Lyubomirsky, 2021). With regard to biological determinants, research from behavioral genetics routinely supports the heritability of momentary and chronic happiness as within a certain set range of subjective well-being scores (Nes & Røysamb, 2017). One's happiness is further affected by life circumstances that may be particularly helpful (e.g., supportive family, safe community) or harmful (e.g., physical health problems, economic challenges, societal prejudice). Within this range of happiness levels, dictated largely by biology and circumstances, well-being can be increased and maintained by intentional actions such as attempts to savor positive circumstantial changes or to engage in activities that evoke positive feelings about one's past, present, or future (Sheldon & Lyubomirsky, 2021). Although clinicians aiming to improve an individual's well-being will have their case conceptualization informed by an understanding of the plausible contributions of genetics and life circumstances, therapeutic supports to improve well-being tend to focus specifically on these intentional positive activities with the goal of evoking more positive emotions for individuals with any potential "room for growth" in their life satisfaction or overall well-being. To this end, understanding one's current level of well-being involves considering their current and potential social, behavioral, and cognitive patterns that can evoke Positive emotions, increase Engagement, strengthen Relationships, cultivate a sense of Meaning and purpose, and/or lead to Accomplishment and achievements (PERMA; Seligman, 2011). Flourishing individuals tend to naturally engage cognitively and relationally in ways that strengthen relationships and enhance their well-being (Lyubomirsky & Layous, 2013; Sheldon & Lyubomirsky, 2021), so it is the goal of a clinician to share this with the students they're working with (i.e., psychoeducation about determinants of happiness) and determine how to encourage these factors for individuals with room for growth related to happiness. Case conceptualization and treatment planning for increasing well-being focuses on: (a) increasing purposeful positive activities to evoke more positive emotions, (b) strengthening relationships, and (c) harnessing motivation to engage in positive activities and strengthen relationships. Integrating these areas of focus within a traditional CBT model allows for direct attention to thoughts, feelings, and behaviors associated with initiating and engaging in positive activities to improve life satisfaction.

An emphasis on understanding and increasing the frequency of one's positive emotions through intentional positive activities is grounded in appreciation for the numerous adaptive functions that positive emotions serve, as illustrated by Fredrickson's (2001) "broaden-and-build" theory. Positive emotions promote psychological wellness by means of upregulating positive affect, which in turn broadens the breadth of our attentional field, creating new opportunities for positive experiences while also alleviating the effects of negative emotions (Frederickson, 2001). Distinguished by increases in cognitive capacity and behavioral flexibility, positive emotions create an upward spiral that allows one to build personal social, psychological, and physical resources, which supports resilience in part through less focus on negative events and limiting harmful negative cognitive patterns (e.g., rumination, catastrophizing) common to anxiety and depression. This theory can inform our understanding of hypothesized causes and contributors to low wellness and/or heightened symptoms of mental illness, as individuals with low well-being are likely experiencing an alternative *downward* spiral of negative emotions and experiences, which can further reinforce their negative core beliefs and limit their ability to access benefits from experiences and resources present in their life. Learning and practicing positive activities is a concrete tool that can be used to change this trajectory by evoking positive emotions and strengthening relationships. When individuals with co-morbid psychopathology shift their attention to more positive events by means of cognitive construal that is evoked from gratitude or optimism interventions, rather than negative events, further benefits may be seen (Xu et al., 2015). In the context of clinical treatment of depression, the adaptive function of positive emotions has been demonstrated by longitudinal research finding that increases in positive emotions predicted concurrent and later improvements in relationship functioning and reductions in symptoms of emotional distress, even after controlling for decreases in negative emotions (McNeil & Repetti, 2022). Such findings in support of the functional benefits of positive emotions lead researchers to suggest clinicians intentionally target induction of positive emotions during therapy, using practices from positive psychology.

Individuals who are directly seeking therapeutic supports related to wellness may arrive with higher motivation to engage in therapy, and to practice specific positive activities, compared to those who are "assigned" to this approach by their caregivers, their school, or other factors. Clinicians operating from a positive psychology lens focus on understanding and increasing individuals' motivation to engage in positive activities and relationship building that would evoke and sustain positive emotions. Understanding personal and circumstantial variables contributing to current levels of motivation is important for case conceptualization, as is determining the positive activities that may be most valuable and feasible for the individual you are supporting. It may also be important to understand and problem-solve barriers to this motivation, which could be related to current or past experiences or relationships, or in the form of cognitive distortions. When conceptualizing positive activities, such as gratitude or optimism interventions, it is important to note that individuals have different preferences and comfort levels for engaging in the range of positive activities yielded from studies within positive psychology (Lyubomirsky & Layous, 2013). Research has demonstrated that not one particular activity will help every individual become happier; thus, honing in on the fit of an activity with the person seeking higher happiness is essential (Lyubomirsky et al., 2005).

Goal setting around improving wellness may first involve helping an individual to understand and estimate their inherited happiness range or setpoint, during the process of psychoeducation about the determinants of happiness. This sets the stage for a goal to increase one's current level of happiness to the upper-end of their potential range and provides an opportunity for reflection on specific activities and feelings associated with happiness in their past. Goal setting should also include increased positive activity use and target specific relationships for strengthening. Given the aforementioned importance of person-activity fit, clinicians should aim to develop skills in a range of positive activities and work collaboratively to identify those that fit best within each individual's preferences and routines as well as detect impact on mood and relationships. We should encourage individuals to "sample" these positive activities and be an emotion detective to find their favorite through self-monitoring and active reflection throughout their practice of these new positive activities. In this way, treatment planning around positive activities is likely to be collaborative and iterative and should be informed by the client's experiences and reactions to practicing new activities.

In sum, when individual youth are referred for targeted mental health supports, clinicians can draw on their knowledge of the determinants of happiness and utilize strengths-based practices to understand why that individual is experiencing diminished mental health. A strengths-based approach to case conceptualization through the combination of traditional CBT infused with PPIs can improve the effectiveness of psychotherapy, as strengths can safeguard against the effects of distress brought on by negative life events, while potentially preventing the development of psychological disorders (Huta & Hawley, 2010; Marques et al., 2011). Treatment goals involve planning for intentional activities that help youth experience PERMA (Seligman, 2011), coupled with attention to positive impact of such activities on social, relational, and academic outcomes in order to harness motivation for continued engagement in behavioral practices that work for them. Selection of activities that may build PERMA will be tailored to the clinician's understanding of the client's goals, values, relational supports, contextual circumstances, and other assets and challenges.

Session Structure When Working with Problem Area (Guiding)

A primary goal across multiple PPIs is to equip students with new skills to support the use of positive activities in their daily life. The emphasis on teaching new skills, with the goal of sustained practice, aligns well with an empirically validated teaching method called Behavioral Skills Training (BST; Kirkpatrick et al., 2019). This instructional approach is based on the principles of applied behavior analysis and includes direct instruction followed by opportunities for modeling, rehearsal, and feedback both within and outside of the training session. This training model can inform the structure of an effective CBT session which may include psychoeducation combined with skill instruction and practice. This approach is commonly used to teach individuals with autism and related disabilities (Erhard et al., 2021) and can also be used to effectively teach new skills to teachers (Kirkpatrick et al., 2019; Slane et al., 2021) and caregivers (Schaefer & Andzik, 2021). Interestingly, Donaldson et al. (2021) reviewed high quality meta-analyses and randomized controlled trial studies of PPIs and found that a very similar structure is used to effectively teach knowledge and skills related to positive psychology. Five specific components were common across the interventions reviewed: (1) learning about and gaining awareness of positive psychology, (2) skills practice, (3) reflection and reinforcement of new skills, (4) relate to peers and clarify understanding to heighten reinforcement of positive outcomes, and (5) plan for sustainable use of skills in daily life. Donaldson and colleagues (2021) suggest that clinicians structure their own PPIs by "following the science" that points to the use of these five components within a flexible training approach. Flexibility can enhance engagement and motivation; past studies demonstrate the value of providing choice in timing, pacing, and scheduling and in reminders or check-ins between counseling sessions. Allowing students to choose to engage in the positive activities that are best suited to their individual preferences and unique contexts can increase the opportunity for natural reinforcement of skills and lead to more positive intervention effects (Lyubormirsky & Layous, 2013) and also aligns with developmentally relevant goals for autonomy and competence.

Taken together, practitioners planning to teach positive activities should ensure that they can clearly describe the rationale for and components of multiple positive activities to their clients, come prepared with specific examples and models to enhance their description, and plan exercises to practice the new positive activity in the session. Routines for sharing about and reflecting on positive activity use should be built into each session, with multiple opportunities for reinforcement and feedback related to use of the new skill within the natural environment and/or within session. In our work with the Well-Being Promotion Program (WBPP; Suldo, 2016, described next section), we describe and practice skills in session individually and with peers, encourage conversations and practice at home through weekly caregiver communication, and incentivize completion of "take home challenges" between sessions with an in-session reward at the beginning of the following session. In this small group setting, students also have access to peers and to group leaders with expertise in positive psychology to get feedback and seek clarification about their positive activity use. Students learn a new positive activity each week, and they are encouraged to self-select their preferred activities for increased practice once they have built their toolbox of positive activities.

Component of Practice and Intervention Modules (Intervening)

This section describes five different interventions relevant to increasing child and adolescent subjective well-being. The theoretical underpinnings of these interventions cut across social-emotional learning (SEL), primary prevention of depression, and positive psychology approaches focused on upregulating positive feelings. The interventions highlighted include MindUP (The Hawn Foundation, 2011), Positivity Project (P2) (The Positivity Project, 2023), Trails to Wellness (TRAILS, 2023a, 2023b), the Penn Resiliency Program (PRP; Gillham et al., 1990), the WBPP (Suldo, 2016), and Positive CBT (Bannink & Geschwind, 2021). The interventions described in this section span multiple levels of intervention ("tiers") as defined within a Multi-Tiered System of Supports (MTSS). MTSS is a theory of proactive and preventative systems of support that use data-based decision-making to allocate school resources to most effectively meet student need across three tiers (Raffaele Mendez, 2017). At Tier 1, interventions address all students in the school or class and generally aim to build skills and competencies to improve outcomes for all students. Practices such as SEL curriculum and positive behavioral interventions and supports (PBIS) are considered Tier 1 strategies (Raffaele Mendez, 2017). At Tier 2, supplemental interventions are offered to a subset of students (about 15% of the population) to address the needs of students whose data suggests they need more support than is provided at Tier 1. Tier 2 aims primarily to prevent larger problems from developing through early intervention and data-based decision-making (Raffaele Mendez, 2017). Tier 3 involves the fewest number of students (about 5%) who are in need of intensive individualized supports. In MTSS, students progress through the tiers based on their data and response to intervention at previous tiers. If a student is struggling despite evidence-based school-wide practices at Tier 1, they may be referred to Tier 2 where they receive more targeted support. Based on their response to that support, they may either return to Tier 1 once their need has been met or progress to Tier 3 for more targeted intervention (Raffaele Mendez, 2017).

MindUP

MindUP is a mindfulness-based Tier 1 SEL curriculum designed to help students (grades K-8) to regulate emotions, promote gratitude and kindness, and increase empathy and relatedness through activities grounded in neuroscience (The Hawn Foundation, 2011). While MindUP contains lessons focused on building traditional core SEL competencies through CBT strategies, it also has a unique focus on upregulating positive emotions through learned optimism, acts of kindness, and gratitude practice. The program consists of 12 weekly SEL lessons combined with daily mindfulness-based practice (~3 minutes a day). MindUP encourages educators to build a positive classroom milieu and reinforce the skills students are learning in lessons to create a more positive and empathetic school and classroom climate that promotes student well-being (Schonert-Reichl et al., 2015).

MindUP is a CASEL SELect program, meaning research of high design quality has shown positive outcomes and evidence-based criteria have been met (Brain Futures, 2023). Positive outcomes of MindUP have been yielded in more than 15 years of independent research, including four randomized control trials (RCTs). Findings from these studies have shown that students participating in the MindUP curriculum have demonstrated increased prosocial behaviors, increased optimism, happiness, and well-being and have shown gains in academic outcomes including performance in math and language arts (The Hawn Foundation, 2023).

Positivity Project

The P2 was developed as a Tier 1 SEL support grounded in positive psychology, the VIA character strengths framework, and the "other people mindset" which refers to the importance of relationship building and relatedness and its role in promoting well-being and positive outcomes in students (Garwood, 2022a). P2 aims to provide schools with a common vocabulary of strengths for students to utilize in their day-to-day lives as well as appreciate and encourage in others. At Tier 1, P2 provides students 15 minute a day classroom lessons that are tied to each of the 24 VIA character strengths. Students are encouraged to build on the lesson's character strength and look for that strength in others in the school community. Some lessons align closely with interventions discussed in the positive psychology literature such as the acts of kindness challenge in the kindness lesson and fostering gratitude through daily reflection. Other lessons incorporate classic CBT techniques oriented toward self-reflection and social awareness, changing thought patterns to foster optimistic thinking, and utilizing a growth mindset with the "power of yet" (The Positivity Project, 2023).

P2 can also be provided at Tiers 2 and 3. P2 partner schools receive implementation supports such as Redirection Guidance and Reflection Questions documents. The Redirection Guidance document provides question stems to prompt students to display appropriate character strengths and get them back on topic. The Reflection Questions can be used to help foster a more in-depth conversation around character strengths and how students can use them to meet expectations at school. Further, at both Tiers 2 and 3, implementation supports include six "toolkits" focused on subjects like anxiety and stress, emotional regulation, and communication. These toolkits provide lessons with more targeted instruction in use of character strengths and traditional CBT skills like cognitive restructuring to target specific areas of concern in small groups or individually. Preliminary studies by Garwood (2022a, 2022b) support the effectiveness of P2 for improving student well-being through targeting positive psychology constructs such as character strengths.

Trails to Wellness

Trails to Wellness is another multi-tiered intervention designed to address student mental health and promote well-being. At the Tier 1 level, Trails to Wellness provides universal SEL through 5 units that address the classic SEL competencies including self-awareness, self-management, social awareness, relationship skills, and responsible decision-making. Available sample SEL lessons (see https://trailstowellness.org/our-programs/social-and-emotional-learning) use "the CBT model" or the cognitive-behavioral triangle to support instruction of social skills such as conflict resolution, problem-solving, and managing strong emotions. While Tier 1 resources are more focused in a traditional approach of down-regulating negative emotions and behaviors, their Tier 2 resources described below focus on upregulating positive emotions and behaviors to improve well-being.

At Tier 2, the TRAILS Coping with COVID-19 and TRAILS CBT and Mindfulness programs are designed to support students in need of more targeted mental health support. The TRAILS Coping with COVID-19 program consists of seven sessions focused on gratitude and self-kindness, managing the physical effects of stress, getting active and practicing positive activities (e.g., using an optimistic explanatory style), coping with anxious thoughts, fostering social connection, and coping with uncertainty. The TRAILS CBT and Mindfulness course has seven to ten sessions spanning mindfulness, relaxation, cognitive coping/cognitive restructuring, behavioral activation, and systematic exposure therapy. At Tier 3, the Trails to Wellness program further addresses mental illness by offering training ("workshops") in suicide prevention, intervention, and postvention for adults at school, home, and in the community. All courses can be found online: https://trailstowellness.org/our-programs/coping-with-covid-19; https://trailstowellness.org/our-programs/cbt-and-mindfulness; https://trailstowellness.org/our-programs/suicide-prevention-and-risk-management.

All three tiers of support in Trails to Wellness are grounded in mindfulness and CBT-based practice, which are evidence-based approaches to improving well-being (van Agteren et al., 2021). Program developers state on their website that RCTs are underway to assess the effectiveness of the Trails to Wellness programs (Trails to Wellness; TRAILS, 2023a, 2023b). However, we were unable to locate any published outcome studies of Trails to Wellness program specifically, underscoring a need for further research.

The Penn Resiliency Program

The PRP intends to help youth learn optimistic thinking, consequently increasing their resilience to stressors (Gillham et al., 1990). The PRP was originally designed to prevent depression symptomology among adolescents and young adults and was expanded to include exercises to bolster strengths such as perspective and optimism (Gillham et al., 1995). This school-based cognitive-behavioral group-based intervention designed for youth ages 10–14 years old was designed to function as a Tier 1 or Tier 2 preventative intervention in hopes of preventing symptoms of depression most likely to emerge a few years later into adolescence (Rashid et al., 2015). It targets the early adolescent developmental period due to youth readiness to develop meta-cognitive skills (i.e., engaging in activities that reflect on their beliefs and the consideration of alternative options; Inhelder & Piaget, 1958).

The PRP is comprised of 12 90–120-minute manualized sessions that are built on two major components, cognitive and social problem-solving, with the intention of making abstract concepts of cognitive behavior accessible and relevant to youth. PRP uses traditional CBT strategies including (a) development of a conceptual framework for each skill, (b) group-wide discussion of hypothetical examples that demonstrate how the learned skills are useful following concept mastery, and (c) application of learned skills to youths' own lives. Through these steps, youth learn to be "detectors" of their own thoughts, specifically, inaccurate thoughts, "evaluators" of those inaccurate thoughts, and "challengers" of those negative thoughts or beliefs by means of considering alternative interpretations. Skills throughout the PRP are learned via role-playing, skits, discussions, and cartoons that illustrate the core concepts, such as self-awareness, self-regulation, strengths of character, connection (i.e., building and maintaining strong and trusting relationships), and optimism. The effects of PRP have been evaluated through several randomized controlled studies with youth ages 9–14 years old. Meta-analytic findings support a positive effect on prevention of depressive symptoms one-year post-intervention (Brunwasser et al., 2009) but without significant effects evident immediate post-intervention (Bastounis et al., 2016). Of note, Cutuli and colleagues (2006) found significant preventative effects on depressive symptoms 24–36 months after the PRP intervention was implemented.

The Well-Being Promotion Program

The WBPP (Suldo, 2016) is a multi-target, multicomponent PPI grounded in Seligman's (2002) framework for increasing subjective well-being through activities that evoke positive feelings about one's past, present, and future experiences, intentional activities that help individuals reach the upper range of their genetic setpoint for happiness (Sheldon & Lyubomirsky, 2021). The activities in the WBPP are developmentally appropriate versions of PPIs that have prior support for efficacy for increasing subjective well-being among adults, through activities that cultivate gratitude, kindness, hope, optimistic thinking, and use of signature character strengths. The WBPP was designed to be a Tier 2 small group intervention, in which school mental health providers lead ten weekly 30–45-minute sessions for small groups of students who have room for growth in life satisfaction. In school-based RCTs when the WBPP was implemented with high fidelity to manual/protocol, improvements were demonstrated in youths' subjective well-being, as well as an observed decreasing trend in externalizing and internalizing symptomology (Roth et al., 2017; Suldo et al., 2014). Currently, we are further evaluating the efficacy, fidelity, feasibility, acceptability of implementation and training, and cost-effectiveness of the WBPP through a five-year multi-site RCT (for details about the study design, see https://sreereg.icpsr.umich.edu/sreereg/ and search under Registry ID # 4600.1). The session goals and activities for the WBPP are outlined in Table 5.1. We describe this intervention in relative detail due to our particular familiarity with it, because of evidence of positive impact on subjective well-being among youth, and to set the stage for understanding the activities from within the WBPP used throughout the case studies presented later in this chapter.

All sessions follow a similar format, namely (a) a review of progress with a homework assignment,[1] (b) group discussion of a new target (e.g., kindness), (c) practice a positive activity that builds the target (e.g., plan to perform five acts of kindness in one day), and (d) assign and plan a take-home challenge for the upcoming week (e.g., perform the five acts of kindness in one day). The caregiver component of the WBPP is intended to keep parents and other caregivers apprised of the student-focused activities and facilitate student discussion and practice of positive activities learned in session to the home context. To accomplish this goal, caregivers are invited to an information session at the start of the WBPP to learn more about the program purpose and flow of activities. Then, weekly caregiver handouts are sent home via hard copy and/or electronically (e.g., email or text message from the leader) that (a) provide a brief overview of the topic covered in group, (b) describe the take-home challenge assigned to students, and (c) suggest how caregivers can apply and make use of the positive activities with their child or across the family. Throughout the group sessions, group leaders encourage students to discuss the information in these handouts with people at home and discuss the impact of family-based use of the positive activities on the wellness of the student and others in their home.

Evoking Positive Emotions about the Past (Sessions 1–3)

The intervention begins with a visualization activity designed to focus attention to positive features of the students' past. In the You at Your Best activity, students reflect and write about a time they felt at their best, allowing youth the opportunity to demonstrate something they are good at. Group leaders encourage students to share aloud these stories to provide a positive introduction of self to others in the group and identify strengths apparent in the student's story. The 1st session then moves into a group discussion on the initial definition and the importance of happiness. Group leaders clarify the purpose of the group (i.e., increase wellness, not address illness) and establish group norms. Group leaders discuss the importance of practicing positive activities between meetings and encourage students to involve someone at home. Students receive their first take-home challenge—review and expand their You at Your Best story—and are encouraged to share it with their caregivers or friends. At the start of the next session, group leaders help students reflect on how completing the take-home challenge and involving family members impacted their mood and relationships. In Session 2, the topic of gratitude is introduced through a discussion of initial definition and its importance to happiness. Research has shown that youth who "count their blessings," also known as "gratitude journaling," experience positive effects on their subjective well-being (Froh et al., 2008). Relatedly, Session 3 introduces a 2nd method for cultivating gratitude, through the gratitude visit positive activity. A gratitude visit involves writing and then delivering (reading aloud) a letter of thanks to an individual. Further details regarding goals for Sessions 2 and 3 can be found in Table 5.1.

Table 5.1 Well-Being Promotion Program (WBPP; Suldo, 2016) Intervention Protocol

Session	*Target*	*Positive Activity*	*Goals of Session*	*Take-Home Challenge (Between-Session Rehearsal and Extension of Positive Activity)*
Caregiver Info Session	Psychoeducation: introduction to the WBPP	Leader choice (e.g., savoring, gratitude list)	• Discuss key concepts in positive psychology. • Overview student sessions in WBPP. • Demonstrate an example of positive psychology activity.	N/A
Student Sessions 1–3: Evoking positive emotions about the past				
1	Positive introduction	You at Your Best	• Establish a supportive group environment. • Increase awareness of subjective well-being. • Introduce students to the broad determinants of happiness and the purpose of the group (learn tools we can use to create positive feelings about our past, present, and future).	You at Your Best review and extension: • Students read their story and think about the strengths they demonstrated in the story. • Students add details and length to the story. • Students can share the story with family members or someone else.
2	Gratitude	Gratitude journaling	• Explore students' current levels of gratitude. • Define gratitude and how it can impact happiness. • Learn a method of using gratitude to focus on positive interpretations of past events. • Decorate gratitude journal, make first entry.	Gratitude journal on a daily basis: • Students set aside five minutes a day to write down five things in their life that they are grateful for that day.

(*Continued*)

Table 5.1 (Continued)

Session	*Target*	*Positive Activity*	*Goals of Session*	*Take-Home Challenge (Between-Session Rehearsal and Extension of Positive Activity)*
3	Gratitude	Gratitude visit	• Explore students' experiences with gratitude journals. • Make connections between grateful thoughts and positive feelings about the past. • Learn to incorporate actions/ expressions of gratitude. • Write a letter of gratitude, plan for delivery.	Carry out the gratitude visit: • Before the next meeting, students carry out the gratitude visit. Continued use of gratitude journal: • Students complete at least one gratitude journal entry at some point during the week.
Student Sessions 4–7: Evoking positive emotions in the present				
4	Kindness	Acts of kindness	• Define kindness (i.e., a character strength), and how it can impact happiness. • Explore students' frequency of kind acts. • Learn a method of using kindness to create positive feelings within present events. • Plan to carry out five acts of kindness on one day.	Perform acts of kindness: • Students perform five acts of kindness on one day in the upcoming week.
5	Character strengths	Introduction to strengths (VIA classification system)	• Define character strengths and virtues, and how use of strengths can impact feelings of happiness in the present. • Explore students' perceived character strengths. • Reinforce acts of kindness.	Continue acts of kindness: • Students perform five acts of kindness on one day in the upcoming week (just like the week prior). Students share character strengths framework with caregivers.
6	Character strengths	Survey assessment of signature character strengths	• Identify students' signature strengths through completion of the online VIA youth survey. • Discuss students' individual signature character strengths. • Explore new ways to use one signature strength. • Develop an individualized plan for new uses of one signature strength.	Use first signature strength in a new way: • Students use their chosen signature strength in new ways daily in the upcoming week and monitor impact on mood. Continued use of acts of kindness or gratitude journaling: • Students continue practicing acts of kindness *or* writing in their gratitude journal.

(*Continued*)

Table 5.1 (Continued)

Session	*Target*	*Positive Activity*	*Goals of Session*	*Take-Home Challenge (Between-Session Rehearsal and Extension of Positive Activity)*
7	Character strengths; savoring	Use signature strengths in new ways; savoring methods	• Reflect on students' use of their signature strengths in new ways, problem-solve barriers. • Make connections between activities that use signature strengths and positive feelings. • Explore new ways to use signature strengths across life domains. • Learn methods of savoring (replay the experience in your mind, share it with someone) to expand positive experiences with use of signature strengths.	Use 2nd signature strength in new ways, with savoring: • Students use a different signature strength in new ways daily, across life domains, monitor mood, and savor positive feelings. Continued use of acts of kindness or gratitude journaling: • Students continue practicing acts of kindness *or* writing in their gratitude journal.
Student Sessions 8–10: Evoking positive emotions about the future				
8	Optimistic thinking	Optimistic explanatory style	• Make connections among activities that use signature strengths, savoring, and positive feelings. • Define optimistic thinking and how it can impact happiness as related to the future. • Learn a method for developing an optimistic explanatory style by thinking about bad events as temporary, specific, and due to external forces, and thinking about good events as permanent, widespread, and due to self.	Optimistic thinking: • Students use an optimistic explanatory style daily in the upcoming week and record their optimistic thoughts along the way. Use 3rd signature strength in a new way: • Students use a different signature strength in new ways daily, across life domains, monitor mood, and savor positive feelings.
9	Hope	Best Possible Self in the Future	• Make connections between optimistic thinking and positive feelings. • Define hope (i.e., goal-directed) and how it can impact happiness as related to the future.	Best Possible Self (Expanded): • Students review their best possible selves in the future story and add thoughts and ideas; focus on ways to achieve future goals.

(*Continued*)

Table 5.1 (Continued)

Session	*Target*	*Positive Activity*	*Goals of Session*	*Take-Home Challenge (Between-Session Rehearsal and Extension of Positive Activity)*
			• Learn a method for developing hope by envisioning goals and paths to achieve goals.	Continued use of acts of kindness, gratitude journaling, using strengths in new ways, or optimistic thinking. • Students practice a 2nd positive activity that they found to be the most meaningful.
10	All positive activities	Termination; review of strategies and plan for future use	• Make connections between goal-directed thoughts and positive feelings. • Review the framework for increasing personal happiness through purposeful activities that evoke positive feelings and build relationships. • Review the activities and exercises learned in the group. • Encourage a personal reflection. • Identify exercises students perceived as most helpful and activities they plan to continue.	Carry out plan for continued use of preferred positive activities Students maintain gains in happiness by using preferred positive activities to evoke positive feelings regularly and during times they detect negative feelings. Caregiver handout summarizes positive activities learned and encourages family to check-in with students about progress with use of preferred positive activities.
Monthly follow-up sessions: Review methods to evoke positive feelings about past, present, and future				
Monthly	All positive activities	Review; spotlight on gratitude, strengths, or optimism	• Review what students recall learning about the happiness framework and positive activities. • Discuss progress with use of positive activities and impact on mood. • Review and practice one to two positive activities that evoke positive feelings about the past, present, or future. • Plan for use of the positive activity and reflection on progress with someone at home.	Continued use of positive activity: • Students complete the positive activity reviewed in the meeting at some point during the month prior to the next follow-up session and share experiences with someone at home or school.

Evoking Positive Emotions about the Present (Sessions 4–7)

To foster positive emotions that can be experienced within the present (e.g., excitement, calm, joy; Seligman, 2002), activities are focused on gratification, as increasing gratifications are related to long-term happiness (Suldo, 2016). To foster increased gratification, Sessions 4 through 7 engage youth in activities that help identify, develop, challenge, and intently engage in character-strengths-related activities (i.e., performing acts of kindness, self-identifying signature character strengths, survey-identified signature character strengths, and planning and intently using signature character strengths in new ways). In Session 4, youth are introduced to a character strength, kindness, and are challenged with performing five acts of kindness in one day, as prior research found that this concentrated dosage increased well-being in adults (Lyubomirsky et al., 2005). Beginning in Session 5, youth are introduced to 24 individual positive traits in the VIA framework (Peterson & Seligman, 2004). Group leaders help students create plans to use their signature character strengths in new ways, monitor the impact of strengths use on mood, and savor positive feelings and experiences.

Evoking Positive Emotions about the Future (Sessions 8–10)

Session 8 shifts into youths' focus on evoking positive emotions about the future, including confidence, faith, trust, and optimism (Seligman, 2002) with its dedication to optimistic thinking. Youth learn how to think optimistically through an explanatory style that is associated with resilience (Suldo, 2016). After practicing and learning how to reframe their thoughts surrounding good and bad events, youth are tasked with using optimistic thinking one time per day for the following week while keeping a record of the use. Session 9 then shifts to the topic of hope (i.e., the perceived ability to set goals, identify pathways to achieving such goals, and motivation to utilize those set pathways; Snyder et al., 1991). Higher levels of hope in youth have been associated with higher success in obtaining their goals, resulting in higher life satisfaction (Brajša-Žganec et al., 2011). Within this session, youth engage in a writing activity, Best Possible Self in the Future, including ways they will achieve their set goal and are challenged with reading their story throughout the upcoming week and adding details to it. Finally, Session 10 focuses on program review and termination. Group leaders guide students to reflect on which positive activities fit best for each student and solicit student feedback on intervention acceptability through completion of a program feedback form.

Maintenance Sessions

After the 10th core session, leaders invite students to engage in monthly follow-up sessions throughout the end of the school year (e.g., two to four times, depending on the school calendar). Session goals are driven by intentional planning for sustained use and rehearsal of the positive activities learned in the core sessions. Monthly booster sessions are carefully organized to allow students to maintain and continue gains in happiness, in line with research that supports individuals have considerable control over their happiness through engaging in purposeful activities to interrupt the hedonic treadmill, in which ceasing use of positive activities would cause a return to baseline levels of subjective well-being (Lyubomirsky et al., 2005).

Positive Cognitive-Behavioral Therapy (CBT)

Individuals with low subjective well-being who need intensive, individualized supports may be good candidates for counseling that utilizes positive CBT (Bannink & Geschwind, 2021). Positive CBT, which can be conceptualized as the fourth wave of CBT, draws on concepts from traditional

CBT, solution-focused therapy (de Shazer et al., 2007), and positive psychology. Similar to traditional CBT, clinicians seek to understand underlying thoughts and feelings that are linked to personal actions, but its focus is on where things are going well, not where they are malfunctioning or bleak, with the desire to help youth gain more substantial benefits from therapy (Bannik, 2017) and long-term maintenance of outcomes reflected in positive subjective well-being. Counter to the traditional emphasis on the analysis of the problem, prominence is put on construction of solutions, tying in solution-focused therapy, and finding a direct route to "what works" for the person at the current moment in their given context. Invitations for conversations regarding what outcomes are wanted, what is working, and what might foster change drive the approach to positive CBT (Bannik & Jackson, 2011). During the intake process, it may be beneficial to directly inform youth about the counselor's approach and its focus on strengths instead of weaknesses and possibilities instead of impossibilities because when youth talk about their problems, clinicians using positive CBT focus on actively and respectfully listening and acknowledging their stories while refraining from asking further details of the problem. After the youth have felt heard by the clinician (10–15 minutes), clinicians begin to encourage the youth to shift their talk from problem talk to solution-focused talk. In positive CBT, interview questions emphasize what changes the youth would like to come to fruition in their lives (i.e., goals) and what is going well with them (i.e., strengths) versus focusing on what is going wrong (i.e., problems) and is perceivably "wrong" with them (i.e., weaknesses).

Another difference between traditional CBT and positive CBT involves the language used within therapy. Positive CBT takes on a social constructivist view, wherein the client's conception of their reality—including their sense of the nature of problems, their abilities, and solutions—is constructed in daily life in communication with others, whereas traditional CBT flows from a logical positivist view. As there are always exceptions to the problem (Wittgenstein, 1968), the language used within positive CBT takes the form of "becoming better at" compared to "learning" and "unlearning" principles. This strength-based approach aims for clients to see themselves as capable, by having the ability within themselves and the environment around them to activate change. A focus on strengths and abilities throughout treatment can enhance therapeutic alliance (Gassmann & Grawe, 2006), which can also enhance youths' motivation to engage with emotionally and cognitively challenging tasks (Wilmots et al., 2020).

Aligned with classic CBT goals of changing thoughts and behavior, therapeutic strategies in positive CBT emphasize hope and optimism. Cultivating skills in optimistic thinking through an explanatory style allows the client to "change the view" of their problems (O'Hanlon, 2000). To change the view, clients are encouraged to acknowledge their past feelings, change what they are focusing on in the problem situation, direct attention to their past or present successes, focus on what they would like in the future (goals) rather than focus on what they did/do not like about their past or current life, challenge discourteous thoughts and beliefs about themselves (fostering adaptive helpful cognitions), and transcend their troubles and draw on resources beyond their usual abilities, by means of the three Cs of spirituality (O'Hanlon, 2000) fostering Connections, Compassion, and Contribution. Another strategy in positive CBT involves use of the upward arrow technique to help clients find and expand on positive emotions. Whereas the traditional model of CBT utilizes a *downward arrow technique* to develop and test new cognitions related to problematic thoughts and behaviors, in positive CBT clients are encouraged to detect core beliefs that seed positive responses to certain situations, allowing the client to think through the best-case scenario in place of the worst-case scenario (Bannink & Geschwind, 2021). Counseling using positive CBT involves assignment of take-home challenges to rehearse methods of changing the thinking, doing, and feeling learned in sessions.

To date, outcome studies of positive CBT have involved samples of adults in treatment for depression. Clients showed larger reductions in depressive symptoms as well as sizeable increases in happiness during treatment that used positive CBT as compared to when treated with traditional CBT

(Geschwind et al., 2019). Interviews with clients who experienced both forms of treatment suggested that acceptability of positive CBT stemmed from clients feeling empowered by a focus on positive experiences and strengths, benefiting from an upward spiral of positive emotions including experiencing further positive experiences as well as resilience from stressors, identifying incremental progress toward goals, and rediscovering optimism which heightened motivation (Geschwind et al., 2020). Research is needed to understand the applicability and efficacy of positive CBT when used with youth clients to increase wellness, reduce illness, or affect both factors.

Assessment of Progress and Outcomes (Monitoring)

To determine impact of the intervention on youth wellness, practitioners can re-administer brief psychometrically sound measures (see section on Interviewing and Assessing Subjective Well-Being) during and at the conclusion of intervention and compare scores from post-intervention to baseline levels recorded during the clinical assessment process. To assess changes in youth subjective well-being, our team frequently uses the SLSS (Huebner, 1991) and PANAS-C-10 (Ebesutani et al., 2012). To assess secondary impact of intervention on indicators of illness, we use measures of psychopathology symptoms that span across internalizing and externalizing problems, such as the Brief Problem Monitor of the Achenbach System of Empirically Based Assessments (ASEBA; Achenbach & Rescorla, 2011). To supplement these quantitative assessments of complete mental health, throughout the intervention process we monitor youth engagement in academic and social domains and extracurricular activities to determine functional improvement in domains of life (PERMA) that support emotional flourishing.

Applications to the School Setting

Schools have long been considered an ideal environment for the provision of social, emotional, behavioral, and mental health services for children. Compulsory attendance and multi-tiered systems of support allow for preventative care and early access to services. Particularly for students identified as having low subjective well-being based on screening data, access to school-based services allows students to receive support for their emotional well-being regardless of the presence of elevated psychopathology levels which are more commonly monitored to identify students in need of more intense traditional mental health treatments.

At Tier 1, schools can provide support for students' well-being by selecting and implementing relevant universal supports discussed above such as Trails to Wellness, MindUP, or the P2's SEL programs. Schools interested in implementing new Tier 1 interventions may consider forming building committees to decide upon curriculums to purchase, individuals to be trained in interventions, and the logistics of bringing a new intervention to the entire school. These committees might include individuals like curriculum directors, teachers, school mental health providers, and building-level administrators. By ensuring all relevant stakeholders are included in these meetings, schools can maximize buy-in for the intervention, helping to ensure a smooth transition. As many school-based practitioners are aware, there can be many barriers to successful implementation of intervention protocols related to cost, time, and cultural fit. Some lessons within a curriculum may not feel appropriate for certain students, or scheduling may limit the number of sessions that can be held. Routine monitoring of student acceptability and outcome data can assist practitioners to tailor interventions to best meet the needs of their students on a case-by-case basis using data-based decision-making to guide intervention.

As discussed in the "Assessing for the Problem" section, students' subjective well-being can be quickly and easily assessed via brief measures of life satisfaction. Schools can conduct school-wide screenings using psychometrically sound measures such as the SLSS or BMSLSS. These measures are available for free in the public domain; primary implementation supports needed involve data collection and scoring methods and access to students (e.g., 10–15 minutes, perhaps during a non-instructional time period such as homeroom or flex periods). Schools can make screening an even more time-efficient process by conducting screening digitally, for example, by having students fill out a Google Form on school-issued Chromebooks and using a Google Sheet to calculate mean scores on a given measure.

School teams can then examine their screening data and decide what their criteria will be for access to focused interventions to target well-being. A team may decide, for example, to invite the bottom quartile, or students with the lowest 25% of well-being scores to more targeted Tier 2 interventions. Such interventions include the WBPP (as described in Case Study 1) or the Trails to Wellness CBT and Mindfulness program. As Tier 2 interventions are often conducted in a small group setting, teams will want to utilize careful consideration of student schedules, personality, and individualized needs. School staff who are familiar with the students (e.g., teachers or school mental health providers) should meet to decide how to form students into groups to receive intervention. They may wish to form groups of students with similar schedules, who have pre-existing commonalities, or who have varied levels of support needs that are manageable for the group leader. School staff will also want to schedule groups for times during the school day that are least disruptive to both students and staff, such as during study halls, specials, or intervention blocks, or rotate when the group meets throughout the day.

Review of post-intervention data can inform which students responded well to the Tier 2 intervention and conversely who may need additional support to address low wellness and/or elevated internalizing and externalizing problems. For students with low subjective well-being, school teams may consider intensive Tier 3 supports discussed earlier such as individual counseling using a method that incorporates PPIs, including manualized interventions such as positive psychotherapy or positive CBT, or a less structured strengths-based CBT counseling approach that integrates activities to increase wellness and reduce illness as described in Case Study 2. While these services may be provided in schools by school-based mental health professionals, schools may also refer to community-based mental health supports provided at the school or within the community. Schools should monitor student progress and plan to decrease the level of support to Tier 2 or universal supports depending on students continued needs.

Case Study of Problem Area—School-Based Fostering of Student Subjective Well-Being

In this section, we will review two such case examples and describe the process of conceptualizing each case and deciding upon a treatment protocol. The first case example describes Derek (pseudonym), a middle school boy on the Autism Spectrum. Derek's educational goals are reviewed, and participation in the WBPP in a small group is selected as an approach well-aligned with his social-emotional goals. Whereas group counseling can be difficult to navigate in private practice or outpatient settings due to client confidentiality or insurance-related concerns, group-based treatment in schools is a time- and resource-efficient way of meeting student needs and can present an opportunity to serve students among groups of peers that they encounter within their daily school routines—this would be much less feasible outside of the school environment and provides natural opportunities to reinforce and sustain the use of positive activities. The second case example illustrates individual counseling services for Ava (pseudonym), a middle school girl with clinically significant psychopathology and familial conflict who is exhibiting conduct issues in school. Ava's history is reviewed, and treatment goals and corresponding PPIs to increase wellness (using specific sessions from the WBPP) are described.

Case Example 1: Group Counseling to Promote Wellness and Peer Relationships

Derek is a 6th-grade student served primarily in general education classes. He receives special education services through an individualized educational plan (IEP), due to eligibility through the category of Autism Spectrum Disorder (ASD). A review of school records indicated that Derek is a high-achieving student with no office disciplinary referrals. His home life is marked by a supportive family who is invested in Derek's success, both in his academic career and social-emotional functioning. Derek's IEP included counseling as a related service, provided through weekly individual counseling with the school counselor to work on reducing emotional and social problems through improving social skills. To help further foster Derek's peer relationships and psychological wellness, the student mental health services team, in consultation with his parents, decided to have him join a small group counseling program, the WBPP. In conjunction with his weekly individual counseling, Derek could further engage with similar-aged peers, while also focusing on increasing his happiness.

To progress monitor Derek's response to the small group counseling intervention, the SLSS and PANAS-C-10 were administered before the program began (i.e., baseline) and at the end of the intervention—after the 10th group session. During baseline, Derek reported a low level of life satisfaction and infrequent positive affect, specifically average scores of 2.3 on the SLSS (range of possible scores: 1–6) and 2.2 on the positive affect scale of the PANAS-C-10 (range of possible scores: 1–5) with higher scores indicating higher levels of subjective well-being. Derek was included in a group of 12 other 6th-grade students who participated in WBPP sessions once a week at 45-minute periods, for ten weeks, followed by three monthly booster sessions (i.e., one session per month). One member of the school mental health team, a school psychologist, and a graduate student in school psychology with prior WBPP facilitation experiences co-led the group. For the purposes of this case study, we discuss sessions from the WBPP where Derek most demonstrated benefit both inside and outside of the group sessions.

Session 1

Following introductions to the group leaders and students in the group, an icebreaker activity asked students to choose if they are a morning person or a night owl and why. With students buzzing with excitement to share their answers, Derek stated that he was a night owl because he is someone who likes to stay up late and analyze the sky and stars. Group norms were then collaboratively established, and focused on maintaining confidentiality, expectations for each student to participate and show respect to others, with a substantive discussion of what kindness/respect looks like to them. All students agreed to uphold these norms for the entirety of the program, both inside and outside of the weekly group meetings; norms were revisited at the beginning of each session. Students then worked on an activity to further get to know one another, by writing a story about a time that they were at their best (i.e., You at Your Best). Group leaders came prepared with their You at Your Best stories and modeled sharing a summary, reflecting on positive feelings, and strength-spotting of themselves and others. After this modeling, students were asked to share their stories. Derek detailed a story in which he felt at his best when playing Minecraft while spending time with his older brother. In response, one group member also expressed interest in Minecraft, and another echoed the importance of spending time with siblings. Next, students learned about the "why" behind the positive psychology lens on which the sessions are built, to provide a rationale for leaning into opportunities to practice and rehearse the intentional ways of thinking, behaving, and striving taught throughout the program.

Session 4

Beginning in Session 4, the program focus shifts from evoking positive feelings about the past to evoking positive feelings in their present lives. The session began by reviewing students' take-home challenge from Session 3, specifically to carry out a gratitude visit to thank someone for something that they had done for them in the past. Derek reported completing a gratitude visit with his math teacher, expressing gratitude for their help in allowing him to retake a math quiz after he had a bad day. He reported that his teacher was "very happy and smiled a whole extra lot" when he read the letter of thanks to them, while also reporting that he felt extremely grateful and happy while reading the letter aloud. One student responded to Derek by strength-spotting his courage to not only ask to retake his math quiz but to also read his letter to a teacher. Derek was enthused to further talk to this student about how he might be able to help them in the future if they were in a situation where they had a bad day and did not perform well on a quiz. Group leaders utilized his response to transition into the positive activity of the day, acts of kindness, and noted how Derek can utilize this positive activity to follow up on that conversation. When students were asked to rate the frequency of their average acts of kindness performed in one week, Derek estimated that on average, he performed two acts of kindness per week and vulnerably stated that he can be selfish. Before the group leaders could respond to this statement, another student jumped in and affirmed Derek by saying, "It's okay to be selfish sometimes, we have to look out for ourselves." The group leaders agreed and reassured Derek that through practicing and engaging in acts of kindness, we can work toward a better balance of helping others and ourselves. The take-home challenge for the week was to perform five acts of kindness in one day. As students planned out what acts they might perform, Derek circled back to the idea of discussing retaking a quiz with his peer and planned to have this conversation during lunch.

Sessions 5 and 6

During the discussion of the acts of kindness take-home challenge, Derek reported completing five acts of kindness in one day, including the follow-up conversation with his peer at lunch about how to courageously speak with a teacher about retaking a quiz. The peer with whom he spoke at lunch confirmed Derek's report and stated his tips were very helpful, along with some further helpful tips on Minecraft. Session 5 focused on defining character strengths and virtues and how the use of strengths can impact feelings of happiness in the present. When asked initially to identify his self-perceived strengths as aided by reviewing strengths evident in the You at Your Best story from Session 1, Derek did not want to share out with the group, as he had difficulty identifying specific strengths. One of the group leaders proceeded to consult with him individually to detect strengths in the story. During this collaboration, Derek blurted out that he wanted to share the strengths demonstrated in his story, such as creativity, love, kindness, and teamwork. He was proud of these identified strengths and stated that he felt "strong" while holding up and flexing his arms. A few students chuckled, and Derek embraced this moment of humor with them.

During Session 6, students completed the VIA Inventory for Youth (VIA-Youth) survey to assess and rank their top five strengths. Derek's signature character strengths were: (1) Humor, (2) Zest, (3) Teamwork, (4) Kindness, and (5) Perseverance. Within an individual conversation with a group leader regarding expected versus survey-identified signature strengths, Derek ruminated on the signature strength Zest and wondered: "Isn't zest related to a lemon…I think my mom uses this for her homemade salad dressing…". The leader directed Derek to the definition Zest provided on the VIA survey results and provide an analogy for Derek to consider, "Lemon zest is generally friendly and bubbly, it provides excitement and energy to your mother's salad dressing, just like you bring energy to our group, you help make the group conversation alive." Derek's face lit up and he responded, "That is so cool, I am full of zest and cannot wait to tell my mom after school!". This week's take-home challenge required students to pick one of their top five character strengths and plan how to use it in new ways each day of the week. Other students within the group disclosed that a few of the strengths did not fit well with them, making it hard to plan out new ways of use. With excitement, Derek reassured others that it is okay if the survey-identified strengths do not feel right at first and that they may grow to like the new signature strengths, referring to his initial and current reactions to his Zest signature strength. Derek's peers responded well to this point, and conversations around this thrived as students worked to plan for new uses of their first signature strength.

Sessions 8 and 9

Students' focus shifted to future-focused activities, where they learned to use an optimistic explanatory style. Students practiced differentiating between a good and a bad event and creating optimistic attributions accordingly. For instance, when thinking about a good event, they would take credit for their role in the positive outcome or view the event as widespread and permanent. In contrast, when a bad event occurred, students learned to consider the external factors that contributed to the outcome or view the event as specific or temporary. When tasked with using optimistic thinking once a day in the upcoming week, Derek stated that this would be very difficult for him because others are not always nice to him, especially on the morning bus ride. The student who Derek had previously behaved kindly to regarding retaking a math quiz stood up from his seat and walked over to Derek to help him problem-solve. The two of them worked together to plan out how they would utilize optimistic thinking for the upcoming week and then walked to their next class together after the bell rang. Session 9 focused on building hope through students envisioning their Best Possible Self in the Future, including writing about what they visualize for themselves, along with generating pathways to reach their personal goals. Derek described his Best Possible Self as involving him no longer being poor or selfish, with goals to become an airplane pilot to enable himself to be among the stars and provide financially for his parents and older brother.

In sum, Derek showed an authentic interest in all nine positive activities learned across the ten-week program. Socially, Derek formed strong relationships with students both inside and outside of the group, as well as with the group leaders. After the 10th session, the SLSS and PANAS-C-10 were re-administered to monitor his response to intervention. His average SLSS score was a 4.2, which is in the positive range of life satisfaction and a substantial improvement from the mean rating of reported 2.3 prior to intervention. The frequency of positive affect reported on the PANAS-C-10 also improved from experiencing positive feelings "a little" at baseline to "moderately" at post-intervention (3.0).

To sustain and continue gains in subjective well-being, the group leaders held monthly follow-up sessions to review and further select positive activities (i.e., gratitude, use of character strengths) for practice. After considering the time gap between the follow-up sessions, Derek asked for more frequent contact with the leaders to show them that he completed take-home challenges regularly. Group leaders created a system for Derek to drop off completed take-home challenge record forms (e.g., documenting how he used a signature strength in new ways and how it made him feel) to a designated person in the school office, who kept the record form for the group leaders to review before the next session. This process further built the student-counselor relationship. During the follow-up sessions, Derek noted that he was no longer bothered on the bus, as he now sits with peers from the group.

Derek's improvement in subjective well-being may be due to several factors, namely strengthened relationships and motivation for sustained use of positive activities. Derek built relationships with, and received peer support from, students who shared their past and current experiences in therapy and who also experienced struggles within their home life, friendships, and academics. Derek also demonstrated a continued eagerness to learn positive activities and intentionally use them in his own life. In this group, students completed the majority of the take-home challenges assigned, including discussion with caregivers about engaging in positive activities. Derek reported sharing and discussing the weekly caregiver handout with family at home on a weekly basis, and on several occasions he stated he was excited to share what he learned with his caregivers after school. The case of Derek demonstrates how participation in the small group WBPP with an intentional caregiver component led to social-emotional gains in a student with ASD, with outcomes that may not have been achieved relying solely on traditional supports (i.e., counseling focused on lowering psychopathology). His gains in social connectedness and subjective well-being further support the importance of incorporating well-being into school mental health interventions.

Case Example 2: Individual Counseling to Address Illness and Wellness

Ava is an 8th-grade female served exclusively through general education. Throughout the 1st week of school, she incurred several office discipline referrals for aggressive and disruptive behavior. Ava was taking psychotropic medication to manage symptoms of bipolar disorder. A review of school records indicated that Ava had been expelled from her previous middle school in 7th grade due to engaging in physical violence against another student. Regarding home life, during her upbringing and childhood, she had been exposed to various traumatic experiences that resulted in her removal from her biological parents' home. Ava and her younger biological brother entered the foster care system, where they were eventually adopted. However, Ava reported significant family discord within the current home (e.g., parent-child relationship challenges, domestic violence). Throughout the intake process, Ava demonstrated strengths in engaging in extracurricular activities within the community and school, fostering new peer relationships, and her continued care for her younger brother. Ava actively and openly spoke about her wishes to improve her mental health and family life, exhibiting strengths in responsibility, motivation, self-awareness, and openness to change.

Upon completion of the intake process, three primary target problems emerged: affective instability and aggressive behavior, family discord, and negative self-esteem. Treatment goals for the first two areas involved reducing symptoms of illness through increasing use of conflict resolution strategies and improving family functioning. Cognitive-behavioral intervention strategies to develop social and communication skills were implemented through individual counseling. Concerning the 3rd problem area, when reflecting on her childhood and current family dynamic, Ava consistently questioned her importance and could not identify any positive attributes. The treatment goal for this area was to increase self-concept by recognizing her positive personal attributes and qualities, decreasing negative self-talk, and increasing time spent in relationships with individuals who value these qualities. Accordingly, the treatment plan for fostering wellness included a blend of traditional and positive cognitive-behavioral techniques that allowed Ava to identify, evaluate, and modify negative automatic thoughts and replace them with optimistic thoughts and positive self-talk.

The counselor selected several session protocols from the WBPP to use with Ava in individual therapy to improve her intentional focus on positive attributes and qualities (i.e., learning her top five signature character strengths), alongside pinpointing life circumstances that were going well (e.g., peer relationships at school) and what had the capacity to improve (family dynamics). Five protocols were utilized directly from the ten core student sessions, including activities from Session 1 (You at Your Best), Session 5 (self-identification of character strengths), Session 6 (identification of top five character strengths from the online VIA Youth survey), Session 8 (optimistic thinking), and Session 9 (Best Possible Self in the Future). Because Ava had previously indicated that written expression provided an outlet for her to process her emotions, we adapted an activity from Session 2 (gratitude journaling) for individual use on a weekly basis. Furthermore, when Ava self-identified kindness as a signature strength, performing acts of kindness (from Session 4) was infused into weekly sessions to encourage further use of this strength and bolster positive interactions with peers, friends, and family. To progress monitor Ava's response to intervention, the SLSS and PANAS-C-10 were administered throughout the treatment phase including at baseline, mid-year, and toward end of year. At intake, Ava also completed the Youth Self-Report of the ASEBA (Achenbach & Rescorla, 2001) to measure levels of psychopathology, consistent with the counselor's use of a dual-factor model of mental health. During baseline, Ava reported a low to neutral level of life satisfaction (i.e., average SLSS score of 3.71 during the initial intake process), moderate positive affect (average score of 3.2), and clinically significant levels of both externalizing and internalizing behaviors.

In all, Ava's treatment plan consisted of a blend of strategies across cognitive-behavioral and PPIs enacted throughout the school year, with less frequent sessions toward the end of the year. The final session ended with the creation of a hope map, which helped her appreciate how far she had progressed in treatment to the point that an exciting future was realistic and supported by identification of steps toward goals and plans for how to address barriers. Despite consistent participation in weekly sessions, several obstacles hindered full engagement and uptake of some skills introduced in sessions due to her complex family history and current psychiatric diagnosis (mood disorder). For instance, when completing the You at Your Best positive writing activity, Ava struggled to identify a time when she was ever doing well. The counselor encouraged Ava to reflect on her recent accomplishment of refraining from drug use for the last year, recently marking her one year of sobriety, a momentous event that she reported during the intake process. Furthermore, when initially asked to self-identify her character strengths, she struggled to think of any positive traits, possibly a sequela of a tumultuous relationship with her adoptive father that included reports of verbal abuse. The counselor modeled and helped Ava use positive self-talk strategies to support the successful completion of this activity. Of note, in a traditional approach to illness-focused treatment, the focus of Ava's initial treatment plan could have been geared toward her aggressive and disruptive behavior as recommended by the school administrator in his referral for counseling services. However, during the intake process, Ava noted that she had not engaged in this behavior for several weeks; she shared that she had an upcoming court date for the incident that led to her expulsion from her prior school and stated strong motivation to not get into further trouble at her current school. Fortunately, in addition to her ability to self-manage her externalizing behaviors, the CBT strategies and positive psychology activities built into her treatment plan allowed her to focus her mindset on signature strengths, optimistic thinking, and hope throughout treatment.

At the end of the fall semester, Ava's average score on the SLSS improved from a 3.7 to a 4.7, and positive affect increased from a 3.2 to the max score of 5.0, indicating clinically significant growth in subjective well-being. Scores remained high at the end of the spring semester (SLSS = 4.7 again, positive affect = 4.4), supporting maintenance of gains. In addition, only internalizing symptoms remained clinically elevated (as measured by the ASEBA; Achenbach & Rescorla, 2001), which may be expected given her ongoing need for support to address symptoms of bipolar disorder and her strong motivation to decrease externalizing behavior problems.

Summary

A modern definition of mental health uses a dual-factor model that recognizes that mental wellness and illness are separable and that both are important targets within psychological care. In this chapter, we operationalized wellness as subjective well-being, reflected in life satisfaction appraisals, along with frequency of positive and negative emotions. A biopsychosocial model of well-being reflects that a combination of genetics, life circumstances, and intentional activities contribute to one's level of personal happiness. There is growing empirical evidence that use of specific activities from research within positive psychology can increase well-being. These activities encourage positive interpretations of the past (e.g., through gratitude), positive behaviors in the present (e.g., though use of signature strengths), and positive thoughts for the future (e.g., through optimistic thinking). To assess for wellness and its determinants, practitioners can use direct measures of life satisfaction and affect, alongside interviews and surveys to identify student assets, resources, and signature character strengths, and use this information to inform case conceptualization, goal setting, treatment planning, and progress monitoring. Practitioners can select from a growing number of evidence-based or promising intervention programs appropriate for school-based practice within a MTSS for student mental health across Tiers 1, 2, and 3. As illustrated in our case studies, school-based interventions drawn from positive psychology can be incorporated within a strengths-based approach to CBT by teaching and practicing purposeful positive activities, strengthening relationships, and harnessing youth motivation to sustain their happiness as a means to promote well-being among youth with diverse backgrounds and presenting concerns.

Reflection Questions

1 How is case conceptualization to understand wellness similar and different to case conceptualization to understand illness/psychopathology?
2 What positive activities described in this chapter do you draw upon or relate to most in your own life? How can you utilize these activities in your personal and professional practice?
3 Clients with which types of presenting problems might be particularly receptive to integration of positive psychology practices in clinical care?

Evidence-Based Treatment Programs for the Problem Area

The following programs foster subjective well-being in children, youth, and young adults, using manualized interventions aligned with principles and practices in positive psychology.

- *MindUP* (The Hawn Foundation, 2011)
- *PRP* (Gillham et al., 1990)
- *Positive CBT* (Bannink & Geschwind, 2021)
- *Positive Psychotherapy (*Rashid & Seligman, 2018)
- *P2* (The Positivity Project, 2023)
- *Strengths-Based Resilience, A Positive Psychology Program* (Rashid et al., 2023)
- *Strengths Gym* (Proctor & Fox Eades, 2016)
- *Trails to Wellness* (TRAILS, 2023a, 2023b)
- *WBPP* (Suldo, 2016)

Note

1 Within the original intervention manual (Suldo, 2016), between-session practice and rehearsal of a positive activity is referred to as "homework"; however, the authors have adapted this terminology to "take-home challenges" to be more youth-friendly and allow them to view these assignments as opportunities to challenge themselves, and ultimately, grow.

References

Achenbach, T. M., McConaughy, S. H., Ivanova, M. Y., & Rescorla, L. A. (2011). *Manual for the ASEBA Brief Problem Monitor (BPM).* Burlington, VT: University of Vermont.
Bannink, F. P. (2017). Positive CBT in practice. In C. Proctor (Ed.), *Positive psychology interventions in practice* (pp. 15–28). Cham, Switzerland: Springer International Publishing. https://doi.org/10.1007/978-3-319-51787-2_2

Bannink, F., & Geschwind, N. (2021). *Positive CBT: Individual and group treatment protocols for positive cognitive behavioral therapy.* Göttingen: Hogrefe Publishing. https://doi.org/10.1027/00578-000

Bannink, F. P., & Jackson, P. Z. (2011). Positive psychology and solution focus: Looking at similarities and differences. *InterAction—The Journal of Solution Focus in Organisations, 3*(1), 8–20.

Bastounis, A., Callaghan, P., Banerjee, A., & Michail, M. (2016). The effectiveness of the Penn Resiliency Programme (PRP) and its adapted versions in reducing depression and anxiety and improving explanatory style: A systematic review and meta-analysis. *Journal of Adolescence, 52*, 37–48. https://doi.org/10.1016/j.adolescence.2016.07.004

Benjamin, C. L., Puleo, C. M., Settipani, C. A., Brodman, D. M., Edmunds, J. M., Cummings, C. M., & Kendall, P. C. (2011). History of cognitive-behavioral therapy in youth. *Child and Adolescent Psychiatric Clinics, 20*(2), 179–189.

Bose, D., Pettit, J. W., Silk, J. S., Ladouceur, C. D., Olino, T. M., Forbes, E. E., Siegle, G.J., Dahl, R. E., Kendall, P. C., Ryan, N. D., & McMakin, D. L. (2023). Therapeutic alliance, attendance, and outcomes in youths receiving CBT or client-centered therapy for anxiety. *Journal of Clinical Child & Adolescent Psychology*, 1–11. https://doi.org/10.1080/15374416.2023.2261547

Brain Futures (2023). *MINDUP*. Retrieved from https://www.brainfutures.org/mind-up-2/

Brajša-Žganec, A., Merkaš, M., & Šverko, I. (2011). Quality of life and leisure activities: How do leisure activities contribute to subjective well-being? *Social Indicators Research, 102*(1), 81–91. https://doi.org/10.1007/s11205-010-9724-2

Brunwasser, S. M., Gillham, J. E., & Kim, E. S. (2009). A meta-analytic review of the Penn Resiliency Program's effect on depressive symptoms. *Journal of Consulting and Clinical Psychology, 77*, 1042–1054.

Bucker, S., Nuraydin, S., Simonsmeier, B. A., Schneider, M., & Luhmann, M. (2018). Subjective well-being and academic achievement: A meta-analysis. *Journal of Research in Personality, 74*, 83–94. https://doi.org/10.1016/j.jrp.2018.02.007

Burckhardt, R., Manicavasagar, V., Batterham, P. J., & Hadzi-Pavlovic, D. (2016). A randomized controlled trial of strong minds: A school-based mental health program combining acceptance and commitment therapy and positive psychology. *Journal of School Psychology, 57*, 41–52.

Cutuli, J. J., Chaplin, T. M., Gillham, J. E., Revich, K. J., & Seligman, M. E. P. (2006). Preventing co-occurring depression symptoms in adolescents with conduct problems: The Penn Resiliency Program. *Annals of the New York Academy of Sciences, 1094*, 282–286.

de Shazer, S., Dolan, Y., Korman, H., McCollum, E., Trepper, T., & Berg, I. K. (2007). *More than miracles: The state of the art of solution-focused brief therapy.* New York: Routledge.

Diener, E., Scollon, C. N., & Lucas, R. E. (2009). The evolving concept of subjective well-being: The multifaceted nature of happiness. In E. Diener (Ed.), *Assessing well-being: The collected works of Ed Diener* (pp. 67–100). Social Indicators Research Series 39. New York: Springer.

DiLeo, L., Suldo, S. M., Ferron, J., & Shaunessy-Dedrick, E. (2022). Three-wave longitudinal study of a dual-factor model: Mental health status and academic outcomes for high school students in academically accelerated curricula. *School Mental Health, 14*, 514–530. https://doi.org/10.1007/s12310-021-09497-9

Donaldson, S. I., Cabrera, V., & Gaffaney, J. (2021). *Following the science to generate well-being: Using the highest-quality experimental evidence to design interventions. Frontiers in Psychology, 12*, 739352. https://doi.org/10.3389/fpsyg.2021.739352

Ebesutani, C., Regan, J., Smith, A., Reise, S., Higa-McMillan, C., & Chorpita, B. F. (2012). The 10-item Positive and Negative Affect Schedule for Children, child and parent shortened versions: Application of item response theory for more efficient assessment. *Journal of Psychopathology and Behavioral Assessment, 34*(2), 191–203. https://doi.org/10.1007/s10862-011-9273-2

Erhard, P., Falcomata, T. S., & Harmon, T. (2021). Behavioral skills training. In F. R. Volkmar (Eds.), *Encyclopedia of autism spectrum disorders.* Cham: Springer. https://doi.org/10.1007/978-3-319-91280-6_102320

Fredrickson, B. L. (2001). The role of positive emotions in positive psychology: The broaden-and-build theory of positive emotions. *American Psychologist, 56*(3), 218–226. https://doi.org/10.1037/0003-066X.56.3.218

Froh, J. J., Sefick, W. J., & Emmons, R. A. (2008). Counting blessings in early adolescents: An experimental study of gratitude and subjective well-being. *Journal of School Psychology, 46*, 213–233. https://doi.org/10.1016/j.jsp.2007.03.005

Furlong, M. J., You, S., Renshaw, T. L., O'Malley, M. D., & Rebelez, J. (2013). Preliminary development of the Positive Experiences at School Scale for elementary school children. *Child Indicators Research, 6*, 753–775. https://doi.org/10.1007/s12187-013-9193-7

Furlong, M. J., You, S., Renshaw, T. L., Smith, D. C., & O'Malley, M. D. (2014). Preliminary development and validation of the Social and Emotional Health Survey for secondary students. *Social Indicators Research, 117*, 1011–1032. https://doi.org/10.1007/s11205-013-0373-0

Garwood, J. D. (2022a). Character education to improve students' sense of relatedness: Preliminary findings from the positivity project. *International Journal of Education, 14*(2), 38–40.

Garwood, J. D. (2022b). Positivity in action: Character education through positivity project. *International Journal of Emerging Trends in Social Sciences, 13*, 46–52. https://doi.org/10.55217/103.v13i2.581

Gassmann, D., & Grawe, K. (2006). General change mechanisms: the relation between problem activation and resource activation in successful and unsuccessful therapeutic interactions. *Clinical Psychology and Psychotherapy, 13*(1), 1–11. https://doi.org/10.1002/cpp.442

Geschwind, N., Arntz, A., Bannink, F., & Peeters, F. (2019). Positive cognitive behavior therapy in treatment of depression: A randomized order within-subject comparison with traditional cognitive behavior therapy. *Behavior Research and Therapy, 116*, 119–130. https://doi.org/10.1016/j.brat.2019.03.005

Geschwind, N., Bosgraaf, E., Bannink, F., & Peeters, F. (2020). Positivity pays off: Clients' perspectives on positive compared with traditional cognitive behavioral therapy for depression. *Psychotherapy, 57*(3), 366–378. https://doi.org/10.1037/pst0000288

Gillham, J. E., Jaycox, L. H., Reivich, K. J., Seligman, M. E. P., & Silver, T. (1990). *The Penn Resiliency Program*. Unpublished manual, University of Pennsylvania, Philadelphia. https://doi.org/10.1002/cpp.442

Gillham, J. E., Reivich, K. J., Jaycox, L. H., & Seligman, M. E. P. (1995). Prevention of depressive symptoms in schoolchildren: Two-year follow-up. *Psychological Science, 6*(6), 343–351. https://doi.org/10.1111/j.1467-9280.1995.tb00524.x

The Hawn Foundation (2011). *The MindUP Curriculum: Grades 6 8: Brain-focused strategies for learning and living* (1st ed). New York: Scholastic.

The Hawn Foundation (2023). *Our research*. Retrieved from https://mindup.org/our-research/

Huebner, E. S. (1991). Initial development of the Students' Life Satisfaction Scale. *School Psychology International, 12*, 231–243.

Huebner, E. S. (1994). Preliminary development and validation of a multidimensional life satisfaction scale for children. *Psychological Assessment, 6*, 149–158.

Huta, & Hawley, L. (2010). Psychological strengths and cognitive vulnerabilities: Are they two ends of the same continuum or do they have independent relationships with well-being and ill-being? *Journal of Happiness Studies, 11*(1), 71–93. https://doi.org/10.1007/s10902-008-9123-4

Inhelder, B., & Piaget, J. (1958). *The growth of logical thinking from childhood to adolescence*. New York: Basic Books.

Kern, M. L., Benson, L., Steinberg, E. A., & Steinberg, L. (2016). The EPOCH measure of adolescent well-being. *Psychological Assessment, 28*(5), 586–597. https://doi.org/10.1037/pas0000201

Kirkpatrick, M., Akers, J., & Rivera, G. (2019). Use of behavioral skills training with teachers: A systematic review. *Journal of Behavioral Education, 28*, 344–361. https://doi.org/10.1007/s10864-019-09322-z

Kuyken, W., Padesky, C. A., & Dudley, R. (2009). *Collaborative case conceptualization: Working effectively with clients in cognitive-behavioral therapy*. New York: The Guilford Press.

Laurent, J., Catanzaro, S. J., Joiner, T. E., Jr., Rudolph, K. D., Potter, K. I., Lambert, S., Osborne, L., & Gathright, T. (1999). A measure of positive and negative affect for children: Scale development and preliminary validation. *Psychological Assessment, 11*, 326–338. https://doi.org/10.1037/1040-3590.11.3.326

Lazarus, P. J., Suldo, S. M., & Doll, B. (2021). *Fostering the emotional well-being of youth: A school-based approach.* New York: Oxford University Press.

Lyubomirsky, S., & Layous, K. (2013). How do simple positive activities increase well-being? *Current Directions in Psychological Science, 22*, 57–62. https://doi.org/10.1177/0963721412469809

Lyubomirsky, S., Sheldon, K. M., & Schkade, D. (2005). Pursuing happiness: The Architecture of sustainable change. *Review of General Psychology, 9*(2), 111–131. https://doi.org/10.1037/1089-2680.9.2.111

Marques, S. C., Pais-Ribeiro, J. L., & Lopez, S. J. (2011). The role of positive psychology constructs in predicting mental health and academic achievement in children and adolescents: A two-year longitudinal study. *Journal of Happiness Studies: An Interdisciplinary Forum on Subjective Well-Being, 12*(6), 1049–1062. https://doi.org/10.1007/s10902-010-9244-4

McNeil, G. D., & Repetti, R. L. (2022). Increases in positive emotions as precursors to therapeutic change. *Clinical Psychology and Psychotherapy, 29*, 1113–1124. https://doi.org/10.1002/cpp.2698

Nes, R. B., & Røysamb, E. (2017). Happiness in behaviour genetics: An update on heritability and changeability. *Journal of Happiness Studies, 18*(5), 1533–1552. https://doi.org/10.1007/s10902-016-9781-6

O'Hanlon, B. (2000). *Do one thing different.* New York: Harper Collins.

The Positivity Project. (2023). Retrieved from https://posproject.org/

Peterson, C., & Seligman, M. E. P. (2004). *Character strengths and virtues: A handbook and classification.* New York: Oxford University Press; Washington, DC: American Psychological Association.

Proctor, C., & Fox Eades, J. (2016). *Strengths gym: Build and exercise your strengths! St Peter Port.* Guernsey: Positive Psychology Research Centre.

Raffaele Mendez, L. M. (2017). *Cognitive behavioral therapy in schools: A tiered approach to youth mental health services.* New York: Routledge.

Rashid, T., Anjum, A., Chu, R., Stevanovski, S., Zanjani, A., & Lennex, C. (2015). Strength based resilience: Integrating risk and resources towards holistic well-being. In G. A. Fava & C. Ruini (Eds.), *Increasing psychological well-being across cultures* (pp. 153–176). The Netherlands: Springer.

Rashid, T., Gillham, J., & Anjum, A. (2023). *Strengths-based resilience, a positive psychology program.* Göttingen: Hogrefe Publishing.

Rashid, T., & Seligman, M. E. P. (2018). *Positive psychotherapy: Manual.* New York: Oxford University Press.

Roth, R., & Suldo, S. M., & Ferron, J. (2017). Improving middle school students' subjective well-being: Efficacy of a multicomponent positive psychology intervention targeting small groups of youth. *School Psychology Review, 46* (1), 21–41. https://doi.org/10.17105/10.17105/SPR46-1.21-41

Rottenberg, J., & Kashdan, T. B. (2022). Well-being after psychopathology: A transformational research agenda. *Current Directions in Psychological Science, 31*, 280–287. https://doi.org/10.1177/09637214221093616

Schaefer, J. M., & Andzik, N. R. (2021). Evaluating behavioral skills training as an evidence-based practice when training parents to intervene with their children. *Behavior Modification, 45*(6), 887–910. https://doi.org/10.1177/0145445520923996

Schonert-Reichl, K. A., Oberle, E., Lawlor, M. S., Abbott, D., Thomson, K., Oberlander, T. F., & Diamond, A. (2015). Enhancing cognitive and social–emotional development through a simple-to-administer mindfulness-based school program for elementary school children: A randomized controlled trial. *Developmental Psychology, 51*(1), 52–66. https://doi.org/10.1037/a0038454

Seligman, M. E. P. (2002). *Authentic happiness: Using the new positive psychology to realize your potential for lasting fulfillment.* New York: Free Press.

Seligman, M. E. P. (2011). *Flourish: A visionary new understanding of happiness and well-being.* New York: Free Press.

Seligson, J. L., Huebner, E. S., & Valois, R. F. (2003). Preliminary validation of the Brief Multidimensional Students' Life Satisfaction Scale (BMSLSS). *Social Indicators Research, 61*, 121–145.

Sheldon, K. M., & Lyubomirsky, S. (2021). Revisiting the sustainable happiness model and pie chart: Can happiness be successfully pursued? *The Journal of Positive Psychology, 16*, 145–154. https://doi.org/10.1080/17439760.2019.1689421

Slane, M., & Lieberman-Betz, R. G. (2021). Using behavioral skills training to teach implementation of behavioral interventions to teachers and other professionals: A systematic review. *Behavioral Interventions, 36*(4), 984–1002. https://doi.org/10.1002/bin.1828

Suldo, S. M., & Doll, B. (2021). Conceptualizing youth mental health through a dual-factor model. In P. J. Lazarus, S. M. Suldo & B. Doll (Eds.), *Fostering the emotional well-being of youth: A school-based approach* (pp. 20–39). New York: Oxford University Press.

Snyder, C. R., Harris, C., Anderson, J. R., Holleran, S. A., Irving, L. M., Sigmon, S. T., Yoshinobu, L., Gibb, J., Langelle, C., & Harney, P. (1991). The will and the ways: Development and validation of an individual-differences measure of hope. *Journal of Personality and Social Psychology, 60*(4), 570–585. https://doi.org/10.1037/0022-3514.60.4.570

Suldo, S. M. (2016). *Promoting student happiness: Positive psychology interventions in schools.* New York: The Guilford Press.

Suldo, S. M., Savage, J. A., & Mercer, S. (2014). Increasing middle school students' life satisfaction: Efficacy of a positive psychology group intervention. *Journal of Happiness Studies, 15*, 19–42. https://doi.org/10.1007/s10902-013-9414-2

Tejada-Gallardo, C., Blasco-Belled, A., Torrelles-Nadal, C., & Alsinet, C. (2020). Effects of school-based multicomponent positive psychology interventions on well-being and distress in adolescents: A systematic review and meta-analysis. *Journal of Youth and Adolescence, 49*, 1943–1960. https://doi.org/10.1007/s10964-020-01289-9

TRAILS (2023a). Retrieved from https://trailstowellness.org/

TRAILS (2023b). *Evaluation and research.* Retrieved from https://trailstowellness.org/our-impact/evaluation-and-research

Trompetter, H. R., Lamers, S. M. A., Westerfhof, G. J., Fedderus, M., & Bohlmeijer, E. T. (2017). Both positive mental health and psychopathology should be monitored in psychotherapy: Confirmation for the dual-factor model in acceptance and commitment therapy. *Behavior Research and Therapy, 91*, 58–63. http://dx.doi.org/10.1016/j.brat.2017.01.008

van Agteren, J., Iasiello, M., Lo, L., Bartholomaeus, J., Kopsaftis, Z., Carey, M., & Kyrios, M. (2021). A systematic review and meta-analysis of psychological interventions to improve mental wellbeing. *Nature Human Behaviour, 5*, 631–652. https://doi.org/10.1038/s41562-021-01093-w

Wilmots, E., Midgley, N., Thackeray, L., Reynolds, S., & Loades, M. (2020). The therapeutic relationship in Cognitive Behaviour Therapy with depressed adolescents: A qualitative study of good-outcome cases. *Psychology and Psychotherapy, 93*(2), 276–291. https://doi.org/10.1111/papt.12232

Wittgenstein, L. (1968). *Philosophical investigations* (3rd ed.). (Original work published 1953). New York: Macmillan.

World Health Organization (WHO) (2022). World mental health report: Transforming mental health for all. Geneva: World Health Organization; 2022. License: CC BY-NC-SA 3.0 IGO.

Xu, Y., Yu, Y., Xie, Y., Peng, L., Liu, B., Xie, J., Bian, C., & Li, Min. (2015). Positive affect promotes well-being and alleviates depression: The mediating effect of attentional bias. *Psychiatry Research, 228*, 482–487. https://doi.org/10.1016/j.psychres.2015.06.011

6

ETHNIC AND RACIAL RESPONSIVENESS IN COGNITIVE-BEHAVIOR THERAPY (CBT)

Ryan C. T. DeLapp and Celenia L. DeLapp

Ethnic-racial identity, or the importance of one's ethnic and racial background within their overall sense of self, is an extremely important part of youth development. And, the development of a positive ethnic-racial self-concept is associated with many metrics of youth adjustment, including prosocial peer relationships, self-esteem, mental wellness, and academic belonging and engagement (Hughes et al., 2016; Neblett et al., 2012). As we will discuss throughout this chapter, Global Majority Youth[1] (GMY) are inundated with societal messages about what it means to be a member of their ethnic-racial group within immediate (e.g., family, neighborhood, schools) and distal (e.g., media coverage, policies, and laws) aspects of their community (Anderson et al., 2022a; Jones et al., 2023). Importantly, school mental health professionals are positioned to help these youth process these societal messages, develop pride and appreciation for who they are, and find ways to confidently express their ethnic-racial identities via their social interactions, academic engagement, and beyond. A significant obstacle to accomplishing these feats is the manifestations and impacts of racism that infiltrate multiple levels of the US society, including educational settings (Anderson et al., 2022a; Jones et al., 2023; Malone et al., 2020). Racism-related stress (RRS), or the social, emotional, and identity-related stresses caused by perceiving that one is being mistreated, unfairly judged, or denied opportunities due to their ethnic-racial background, can thwart healthy ethnic-racial identity development and cause negative emotional and academic consequences for youth (Anderson et al., 2022a). Furthermore, RRS can be subtle, pervasive, and chronic within educational settings, resulting from one-on-one and group interactions, from witnessing or hearing about incidents of racism toward others, and from youth and their families trying to navigate larger systems of oppression directly (e.g., finding adequate academic resources within one's school system) or indirectly (e.g., finding affordable, quality housing) related to educational settings. Also, it is important to remember that youth often spend more waking hours in a school context, thus making educational settings an environment where GMY has the greatest potential to experience prejudice and discrimination (Saleem & Byrd, 2021).

In light of the varied ways RRS can impact the daily experiences of GMY, this chapter will provide guidelines for how mental health professionals can support GMY in making decisions that can cultivate a sense of self-pride, appreciation, and agency within educational settings while supporting their decision-making when RRS creates a stressful academic environment. Specifically, the authors will discuss how to adapt Cognitive-Behavioral interventions to promote the Empowered Decision-Making of GMY within these settings.

 DOI: 10.4324/9781003392439-8

What Is Empowered Decision-Making?

Empowered Decision-Making describes one's ability to identify and implement accessible and meaningful coping decisions that address the perceived impacts of a stressful life event (such as encountering RRS). Such decision-making is a quite complex process, as it necessitates that youth are able to (1) identify the specific demands placed upon them by the stressful experience, (2) have learned and be able to identify coping resources available to them in that moment, and then (3) make a coping decision that meaningfully addresses some degree of the demands and impacts of the stressful experience.

The components of this Empowered Decision-Making process have been conceptualized and studied by scholars for decades (Anderson & Stevenson, 2019; DeLapp & Williams, 2019). From this work, we have learned that RRS coping is enhanced when persons of color experience racial coping self-efficacy—meaning they feel capable of identifying a set of coping skills they can use, feel a sense of hope and optimism that these coping skills will be effective, and then are able to experience the effective resolution of the stressful situation when using their coping skills (Anderson & Stevenson, 2019; DeLapp & Williams, 2019). Importantly, such perceived self-efficacy is believed to enhance the ability to brainstorm options for persisting toward goal attainment and "increase[es] the likelihood that [a person] will be able to match any given stressor with an appropriate coping strategy." (Danoff-Burg et al., 2004, p. 210). It is also important to note that the lack of self-efficacy (or the absence of perceived self-control, optimism, or goal attainability) when faced with RRS is linked with thwarted coping decision-making and negative health outcomes (DeLapp & Williams, 2019, 2021). And, given that racial coping self-efficacy is conceptualized to mediate the relationship between perceived RRS and coping decision-making (Anderson & Stevenson, 2019; DeLapp & Williams, 2021), mental health professionals must be aware of strategies to inspire growth in racial coping self-efficacy when working with GMY who disclose experiences of RRS.

Also, Empowered Decision-Making describes how persons of color translate their racial coping self-efficacy into actionable coping decisions (Anderson & Stevenson, 2019; DeLapp & Williams, 2021; Rollins & Valdez, 2006). There is an array of coping responses that have been empirically studied and identified as strategies that promote healthy adjustment within racially stressful contexts (see DeLapp & Williams, 2019; Jacob et al., 2023; Neblett et al., 2012; Williams et al., 2022a, 2022b for reviews of the racial coping literature). However, a pivotal question remains for GMY's racial coping self-efficacy, "How can they translate what is empirically shown to be effective within research studies into their daily living?" Beyond simply knowing what has been shown broadly to be effective, it is arguably most important that GMY know how to select coping strategies that effectively resolve the specific stressful demands placed upon them by RRS in a way that is personally meaningful to them (Anderson & Stevenson, 2019).

As such, when youth perceive RRS, Empowered Decision-Making characterizes the synthesis of coping awareness ("I know what I can do"), optimism and control ("I believe my coping responses will help"), and competency ("I can use a coping response to resolve at least some aspects of the stressful experience in a way that is meaningful to me").

How Can Youth Develop Empowered Decision-Making?

Ethnic-racial socialization, or the messages communicated to youth about the significance of their racial and ethnic background, is one of the conduits by which the components of Empowered Decision-Making are introduced and strengthened among GMY (Anderson et al., 2022a; Anderson & Stevenson, 2019). The acquisition of this "ethnic-racial self-knowledge" begins at an early age but notably becomes more critical during adolescence, as this is a developmental stage when youth become more conscious of their self-concept and are gaining socio-cognitive abilities to critically evaluate how their ethnic-racial backgrounds are responded to by the world around them (Hughes et al., 2016; Jones et al., 2020; Xie et al., 2021). During its earliest conceptualization, ethnic-racial socialization described the communication strategies used by parents and caregivers to instill cultural pride, inspire a sense of self-worth, and orient youth to the existence of racial bias within certain relationships and throughout their communities (Hughes et al., 2016). Furthermore, a key aspect of this ethnic-racial socialization process includes introducing youth to the available resources that can be used to cope with RRS and modeling how to use these resources effectively (Anderson & Stevenson, 2019; DeLapp & Williams, 2019)—all important ingredients for developing Empowered Decision-Making skill sets.

Research has moved beyond studying parents/caregivers as the primary socializing agents within their children's upbringing (Anderson et al., 2022a; Jones et al., 2023). In fact, all aspects of a child's environment (including their school counselors and clinicians—Bentley-Edwards et al., 2020; Saleem & Byrd, 2021) can actively and beneficially participate in this socialization process. Despite the great potential for non-parental socializing agents to have this impact on GMY, there remains a lack of prevention and intervention programming that offers a guide for non-parental figures, particularly those within the school context, to engage GMY in an ethnic-racial socialization process that promotes growth in Empowered Decision-Making (Anderson et al., 2022a; Saleem et al., 2020).

Preparing to Support Empowered Decision-Making

When working with GMY to promote their Empowered Decision-Making, it is imperative that socializing agents[2] embody a culturally responsive (CR) approach that seeks to promote GMY's cultural strengths, hold space for cultural stressors impacting their daily life, and acknowledge the dynamic interaction between GMY and their surrounding environment. This CR approach requires more than a set of step-by-step instructions that socializing agents rigidly adhere to. Rather, this approach necessitates effortful turning of the mind away from the status quo and toward an idiographic understanding of each student. Before thoroughly reviewing the guidelines for promoting Empowered Decision-Making with GMY, it is important for socializing agents to engage in proactive, ongoing self-education and introspection to enhance their utilization of the forthcoming guidelines. Specifically, this section of the chapter will provide recommendations for expanding one's *community consciousness* and capacity for *cultural humility*—as both are important factors in the provision of CR support to GMY.

Promoting Community Consciousness

Community consciousness, or a socializing agent's awareness of the historical and current social, political, and economic events relevant to a specific community, is a key component of offering CR support to GMY. Each level of a GMY's community (e.g., immediate family, peers, school, neighborhood, and country of origin) can impact GMY's daily experiences and life trajectory (Jones et al., 2023). And, given that Empowered Decision-Making prioritizes first acknowledging the environmental demands that are influencing one's decision-making, socializing agents must develop a degree of community consciousness that enables them to express humility toward the community strengths and stresses that influence the types of environmental demands placed on GMY. Table 6.1 offers a list of self-education prompts that can guide the development of this community consciousness. Using these prompts to guide self-education can enhance the ability of socializing agents to appreciate the historical roots of any social and academic inequities impacting GMY while also providing an opportunity to highlight aspects of resilience among students (and their families) who have found ways to navigate systems-level barriers effectively. And, from the information learned from self-education, socializing agents are encouraged to engage in proactive introspection in an effort to examine their personal responses to what they have learned, to consider the relevance of this information to their efforts to support GMY, and, finally, identify if there are any social actions they would like to make to fight for systemic change within their school's community.

Table 6.1 Self-Education Prompts for Enhancing Community Consciousness

System-Level	*Self-Education Prompts*
Immediate family	1 What are the common demographics of the families whose children attend your school? 2 Have these demographics remained stable or evolved throughout the history of the school's existence? 3 What factors have contributed to the stable or evolving nature of these demographics?
Peer-to-peer relationships	1 Is there ethnic-racial diversity within peer-to-peer relationships within the school environment? If so, what has helped this diversity to exist within the school environment? 2 Is there a history of racism-related stress within peer-to-peer interaction within the school environment? If so, how has this historically been handled with the victim(s), perpetrator(s), and administratively? 3 What opportunities are offered within school curriculum or programming for students to develop positive multicultural relationships within peers within or outside of the school? 4 Does your school offer affinity spaces for GMY to process their unique cultural experiences? If not, what has interfered with the development of these affinity spaces for GMY?
Student-to-school staff relationships	1 How have school staff (e.g., teachers, counselors, administrators) historically treated GMY and their families? 2 Is there a history of racism-related stress in student-to-school staff interactions within the school environment? If so, how has this historically been handled with the victim(s), perpetrator(s), and administratively? 3 Does it seem that GMY and their families have developed a sense of trust in school staff? Also, what has helped or hindered the development of their trust in school staff? 4 Does your school offer any trainings or resources to school staff to enhance their ability to support GMY and their families? If so, what has been the effectiveness of these trainings or resources?
Academic resources	1 Are you aware of the current systems that divide children into accelerated (e.g., gifted and talented), regular, or special education? How might these systems impact the life trajectories of the student you are serving? 2 What have you learned about students who speak a language other than English and what supports your school has or has not offered to such students? 3 Has your school adopted an educational curriculum that represents the cultural experiences and celebrates the contributions of People from the Global Majority? If so, how has your school community responded to this curriculum?
Past school context	1 Are you aware of the history of educational segregation and integration and its current effects on your students (and their families)? 2 If you work in a private, parochial, or Montessori school, do you know when, why, and how your school was founded?

(*Continued*)

Table 6.1 (Continued)

System-Level	*Self-Education Prompts*
Neighborhood context	1 What kinds of resources (or lack thereof) are offered to students within their neighborhoods? Examples can include access to physical and mental health, recreation, libraries, or transportation resources. 2 Do students experience a sense of physical and emotional safety within the neighborhoods they live in? What factors influence their sense of safety? 3 Who are the most prominent community stakeholders (e.g., faith leaders, politicians, social activists) within their neighborhoods? How do these stakeholders influence the neighborhood context?
Cultural trends	1 What current events are influencing the social, emotional, and political climate of the community surrounding your school? Are there any historical events that influence community surrounding your school? 2 What social justice movements or initiatives are currently impacting the community surrounding your school? Are there past social justice movements or initiatives that continue to influence the community surrounding your school?

Note: This is not an exhaustive list of prompts. Consider reviewing Malone et al. (2020) and Stern et al. (2022) for further discussion of socio-ecological systems that can influence the ethnic-racial socialization of GMY within educational settings and beyond.

Promoting Cultural Humility

Cultural humility is defined as "a way of being that involves a willingness, an openness and desire to (a) reflect on oneself as an embedded cultural being and (b) hear about and strive to understand others' cultural backgrounds and identities" (Zhang et al., 2022, p. 2). As this definition alludes to, cultural humility is not a finite list of self-preparatory actions that will lead to definitive cultural competence. Instead, such humility represents a lifelong commitment to "critical reflection, self-awareness, and the development of personal attitudes that allow practitioners to build stronger working relationships and to more fully engage with diverse populations" (Fisher, 2020, p. 54). When socializing agents embark on the journey of practicing cultural humility, it can increase the likelihood that cultural topics (e.g., cultural strengths and stresses) are broached within therapeutic spaces and strengthen the therapeutic alliance with individuals of diverse cultural backgrounds (Zhang et al., 2022). To support one's growth in developing cultural humility, socializing agents are encouraged to (1) thoughtfully examine their own cultural background, (2) engage in actions that lead to bias awareness and reduction, and (3) strengthen their ability to engage in sensitive race-related discussions.

First, it is imperative that socializing agents engage in proactive and ongoing exploration of their own cultural background, as this can improve their multicultural interactions (Atkins & Lorelle, 2022) and enhance cultural humility within race-related conversations and intervention for adults (Anderson et al., 2022b). Such self-examination can include a mapping of one's cultural identities, identifying how these identities have shaped one's beliefs, worldviews, and social interactions, and how these identities intersect with power and privilege (Fisher, 2020). There are several resources that socializing agents can utilize to support their self-exploration, including reviewing the ADDRESSING model (Hays, 1996, 2008) or answering questions about their identity and upbringing from the Cultural Formulation Interview in the Diagnostic and Statistical Manual, 5th edition (APA, 2013).

Additionally, there must be an exploration of the type of biases that exist toward others with shared or nonshared cultural backgrounds (Fisher, 2020). Biases can be thought of as mental shortcuts that have the potential to be harmful in certain contexts if enacted without careful consideration. For example, consider the case of a student whose family is known to be very wealthy. A possible bias could be that such a student will never have an issue paying for school trips or clothing. However, the synthesis of community consciousness (e.g., there is a culture of lavish spending among students and their families within the school) and cultural humility (e.g., curiosity about the impact of this spending culture on each student and their family) can help challenge any assumptions about the financial security of the student and reveal opportunities for offering support that is idiosyncratic and customized to the student's true current experience (e.g., exploring the possibility of financial distress within the home). One way socializing agents can begin examining their implicit biases is by completing free-to-access Implicit Association Tests via Harvard University's website (Greenwald et al., 1998). And, with any newfound bias awareness, socializing agents may experience negative reactions (e.g., guilt, shame, defensiveness), as it may be difficult to confront implicit biases that conflict with personal beliefs about oneself. In response to these emotions, it is important to foster self-compassion (Neff, 2023) and to turn one's mind back to a spirit of openness and nonjudgmental self-discovery. In part, such self-compassion can be derived from acknowledging that every person is socialized to develop strong beliefs and attitudes toward various aspects of our society; everyone has some in-group preference because it is a biological necessity and has contributed to human survival (Thompson & Wildavsky, 2008). And, while compassionately and nonjudgmentally acknowledging the various aspects of one's own bias, socializing agents can reduce the impacts of these biases by (1) engaging in multicultural social interactions that provide counterexamples to the prevailing stereotypes held about ethnic-racial backgrounds represented among GMY within one's educational setting (Devine et al., 2012), (2) seeking and actively participating in supervision/consultation that promotes critical analysis of the ways bias is impacting one's therapeutic practices (DeLapp & DeLapp, 2021), (3) proactively and regularly attending structured learning activities to enhance one's ability to practice within culturally diverse settings (Fisher, 2020), and (4) engaging in anti-racist social actions (Williams et al., 2022a).

Finally, offering CR support to GMY requires socializing agents to create interpersonal safety within therapeutic relationships, especially when hoping that GMY confide in such professionals with their experiences of RRS (DeLapp & DeLapp, 2021). Strategies for promoting such safety include obtaining consent from GMY before initiating discussion about GMY cultural experiences, showing willingness and openness to race-related discussions with GMY, actively listening to GMY disclosures without immediately jumping to problem-solving, normalizing the discomfort of disclosing certain cultural experiences within therapeutic settings, naming and honoring power imbalances within the therapeutic relationship, and stating the limitations of the socializing agent's role and social influence (Bentley-Edwards et al., 2020; DeLapp & DeLapp, 2021). Undoubtedly, these discussions may result in socializing agents experiencing discomfort or doubt regarding their ability to engage with GMY on topics of race and culture effectively. Thus, there may be a reluctance to broach topics related to race or culture (regardless if GMY perceive the space to be safe or not—Naz et al., 2019). As such, it is important that socializing agents engage in race-related conversations beyond their interactions with GMY, as doing so can help agents develop the interpersonal effectiveness and distress tolerance skills to navigate these discussions with openness, humility, and sensitivity when working with GMY (see for additional recommendations DeLapp & DeLapp, 2021).

Introducing the REACH UP: A Model for Teaching Empowered Decision-Making

The Racial, Ethnic, And Cultural Healing Unifying Principles (or REACH UP—DeLapp & Gallo, 2022) is a therapeutic framework designed to help socializing agents utilize their community consciousness and cultural humility to support youth in building the necessary skills to feel empowered in their decision-making. Specifically, this model provides a flexible framework for proactively and reactively promoting Empowered Decision-Making using a 3-pronged approach: (1) helping youth clarify a personal definition of empowerment, (2) exploring how RRS obstructs a sense of empowered decision-making, and (3) supporting youth in strengthening empowered coping responses to RRS.

Defining Empowerment

Youth are tasked with making a variety of decisions within educational settings, including what they can do to achieve desired academic goals, how to interact with classmates and teachers, and even which extracurriculars they would like to participate in. Often, these decisions are strongly influenced by the values imposed on youth by the adults in their lives and the opportunities afforded to them by their educational environment. However, as youth vie for more independence and autonomy as they mature, their decision-making begins to reflect their development of personal values and intrinsically defined goals. This normative developmental progression toward independent decision-making represents an invaluable opportunity for socializing agents to engage youth in exercises that help them clarify how their personal values and goals can translate into *meaningful* decision-making. To support their self-exploration, Table 6.2 offers a list of values and goal clarification activities often utilized within evidence-based interventions, such as ACT (Hayes et al., 2011) and adolescent DBT (Rathus & Miller, 2014), that can be incorporated within counseling services. Importantly, these activities enable youth to explore their personal values and goals while acknowledging influences from family and their broader community on these attributes of themselves; an important consideration when aspiring to be CR during such exercises.

Practically, the information gained from any of these activities in Table 6.2 can be used to support GMY in (1) establishing school-related goals that align with their values (e.g., what academic and relationship goals does the student feel compelled to achieve due to strongly valuing filial piety), (2) carefully considering how their daily decision-making is already helping them progress toward these valued goals (e.g., what decisions is the student already making toward their academic and relationship goals), (3) brainstorming options for enhancing such values-aligned decision-making (e.g., helping the student clarify options for honoring and respecting their family via school activities), and (4) supporting youth in resolving any values conflict that may be complicating their decision-making (e.g., helping the student navigate decision-making when there are conflicts between filial piety and individualism). And, from these interventions, it is anticipated that GMY will learn to use their values and goals to identify decisions that promote a general sense of empowered and meaningful decision-making.

Barriers to Empowered Decision-Making

The nebulous, ever-evolving, chronic, and systemic dwellings of RRS can make the development of Empowered Decision-Making extremely challenging (Anderson et al., 2022a). In an effort to honor the complexity and challenging task of GMY practicing Empowered Decision-Making within educational settings, the REACH UP model "embodies a dialectical perspective in that [socializing agents] seek to enhance an awareness of the 'I can' and acknowledge (and at times support the grieving of) the 'I can't right now.'" (DeLapp & Gallo, 2022, p. 4) To this end, the "Barriers to Empowered Decision-Making" step of the REACH UP model is about orienting GMY to the potential ways RRS may impede their Empowered Decision-Making and then helping them identify the specific barriers they are facing in any given moment.

Specifically, this model translates RRS into four types of barriers to Empowerment. As shown in Table 6.3, there are two external barriers: Community Stress (or the ways systemic and cultural racism limit access to important resources and opportunities) and Relationship Stress (or the ways

Table 6.2 Strategies for Supporting Values Clarification and Goal Definition

Exercise	*Description*	*Examples*
Values card sort	Prompt student to sort an array of cards displaying values (and their definitions) according to degree of personal importance. Use the student's sorting to guide discussion of empowered responses to RRS.	Student completes a sorting task and identifies "justice, multicultural connection, health/wellness and mindfulness" as top four most important values. Student expresses interest in learning to balance personal wellness while trying to stand up for what's right within their school. Finally, clinician helps student identify goals both in and outside of school that align with these values.
Defining importance of coping goals	Identify coping goal 1st, then explore the meaning/ importance of the goal (clarify values)	Student desires to be more confident displaying authentic attributes of their identity at school. Clinician and student then discuss the importance of this goal, which leads to clarification of student's values related to increasing confident expressions.
Valued role models	Identify role model (family member, character, athlete, historical figure), then explore admired characteristics	During initial meetings, student and clinician discuss revered athletes and identified attributes of the athletes that are personally relevant to the student. When RRS onsets, student would express how their coping goals were to emulate certain characteristics of the role models we discussed.
Values within a concept	Identify a concept (e.g., "I want to be a social justice warrior"), then explore different values/ characteristics that make up this concept	Student aspires to be an activist so clinician prompts student to identify characteristics of activism that the student feels are personally relevant and explores student's vision for prioritizing activism within their daily life.
Values venn diagram	Create Values Venn Diagram where student contrasts personal values with another entity (e.g., family member, job/school setting), which allows clinician and student to explore how definition of empowerment may shift between different environments	Student identifies that multicultural connection and non-conformity are important values, which conflict with their family values of familial harmony and cultural tradition. Student and clinician discuss how empowered responses may differ depending on the student's environment, identify contexts where non-conformity and multicultural connection can be prioritized, and explore whether the student is willing to accept any unwanted consequences associated with prioritizing these values when around family.
Values within a narrative	Discussion of individual and/ or family narratives with an emphasis on identifying values reflected within the narrative	Student narrates a history of their family prioritizing generosity toward community despite their family encountering countless hardships. The student and clinician then explore what values are emphasized within this narrative and then explore the degree to which they find these values personally relevant. Student then identifies empowered responses that may align with generosity that can be incorporated into their daily life.
Exploring interests to clarify values	Explore personal interests (e.g., music/art/poetry/books/ movies/games) in order to gain insight into what is meaningful or important to patient	Student has expressed interest in reading and poetry, and the clinician asks the student to share a piece that is meaningful to them. Patient selects and reads Audre Lorde's poem "Power" in session to clinician. This leads to exploring the experience of anger and rage regarding racism and personal desire to pursue values of empowerment and activism.

Adapted from DeLapp and Gallo (2022).

prejudice, stereotyping, and discrimination make knowing how to exist within certain relationships challenging). In contrast, Table 6.3 identifies two internal barriers: Emotional Stress (or the physiological and emotional discomforts that are difficult to cope with when exposed to RRS) and Identity Stress (or the difficulty developing and preserving a sense of self-love and -pride due to exposure to RRS). Table 6.3 also includes a list of assessment prompts that can be used to help youth evaluate the relevance of any of these RRS barriers. Importantly, socializing agents can explore the relevance of these barriers as a form of *prevention* (e.g., exposing youth to these barriers and supporting them in coping ahead if they ever perceive any barriers as posing a threat to their Empowered Decision-Making) or *intervention* (e.g., assessing the degree to which any of these barriers are perceived as interfering with their coping efficacy following an experience of RRS and then exploring options for Empowered Decision-Making). Ultimately, acknowledging the existence of these barriers to empowerment enables socializing agents to validate the intricacy of the RRS coping process while helping youth establish clear yet realistic expectations for what their Empowered Decision-Making can help them achieve when faced with RRS (DeLapp & Gallo, 2022).

Strengthening Empowered Decision-Making

When trying to cope with RRS, the REACH UP model proposes that GMY experience empowerment when they are able to make decisions that preserve their *self-acceptance* (or "learning to embrace what is appreciated and loved about themselves while protecting this sense of self from being degraded by the culturally stressful aspects of one's environment") and promote their *healing* (or "learning to recover from moments of perceived powerlessness and identifying effective coping responses that bolster a sense of empowerment"—DeLapp & Gallo, 2022, p. 5). Below are recommendations for how socializing agents can use evidenced-based interventions to strengthen Empowered Decision-Making in response to each RRS-related barrier.

Table 6.3 Clinician Prompts for Assessing Barriers to Empowered Decision-Making with Global Majority Youth

Internal and External Barriers to Empowerment		
Barrier	*Description*[a]	*Assessment Examples*
Community stress	*Community stress* is caused when parts of one's community (e.g., schools, job, housing, laws) limits their access to important resources and opportunities. These resources/opportunities can include lacking access to a sense of safety, emotional and social support, the ability to confidently express one's identity in certain parts of their community, and financial stability within one's community. Importantly, the lack of access to these resources within one's community can interfere with their ability to pursue certain goals they have.	1 Do you feel like you have access to any of the following resources in your school: a sense of safety, emotional and social support, or the ability to confidently express your racial identity? 2 Have you ever felt unfairly denied access to a resource or an opportunity within your school? If so, can you explain? 3 Do you feel as if you have the resources needed to pursue your academic, relationship, or wellness goals? If not, can you share the impact of not having access to these resources? 4 Have you (or your family) ever tried to get access to needed resources? If so, can you tell me about what happened when you tried to do so?

(*Continued*)

Table 6.3 (Continued)

Internal and External Barriers to Empowerment		
Barrier	*Description*[a]	*Assessment Examples*
Relationship stress	*Relationship stress* can occur in one's relationships with other people, both people with shared and nonshared backgrounds. When people show their negative beliefs about one's cultural background(s)/identity or show disrespect toward someone's cultural values, it can make it difficult to know how to remain within these types of relationships. Also, being around these negative beliefs or the lack of respect for one's values can lead to interpersonal conflicts and various forms of mistreatment. Examples of Relationship Stress can include exposure to interpersonal racism, racial microaggressions, and bicultural stress.	1 What positive and uplifting messages have you heard about your identity from family/ friends/peers/community members? 2 What negative and hurtful messages have you heard about your identity from family/ friends/peers/community members? 3 If you are willing, can you share with me a recent situation in which you felt you were treated with less respect and courtesy because of your identity? 4 Can you tell me about a relationship that is important to you in which this person holds a different set of beliefs about an aspect of your identity that is important to you?
Emotional stress	*Emotional stress* describes the strong and hurtful emotions (e.g., anger, anxiety, sadness, numbness) felt when someone questions if they have been judged, mistreated, or denied an opportunity because of some part of their identity. Unfortunately, it can be hard to recognize these emotions or know what to do when feeling them.	1 How challenging do you find it to stay present and aware when you are being faced with a race-related stress? 2 When you are faced with a cultural stressor, what emotions tend to show up for you? 3 Are you accepting and/or welcoming toward your emotions? 4 What emotions do you find most challenging to cope with when they arise? 5 How do you cope when you are faced with a cultural stressor? Do you feel this way of coping is working for you? If so, how? If not, what would you like to change?
Identity stress	*Identity stress* is caused when someone witnesses negative or critical messages from their surroundings that they are "less than" someone else because of who they are. Such messages can be communicated directly within relationships and by witnessing how others who have a similar background are treated—especially via different forms of media (e.g., news, social media, TV/Movies). As one matures and learns about themselves, it can be difficult to develop self-love, self-pride, and self-confidence when exposed to these negative messages about one's identity and cultural background(s). Struggling to have self-love, self-pride, and self-confidence can be hard to cope with and can make it seem less possible to achieve important life goals.	1. What kind of messages do you get about who you are or should be from family/ friends/peers/community members? How does this impact your thoughts about your racial/ethnic background? 2. What kind of messages do you get about who you are or should be from movies, music, social media? How does this impact your thoughts about your racial/ethnic background? 3. Do you ever find any of the negative and hurtful messages about your identity from family/friends/peers/community members/ social media believable? 4. Are there aspects of your identity that you dislike? If so, can you tell me about that, and where you think those beliefs come from?

Adapted from DeLapp and Gallo (2022).

[a] Descriptions are phrased conversationally to provide examples of how clinicians can introduce each barrier type. Wording is based on phrasing used with preteens and teens of color.

Promoting Empowered Decision-Making in Response to Emotional Stress

It is well documented that RRS carries significant psychological consequences, including intense and, at times, chronic emotional distress (Hope et al., 2021; Gibson et al., 2022). And, these emotional impacts of RRS may differ based on GMY's anticipation of, present exposure to, and post-event processing of RRS (Wilson & Gentzler, 2021). For example, the anticipation of experiencing RRS-oriented Relationship Stress, such as thinking about presenting in front of peers suspected of being racially prejudiced, may prompt anxiety and heightened physiological arousal that causes the student to consider not attending class. In contrast, emotions felt in the heat of the moment, such as surprise, shock, or rage in response to a racially insensitive comment during the presentation, may feel sudden, intense, and cause the student to be unsure what to say or do. And, after encountering RRS, youth may experience lingering emotional discomforts that are intermittently triggered by reminders of the encounter and that disrupt their efforts to remain socially and academically engaged within their educational setting. Altogether, exposure to RRS can provoke a complex emotional experience and thus socializing agents need to be able to support youth in exploring their options for mindfully, compassionately, and effectively responding to their emotional experiences. Table 6.4 provides a summary of the coping decisions that youth can choose from to identify empowered responses to Emotional Stress—Mindfulness, Opposite Action, Soothing My Emotions, and Taking Care of My Emotions Over Time.

Table 6.4 Coping Decisions for the Emotional Stress

Coping Category	*Examples of Coping Decisions*	*Description*
Mindfulness	Mindfulness	Observing and describing their BEAT[a] before, during, or after race-related event
	Self-compassion	Practicing acceptance, kindness, and understanding toward their BEAT
Opposite action	Notice the urge(s)	Proactively identifying any unhelpful urges and using mindfulness to notice when the urges are present
	Resist any unhelpful urge(s)	Choosing to resist these urges when acting on the urges do not seem helpful
	Mindfully engage in an alternate response	Choosing to mindfully engage in a different, more helpful action
Soothe my emotions	Soothing activity	Choosing a calming activity to tolerate discomfort and act opposite to unhelpful urges
	Body-focused coping	Choosing a body-focused activity to tolerate discomfort and act opposite to unhelpful urges
	Seeking social connection and support	Choosing to express emotions or asking for help coping with emotions from a trusted ally
Take care of myself over time	Physical well-being	Investing time into activities or tasks that promote physical wellness
	Social connection	Investing time in growing and keeping relationships with trusted allies
	Fun/enjoyment	Investing time in activities or tasks that give you opportunities to have fun/enjoyment
	Accomplishment/mastery	Investing time in activities or tasks that give you opportunities to feel accomplished

[a] BEAT = Body sensations, Emotions, Action urges, and Thoughts.

MINDFULNESS

When emotionally triggered by exposure to RRS, a goal can be to identify coping resources that can help GMY regulate the intense and uncomfortable body sensations, emotions, action urges, and thoughts. As emphasized in many evidence-based interventions (e.g., ACT and DBT—Hayes et al., 2011; Rathus & Miller, 2014), an important precursor to engaging in such emotion-focused coping is mindfulness, or the ability to orient one's attention to internal responses (e.g., emotion or action urges) and then nonjudgmentally describe what is being experienced. Such awareness is vital for learning how to respond to (rather than react to or make efforts to avoid) uncomfortable emotional states according to one's values and goals (Williams et al., 2022a, 2022b). Said differently, equipping youth with foundational mindfulness skills can help GMY select empowered coping decisions that enable them to meaningfully regulate emotions triggered by RRS. Practically, mindfulness training can include engaging youth in non-racism-related activities (e.g., playing games, listening to music, watching media) and prompting them to notice and describe their in-the-moment body sensations, emotions, action urges, and thoughts. If youth experience difficulty with labeling these aspects of their internal experience, then they may benefit from foundational emotion recognition and expression activities (e.g., using Feelings Charts, playing Emotion Charades, or reading stories and then discussing the emotional responses of the characters). And, once these foundational mindfulness skills are established, GMY can be supported in observing and describing their thoughts, feelings, and action urges in response to racially stressful events that have occurred both in and outside of academic settings.

Furthermore, increasing mindfulness without strengthening self-compassion, or the ability to express openness and acceptance toward one's experience of emotions, can thwart emotion-focused coping efforts. When youth are overly critical of their emotions, feel alone in their emotional pain, or feel stuck and unable to escape their emotional pain, it can increase emotional distress following encounters with RRS (Watson-Singleton et al., 2021). Moreover, the temptation to engage with any negative self-criticisms (e.g., "You are being weak" or "You should be over this by now") can ultimately interfere with both self-acceptance and emotional healing. As such, socializing agents should consider orienting youth to the concept of self-compassion, which can include exercises such as prompting GMY to "speak to yourself like you would a friend," normalizing their emotional response by discussing the possible emotions other GMY might feel if in a similar situation, and externalizing the blame to outside factors rather than aspects of the self. And, though not created solely for youth experiencing RRS, socializing agents may benefit from reviewing the work of Drs. Kristen Neff and Christopher Germer to learn more about experiential exercises for helping to strengthen self-compassion—particularly publications about their Mindful Self-Compassion Program (Germer & Neff, 2019). Also, there have been adaptations of ACT (Banks et al., 2021) and cognitive-behavior therapy (CBT) (Steele, 2020) for internalized racism that offer therapeutic approaches for increasing awareness of negative self-judgments caused by RRS and cognitive techniques for reducing the impact of these judgments on youth's emotion regulation processes.

OPPOSITE ACTION

When GMY choose to practice mindful self-compassion, they can also gain awareness of the emotion-action urge relationship. Such awareness is crucial to the Empowered Decision-Making process, as increasing one's ability to nonjudgmentally notice the present-moment emotions that are associated with certain action urges (e.g., anxiety and avoidance, sadness and withdrawal, anger and confrontation) is a vital 1st step to enhancing emotion regulatory decision-making in many CBT-oriented interventions (adolescent DBT—Rathus & Miller, 2014; Unified Protocol—Ehrenreich et al., 2009).

To this end, evidence has associated exposure to RRS with the following unhealthy action urges: substance use, self-harm, suicidal ideation, and disordered eating (Williams et al., 2022a, 2022b). And, while it is clear that each of these actions can have a myriad of negative consequences, it is important to not pre-emptively categorize coping responses as either "good" or "bad" (DeLapp & Williams, 2019; Williams et al., 2022a, 2022b). Rather, it is imperative that youth be encouraged to consider whether certain action urges are more or less helpful in supporting their effort to live according to the values and goals they acknowledged in the "Defining Empowerment" component of the REACH UP model. Importantly, by using GMY's values and goals in this way, it promotes cultural responsiveness and provides a safeguard from socializing agents infusing their personal biases into the GMY's selection of empowered coping decisions.

SOOTHING MY EMOTIONS

As youth gain better awareness of and the ability to resist values-incongruent actions, it is imperative that socializing agents also support their awareness and use of values-congruent soothing activities. Self-soothe activities are not to be confused with activities that rid youth of the uncomfortable emotions they are experiencing. Importantly, Jacob and colleagues (2023) discuss that the effectiveness of these skills is often limited to short-term stress management (e.g., youth feel able to tolerate the momentary emotional impact of racism) and is not focused on long-term change (e.g., self-soothe skills do not change the source of RRS and thus future opportunities remain for further Emotional Stress). As such, when socializing agents are exploring these decision-making abilities with youth, they should maintain a dialectical framework by acknowledging both the strengths (e.g., these are activities that enable youth to "ride the wave" of their emotional pain) and limitations (e.g., self-soothe skills do not change the systems or interpersonal dynamics that perpetuate RRS).

Practically, socializing agents can draw from existing emotion regulation skills created by DBT to help youth identify their personal self-soothe toolkit (e.g., Distract with ACCEPTS, Self-Soothe, IMPROVE, TIPP—Johnson & Melton, 2020; Rathus & Miller, 2014). And, given the healing role that faith and spirituality play within many communities of color (DeLapp & Williams, 2019), socializing agents should inquire if youth ascribe to any religious or spiritual belief systems and if they would like to add any element of their religious or spiritual practice within their self-soothe toolkit (e.g., scriptures, prayers, a list of social supports within their faith community). In summary, socializing agents can use the acronym "BASICS" to help youth identify Empowered Decisions that can fulfill a self-soothing function (DeLapp & Gallo, 2022): Body-focused coping (e.g., paced breathing, progressive muscle relaxation, grounding, or intense exercise); Activism (e.g., any effort to channel emotional pain into system change or resistance); Social support seeking (e.g., utilizing family, friends, or trusted allies to express and receive validation for emotional pain); Investing in self (e.g., making an effort to act on "Taking Care of My Emotions Over Time" recommendations below); Calming activities (e.g., riding the wave of discomfort by mindfully participating in activities that strongly engage at least one of the five senses); Spiritual connection (e.g., engaging in a spiritual or faith-oriented healing practice).

TAKING CARE OF MY EMOTIONS OVER TIME

Healing-focused decision-making is more than solely learning how to cope with the direct emotional impacts of RRS. It also includes investing in a lifestyle or daily routine that buffers the development of an overriding sense of powerlessness and hopelessness. The essence of empowerment entails feeling able to achieve important life goals, such as establishing close friendships, promoting physical or spiritual wellness, and progressing toward important life achievements (e.g., education, personal hobbies, careers). And, while the aforementioned coping skills are directly focused on managing the intensity and immediate consequences of Emotional Stress, there is also a need to help youth maintain a broader perspective on their overall well-being. A perspective that keeps their values-congruent goals in mind, that motivates daily efforts toward achieving these goals, and that supports their celebration of accomplishments along the way to their goal attainment. This recommendation draws upon literature identifying the distal impacts of RRS, such as social withdrawal and reduced goal attainment (Goodrum et al., 2023); all impacts that can reduce the overall quality of life and a broader sense of empowerment.

Practically, socializing agents can look to racial socialization-oriented behavioral activation approaches (Saleem & Byrd, 2021) to help youth identify activities that represent achievable and values-congruent investments in their *physical wellness*, *social connection*, *fun/enjoyment*, and sense of *mastery/accomplishment* (as shown in Table 6.4). For example, socializing agents could help GMY generate list of activities that fall under each of these categories and then explore the degree to which they are choosing to routinely invest in their emotional wellness via these activity targets. If they are experiencing difficulty engaging in these activities, it may be important to revisit the assessment approaches in Table 6.3 to explore whether external (e.g., inaccessible resources or ongoing interpersonal mistreatment) or internal (e.g., chronic anxiety and fear, or a lack of self-confidence) barriers are interfering with their efforts to invest in these goal-oriented initiatives (Williams et al., 2022a, 2022b). And, when youth present with ongoing anxiety and avoidance of investing in these initiatives, it is recommended that socializing agents consider evaluating GMY for symptoms of racial trauma and refer to a clinician who is well-trained in a TF-CBT adaption for racial trauma (Metzger et al., 2021).

Promoting Empowered Decision-Making in Response to Community and Relationship Stress

While the aforementioned decision-making focused on Emotional Stress can inspire self-acceptance and healing toward internal responses to RRS, Empowered Decision-Making also includes strengthening how youth can inspire healing via acting on their self-agency to shape and mold their relationships and parts of community to be more promoting of their wellness and goal attainment (Williams et al., 2022a, 2022b). Socializing agents should invest time in helping GMY understand the relevance of systemic, cultural, and interpersonal racism within the social stratosphere of their school or broader community and then help them identify empowered decisions related to changing the dynamics of their social or community spaces (or Situation-focused Coping) or learning to meaningfully navigate these stressors as they pursue important life goals within these spaces (or Self-focused Coping). Table 6.5 provides a summary of the coping decisions that youth can choose from to identify and empower responses to Community and Relationship Stress—Mindfulness, Situation-focused Coping, and Self-focused Coping.

MINDFULNESS

Previously, mindfulness was described as the decision to pause, notice, and nonjudgmentally describe one's internal responses at any given moment. Such mindfulness is also vital for understanding how the educational environment has or is impacting GMY's momentary sense of agency. In order to apply their mindfulness skills as described, GMY may benefit from identifying sources of Community or Relationship Stress within their environment and then using their mindfulness skills to explore the cognitive, emotional, and behavioral impacts of these experiences.

Table 6.5 Coping Decisions for Community and Relationship Stress

Coping Category	*Examples of Coping Decisions*	*Description*
Mindfulness	Mindfulness	Noticing how the Community or Relationship Stress has impacted their BEAT[a]
	Self-compassion	Showing acceptance, kindness, and understanding toward their BEAT
Situation-focused coping	Assertiveness	Confidently communicating what they want or need (including setting boundaries, educating others, or saying "No") to perpetrators of RRS or their trusted allies
	Seeking advocacy	Asking trusted allies to pursue change with them or on their behalf
	Activism	Investing time in projects, activities, or acts of self-expression intended to address injustice
Self-focused coping	Information seeking	Seeking information about the quality of the people and the rules/ policies in an environment
	Self-expression	Selectively investing their time, energy, and self-expression within certain relationships or activities
	Seeking support and connection	Investing time in growing and keeping relationships with trusted allies in the environment causing Community and Relationship Stress
	Selective compromise	Selectively choosing when to engage in resistance and when to adhere to policies, requests, or demands in order to preserve energy and wellness
	Goal attainment	Maintaining efforts toward important relationship, wellness, and achievement goals

[a] BEAT = Body sensations, Emotions, Action urges, and Thoughts.

Practically, socializing agents may choose to begin with psychoeducation about the different sources of RRS—possibly by administering self-report inventories that prompt youth to rate their exposure to a list of racism-related events (e.g., Perceptions of Racism in Children and Youth—Pachter et al., 2010) or by prompting youth to reflect on their access to important community resources and the impacts of interpersonal racism within their communities using a community mapping exercise (Mapping Vulnerability and Privilege tool; Siber-Sanderowitz et al., 2022). Next, youth can be provided psychoeducation about different belief systems that can emerge in response to Community and Relationship Stress, which would allow youth to monitor the occurrence and impact of these beliefs. For example, GMY can be oriented to the following thought patterns:

> unsafe world thoughts (or a belief that their environment is unsafe for them to confidently express their identity), unjust world thoughts (or belief that their environment has different standards of fairness for people who share their identity), or general powerlessness (or a low sense of efficacy or motivation to engage in empowered responses—DeLapp & Gallo, 2022, p. 7).

Furthermore, Williams and colleagues (2022a, 2022b) recommend that persons of color monitor causal attributions about why Community and Relationship Stresses occur. For example, some youth may believe that inaccessible resources, interpersonal conflicts, or unwanted outcomes are due to personal flaws or inadequacies (e.g., "I was not accepted into the gifted and talented program because I didn't work hard enough"). And, while such beliefs may inspire increased hard work in the short-term for some, the long-term consequences can include chronic self-blame that inhibits self-compassion, diminished psychological and physical wellness, and an inability to set realistic, achievable goals within life domains greatly impacted by racism (Williams et al., 2022a, 2022b). Finally, with a knowledge of these belief systems, youth may benefit from practice with nonjudgmentally observing and labeling the occurrence of such belief systems. For example, students might use their mindfulness skills to notice and verbalize when they have the following thoughts, "I am noticing the thought that 'I don't think this school is safe place for people like me'" or "I noticed the thought that 'Things don't usually go well for us [people of color].'" And, when seeking to support students' Empowered Coping responses to Community and Relationship Stress, youth can be encouraged to observe whether the presence of such thoughts is associated with any emotions (e.g., hopelessness, helplessness) or action urges (e.g., giving up or avoidance) that may influence their Empowered Decision-Making process.

SITUATION-FOCUSED COPING

This category of coping decisions focuses on the efforts GMY can make to confront (and, if possible, change) the causal factors that lead to repeated exposure to Community and Relationship Stress. It is about helping youth "feel empowered to use their voice in a manner that is fitting their personality and values" and doing so in a way that enhances their sense of control and ability to be their authentic selves within their environment (Jacob et al., 2023; Williams et al., 2022a, 2022b, p. 13). And, though there are legitimate barriers that may hinder any one person's effort to eradicate the existence of Community or Relationship Stress, it does not mean socializing agents cannot help GMY explore their options for pursuing change and resistance within certain relationships or parts of their community. Moreso, the emphasis of this coping category is to explore the range of GMY agency and control while maintaining a healthy respect for the ways individual autonomy can be limited by systemic, cultural, and interpersonal manifestations of racism.

Practically, socializing agents should first help youth clarify which goals they hope to achieve via resistance and change along with how their efforts to achieve their goals would align with their values (see Table 6.2 for strategies to support this clarification process). Goals might include confronting a perpetrator of Relationship Stress, setting boundaries within relationships to reduce the incidence of RRS, educating people about one's race-related experiences in an effort to foster greater understanding and compassion, seeking justice and accountability from authority figures, advocating for or creating increased access to desired resources within the academic community, or participating in activities that enhance the overall wellness of the academic community. Also, GMY may need support identifying which of their personal abilities and social resources can be used to achieve the specific goals they clarified. In particular, socializing agents can help youth consider when to use assertive communication or participation in activism while also knowing when to invest their efforts in seeking advocacy from peers and authority figures to join them in their fight for change. Of note, aside from coping with the personal impacts of Community and Relationship Stress, GMY may also be curious about Situation-focused Coping Decisions that pertain to allyship or advocacy on behalf of another person within their educational setting who has been impacted by RRS (Heard-Garris et al., 2021). Finally, it is recommended that socializing agents engage youth (and their families when there is potential for significant consequences) in a cost-benefit analysis for any Situation-focused Coping Decisions. Specifically, such cost-benefit analysis holds space for how their decision aligns with their goals and values while acknowledging potential negative consequences associated with their chosen method to fight for change. For instance, it is not uncommon for persons of color to encounter adverse social (e.g., retaliation, dismissiveness, invalidation, or criticism from systems or individuals being confronted) and emotional consequences for publicly acknowledging the existence of racism and fighting for social change (DeLapp & Williams, 2019; Jacob et al., 2023). As such, it is important that youth are supported with exploring these real possibilities and with developing a "coping ahead" plan for any anticipated adverse outcomes that may result from Situation-focused Coping (DeLapp & Gallo, 2022). For additional considerations for using assertiveness and activism to fight for change, see Heard-Garris et al. (2021), Jacob et al. (2023), and Williams et al. (2022a, 2022b).

SELF-FOCUSED COPING

Unfortunately, Situation-focused Coping Decisions often do not result in immediate changes to relationships and communities influenced by racism. Also, such coping decisions may not seem readily available or within the youth's best interest, given the possible social and emotional consequences that are anticipated. As such, socializing agents should help youth explore what other empowered decisions are available for them to remain in this environment in a way that is as meaningful as possible. Often, GMY will be tasked with utilizing Self-focused Coping to manage the manifestations of RRS in educational settings, as the frequent sources of this stress (e.g., peers, teachers, and authority figures) may be beyond their direct and immediate influence.

Practically, socializing agents should help youth utilize their mindfulness skills to notice their internal responses to Community or Relationship Stresses that lack clear and immediate options for swiftly changing. And, in an effort to counterbalance this acknowledgment of the "I can't right now," it is important to explore the options that remain within the student's locus of control. As shown in Table 6.5, such choices can include *information gathering* (e.g., monitoring social norms and behavior of peers, teachers, and other authority figures to determine how the student wants to approach these relationships), *building social support and connection* (e.g., cultivating close and supportive relationships with trusted peers who may have similar lived experiences, or connecting them with extracurricular activities or social events that are more promoting of their agency and authentic self-expression), *selective self-expression* (e.g., helping them explore how much energy and time they choose to invest within their educational setting, or how much information they share about themselves within certain relationships), and *maintaining progress toward desired goals* (e.g., helping youth see avenues for still achieving important life goals related to their relationship, well-being, and overall life satisfaction). As aforementioned, Empowered Decision-Making does not only include knowing what coping decisions you can make but also being able to select a coping decision that feels most accessible and effective for the stressful moment. As such, when supporting GMY with identifying Self-focused Coping Decisions, socializing agents may find it beneficial to help them evaluate the degree to which the coping decisions under consideration align with their personal values and goals. And, if students struggle to have such clarity, they may benefit from utilizing one of the exercises from Table 6.2 to gain clarity regarding the values and goals they want to pursue using the available coping decisions.

Promoting Empowered Decision-Making in Response to Identity Stress

GMY are exposed to a variety of socialization messages about their racial and ethnic backgrounds from family, peers, authority figures, and more broadly via a variety of media sources. Such messages engage youth in a developmental process of discerning how their ethnic-racial knowledge (or understanding of what it means to be a member of their ethnic or racial group within America—Xie et al., 2021) will influence how they want to carry themselves, who they want to be surrounded by, and even what they feel capable of achieving. As GMY mature and develop through adolescence, they develop more sophisticated metacognitive abilities that enable them to better evaluate the significance of these societal messages (Hughes et al., 2016). And, with the increased salience of clarifying their

Table 6.6 Coping with Identity Stress

Coping Category	*Examples of Coping Decisions*	*Description*
Mindfulness	Mindfulness	Noticing how the Identity Stress has impacted their BEAT[a]
	Self-compassion	Showing acceptance, kindness, and understanding toward their BEAT
Identity exploration	Self-reflect	Thinking about the people, places, and events that influence their racial/ethnic identity
	Research	Seeking information that would help them better understand their racial/ethnic identity
	Activity scheduling	Attending events or engaging in activities that would help you better understand your racial/ethnic identity
Identity expression	Find safe spaces for expression	Identifying relationships or parts of their community that supports their confident self-expression
	Express and tolerate discomfort	Choosing to express a part of their racial/ethnic identity even though they feel discomfort
	Code switching	Choosing to selectively express part of their racial/ethnic identity in different relationships and parts of their community
Identity protection	Characterize the negative messages	Choosing a label and character to represent the negative messages they most often experience from others or themselves
	Cope with emotional impact	Choosing to use Opposite Action and Soothing My Emotions skills (see Table 6.4) to cope with emotional impact from the negative message(s)
	Use my reframing questions	Using their values, goals, and counterfactual examples to evaluate the validity and personal significance of negative messages
	Live in my self-affirmation	Choosing to build self-love and self-acceptance by using Identity Exploration and Expression (see above)

[a] BEAT = Body sensations, Emotions, Action urges, and Thoughts.

sense of "Who Am I," many adolescents, more so than younger children, tend to think more critically and carefully about the significance of their ethnic-racial identity relative to their overall sense of self. Furthermore, research has shown that adolescent well-being (including their mental and physical health) can be significantly influenced by their ethnic-racial identity development (see, for reviews, Hughes et al., 2016; Neblett et al., 2012).

And, given that a strong ethnic-racial identity can be a protective factor for youth of color when they are exposed to RRS (Gibson et al., 2022), it is imperative that socializing agents are able to help youth make Empowered Decisions for exploring the significance of ethnic-racial identity, navigating contexts when their ethnic-racial identity becomes salient, and expressing the aspects of their identity that are most important to them. Table 6.6 provides a summary of the coping decisions that youth can choose from to identify empowered responses to Identity Stress—Mindfulness, Identity Exploration, Identity Expression, and Identity Protection.

MINDFULNESS

In order to support youth's ability to identify when Identity Stress is a relevant stressor to cope with, a key 1st step is developing an understanding of the self-narrative they have constructed about themselves and, in particular, how this narrative is influenced by their ethnic-racial background. Specifically, socializing agents can help youth use their mindfulness skills to become curious about their thoughts, feelings, and behavioral responses to moments when their ethnic-racial background becomes a more salient aspect of their identity. Moreover, the Multidimensional Model of Racial Identity (or MMRI; Sellers et al., 1998) proposes that racial identity becomes most influential to one's daily experiences when someone is in a context where their ethnicity/race is perceived as a more visible or salient quality of themselves.

Practically, GMY can be supported in mindfully considering when and where they are most conscious of their ethnic-racial identity (also referred to as Salience—Sellers et al., 1998). For example, GMY may find that there are moments within their school day or while they are navigating certain communities when they feel more or less aware of their ethnicity/race—possibly when noticing a particular race-related comment by a teacher or peer, when content related to race is covered within their curriculum, or broadly when any similarities or differences between themselves and their peers are accentuated. And, after developing an awareness of the situational contexts where their identity feels most salient, socializing agents can help youth monitor their cognitive, emotional, and behavioral responses within these contexts. Regarding cognitive-emotional responses, youth may benefit from noticing whether they experience the salience of their ethnic-racial identities as a positive experience—either because such salience engenders a sense of pride and appreciation (positive private regard) or because they anticipate the people around them will have positive judgments about the parts of their ethnic-racial identity (positive public regard—Sellers et al., 1998). Alternatively, such salience may be experienced as stressful, uncomfortable, and possibly unwanted if youth perceive such situations as shedding light on an aspect of themselves that they feel a sense of dislike or discomfort toward (negative private regard) or that they perceive others to hold negative judgments or attitudes about (negative public regard—Sellers et al., 1998). And, regarding their behavioral responses, socializing agents can help youth explore how the combination of these cognitive-emotional experiences influence their actions (particularly their self-expression) within the salient moments. Importantly, the development of such mindful awareness can help youth (and their supporting socializing agents) clarify the nature of their Identity Stress (e.g., are they struggling to develop positive private regard or having difficulty existing in spaces where they perceive negative public regard) and begin to understand how youth are trying to navigate the experience of Identity Stress (e.g., are cognitive and behavioral responses to their Identity Stress aligning with their goals or values).

IDENTITY EXPLORATION

For GMY who are able to at least acknowledge an interest in discovering the personal significance of their race and ethnicity, socializing agents can support them with generating Empowered Decisions for Identity Exploration or intentional efforts to obtain information that would enhance their understanding of their ethnic-racial identity. Importantly, Identity Exploration can be conceived as both a proactive and reactive process. The concept of "salience" implies the conscious relevance of one's ethnic-racial identity only occurs in response to a prompting event or situation. And, when racism-related events are the prompting events, Identity Exploration, in this context, would occur while youth are contending with the uncomfortable cognitive-emotional responses to the event. Additionally, it is important for socializing agents to also help students proactively identify exploration opportunities that permit exposure to positive and affirming messages about one's ethnic-racial background.

Practically, Identity Exploration can be pursued in three ways: *reflection, research, and activity scheduling* (as shown in Table 6.6). *Reflection* activities describe any effort students make to pause and reflect on the personal significance of particular relationships (e.g., living and deceased family), role models (e.g., lauded community and spiritual leaders), and community impacts (e.g., community strengths and stresses) that have a connection to their ethnic-racial background. Moreover, GMY can reflect on how these influences have impacted their distant (e.g., "I want to be a doctor because I want to honor the sacrifices of my family") and immediate goals (e.g., "I am working hard to be kind within my friendships because 'sacrificial love' is a big thing in my faith community"), their values (e.g., "It is important for me to serve my community because of how my family has always served the community"), and their personal strengths (e.g., "I am a good storyteller because all my family seems to do is sit around and tell stories"). Such reflection can be prompted via informal Socratic questions about how GMY think about certain cultural representations of their ethnic-racial background and via formal, structured exercises (e.g., "The Tree of Life" exercise—Denborough, 2018). Socializing agents can also utilize the assessment prompts in Tables 6.2 and 6.3 for the purpose of supporting youth with engaging in such self-reflection.

Upon being prompted to engage in self-reflection about their ethnic-racial backgrounds, youth may realize gaps in their understanding (e.g., "I don't really know where my grandparents are from" or "I really don't know why my family cares so much about this particular tradition"), which in turn may interfere with their internal resolution about how a specific aspect of their ethnic-racial background fits into their overall self-concept. Moreover, youth may also disclose uncertainty about how they want to express or represent aspects of their background (e.g., "I don't know if I really want to wear my natural hair" or "I don't really know if I am all that religious"). Finally, some youth may find it difficult to derive meaning and clarity from only engaging in these self-reflection activities. In these cases, GMY may benefit from a more hands-on self-exploration process that includes more active information gathering or possibly experimentation with certain forms of Identity Expression before obtaining a clearer sense of what their race or ethnicity means to them.

Practically, the *research and activity scheduling* components of Identity Exploration can include the following: consuming some form of identity-affirming media (e.g., books, movies, poetry), interviewing family members about genealogy and family history, participating in cultural traditions, or attending cultural events. It is important that youth are prompted to thoughtfully engage in these activities as an opportunity for greater self-reflection and discovery. Again, youth can be encouraged to consider how their experiences with identity-related research and activity engagement are shaping their ethnic-racial knowledge and their understanding of their personal goals, values, and strengths. Of note, socializing agents should inquire about similarities and differences in the acculturative experiences of the family that are involved in such research and activity scheduling (e.g., do they have similar values or beliefs as GMY, or do they have a similar ethnic-racial identity as the GMY), as some GMY (particularly those who are 1st- or 2nd-generation residents of the United States) may receive socializing messages that conflict with their daily experiences, values, and worldviews. In such instances, GMY may benefit from using the Venn Diagram exercise within Table 6.2 to support their processing of any similarities and conflicting differences. Collectively, this framing of Identity Exploration is intended to provide a means for socializing agents to help GMY consciously, critically, and compassionately examine the personal significance of their ethnic-racial group in ways that promote increase self-acceptance and pride.

IDENTITY EXPRESSION

As GMY discover the most appreciated and meaningful parts of their ethnic-racial identity, it is important to examine how comfortable and confident they are in their expression of their identity. Understandably, Identity Expression is often dependent on the trustworthiness of people youth are surrounded by and the perceived level of physical and emotional safety associated with being one's authentic self. Unfortunately, the negative impacts of RRS show itself as youth negotiate when, where, and how to engage in Identity Expression. Specifically, authentic self-expression can be impeded by experiencing (or even anticipating) judgment or mistreatment for accentuating one's ethnic-racial identity or by embodying internalized negative and critical social messages about their self-expression (e.g., "Wearing my natural hair is unprofessional").

Practically, socializing agents can support youth in clarifying the parts of the ethnic-racial identity that, in an ideal world, they would want to share more openly. Such self-expression can include the types of clothing worn, speaking native languages, publicly eating cultural foods, or even correcting others when they mispronounce a student's name. Next, GMY can be supported in identifying the persons and places where each form of self-expression has the greatest likelihood of being affirmed (or at least being met with the least resistance, judgment, or mistreatment). And, with this information, socializing agents can utilize an exposure-based framework for helping GMY to practice *Expressing and Tolerating Discomfort* (DeLapp & Gallo, 2022), especially for youth whose anxiety and avoidance are significantly interfering with such self-expression (Kline et al., 2021). Also, GMY can be supported in exploring how these forms of Identity Expression might align with personal values and permit achievement of important goals (e.g., Table 6.2 from "Defining Empowerment"), as doing so might enhance motivation for such Identity Expression despite the anticipated emotional discomfort of doing so. Finally, socializing agents can help youth process their learning following decisions to prioritize Identity Expression—specifically examining thoughts about the personal significance of prioritizing self-expression, any feelings of pride and gratitude for such self-expression, any increased distress tolerance for such self-expression, and whether they feel continued self-expression would be beneficial moving forward.

IDENTITY PROTECTION

While Identity Exploration and Expression describe Empowered Decisions that GMY can make to increase their love and appreciation for their ethnic-racial identity, Identity Protection features Empowered Decisions youth can make to guard themselves from negative social messages denigrating the love and appreciation they are trying to cultivate. Such decisions describe intentional efforts that youth make to navigate both their own negative self-judgments along with the disparaging societal messages they are exposed to.

Practically, socializing agents can support youth in using their mindfulness skills, as described earlier, to notice when they are perceiving any negative internal (e.g., "People like me are just not good at these types of things") or external (e.g., "My classmates don't think people like me are good at these types of things") messages that are impactful. To aid GMY's awareness of such messages, it may be helpful to *Characterize the Negative Messages* with a label (e.g., catching phrase) or character (e.g., selecting a pop culture reference as a personification of this message—Banks et al., 2021). And, given the emotionally painful impact that these messages can have, consider exploring the relevance and benefits of the Coping Decisions outlined in Table 6.4 to support GMY in processing and coping with any Emotional Stress triggered by these messages. Finally, in order to help youth protect themselves from these negative messages becoming chronic internalized self-beliefs (e.g., "I tend to think I am not good at things like this"), GMY should be supported in reframing these negative messages in ways that foster greater self-compassion (Williams et al., 2022a, 2022b). To this end, GMY may benefit from creating a list of *Reframing Questions* that prompt them to question how trustworthy the source of the negative message is, to acknowledge counterfactual information that dispels the validity of the negative messages, and to reflect on the self-truths they learned about themselves from the Identity Exploration and Expression (e.g., their goals, values, personal and cultural strengths). Of note, such reframing efforts should not focus on whether students perceived the right or wrong messages from their environment. For example, if GMY express that they feel a specific teacher treats them as if they are not smart, socializing agents should not focus on whether the student's perception of the teacher's actions was justified or not. Rather, the focus should be on how the student's perception has impacted them emotionally and how they can protect themselves from this perceived message becoming an internalized self-belief that interferes with their self-love and self-expression. And, if the GMY were to have questions about how to interact with or confront this teacher about their perception of them, then socializing agents can support students in identifying which Coping Decisions from Table 6.5 would help them address their teacher in a way that aligns with their goals and values. For additional details on how to help GMY cope with internalized negative beliefs, see Banks et al. (2021), Steele (2020), and Williams et al. (2022a, 2022b).

Conclusion

Empowered Decision-Making captures how GMY choose to navigate the stressful demands of their environment according to their values and goals. This chapter describes how socializing agents can offer CR support to GMY by helping them develop such decision-making abilities within educational settings. Specifically, this chapter draws upon the REACH UP model (DeLapp & Gallo, 2022) to provide a framework for helping GMY understand how to use their values and goals to aid Empowered Decision-Making (Definition of Empowerment), examine how RRS interferes with such decision-making (Barriers to Empowered Decision-Making), and make Empowered Decisions that promote their emotion regulation, conflict resolution, and identity development (Strengthening Empowered Decisions-Making). Importantly, the utilization of the REACH UP model necessitates that socializing agents proactively invest time and energy into self-educating and introspective activities that promote their own community consciousness, cultural humility, and overall cultural responsiveness. And, while this chapter primarily focuses on the psychotherapeutic support offered by school mental health professionals to GMY, there remains a broader responsibility for school staff, administrators, and the local, state, and federal government to revise laws and policies that perpetuate the very impacts from racism GMY are trying cope with. Said differently, the onus of resilience and RRS coping should not rest solely on the shoulders of GMY and their families (Jones et al., 2023). However, given that such systemic progress is unlikely to yield immediate and swift change, socializing agents, such as mental health professionals, are encouraged to continue supporting GMY with the complex task of learning to practice Empowered Decision-Making to navigate such environments.

Reflection Questions

1 How can school-based mental health professionals integrate the concepts of ethnic-racial identity and racism-related stress (RRS) into their work with Global Majority Youth (GMY)?
2 What strategies can be employed to enhance a clinician's ability to promote Empowered Decision-Making among GMY facing RRS in educational settings?
3 In what ways can school-based mental health professionals collaborate with educators and other school staff to create a more inclusive and supportive environment for GMY to explore and express their ethnic-racial identities?

Notes

1 Given that language is ever evolving and to remain consistent with current APA recommendations on inclusive language, this chapter will refer to youth who identify with an ethnic or racial identity other than Caucasian or white as Global Majority Youth (GMY) (American Psychological Association [APA], 2023). Such terminology is considered more inclusive relative to previous language that has included terms like BIPOC (Black, Indigenous, People of Color).

2 The term "socializing agent" will be used to refer to school-based mental health professionals throughout the remainder of the chapter. Such terminology seeks to highlight the unique role these professionals have in participating in the ethnic-racialization of GMY.

References

American Psychiatric Association. (2013). *Diagnostic and statistical manual of mental disorders* (5th ed.). American Psychiatric Publishing, Washington, DC.

American Psychological Association (2023). *Inclusive language guidelines* (2nd ed.). https://www.apa.org/about/apa/equity-diversity-inclusion/language-guide.pdf

Anderson, R. E., Heard-Garris, N., & DeLapp, R. C. (2022a). Future directions for vaccinating children against the American endemic: Treating racism as a virus. *Journal of Clinical Child & Adolescent Psychology, 51*(1), 127–142.

Anderson, A. J., Riordan, A., Smith, L., Hillard, B., & Sánchez, B. (2022b). Cultural humility training for mentors: Lessons learned and implications for youth programs. *Journal of Youth Development, 17*(3), 21–38.

Anderson, R. E., & Stevenson, H. C. (2019). RECASTing racial stress and trauma: Theorizing the healing potential of racial socialization in families. *American Psychologist, 74*(1), 63.

Atkins, K., & Lorelle, S. (2022). Cultural humility: Lessons learned through a counseling cultural immersion. *Journal of Counselor Preparation and Supervision, 15*(1), 9.

Banks, K. H., Goswami, S., Goodwin, D., Petty, J., Bell, V., & Musa, I. (2021). Interrupting internalized racial oppression: A community based ACT intervention. *Journal of Contextual Behavioral Science, 20*, 89–93.

Bentley-Edwards, K. L., Stevenson, H. C., Thomas, D. E., Adams-Bass, V. N., & Coleman-King, C. (2020). Teaching scared: Pre-service teacher appraisals of racial stress, socialization and classroom management self-efficacy. *Social Psychology of Education, 23*, 1233–1257.

Danoff-Burg, S., Prelow, H. M., & Swenson, R. R. (2004). Hope and life satisfaction in Black college students coping with race-related stress. *Journal of Black Psychology, 30*(2), 208–228.

DeLapp, C. L., & DeLapp, R. C. T. (2021). Talking racial stress: Clinician recommendations for exploring racial stress with BIPOC patients. *The Behavior Therapist, 44*(2), 75–79.

DeLapp, R. C., & Gallo, L. (2022). A flexible treatment planning model for racism-related stress in adolescents and young adults. *Journal of Health Service Psychology, 48*(4), 161–173.

DeLapp, R. C. T., & Williams, M. T. (2019). Preparing for racial discrimination and moving beyond reactive coping: A systematic review. *Current Psychiatry Research and Reviews Formerly: Current Psychiatry Reviews, 15*(1), 58–71.

DeLapp, R. C. T., & Williams, M. T. (2021). Preparing for racial microaggressions: The role of cognition and emotion in the proactive coping process of African American college students. *New Ideas in Psychology, 63*, 100897.

Denborough, D. (2018). *Do you want to hear a story?: Adventures in collective narrative practice*. Adelaide: Dulwich Centre Publications.

Devine, P. G., Forscher, P. S., Austin, A. J., & Cox, W. T. (2012). Long-term reduction in implicit race bias: A prejudice habit-breaking intervention. *Journal of Experimental Social Psychology, 48*(6), 1267–1278.

Ehrenreich, J. T., Goldstein, C. R., Wright, L. R., & Barlow, D. H. (2009). Development of a unified protocol for the treatment of emotional disorders in youth. *Child & Family Behavior Therapy, 31*(1), 20–37.

Fisher, E. S. (2020). Cultural humility as a form of social justice: Promising practices for global school psychology training. *School Psychology International, 41*(1), 53–66.

Germer, C., & Neff, K. (2019). *Teaching the mindful self-compassion program: A guide for professionals*. New York: Guilford Publications.

Gibson, S. M., Bouldin, B. M., Stokes, M. N., Lozada, F. T., & Hope, E. C. (2022). Cultural racism and depression in Black adolescents: Examining racial socialization and racial identity as moderators. *Journal of Research on Adolescence, 32*(1), 41–48.

Goodrum, N. M., Cooper, D. K., Edmunds, S., Wippold, G. M., Bradshaw, J., Nguyen, J. K., Milburn, N. & Are, F. (2023). Achieving equity in child and adolescent mental health by addressing racism through prevention science. *Adversity and Resilience Science, 5*(1), 1–10.

Greenwald, A. G., McGhee, D. E., & Schwartz, J. L. (1998). Measuring individual differences in implicit cognition: The implicit association test. *Journal of Personality and Social Psychology, 74*(6), 1464.

Hayes, S. C., Strosahl, K. D., & Wilson, K. G. (2011). *Acceptance and commitment therapy: The process and practice of mindful change*. New York: Guilford press.

Hays, P. A. (1996). Addressing the complexities of culture and gender in counseling. *Journal of Counseling & Development, 74*(4), 332–338.
Hays, P. A. (2008). *Addressing cultural complexities in practice* (2nd ed.). Washington, DC: American Psychological Association.
Heard-Garris, N., Ekwueme, P. O., Gilpin, S., Sacotte, K. A., Perez-Cardona, L., Wong, M., & Cohen, A. (2021). Adolescents' experiences, emotions, and coping strategies associated with exposure to media-based vicarious racism. *JAMA network Open, 4*(6), e2113522–e2113522.
Hope, E. C., Brinkman, M., Hoggard, L. S., Stokes, M. N., Hatton, V., Volpe, V. V., & Elliot, E. (2021). Black adolescents' anticipatory stress responses to multilevel racism: The role of racial identity. *American Journal of Orthopsychiatry, 91*(4), 487–498.
Hughes, D. L., Watford, J. A., & Del Toro, J. (2016). A transactional/ecological perspective on ethnic-racial identity, socialization, and discrimination. *Advances in Child Development and Behavior, 51*, 1–41. https://doi.org/10.1016/bs.acdb.2016.05.001
Jacob, G., Faber, S. C., Faber, N., Bartlett, A., Ouimet, A. J., & Williams, M. T. (2023). A systematic review of Black People coping with racism: Approaches, analysis, and empowerment. *Perspectives on Psychological Science, 18*(2), 392–415.
Johnson, M. M., & Melton, M. L. (2020). *Addressing race-based stress in therapy with black clients: Using multicultural and dialectical behavior therapy techniques.* New York: Routledge.
Jones, S. C., Anderson, R. E., Gaskin-Wasson, A. L., Sawyer, B. A., Applewhite, K., & Metzger, I. W. (2020). From "crib to coffin": Navigating coping from racism-related stress throughout the lifespan of Black Americans. *American Journal of Orthopsychiatry, 90*(2), 267.
Jones, S. C., Simon, C. B., Yadeta, K., Patterson, A., & Anderson, R. E. (2023). When resistance is not enough: Imagining novel approaches to supporting Black youth navigating racism. *Development and Psychopathology, 35*(5), 2132–2140.
Kline, E. A., Warner, C. M., Grapin, S. L., Reyes-Portillo, J. A., Bixter, M. T., Cunningham, D. J., Mahmud, F., Singh, T., & Weeks, C. (2021). The relationship between social anxiety and internalized racism in Black young adults. *Journal of Cognitive Psychotherapy, 35*(1), 53–63.
Malone, C. M., Wycoff, K., & Turner, E. A. (2020). Applying a MTSS framework to address racism and promote mental health for racial/ethnic minoritized youth. *Psychology in the Schools, 59*(12), 2438–2452.
Metzger, I. W., Anderson, R. E., Are, F., & Ritchwood, T. (2021). Healing interpersonal and racial trauma: Integrating racial socialization into trauma-focused cognitive behavioral therapy for African American youth. *Child Maltreatment, 26*(1), 17–27.
Naz, S., Gregory, R., & Bahu, M. (2019). Addressing issues of race, ethnicity and culture in CBT to support therapists and service managers to deliver culturally competent therapy and reduce inequalities in mental health provision for BAME service users. *The Cognitive Behaviour Therapist, 12*, E22.
Neblett Jr, E. W., Rivas-Drake, D., & Umaña-Taylor, A. J. (2012). The promise of racial and ethnic protective factors in promoting ethnic minority youth development. *Child Development Perspectives, 6*(3), 295–303.
Neff, K. D. (2023). Self-compassion: Theory, method, research, and intervention. *Annual Review of Psychology, 74*, 193–218.
Pachter, L. M., Szalacha, L. A., Bernstein, B. A., & Coll, C. G. (2010). Perceptions of Racism in Children and Youth (PRaCY): Properties of a self-report instrument for research on children's health and development. *Ethnicity & Health, 15*(1), 33–46.
Rathus, J. H., & Miller, A. L. (2014). *DBT skills manual for adolescents*. New York: Guilford Publications.
Rollins, V. B., & Valdez, J. N. (2006). Perceived racism and career self-efficacy in African American adolescents. *Journal of Black Psychology, 32*(2), 176–198.
Saleem, F. T., Anderson, R. E., & Williams, M. (2020). Addressing the "myth" of racial trauma: Developmental and ecological considerations for youth of color. *Clinical Child and Family Psychology Review, 23*(1), 1–14.
Saleem, F. T., & Byrd, C. M. (2021). Unpacking school ethnic-racial socialization: A new conceptual model. *Journal of Social Issues, 77*(4), 1106–1125.
Sellers, R. M., Smith, M. A., Shelton, J. N., Rowley, S. A., & Chavous, T. M. (1998). Multidimensional model of racial identity: A reconceptualization of African American racial identity. *Personality and Social Psychology Review, 2*(1), 18–39.
Siber-Sanderowitz, S., Glasgow, A., Chouake, T., Beckford, E., Nim, A., & Ozdoba, A. (2022). Developing a structural intervention for outpatient mental health care: Mapping vulnerability and privilege. *American Journal of Psychotherapy, 75*(3), 134–140.
Steele, J. M. (2020). A CBT approach to internalized racism among African Americans. *International Journal for the Advancement of Counselling, 42*(3), 217–233.

Stern, J. A., Barbarin, O., & Cassidy, J. (2022). Working toward anti-racist perspectives in attachment theory, research, and practice. *Attachment & Human Development, 24*(3), 392–422.

Thompson, M., & Wildavsky, A. (2008). A cultural theory of information bias in organizations. In P. Six & G. Mars (Eds.), *The institutional dynamics of culture*, Volumes I and II (pp. 704–717). London, UK: Routledge.

Watson-Singleton, N. N., Womack, V. Y., Holder-Dixon, A. R., & Black, A. R. (2021). Racism's (un) worthiness trap: The mediating roles of self-compassion and self-coldness in the link between racism and distress in African Americans. *Cultural Diversity and Ethnic Minority Psychology. 28*(4), 557–568.

Williams, M. T., Faber, S. C., & Duniya, C. (2022a). Being an anti-racist clinician. *The Cognitive Behaviour Therapist, 15*, e19.

Williams, M. T., Holmes, S., Zare, M., Haeny, A., & Faber, S. (2022b). An evidence-based approach for treating stress and trauma due to racism. *Cognitive and Behavioral Practice, 30*(4), 565–588.

Wilson, T. K., & Gentzler, A. L. (2021). Emotion regulation and coping with racial stressors among African Americans across the lifespan. *Developmental Review, 61*, 100967.

Xie, M., Fowle, J., Ip, P. S., Haskin, M., & Yip, T. (2021). Profiles of ethnic-racial identity, socialization, and model minority experiences: Associations with well-being among Asian American adolescents. *Journal of Youth and Adolescence, 50*, 1173–1188.

Zhang, H., Watkins Jr, C. E., Hook, J. N., Hodge, A. S., Davis, C. W., Norton, J., Wilcox, M. M., Davis, D. E., DeBlaere, C., & Owen, J. (2022). Cultural humility in psychotherapy and clinical supervision: A research review. *Counselling and Psychotherapy Research, 22*(3), 548–557.

7

AFFIRMATIVE CBT FOR LGBTQ+ STUDENTS

Emily S. Fisher, Barbara Katic and Dawn M. Richards

Introduction and Overview

We live in a society in which the basic human rights of lesbian, gay, bisexual, transgender, and questioning (LGBTQ+) individuals are the subject of debate, media sound bites, ever-changing legislation, and religious and political persecution. Given this larger sociopolitical context, it is not surprising that LGBTQ+ students experience high rates of discrimination, rejection, and oppression, often leading to poorer mental health, academic, and behavioral outcomes than their heterosexual and cisgender peers (Kosciw et al., 2022; The Trevor Project, 2022). Certainly, many LGBTQ+ students have the necessary social support and coping skills to demonstrate resilience in the face of systemic and interpersonal discrimination, but others may need targeted counseling interventions to support healthy development and coping. This chapter highlights the lived experiences of LGBTQ+ students and, through a cognitive-behavioral therapy (CBT) lens, offers clinicians strategies to affirm LGBTQ+ students' identities, help them manage the negative impact of discrimination and oppression, and promote positive development, mental health, and well-being.

For this chapter, the acronym LGBTQ+ is meant to be respectful and inclusive of the wide-range of minoritized sexual orientations and gender identities, recognizing that terminology often is limited and fails to keep pace with our ever-developing understanding of the individual nuances of sexuality and gender identity. It is recommended that clinicians stay abreast of terminology related to their student populations, such as can be found from the Human Rights Campaign (https://www.hrc.org/resources/glossary-of-terms) or the It Gets Better Project (https://itgetsbetter.org/glossary/), always allowing students to name their own experiences of their sexuality and gender identity.

Lived Experiences and Mental Health Outcomes

Two large-scale studies conducted in the United States (U.S.) help us understand the lived experiences of LGBTQ+ youth. The 1st, conducted by The Trevor Project (2022), surveyed almost 34,000 LGBTQ young people aged 13–24. Almost half of the sample identified as youth of color, and almost half identified as transgender or gender nonbinary. Overall, researchers found that 73% of LGBTQ youth reported symptoms of anxiety, 58% reported symptoms of depression, 45% reported seriously considering suicide in the past year, and 14% reported attempting suicide in the past year. These statistics were generally higher for school-aged LGBTQ youth. Researchers couched these findings

DOI: 10.4324/9781003392439-9

within youth's lived experiences, highlighting the negative impact of anti-LGBTQ victimization, discrimination, and political attacks on youth's overall mental health and well-being.

The 2nd study, conducted by GLSEN (Kosciw et al., 2022), surveyed over 22,000 students aged 13–21 about their school experiences, with approximately 29% of the sample identifying as gay or lesbian, 30% identifying as bisexual, 31% identifying as nonbinary, and 33% identifying as students of color. Overall, researchers found that almost all LGBTQ+ students heard "gay" being used in a derogatory manner at school, along with high numbers hearing other anti-LGBTQ remarks. Over 76% of LGBTQ+ students reported experiencing verbal harassment at school due to their sexual orientation, gender identity, and/or gender expression; 31% experienced physical harassment, and 12% were physically assaulted, leading the majority of LGBTQ+ students (68%) to feel unsafe at school. Experiences of victimization were associated with more days of missed school, higher rates of school discipline, poorer academic performance, lower self-esteem, and higher rates of depression.

Research conducted outside the U.S. highlights similar experiences for LGBTQ+ students. For example, Peter et al. (2021) conducted a school climate survey across Canada, finding high rates of discrimination, harassment, and bullying and corresponding mental health challenges and feelings of unsafety at school. Wei and Liu (2019) examined the experiences of LGBTQ students across Mainland China, finding schools were not inclusive, and LGBTQ students reported high rates of depression and suicidality. Fernandes and colleagues (2022) examined the experiences of LGBTQ students in Portugal, highlighting high levels of anti-LGBTQ bullying and victimization at school.

Across the research, certain groups of LGBTQ+ students experience even higher rates of victimization and the associated negative outcomes, highlighting the extreme vulnerability of this group of young people and the need for intervention. Overall, transgender and gender non-conforming students experience the most hostile school climates (Kosciw et al., 2022) and the highest rates of anxiety, depression, and suicidality (The Trevor Project, 2022). Similarly, pansexual students and questioning students, as compared to students of other sexual orientations, report higher rates of victimization (Kosciw et al., 2022) and mental health challenges (The Trevor Project, 2022). LGBTQ+ students who also identify with a racially/ethnically minoritized group, except for those who identify as Asian American/Pacific Islander, report greater depression and suicidality than their White peers, with Indigenous/Native students experiencing the highest rates of victimization at school and reporting the highest rates of suicidality (Kosciw et al., 2022; Peter et al., 2021; The Trevor Project, 2022).

Yet, schools can also serve as places of acceptance, inclusion, and protection for LGBTQ+ students. Specifically, Kosciw et al. (2022) found that LGBTQ+ students who attended schools with inclusive school policies, a gender-sexuality alliance or similar club, supportive educators, and LGBTQ-inclusive curriculum experienced lower levels of discrimination and harassment, felt safer, and had better psychological well-being. Similarly, Hatchel et al. (2019) found that feelings of school connectedness were associated with lower suicidality among LGBTQ youth, and Fields and Wotipka (2022) found that "sexual minority students in states with more extensive LGBT anti-discrimination policy report more safety in schools and better academic outcomes" (p. 320).

Families also play a critical role in the experiences of LGBTQ+ young people. The Trevor Project (2022) found that 37% of LGBTQ+ young people identified their home as an affirming space; similarly, McConnell et al. (2015) found that about 40% of LGBT youth surveyed reported high levels of family support. Not surprisingly, affirming and supportive families were associated with more positive mental health outcomes, while low family support and rejection were associated with poorer mental health outcomes (McConnell et al., 2015; Ryan et al., 2010; The Trevor Project, 2022). Family support is also related to housing stability and homelessness. In a research brief focused on LGBTQ youth homelessness, Morton et al. (2018) reported that LGBTQ youth were twice as likely to experience homelessness than their non-LGBTQ peers, with these rates even higher for Black and multiracial LGBTQ youth. LGBTQ youth described the pathway to homelessness as "a gradual escalation of the parent-child conflict over time, or a growing sense of rejection in the home, rather than an immediate reaction to the disclosure" (Morton et al., 2018, p. 11). Further, preexisting family stress, such as poverty, housing troubles, and mental health problems, were associated with eventual homelessness among many LGBTQ youth (Morton et al., 2018).

Research clearly demonstrates that LGBTQ+ students' mental health and well-being are impacted by their experiences of discrimination and oppression (e.g., Kosciw et al., 2022; The Trevor Project, 2022), indicating a clear need for identity-affirming counseling services. Further, the majority of LGBTQ+ youth (82%) expressed a desire for mental health care, but most (60%) were unable to access this support (The Trevor Project, 2022). Barriers identified by those wanting counseling included fear of non-affirming care (e.g., being outed, not being taken seriously, or having identity misunderstood) and concerns with parental permission needed for counseling. Clinicians working in schools have a unique opportunity to reduce barriers to counseling services for LGBTQ+ students by providing affirmative counseling within the school context.

Empirical Support of CBT with LGBTQ+ Youth

The field of psychology is committed to the integration of science and practice, and clinicians are tasked with selecting and implementing interventions that have demonstrated effectiveness for the populations they serve (American Psychological Association [APA], 2006). Given this emphasis, the development and evaluation of CBT-based intervention and programming continues to grow, and empirical support for affirmative CBT tailored toward LGBTQ+ individuals has expanded in the last two decades. Current studies evaluate CBT-based interventions ranging from manualized programs, which are implemented in-person, to computerized programming which students themselves complete.

As the research on affirmative CBT for the LGBTQ+ community progresses, it is critical for clinicians to be aware of not only interventions that have demonstrated effectiveness but also those that have the potential to cause harm. "Conversion" or "reparative" interventions, which are designed to change one's sexual orientation or gender identity, are associated with harmful client outcomes (e.g., depression and suicide attempts) and have been discredited by the APA (APA 2009; Ryan et al., 2020). However, these practices continue to be practiced by clinicians and religious leaders across the globe, including the U.S. (APA, 2009). Regardless of one's theoretical orientation, it is imperative for clinicians to be able to discern interventions that demonstrate effectiveness/promote positive outcomes for LGBTQ+ clients from those that cause harm (i.e., conversion, reparative therapy). While not an exhaustive list, the following section presents highlights of the current empirical support of affirmative CBT interventions tailored toward LGBTQ+ individuals.

AFFIRM

AFFIRM is an eight-module cognitive-behavioral coping skills intervention developed for youth with sexual and/or gender minority identities (Austin et al., 2018; Craig & Austin, 2016). Preliminary pilot data indicates the potential effectiveness of AFFIRM in promoting positive mental health outcomes among LGBTQ+ youth. In a study by Craig and Austin (2016), the AFFIRM program was provided to a diverse sample of sexual and gender minority youth (n = 30). The study implemented a one-group pre-post design and assessed the effectiveness of AFFIRM on participant levels of depression, reflective coping, and stress appraisals across three time points (pre-intervention, post-intervention, and follow-up). Depressive symptoms were measured using the Beck Depression Inventory (BDI-II), reflective coping was measured using the Reflective Coping Subscale (RCS), and stress appraisal was measured through the Stress Appraisal Measure for Adolescents (SAMA). Results indicated significant reductions in depression and stress appraisal across time. Moreover, there were significant increases in reflective coping across time.

Similarly, another pilot study by Austin and colleagues (2018) evaluated the effectiveness and acceptability of AFFIRM to a small subsample ($n = 8$) of transgender youth between the ages of 16 and 18. To assess the impact of AFFIRM on participants, data were collected on (a) depressive symptoms, measured using the BDI-II; (b) reflective coping skills, measured using the RCS; and (c) participant satisfaction, measured through a 17-item self-report questionnaire. Paired sample t-tests were conducted to assess change across depression and coping skills during pre-intervention, post-intervention, and at a three-month follow-up. Results indicate that while there were significant reductions in depression scores, there were no significant improvements in coping skills. In terms of program satisfaction, participants responded to the program positively.

Proud & Empowered

Another program available for supporting LGBTQ+ students in school settings is Proud & Empowered (Goldbach et al., 2023). Proud & Empowered is a ten-session school-based program developed to support sexual and gender minority adolescents in coping with minority stress experiences using psychoeducation, didactic discussion, and opportunities for interactive activities (Goldbach et al., 2021). The program is guided by a facilitator manual, includes facilitator training, and addresses fidelity monitoring (Goldbach et al., 2021). Although in its early stages of evaluation, both the development process and preliminary results demonstrate program potential. To illustrate, the development of Proud & Empowered is aligned with the NIH Intervention Stage Model for Behavioral Intervention Development (Goldbach et al., 2021), which provides guidance on best practices for developing, implementing, and evaluating effective behavioral interventions to be delivered in real-world settings, including schools (Onken et al., 2014).

One randomized controlled trial has been conducted to evaluate the effectiveness of Proud & Empowered (Goldbach et al., 2021). The study included 44 student participants (across four high schools), with 26 randomly assigned to the intervention group and 18 to the control group (Goldbach et al., 2021). Measures included demographic characteristics, hypothesized mechanisms of change (e.g., minority stress), and mental health symptoms (including anxiety, depression, PTSD, and suicidality). Through moderation analysis, findings demonstrated that Proud & Empowered was significant in moderating the relationship between minority stress and PTSD ($b = -1.28$, $p = .032$), depression ($b = -0.79$, $p = .023$), and suicidality ($b = 0.14$, $p = .012$) symptoms. Compared to the control group, students who received the intervention reported lower rates of minority stress and victimization experiences and decreased mental health symptoms. Moreover, students in the intervention group were less likely to report PTSD, depression, and suicidality even when they did experience minority stressors. Overall, Proud & Empowered holds promising results for LGBTQ+ students through the reduction of mental health symptoms (associated with minority stress experiences) and the improvement of coping skills.

ASSET: Affirmative Supportive Safe and Empowering Talk

Affirmative Supportive Safe and Empowering Talk (ASSET) is an affirmative cognitive-behavioral group intervention geared toward LGBTQ+ students in the school setting (Craig, 2013). In a one-group pretest-posttest pilot study by Craig and colleagues (2014), ASSET was provided to 15 urban high schools. Each school received approximately eight to ten sessions with groups of 6–12 students. Measures of proactive coping, self-esteem, social connectedness, and program acceptability were assessed. Results indicated statistically significant increases in self-esteem and proactive coping from baseline to posttest. However, there were no significant differences in social connectedness. Responses to program acceptability surveys indicated that participants found the treatment to be helpful and satisfactory (Craig et al., 2014).

Digital Health Interventions

Amid the ongoing advancement of technology, programs that were initially developed to be delivered in-person, such as AFFIRM, are now being implemented online (Craig et al., 2021). Moreover, digital health interventions have been developed and adapted for LGBTQ+ youth. One such program, Rainbow SPARX, is a seven-session computerized program based on cognitive-behavior therapy principles. Adapted from SPARX, a computerized program developed to support adolescents with depression, Rainbow SPARX has been specifically adapted for sexual minority youth (Lucassen et al., 2015). Lucassen and colleagues (2015) implemented a pilot study to evaluate the effectiveness of Rainbow SPARX. The participants receiving the program ($n = 21$) identified as sexual minority youth, were between the ages of 13 and 19 years, and had significant depressive symptoms. Depressive symptomatology was assessed at pre-intervention, post-intervention, and follow-up using the Depression Rating Scale-Revised (CDRS-R). Preliminary data demonstrated that depressive symptoms decreased significantly from pre- to post-intervention, and the positive change was maintained at follow-up.

ESTEEM: Effective Skills to Empower Effective Men

Evidence-based programming is available to support students' transition to young adulthood. The Effective Skills to Empower Effective Men (ESTEEM) program has been linked to positive outcomes for LGBTQ+ individuals, particularly for gay and bisexual men aged 18–35 who have experienced mental health and behavioral concerns (Pachankis et al., 2015, 2022). ESTEEM is a ten-session, individually delivered CBT-based intervention which aims to reduce mental health concerns of participants through the improvement of emotional regulation skills and subsequent facilitation of behavior change (Keefe et al., 2023). The ESTEEM program has been adapted from the Unified Protocol for the Transdiagnostic Treatment of Emotional Disorders (Barlow et al., 2010) and has been tailored to address maladaptive behavior patterns (e.g., depression, anxiety, and substance use) related to minority stress (Burton et al., 2019).

ESTEEM is one of the first LGBQ-affirmative CBT programs to have been tested in a randomized controlled trial (Keefe et al., 2023). Pachankis and colleagues (2015) tested the efficacy of the ESTEEM program for improving depression and co-occurring health risks among young gay and bisexual men. When compared to the waitlist condition, the participants who received the ESTEEM program demonstrated significantly lower levels of depressive symptoms and health risks, including reductions in alcohol-use problems and sexual compulsivity. Further, those who received the ESTEEM program demonstrated moderate to marginally significant improvements in anxiety symptoms.

Keefe and colleagues (2023) set out to identify potential treatment moderators of the ESTEEM program's efficacy. Participants included over 250 gay and bisexual men with mental health and behavioral concerns who were randomized into the ESTEEM program or the control group. The control group consisted of two conditions: (a) LGBQ-affirmative community treatment and (b) HIV testing and counseling. A comorbidity index was developed and measured outcomes pertaining to depression, anxiety, alcohol/drug problems, and HIV risk behaviors. Each outcome was measured at 4-month, 8-month, and 12-month follow-up. Results indicated that at the eight-month follow-up, participants receiving the ESTEEM program had lower comorbidity index scores when compared to the control group. Moreover, when participants identified as a racial and/or ethnic minority, the effects of the ESTEEM program were greater. For example, Black/African American participants who received ESTEEM had significantly greater improvements when compared to the control condition.

Future Directions

In order to implement evidence-based practices, clinicians must be updated on the current literature on providing mental health services for LGBTQ+ individuals, and the research surrounding affirmative CBT for LGBTQ+ students indicates that, while there are several one-group pilot studies, there is a need for larger scale research, particularly for studies including comparison/control conditions. To illustrate, the results of a systematic review by O'Shaughnessy and Speir (2018), who evaluated 49 empirical studies (published between 2000 and 2015) on affirmative therapy available to LGBQ individuals, found that, although there were limited, large-scale studies (e.g., randomized controlled trials), LGBTQ+-affirmative therapy presents promising outcomes and warrants further research.

Relational Considerations for Affirmative CBT

The clinician is at the heart of what makes CBT, or any counseling, affirmative for LGBTQ+ students. To be affirmative, clinicians recognize LGBTQ+ identities as a natural aspect of diversity, respect the value and dignity of LGBTQ+ individuals, and support LGBTQ+ human rights. Moradi and Budge (2018) suggest that affirmative clinicians embrace LGBTQ+-affirming attitudes, recognize the ubiquitous nature and impact of their own and others' heteronormativity and cisgendernormativity, gain knowledge about LGBTQ+ lived experiences, and integrate these into counseling interventions. One important aspect of affirmative counseling is for clinicians to recognize that LGBTQ+ students are greatly impacted by environmental factors, such as discrimination and oppression, which are strongly correlated with mental health challenges (de Lange et al., 2022; Dürrbaum & Sattler, 2020). Another important consideration is recognizing when a student's presenting problem is related to, is exacerbated by, or is not related to the student's sexual orientation or gender identity (Israel et al., 2008). In a study of therapy experiences, Israel and colleagues (2008) found that clinicians who were rated as "affirming, validating, and knowledgeable regarding sexual orientation" (p. 301) were found to be more helpful for LGBTQ+ clients, while clinicians who "focused inappropriately on sexual orientation or tried to persuade LGBT clients to change or hide their sexual orientation or gender identity" (p. 301) were unhelpful to clients.

Confidentiality is a major relational consideration in counseling LGBTQ+ students, as this is the foundation of a trusting therapeutic alliance. As reviewed by Fisher and Kennedy (2016), clinicians must take every measure possible within the bounds of the law to protect a student's confidentiality related to their sexual orientation or gender identity. This includes ensuring notes and records are secure, information about the student's LGBTQ+ identity is not included in the student's school file, and in discussions with parents, who may hold privilege, clinicians protect the student's privacy. As the foundation of trust, clinicians should "emphasize reasonable expectations of privacy in the clinical relationship with sexual and gender minority youth—not to express shame, but to permit the exploration of sexual identity free from fear and with a sense of control over disclosure" (Adelson & The American Academy of Child and Adolescent Psychiatry Committee on Quality Issues, 2012, p. 965). Relatedly, laws about the age of consent for the type of counseling sought differ by state and type of clinician, and clinicians must be informed about these specific legal mandates for their profession in their state. When seeking parental consent, clinicians must ensure they do not disclose the student's LGBTQ+ identity if the student is not out at home, instead focusing on the issue of concern.

For example, the clinician may seek consent by saying, "Jason came to talk with me about some peer issues that have been bothering him, and, with your permission, I'd like to talk with him more so we can develop some strategies to manage these issues." Or, "Sam's teachers have noticed that she has been more disengaged lately. I'm wondering what you're noticing at home and if it might be helpful for me to talk with Sam about what's going on." Students need to be made aware of the legal requirements and may have ideas about how to best obtain consent from parents.

Self-disclosure is not a typical part of CBT, yet there may be times that clinician self-disclosure benefits the student and enhances the therapeutic relationship. Two examples are provided here for consideration. First, although clinicians do not need to identify as LGBTQ+ to work effectively with LGBTQ+ clients (Israel et al., 2008), there may be times when it is beneficial for the clinician to disclose their own sexual orientation or gender identity to enhance the counseling relationship. An example of this might be in working with an LGBTQ+ student who does not have any real-life adult role models. In this scenario, the clinician must ensure that the focus of counseling stays on the student and the student's experience. Second, there may be situations in which the clinician discloses their affirmative beliefs about sexual orientation and gender identity. For example, a clinician is working with a 7th-grade girl who identifies as bisexual. The student's parents discovered her sexual identity by reading her text messages, and, being a very religious family, were not accepting. Through open questions, the clinician helped the student explore her own beliefs about the nature of sexual orientation in general and her sexual orientation in particular, with the student sharing that she believed she was normal and that being bisexual was not wrong or a sin. After a pause in the conversation, the clinician said, "I share your beliefs that being LGBTQ+ is natural and normal." The clinician decided to self-disclose to ensure the student knew she was safe and fully accepted when talking about her sexuality in counseling.

Interviewing and Assessing LGBTQ+ Students

The intake and assessment phase of counseling sets the stage for communicating that the counseling office is a safe space and the clinician is a supportive, affirmative ally. In order to create a safe and approachable therapeutic environment for LGBTQ+ students, clinicians should reassure students of confidentiality, review limits to confidentiality, maintain a nonjudgmental attitude, be sensitive to the experience of LGBTQ+ clients, and demonstrate transgender awareness (Holman & Goldberg, 2006). Attention to the therapeutic environment is also important in creating a physically safe space. Clinicians may consider having magazines or articles related to LGBTQ+ identity, LGBTQ+-affirmative posters, and inclusion statements, making it clear that LGBTQ+ students are welcome and supported in the therapeutic space (Holman & Goldberg, 2006).

During the intake process for all students, clinicians need to include questions about sexual orientation and gender identity, as many students may not be out or may not know how to articulate their experiences. It is well documented that students who belong to the LGBTQ+ community may have had difficulty in the past accessing high-quality mental health support (Oh et al., 2019); therefore, it is important to create an affirmative therapeutic environment for all students. Holman and Goldberg (2006) suggest adding a brief question about gender into the intake process with all students, not just with those students who appear to be LGBTQ+ as this creates space for students to disclose their identity. It is also recommended that clinicians use affirmation throughout the initial interview by using gender-neutral language (i.e., partner instead of boyfriend or girlfriend), using the student's own language in defining their sexuality and gender identity, being nonjudgmental, and normalizing the student's feelings (Holman & Goldberg, 2006).

Table 7.1 represents intake categories and sample questions drawing on the works of Oh and colleagues (2019), who outline the process of conducting multiculturally competent intakes with

Table 7.1 Intake Categories and Sample Questions

Category	*Purpose*	*Sample Questions*
Individual identity and lived experiences	To understand the student's intersectional identity and lived experiences, clinicians can ask questions about the student's age, race/ethnicity, language, sexual orientation, gender identity, disability, cultural identities, etc.	• Which identities are most important to you? • How do your different identities affect your perception of yourself? • Have you experienced any personal challenges or difficulties because of your identities? • Do you have questions about your sexuality and/or gender identity? • Do you ever worry that others will find out about your sexuality and/or gender identity? • Have you dated anyone who is aware of your sexuality and/or gender identity? How did they find out and how did they react?
Important relationships/ contexts	To understand the student's interpersonal relationships within key contexts, clinicians can ask questions about important people in the student's life, social activities that the student may be involved in, experiences at school, etc.	• Who do you live with? Are they aware of your sexuality and/or gender identity? How did they find out and how did they react? • How do you think your family and/or friends perceive your sexuality and/or gender identity? • Do you have friends who know about your sexuality and/or gender identity? • Do you feel like you can be yourself around friends and family? • Do you have friends who support you? • What social activities at school or outside of school? • Who at school is aware of your sexuality and/or gender identity? • Who at school can you talk to about your sexuality and/or gender identity? • Who are adults on campus you trust? • What kind of help of support would be the most beneficial for you? • Have you ever been harassed, bullied, or treated unfairly at school because of your sexuality and/or gender identity? • Have you ever felt isolated from your family or friends because of your identities?
Understanding of the problem	To understand what brought the student to counseling, clinicians can ask questions about how the student understands or perceives their own experiences and what their presenting concerns are.	• What made you want to come to counseling? • Why do you think your caregiver/loved one encouraged you to come to counseling? • How do you think your family would describe your presenting concern? • What do you hope to get out of our time working together? • Does identifying as LGBTQ+ contribute to the presenting problem?

(*Continued*)

Table 7.1 (Continued)

Category	*Purpose*	*Sample Questions*
Psychosocial stressors and risk factors	To understand the student's psychosocial stressors and risk factors, clinicians can ask questions about the student's social, environmental, and systemic distress and maladaptive coping strategies.	• Have you ever thought about or attempted to harm or kill yourself? • Have you ever felt/do you feel hopeless? • Do you worry about people finding out about your identity? • Has anyone ever threatened to out you without your permission? • Have you ever used alcohol or drugs to cope with negative feelings? How often do you use? • Have you ever been threatened or attacked because of your identity? • How do you feel about the way you look? • Do you wish you looked different? In what ways? • Do you eat more or less than you used to? • Has anyone ever offered your money, alcohol, drugs, etc., in exchange for sex/sexual activity?
Resilience and protective factors	To understand the student's protective and resilience factors, clinicians can ask questions about the student's positive coping skills and supportive communities.	• Do you know any other people who identify in the same or in similar ways as you? How did you meet them? How much time do you spend with them? • What are some positive ways you cope when feeling stressed? • What are some communities that provide you with support? • Where do you feel most safe? • With whom do you feel most safe? • What individuals can you identify both inside and outside of school who are safe?

LGBTQ+ clients, and Holman and Goldberg (2006), who adapted the HEEADSSS psychosocial interview tool (Goldenring & Rosen, 2004) to specifically address transgender adolescents. This provides guidance for clinicians and can be adapted depending on students' responses and the purpose of counseling.

The intake allows us to assess better what role, if any, the student's sexual orientation and/or gender identity play in their presenting problem. As counseling progresses, some of these topics and questions may be discussed in more detail.

Case Conceptualization and Treatment Planning

The concept of minority stress centers conceptualization of LGBTQ+ students' lived experiences and mental health needs. LGBTQ+ students experience increased stress (minority stress) due to interpersonal and systemic discrimination and oppression, which leads to greater mental health challenges (Meyer & Frost, 2013). Results from meta-analyses support this, with Dürrbaum and Sattler (2020) reporting a positive correlation between minority stress and mental health difficulties, especially depression, for sexual minority youth, and de Lange and colleagues (2022) reporting "a significant association between minority stressors and suicidal ideation and suicide attempts for LGBT adolescents and young adults" (p. 233). In reviewing the literature on minority stress and LGBTQ youth,

Heck (2015) outlines four intersecting stressors impacting LGBTQ+ youth's mental health. First, as previously documented in this chapter, LGBTQ+ youth experience high levels of prejudice, such as bullying and harassment at school and family rejection. Second, based on these experiences of prejudice, LGBTQ+ youth anticipate experiencing prejudice or rejection in future interactions. Third, LGBTQ+ youth experience increased minority stress when they feel they must conceal their identity and conform to heterosexual or cisgender norms. Lastly, LGBTQ+ youth internalize negative societal views, leading to internalized homophobia or transphobia.

Drawing on the research on minority stress and LGBTQ+ people, Hall and colleagues (2019) outline six assumptions that help clinicians conceptualize minority stress to assist with counseling interventions:

> (1) LGBTQ people are not abnormal but represent normal and natural variation in sexuality and gender among humanity; (2) social systems of oppression facing LGBTQ people (i.e., heterosexism and cisgenderism) are pervasive in society; (3) these systems of oppression lead to added stress for LGBTQ people in terms of hostile environments, negative interpersonal interactions, and discriminatory or inequitable policies and institutional systems; (4) because heterosexism and cisgenderism are pervasive in society, LGBTQ [people] internalize heterosexist and cisgenderist attitudes and beliefs, which negatively affect their mental health; (5) this internalized oppression is a primary contributing factor to depression among LGBTQ people; and (6) interventions aimed at modifying cognition (e.g., CBT) can be used to target internalized oppression.
>
> *(p. 5)*

With this understanding of the impact of minority stress on LGBTQ+ youths' well-being, treatment planning and goal setting revolves around the question: what does this student need to develop a healthy, integrated identity that includes a positive sense of self related to their sexual orientation and/or gender identity? The answers to this question, and thus the focus of counseling, depend on many factors, including where the student is in understanding their sexuality and gender identity, their lived experiences, their strengths and resources, and their understanding of and ability to cope with interpersonal and systemic discrimination and oppression (Crisp & McCave, 2007). The information gleaned from the interview and assessment phase of counseling provides a starting point to understand who the student is, what is affecting their well-being, and what types of interventions may be impactful.

Components of LGBTQ+-Affirmative Cognitive-Behavioral Therapy

Cognitive-behavioral therapy is a promising intervention for LGBTQ+ students as "skillful delivery of CBT places substantial emphasis on clarifying which part of the problem is environmental and which part is cognitive (internal)" (Craig et al., 2013, p. 260). Affirmative CBT considers the unique experiences and needs of LGBTQ+ students when implementing common CBT interventions, such as psychoeducation and cognitive restructuring. These considerations affirm a positive LGBTQ+ identity, recognize the impact of minority stress, and support students in learning new strategies to cope with negative experiences and improve their well-being.

Foster Trust through Collaboration, Psychoeducation, and Validation

Trust is a critically important component of counseling with LGBTQ+ students. As highlighted earlier in this chapter, clinicians can begin building trust by demonstrating an affirming stance in early interactions with all students, including during the intake and assessment process. Trust is further enhanced through the collaborative nature of CBT, with the clinician providing "a clear description of the rationale and process of the sessions" (Craig et al., 2013, p. 261). This type of transparency demonstrates respect for the student, recognizes them as being an expert on themselves, and empowers them to be active agents in the counseling process (Craig et al., 2013). This collaborative approach is critical throughout counseling to ensure students feel safe and supported by the clinician and, ultimately, see the clinician as an ally.

The trusting therapeutic alliance is further enhanced through psychoeducation and discussions about the student's experiences. Psychoeducation can demonstrate the clinician's awareness of and sensitivity to LGBTQ+ issues and begins by recognizing where the student is in their identity development. For students in the early stages of understanding their sexuality or gender identity, psychoeducation may include talking about common feelings associated with early awareness, such as uncertainty, anxiety, curiosity, or fear, and can help normalize students' experiences. Further, psychoeducation may help students learn new identity terminology and find words to put to their internal experiences. For example, a clinician might say, "Sometimes students use the word 'questioning' to describe not yet being sure about their attractions. In what ways does this fit or not fit for you?" For students who are more certain about their sexual or gender identity, psychoeducation may focus on how growing up in an environment in which heterosexism and cisgenderism are the norm contributes to minority stress and mental health difficulties for many LGBTQ+ individuals, which can open a discussion about the student's lived experiences and help them contextualize their experiences of depression, anxiety, and hopelessness (Austin & Craig, 2015). Psychoeducation helps students "move away from a view of themselves as 'disordered' and 'pathological' toward an affirming view of themselves as 'doing their best to cope with complex and often hostile external circumstances'" (Austin & Craig, 2015, p. 24). This seemingly simple intervention sends a powerful message to the student about their worth and the clinician's affirming, nonjudgmental stance, which can deepen the counseling alliance.

When LGBTQ+ students talk about experiences of discrimination, rejection, or homophobia/transphobia, it is critical that clinicians respond in a validating manner to maintain trust, which may necessitate a different approach than typically used in CBT. Craig and colleagues (2013) suggest clinicians refrain from universalizing the experience or seeking alternative explanations and instead validate what was shared and ask questions to understand the impact of the experience on the student. For example, a 13-year-old female student who recently came out to her parents as lesbian shares that she feels her coming out has made her father more distant. Statements such as "A lot of fathers are uncomfortable thinking about their daughter as a sexual being" or "I wonder if there might be other reasons for the distance you're feeling rather than your sexual orientation" may invalidate her experience. Instead, the clinician might respond with statements that focus on the student's experience, such as "Tell me more about your relationship with your father," "What thoughts or feelings does this bring up for you?", or "How are you managing this change in the relationship?" What is important is to honor the student's experience rather than potentially minimize it, explore the impact on the student, and begin to understand it within the context of the student's LGBTQ+ identity.

Help Students Cope with Systemic and Interpersonal Oppression

Drawing on the minority stress model, it is important to overtly acknowledge that LGBTQ+ students experience many situations over which they have little or no direct control but greatly impact their mental health and well-being (e.g., parental rejection and school bullying; Craig et al., 2013). Frequently, LGBTQ+ students are dependent on their families for material support and have little choice of where they attend school, which can lead to feelings of frustration, helplessness, and hopelessness.

In the counseling session, clinicians can help students recognize their level of control/influence over the situation, validate students' feelings, and provide hope that there are strategies that can help the student tolerate or cope with the situation until they have more autonomy. For example, a 14-year-old male student who is uncertain about his sexuality shares that he is frequently bullied at school for being perceived as gay and feels pressure from his father to be more masculine. He shares feelings of hopelessness about his situation. The clinician responds by validating his experience and recognizing that he feels "stuck" at home and school. The discussion eventually leads to the student's older brother, who is in college, and with questioning from the clinician, the student begins to talk about what might be different in his life once he is old enough to make decisions for himself. The clinician might say something like,

> Right now, you feel really stuck at home and school, but you can see some light in the future. Our job is to find ways, even little ways, for you to find some of that light now. I can help you with that.

Assertiveness Training

Assertiveness training is one of the topics in the ESTEEM intervention, based on the premise that in safe situations, LGBTQ+ individuals "have the right to stand up to stigma or to articulate their needs or preferences" (p. 292) instead of silencing themselves in interpersonal interactions to avoid rejection or other negative responses (Burton et al., 2019). Burton and colleagues (2019) outline the steps for assertiveness training. First, the clinician and student collaborate to recognize situations in which they may have avoided standing up for themselves due to fear of negative reactions from others, perhaps even recognizing situations in which the student attempted to stand up for themselves only to be harassed or rejected. For example, a 16-year-old male student who identifies as bisexual shared that he was at a sporting event with a large group of students from his school, and many of the students, especially the boys, were using phrases like "that's so gay" and "no homo." While he is out to some of his friends, he is not out globally at school, and although he wanted to say something, he was worried about how people would respond. Next, the clinician and student explore the student's thoughts in a real or imagined safe situation. Using the same example, the clinician might ask, "What went through your head when you first heard that?" "Did those thoughts change the more they said those derogatory comments?" "What feelings came up for you during that experience?" "What do you think would have happened if you said something?" "How do you think your closer friends would have reacted? The other students?" In this step, the clinician can help the student explore the usefulness of the thoughts and help reframe any unhelpful thoughts (see "Restructure Unhelpful Thoughts and Beliefs" section below for specific affirmative strategies for reframing). Next, the clinician can encourage the student to practice being assertive in the safety of the counseling office. This is an opportunity to practice wording, tone, volume, body language, etc. For example, the student might decide to start with a firm statement like, "Saying things like that isn't cool with me," practicing it until he feels comfortable saying it. The clinician can provide positive praise and feedback during this step. Finally, the clinician and student can collaboratively decide on a safe situation in which the student will try being more assertive, which can be a situation that has nothing to do with the student's LGBTQ+ identity. For example, the student decides to tell his friend, who always brings him a latte in the morning, that he prefers his coffee black. As the student becomes more comfortable with these burgeoning assertiveness skills, he can report back each week as he uses them in more situations.

In discussing assertiveness training with LGBTQ+ individuals, Carvalho and colleagues (2022) highlight the importance of assertiveness in creating healthy interpersonal and sexual boundaries and further stress that "part of assertiveness training is also learning to recognize when it is safe to act assertively" (p. 12). They frame assertiveness through the lens of courage, recognizing that standing up for oneself in the face of anticipated social consequences helps empower LGBTQ+ individuals to feel in control and live authentically (Carvalho et al., 2022).

Mindfulness and Self-Compassion

Self-compassion, a component of mindfulness, is associated with positive well-being for LGBTQ+ youth (Hatchel et al., 2019; Helminen et al., 2023). Yet general mindfulness interventions that do not consider the unique needs and experiences of LGBTQ+ youth have not demonstrated effectiveness (Sun et al., 2021). Thus, to foster self-compassion, clinicians need to consider LGBTQ+-specific adaptations to mindfulness activities. Iacono and colleagues (2022) conducted focus groups and interviews with LGBTQ+ youth to develop affirmative mindfulness interventions, finding that youth reported greater benefits when mindfulness interventions were framed through an LGBTQ+-affirmative lens. The following recommendations stem from this study: mindfulness activities need to be framed with discussions of minority stress and LGBTQ+ identity, making it more meaningful and relevant for LGBTQ+ students. Affirmative mindfulness activities can be woven throughout counseling, such as "through psychoeducation, coping skills development (e.g., grounding, mindful assertive communication, reaching out to one's affirming support network), and problem-solving" (p. 233). Mindfulness activities need to be introduced slowly, with special consideration for activities that focus on the body and physical sensations, checking in frequently to ensure youth feel safe and comfortable with this approach. In fact, for LGBTQ+ youth who have experienced trauma, mindfulness interventions should focus on other senses, such as sight or sound, rather than on bodily sensations. Finally, mindfulness activities that intentionally focus on self-compassion, such as helping students develop an awareness of tensions or unhelpful thinking in different situations and mindfulness strategies they can use during these experiences, were highlighted as a crucial aspect of coping. In sum, general mindfulness activities (e.g., loving-kindness meditation) framed through LGBTQ+-affirmative discussions made these interventions more impactful for LGBTQ+ youth.

Behavioral Activation

The primary purpose of behavioral activation for LGBTQ+ students is to increase social connection (Austin & Craig, 2015; Carvalho et al., 2022). Affirmative behavioral activation also can promote positive identity development, self-advocacy, and joy (Carvalho et al., 2022; The Trevor Project, 2022). LGBTQ+ students can become more isolated as they have negative experiences or anticipate negative reactions to them and their LGBTQ+ identity (Austin & Craig, 2015). The steps for behavioral activation are similar to those for general CBT, yet clinicians must help students consider the safety of the situation to increase the likelihood of affirming interactions. First, the clinician can work collaboratively with the student to identify situations or people the student is avoiding. Then, they can identify safe situations for the student to engage with others and create a plan for how the student feels comfortable engaging. Finally, as the student takes small steps to engage, they can evaluate if the engagement benefited the student. Specific to LGBTQ+ students, behavioral activation focuses on engagement with affirming people and activities, which can be in person or through reputable online forums. In their survey of LGBTQ+ youth mental health, The Trevor Project (2022) reported on sources of joy that included social connection (e.g., accepting and affirming friends, family and parental support, and supportive teachers), identity-affirming activities (e.g., learning about LGBTQ history, gender-affirming clothing, and queer role models), and involvement in the LGBTQ+ community (e.g., LGBTQ clubs on campus, victories for LGBTQ rights, and online communities and support). LGBTQ+ students should be encouraged to start with a low-risk activity, such as watching a movie featuring LGBTQ+ characters and moving to more engaged activities, such as going to an LGBTQ+ community event, as they gain comfort and experience success (Austin & Craig, 2015).

Building on this, Robinson and Schmitz (2021) highlight the idea of resistance, or challenging systemic oppression, as a way for LGBTQ+ youth to feel engaged and empowered in changing the dominant narrative about LGBTQ+ identity. Resistance can be particularly empowering for LGBTQ+ youth who experience intense frustration with the heteronormative and cisgendernormative social and political institutions, and clinicians can use the concept of resistance to help LGBTQ+ youth channel their energy into activities that challenge oppressive forces. For example, Robinson and Schmitz (2021) discuss school as an often LGBTQ+-oppressive institution, documenting resistance activities such as refusing to use pronouns to disrupt the notion of a gender binary, starting a gender-sexuality alliance to educate and advocate at school, promoting LGBTQ+ visibility through pride activities, and choosing LGBTQ+ topics for class assignments, among many others. "Resistance allows the youth to define what is causing oppression and what needs to be changed" (p. 11), centering and uplifting student voice.

Restructure Unhelpful Thoughts and Beliefs

Cognitive restructuring is a common CBT technique that can be used effectively with LGBTQ+ students by attending to specific considerations. First, clinicians must avoid using terms like "irrational" or "invalid," as these may inadvertently pathologize LGBTQ+ students or contribute to the social message that something is wrong with them. Instead, thoughts can be framed as being "helpful" or "unhelpful" (Craig et al., 2013). Similarly, clinicians must be mindful when using Socratic questioning with LGBTQ+ students, as these types of challenges may exacerbate real fears (Craig et al., 2013). For example, Craig and colleagues (2013) provide the example of the clinician asking, "what's the worst thing that could happen if you disclose your sexuality to your family?" which is highly insensitive to many LGBTQ+ students' lived experiences of rejection and abuse from family members. Instead, they suggest clinicians help clients list their different thoughts about coming out to their family, label each thought as helpful/useful or unhelpful/unuseful, and discuss how holding onto unhelpful thoughts relates to emotional distress. Next, when working with LGBTQ+ students to identify more helpful replacement thoughts, clinicians can draw on students' strengths and past successes to help students develop more positive self-statements such as, "I am strong and I can manage this challenge," "I love myself and others will love me for who I am," or "I am learning more about who I am every day, and I'm excited to become more myself" (Craig et al., 2013).

Clinicians need to be sensitive to the unique experiences of transgender and gender-diverse students when using cognitive restructuring, recognizing the cognitive dissonance that occurs when one's gender identity does not align with one's assigned sex at birth (Joseph et al., 2020). Joseph and colleagues (2020) recommend an approach to cognitive restructuring with transgender and gender-diverse youth that simultaneously validates the difficulties inherent in being gender diverse in our society and provides hope that they can choose to think and feel differently about themselves. For example, a 6th-grade transgender girl who has made a social transition frequently becomes distraught in counseling, saying things like, "It's not fair! Why was I born like this? I don't want to be transgender; I want to be a real girl." An affirmative response from the clinician might include, "You're right, it's not fair. You have to navigate things that other kids don't. I also see how much strength you have and how loved you are by your family and friends." The clinician can go on to help the student identify affirming replacement thoughts, focusing on the idea that "things can be hard and I can be happy." As part of cognitive restructuring, transgender and gender-diverse students may benefit from psychoeducation about gender as a social construct and minority stress, and as their awareness increases, clinicians can gently challenge them to redefine what it means to be a "real" girl/woman or boy/man (Carvalho et al., 2022).

Support Identity Development and Coming Out at the Student's Pace

A primary goal of counseling with LGBTQ+ students is to support healthy identity development that includes students' sexuality and gender identity (Crisp & McCave, 2007). Students are invariably going to be at different points in understanding and integrating their LGBTQ+ identity, including disclosure of that identity to others (i.e., coming out). Coming out is a process, as LGBTQ+ individuals must first become aware of their own LGBTQ+ identity and then make a decision whether or not to disclose their LGBTQ+ identity within each new situation and with each new person (Ali & Barden, 2015). Although coming out is associated with more positive mental health outcomes and may be a marker of positive identity development, students may choose not to come out globally due to very real risks to their physical and mental health (Ali & Barden, 2015). Thus, what is important for clinicians is to support students' LGBTQ+ identity development and help them explore the benefits and risks associated with coming out within their different social networks (e.g., family, friends, and school). Ali and Barden (2015) offer clinicians a three-phase framework for supporting LGBTQ+ youth in understanding their LGBTQ+ identity and making informed decisions about disclosure. The 1st phase, awareness, involves the student's awareness of their LGBTQ+ identity and awareness of an opportunity or desire to disclose their identity. In this phase, clinicians can support the student by asking questions to explore the student's identity, any previous experiences with identity disclosure, and what is prompting the student to consider disclosing their identity at this time. The 2nd phase, assessment, involves understanding the risks and benefits of identity disclosure, with a focus on ensuring the student's safety. In this phase, clinicians can support the student by helping them explore the importance of disclosure and their motivation for disclosure, how the student believes disclosure will benefit them, and what perceived or real risks may be involved with disclosure. The final phase, decision, involves the student's choice to disclose or not disclose their LGBTQ+ identity. Clinicians can support the student in this phase by ensuring they have fully considered the benefits and risks, they have a safety plan if there is the possibility of physical danger after disclosure (such as disclosure to religiously conservative family members), and they have identified supportive allies who they can turn to if needed.

Ali and Barden (2015) note that this three-phase model may not apply to transgender and gender-diverse students and their coming out process. Holman and Goldberg (2006) offer strategies for clinicians in working to support identity development for gender-diverse students. For students in early stages of gender identity awareness, clinicians can help students explore and experiment with activities such as journaling, watching videos with gender-diverse characters, and trying different names and pronouns within the counseling setting. For students who are more certain about their gender identity, clinicians can support students in exploring the fluidity of gender and "experimenting as a way of deciding who they are and what feels right" (p. 104), such as trying different clothes, hair styles, and makeup. For example, in the safety of the counseling office, the student can try interacting with the clinician in different ways and process how it feels to do so. As the student becomes more confident in their gender identification, clinicians can help the student find ways to integrate their gender identity and expression into their daily life, including exploring disclosure. Similar to the framework proposed by Ali and Barden (2015), Holman and Goldberg (2006) highlight the need to discuss potential benefits, potential risks, and student safety related to coming out. They also suggest that the clinician help the student make a plan for "involuntary discovery" (p. 105) of their gender identity to ensure the student's physical and emotional safety.

Address Suicide

As previously discussed, LGBTQ+ students are at increased risk for depression, feelings of hopelessness, and suicidal ideation due to minority stress (de Lange et al., 2022; Hatchel et al., 2021). In the absence of research on effective treatments to address suicide for LGBTQ+ youth (Russon et al., 2022), clinicians can assess risk factors and promote protective factors to support students. In a meta-analysis and systematic review conducted by Hatchel and colleagues (2021), the risk factors most strongly correlated with increased suicidal thoughts and behaviors among LGBTQ+ youth include perceived burdensomeness (the feeling that others wish the student were gone or would be better off if the student was not around), self-harm, and sexual risk behaviors. Other risk factors demonstrate small to medium effect sizes, including depression, thwarted belongingness (rejection), and family conflict. Protective factors associated with lower levels of suicidal thoughts and behaviors include self-compassion, self-esteem, school belonging, supportive families, and being out/open about LGBTQ+ identity.

During the interviewing and assessing phase of counseling, clinicians can ask questions to determine levels of risk and protective factors, and it is recommended that clinicians ask questions about these factors and suicidal ideation as topics arise in counseling (e.g., experiences of rejection) to create an open, safe space for students to share their thoughts and feelings. For LGBTQ+ students expressing suicidal thoughts and behaviors, clinicians can help students understand how minority stress impacts their mental health (psychoeducation; de Lange et al., 2022), focus on building strong, affirmative social support networks (Austin & Craig, 2015), and address unhelpful, harmful thinking, such as that nobody wants the student around (cognitive restructuring; Craig et al., 2013). It is important to note that family relationships can exacerbate risk or serve as a protective factor. When engaging with families, it is critical that clinicians know the student's outness with different family members so as not to inadvertently disclose the student's LGBTQ+ identity. For example, an 8th-grade male student who identified as gay with select peers at school was not out to his mother. He began to express suicidal ideation at school and was seen by the school psychologist. The school psychologist determined he was actively at risk (i.e., was despondent and had a plan), necessitating that his mother be involved for follow-up and development of a safety plan. In discussion with the student's mother, the school psychologist was careful to respect the student's privacy about his sexuality, instead focusing on the student's symptoms and assessment of risk for suicide. The mother shared that she had noticed that the student was depressed at home, and she had begun to look into counseling at a local community clinic. The student, mother, and school psychologist collaboratively discussed a safety plan, including who outside of the home the student could call for support (an aunt), a plan for counseling to begin at school the next day, and a plan for counseling outside of school.

Several reputable online resources are available to support LGBTQ+ students experiencing suicidal thoughts and behaviors. For example, The Trevor Project has chat, text, and call access to counselors 24 hours a day, seven days a week (https://www.thetrevorproject.org/get-help/), and the LGBT Youth Talkline offers phone support Monday through Saturday in the afternoons and evenings (https://www.lgbthotline.org/national-hotline). Clinicians are encouraged to provide these resources to students, adding these numbers to their mobile phones to ensure quick access.

Assessment of Progress and Outcomes

As clinicians providing affirmative CBT to LGBTQ+ students, it is imperative to assess the progress of students and the effectiveness of the intervention during treatment. At the start of treatment, the clinician and student should collaboratively identify the goals for counseling and subsequently develop

Table 7.2 Formal Assessment Methods

Domain	*Assessment Tool Examples*
Depression	• Beck Depression Inventory (BDI-II; Beck et al., 1996) • Children's Depression Inventory (CDI; Kovacs, 1978) • Reynolds Adolescent Depression Scale (RADS-2; Reynolds, 2004)
Anxiety	• Generalized Anxiety Disorder 7-Item Scale (GAD-7; Spitzer et al., 2006) • Screen for Child Anxiety Related Disorders (SCARED; Birmaher et al., 1997) • Spence Children's Anxiety Scale (SCAS; Spence, 1998)
Coping skills/ quality of life	• Reflective Coping Subscale (RCS) of the Proactive Coping Inventory (PCI; Greenglass et al., 1999) • Rosenberg Self-Esteem Scale (RSE; Rosenberg, 1965) • The Social Connectedness Scale-Revised (SCS-R; Lee & Robbins, 1995) • Stress Appraisal Measure for Adolescents (SAMA; Rowley et al., 2005)

a plan for how to assess whether progress is being made toward these goals. Considering that the goals of treatment will likely vary among students, it is beneficial for clinicians to have an awareness of the different assessment tools available to them. Tools for assessing progress and outcomes may range from informal to formal. Informal assessment tools may include clinician-developed rating scales (e.g., mood meter) and unstructured interview questions. Formal assessment measures are standardized instruments that have been evaluated through rigorous scientific research (e.g., assessed for reliability and validity). Table 7.2 provides examples of formal assessment tools according to each potential outcome domain. Lastly, an opportunity should be given to students to evaluate the treatment process themselves (e.g., AFFIRM Acceptability Survey). Feedback from students may be beneficial as it may help improve program implementation for future students.

Applications to the School Setting

Schools may be an ideal location for affirmative counseling for LGBTQ+ students, as counseling at school can reduce barriers and increase access (Ormiston et al., 2021). Research has consistently demonstrated that youth, especially marginalized youth who are typically underserved, are significantly more likely to engage in mental health services when offered at school than in community mental health settings (Cummings et al., 2010; Juszczak et al., 2003). School-based mental health services decrease barriers such as time, transportation, and cost and increase students' ability to access counseling as most students attend school (Ormiston et al., 2021). As previously mentioned, a large portion of LGBTQ+ youth who want counseling are unable to access it and fear that counseling will replicate other unaffirming experiences (The Trevor Project, 2022). Thus, clinicians can take steps to ensure that all students, including LGBTQ+ students, know how to access counseling services at school and ensure that their counseling office and materials demonstrate LGBTQ+ inclusivity (e.g., stickers, posters, images).

In addition to providing greater access to affirming mental health services for individual students, clinicians can impact the school system to create more inclusive, supportive climates for LGBTQ+ students. Key school climate indicators associated with more positive outcomes for LGBTQ+ students are summarized here, and readers are encouraged to visit the GLSEN website (https://www.glsen.org/) for more comprehensive information. Reporting on the results of GLSEN's biannual school climate survey, Kosciw and colleagues (2022) highlight four aspects of school climate that are amenable to change and consistently associated with more positive outcomes for LGBTQ+ students: (a) schools with anti-bullying policies that specifically protect students based on actual or perceived sexual orientation and gender identity are associated with lower levels of harassment and victimization and higher levels of intervention by school personnel; (b) schools with a gender-sexuality alliance or similar student organization are associated with lower levels of victimization and higher experiences of safety and school connectedness; (c) schools with many visible supportive educators are associated with higher levels of school belonging and overall better psychological well-being; and (d) schools with curriculum inclusive of LGBTQ+ topics are associated with less victimization, greater peer acceptance, and better overall psychological well-being.

Case Study: Affirmative CBT

Jenny is a 9th-grade Caucasian student. Jenny was assigned male at birth and, with the support of her parents and school personnel, made a social transition in 5th grade. Prior to her transition, Jenny and her parents worked with a clinician, but she has not been in counseling since that time. Jenny began taking puberty-blocking medication in middle school, and she and her parents have spoken with doctors about the timing of hormone treatment and gender alignment surgery. Jenny and her parents felt very supported during her transition in 5th grade, and they were very thoughtful to choose a high school where they believed she would be accepted. Jenny is a high-achieving student and has a core group of friends at school. Jenny lives in a state in which transgender rights are consistently upheld.

Reason for Referral

Jenny's mother reached out to the clinician due to concerns about Jenny's increasing emotionality at home. She reported that since starting 9th grade, Jenny has become more "moody" and "angry," seems to be focusing more on her appearance, and gets frustrated when her parents try to talk with her, saying things like, "you just don't get it." Jenny's mother shared that Jenny is aware that her mother is talking with the school clinician, and Jenny expressed a willingness to meet with the clinician. The clinician spoke with Jenny's mother about the importance of confidentiality in the counseling relationship, and they agreed that Jenny should have absolute confidentiality in talking with the clinician, with the typical limits of harm to self, harm to others, and abuse.

Initial Interview and Impressions

During the intake interview, after reviewing confidentiality, Jenny expressed frustration and distress that the transition to high school did not go as she hoped. She wanted to be seen as "just a girl," and she had hoped that all the new students in high school would not know she was transgender. However, within the 1st week of the year, she felt like all the students at school knew she was transgender. Jenny shared that she has a couple of close friends who she spends time with outside of school, and with these friends, she can "forget" for a while that she is transgender. At school, however, she always feels "on the outside" because she is the "transgender kid." When asked follow-up questions, Jenny shared that she does not feel bullied or excluded; rather, she never feels fully relaxed and able to be fully herself at school. Jenny said that this is the way she has always felt at school—before her transition, she knew she was different and could not be herself; after her transition, she always felt different as the transgender kid, and now, she still feels different. Jenny reported that she feels supported by her parents, but because they are involved in her medical care, in which she has to talk about very personal things, she craves privacy and does not want to share everything with them. When the clinician prompted her with, "I wonder if there is something, in particular, you don't want to talk about with your parents," Jenny blushed and then looked at the clinician and said, "I like someone, but who is going to like me?" and then she started to cry. The clinician demonstrated understanding, saying,

> You've been holding on to a lot. High school can be hard enough, and you have some very real additional stressors. But Jenny, you clearly have a lot of strength, and I really appreciate how open you've been with me. I think there are some things we can talk about together that will be helpful for you. Would you be open to that?

Jenny nodded, and they scheduled an appointment together for the following week.

The clinician's initial impressions were as follows: Jenny demonstrates a lot of resilience and has a strong support network. She is generally managing the typical stresses of adolescence but is experiencing negative feelings about her gender identity, the meaning of her gender identity in her peer relationships, and considering her future as a transgender person—all components of minority stress. In her desire to be "just a girl" and not be seen as the "transgender kid," she has distanced herself from other gender-diverse students and the larger LGBTQ+ community at school. Jenny is also experiencing age-typical distancing from her parents, but due to her unique circumstances as a transgender individual, her parents must be more involved in her medical care and decision-making. Although not discussed in depth, Jenny alluded to "laws that make me feel like there is something wrong with me," which further speaks to the impact of minority stress on Jenny's overall well-being.

Goals and Treatment Plan

Two initial counseling goals were developed for Jenny: (1) Jenny will recognize experiences of minority stress, understand the impact on her mood, and develop at least three strategies she can use to feel better and (2) Jenny will recognize when she is having an unhelpful thought about herself and/or her transgender identity and will replace it with a more helpful, compassionate thought.

The eight-week treatment plan was designed to focus first on aspects of minority stress to help Jenny contextualize and understand her experiences as a transgender student in a transphobic society. Even with supportive parents and teachers, Jenny experiences intense feelings of "differentness" and "being on the outside," and her life is undoubtedly harder due to having to navigate the additional challenges of being transgender. By focusing first on external factors that are impacting her well-being, the clinician aimed to display empathy and validate Jenny's lived experiences while helping Jenny build self-compassion for her unique challenges as a transgender individual in society. Next, treatment focused on increasing affirming experiences and coping strategies to improve Jenny's mood. Finally, the treatment helped Jenny explore her unhelpful thoughts and replace them with more affirming and compassionate thoughts. Progress was monitored informally through homework and formally using the BDI. Table 7.3 outlines the treatment plan.

Treatment Summary

Overall, Jenny responded well to the treatment plan. At intake, she scored in the Moderate range on the BDI-II, and at the end of the eight-week intervention, she scored in the Mild range. Additionally, Jenny demonstrated progressive growth in her understanding of and ability to cope with stress as measured by her homework assignments. Jenny had not heard the term minority stress before but quickly talked about how she has experienced stress due to her gender identity and perceived sexual orientation at different times in her life. With gentle questioning, Jenny was able to share her thoughts and feelings with each of these experiences. In certain situations, Jenny was able to identify specific things that increased her stress like her friends talking about boys they like at school. In other

Table 7.3 Treatment Plan

	Key Topics/Agenda	*Homework*
Session 1	• Review confidentiality • Share key takeaways from intake and solicit feedback from Jenny on goals for counseling • Psychoeducation on minority stress • Exploration of Jenny's experiences as a transgender student in our society	Log of times feeling high stress or distress, noting the situation if applicable.
Session 2	• Review homework and ask questions to better understand Jenny's experiences of stress/distress and situational factors • Discuss current coping strategies and assess their effectiveness • Introduce mindfulness and self-compassion, starting with breathing techniques, and assess Jenny's comfort with this activity	Continue to keep a log of stress and distress, adding a note of coping strategies used. Practice breathing activity.
Session 3	• Review homework and ask questions to learn more about Jenny's experiences and coping techniques • Assess level of comfort with mindful breathing and decide if this should continue, possibly adding a positive mantra (e.g., I am strong) • Psychoeducation about behavioral activation • Discussion of past and current activities in which Jenny feels she can be fully herself	Log of situations in which the student feels "fully herself."
Session 4	• Review homework, providing validation and encouragement to Jenny, noting times she feels fully herself • Check in about mindful breathing and consider adding another component, such as a listening meditation • Psychoeducation about the possible benefits of connection with a supportive LGBTQ+ community • Exploration of Jenny's past and current experiences interacting with LGBTQ+ students, adults, and organizations, focusing on her thoughts about these interactions • Developing a plan to add one additional affirming activity in Jenny's week	Activity and mood monitoring.
Session 5	• Review homework and discuss how activities impacted Jenny's mood • Check in about mindfulness activities and what is working for Jenny; consider adding a loving-kindness meditation • Revisit Jenny's interactions with other LGBTQ+ individuals and identify one activity she will try this coming week • Provide psychoeducation about the ABCs of CBT, with a focus on how our thoughts impact our feelings and behaviors • Introduce automatic thoughts and thought tracking	Activity and mood monitoring, including an activity engaged with LGBTQ+ peers, and thought tracking worksheet.

(*Continued*)

Table 7.3 (Continued)

	Key Topics/Agenda	*Homework*
Session 6	• Review homework • Engage in discussion about thought tracking • Introduce replacement thoughts • Provide psychoeducation on the concept of internalized transphobia and how that impacts our self-talk • Work through several examples based on Jenny's week, helping Jenny identify more helpful replacement thoughts	Thought tracking and replacement thought worksheet.
Session 7	• Review homework, providing support and praise for Jenny's attempts at cognitive restructuring • Continue cognitive restructuring activities with current and past stressful situations • Check in regarding overall mood, strategies, experiences to determine if goals have been met or if new goals are needed	Reflect on new coping strategies as counseling draws to an end.
Session 8	• Review homework and use this to frame review of the previous seven weeks • Discuss Jenny's strengths and harnesses strengths when encountering challenges • Plan for a check-in in two weeks to ensure continued progress • Discuss Jenny's comfort with the clinician sharing progress report with parents, ensuring that anything Jenny is not comfortable sharing is kept private	

situations, Jenny felt stressed or distressed but was not sure why. Jenny had previous experience with mindfulness activities and willingly engaged with them as part of counseling. Jenny was open to behavioral activation and had fun talking about different activities she could add into her week. She was initially more hesitant to engage with LGBTQ+ peers, voicing a fear of being perceived as even more different, but she agreed to try joining an online community and found herself logging on almost daily. Jenny struggled a bit with identifying helpful replacement thoughts, initially saying things like, "but I'm always going to be transgender, so I'll always be different." With support and connecting with the concept of internalized transphobia, she was able to slowly find ways to shift her thinking to be more compassionate and affirming. Jenny may need additional support in using cognitive restructuring effectively, which will be reviewed at the two-week check-in.

Postscript

At the check-in, Jenny arrived visibly upset and shared an incident that had happened at lunch that day. A group of her friends were talking about boys they thought were cute, and throughout the conversation, not one friend included Jenny in the conversation or asked Jenny her opinion. Jenny chose not to spontaneously share as she was uncertain how it would be received. The interaction left her feeling excluded and uncomfortable and brought up unhelpful thoughts about herself as a transgender individual in the dating scene of high school. During the original eight-week counseling intervention, the clinician brought up the idea of crushes or liking someone several times, but each time, Jenny did not engage. To respect Jenny's boundary and autonomy, the clinician did not push her to talk about it;

rather, the clinician provided the space, demonstrated openness, and trusted Jenny would talk about it when she was ready. Now seemed to be the time to gently delve into this important milestone in Jenny's development. Jenny and the clinician agreed to meet for four more weeks, which would lead to a natural break in the school year, and then together assess how Jenny was feeling and if she needed continued support during the break.

Summary

This chapter overviews current research highlighting the inequities and injustices LGBTQ+ individuals face daily while emphasizing a clear need for identity-affirming counseling and mental health care, including affirmative CBT. Although the research on CBT with LGBTQ+ students is in its infancy, the interventions provided have been documented to reduce symptoms of depression, stress, and anxiety while increasing coping and self-compassion. Affirmative clinicians recognize the unique identities of the students they work with while bringing attention to minority stress, respecting the rights of their clients, seeking knowledge, and using this knowledge in counseling sessions. Clinicians acknowledge the discrimination and oppression that LGBTQ+ students face and strive always to provide a safe therapeutic space and maintain confidentiality. Using affirmative CBT includes fostering trust, providing psychoeducation, validating client experiences, providing hope, facilitating assertiveness training, engaging in affirmative mindfulness to promote self-compassion, encouraging clients to increase social connection, utilizing cognitive restructuring supporting identity development, and addressing risk for suicide. Using affirmative CBT, clinicians can help support LGBTQ+ youth in learning positive coping strategies and help improve overall well-being. Lastly, assessing the progress of the affirmative CBT intervention is crucial. This can be done formally and/or informally and should include gaining client feedback to inform future interventions and practice.

Reflection Questions

1 In what ways can clinicians communicate an LGBTQ+-affirming approach during the intake and throughout the counseling process?
2 How can the concept of minority stress inform case conceptualization and support affirmative interventions?
3 What are some specific ways clinicians can make CBT more affirmative for LGBTQ+ students?

References

Adelson, S. L., & The American Academy of Child and Adolescent Psychiatry Committee on Quality Issues (2012). Practice parameter on gay, lesbian, or bisexual sexual orientation, gender nonconformity, and gender discordance in children and adolescents. *Journal of the American Academy of Child and Adolescent Psychiatry, 51*(9), 957–974. https://doi.org/10.1016/j.jaac.2012.07.004

Ali, S., & Barden, S. (2015). Considering the cycle of coming out: Sexual minority identity development. *The Professional Counselor, 5*(4), 501–515. https://doi.org/10.15241/sa.5.4.501

American Psychological Association, Presidential Task Force on Evidence-Based Practice (2006). Evidence-based practice in psychology. *American Psychologist, 61*(4), 271–285. https://doi.org/10.1037/0003-066X.61.4.271

American Psychological Association, Task Force on Appropriate Therapeutic Responses to Sexual Orientation (2009). *Report of the American Psychological Association task force on appropriate therapeutic responses to sexual orientation.* Retrieved from http://www. apa.org/pi/lgbc/publications/therapeutic-resp.html

Austin, A., & Craig, S. L. (2015). Transgender affirmative cognitive behavioral therapy: Clinical considerations and applications. *Professional Psychology: Research and Practice, 46*(1), 21–29. http://doi.org/10.1037/a0038642

Austin, A., Craig, S. L., & D'Souza, S. A. (2018). An AFFIRMative cognitive behavioral intervention for transgender youth: Preliminary effectiveness. *Professional Psychology: Research and Practice, 49*(1), 1. http://doi.org/10.1037/pro0000154

Barlow, D. H., Ellard, K. K., & Fairholme, C. P. (2010). *Unified protocol for transdiagnostic treatment of emotional disorders: Workbook*. New York: Oxford University Press.

Beck, A. T., Steer, R. A., & Brown, G. (1996). *Beck Depression Inventory–II (BDI-II)* [Database record]. APA PsycTests. https://doi.org/10.1037/t00742-000

Birmaher, B., Khetarpal, S., Brent, D., Cully, M., Balach, L., Kaufman, J., & Neer, S. M. (1997). The screen for child anxiety related emotional disorders (SCARED): Scale construction and psychometric characteristics. *Journal of the American Academy of Child & Adolescent Psychiatry, 36*(4), 545–553. https://doi.org/10.1097/00004583-199704000-00018

Burton, C. L., Wang, K., & Pachankis, J. E. (2019). Psychotherapy for the spectrum of sexual minority stress: Application and technique of the ESTEEM treatment model. *Cognitive and Behavioral Practice, 26*(2), 285–299. https://doi.org/10.1016/j.cbpra.2017.05.001

Carvalho, S. A., Castilho, P., Seabra, D., Salvador, C., Rijo, D., & Corona, C. (2022). Critical issues in cognitive behavioural therapy (CBT) with gender and sexual minorities (GSMs). *The Cognitive Behaviour Therapist, 15*(3), 1–20. https://doi.org/10.1017/S1754470X21000398

Craig, S. L. (2013). Affirmative Supportive Safe and Empowering Talk (ASSET): Leveraging the strengths and resiliencies of sexual minority youth in school-based groups. *Journal of LGBT Issues in Counseling, 7*(4), 372–386. https://doi.org/10.1080/15538605.2013.839342

Craig, S. L., & Austin, A. (2016). The AFFIRM open pilot feasibility study: A brief affirmative cognitive behavioral coping skills group intervention for sexual and gender minority youth. *Children and Youth Services Review, 64*, 136–144. https://doi.org/10.1016/j.childyouth.2016.02.022

Craig, S. L., Austin, A., & Alessi, E. (2013). Gay affirmative cognitive behavioral therapy for sexual minority youth: A clinical adaptation. *Clinical Social Work Journal, 41*, 258–266. https://doi.org/10.1007/s10615-012-0427-9

Craig, S. L., Austin, A., & McInroy, L. B. (2014). School-based groups to support multiethnic sexual minority youth resiliency: Preliminary effectiveness. *Child and Adolescent Social Work Journal, 31*, 87–106. https://doi.org/10.1007/s10560-013-0311-7

Craig, S. L., Iacono, G., Pascoe, R., & Austin, A. (2021). Adapting clinical skills to telehealth: Applications of affirmative cognitive-behavioral therapy with LGBTQ+ youth. *Clinical Social Work Journal, 49*(4), 471–483. https://doi.org/10.1007/s10615-021-00796-x

Crisp, C., & McCave, E. L. (2007). Gay affirmative practice: A model for social work practice with gay, lesbian, and bisexual youth. *Child and Adolescent Social Work Journal, 24*, 403–421. https://doi.orh/10.1007/s10560-007-0091-z

Cummings, J. R., Ponce, N. A., & Mays, V. M. (2010). Comparing racial/ethnic differences in mental health service use among high-need subpopulations across clinical and school-based settings. *Journal of Adolescent Health, 46*(6), 603–606. https://doi.org/10.1016/j.jadohealth.2009.11.221

de Lange, J., Baams, L., van Bergen, D. D., Bos, H. M. W., & Bosker, R. J. (2022). Minority stress and suicidal ideation and suicide attempts among LGBT adolescents and young adults: A meta-analysis. *LGBT Health, 9*(4), 222–237. https://doi.org/10.1089/lgbt.2021.0106

Dürrbaum, T., & Sattler, F. A. (2020). Minority stress and mental health in lesbian, gay male, and bisexual youth: A meta-analysis. *Journal of LGBT Youth, 17*(3), 298–314. https://doi.org/10.1080/19361653.2019.1586615

Fernandes, T., Alvez, B., Ioverno, S., & Gato, J. (2022). Somewhere under the rainbow: LGBTQ youth and school climate in Portugal. *Portuguese Journal of Social Sciences, 20*(3), 203–218. https://doi.org/10.1386/pjss_00042_1

Fields, X., & Wotipka, C. M. (2022) Effect of LGBT anti-discrimination laws on school climate and outcomes for lesbian, gay, and bisexual high school students. *Journal of LGBT Youth, 19*(3), 307–329. https://doi.org/10.1080/19361653.2020.1821276

Fisher, E. S., & Kennedy, K. (2016). *Counseling special populations in schools*. Oxford University Press. https://doi.org/10.1093/med:psych/9780199355785.001.0001

Goldbach, J. T., Rhoades, H., Mamey, M. R., Senese, J., Karys, P., & Marsiglia, F. F. (2021). Reducing behavioral health symptoms by addressing minority stressors in LGBTQ adolescents: A randomized controlled trial of Proud & Empowered. *BMC Public Health, 21*, 1–10. https://doi.org/10.1186/s12889-021-12357-5

Goldbach, J. T., Rhoades, H., Rusow, J., & Karys, P. (2023). The development of Proud & Empowered: An intervention for promoting LGBTQ adolescent mental health. *Child Psychiatry & Human Development*, 1–12. https://doi.org/10.1007/s10578-021-01250-2

Goldenring, J. M., & Rosen, D. S. (2004). Getting into adolescent heads: An essential update. *Contemporary Pediatrics, 21*(1), 64–90. Retrieved from https://renaissance.stonybrookmedicine.edu/sites/default/files/HEADSSS%20by%20Goldenring%202004.pdf

Greenglass, E., Schwarzer, R., Jakubiec, D., Fiksenbaum, L., & Taubert, S. (1999, July). *The proactive coping inventory (PCI): A multidimensional research instrument* [Paper presentation]. The 20th International Meeting of the Stress and Anxiety Research Society (STAR). Cracow, Poland.

Hall, W. J., Rosado, B. R., & Chapman, M. V. (2019). Findings from a feasibility study of an adapted cognitive behavioral therapy group intervention to reduce depression among LGBTQ (lesbian, gay, bisexual, transgender, or queer) young people. *Journal of Clinical Medicine, 8*(7), 949. https://doi.org/10.3390/jcm8070949

Hatchel, T., Merrin, G. J., & Espelage, D. (2019). Peer victimization and suicidality among LGBTQ youth: The roles of school belonging, self-compassion, and parental support. *Journal of LGBT Youth, 16*(2), 134–156. https://doi.org/10.1080/19361653.2018.1543036

Hatchel, T., Polanin, J. R., & Espelage, D. L. (2021). Suicidal thoughts and behaviors among LGBTQ youth: A meta-analysis and systemic review. *Archives of Suicide Research, 25*, 1–37. https://doi.org/10.1080/13811118.2019.1663329

Heck, N. C. (2015). The potential to promote resilience: Piloting a minority stress-informed, GSA-based, mental health promotion program for LGBTQ youth. *Psychology of Sexual Orientation and Gender Diversity, 2*(3), 225–231. http://doi.org/10.1037/sgd0000110

Helminen, E. C., Ducar, D. M., Scheer, J. R., Parke, K. L., Morton, M. L., & Felver, J. C. (2023). Self-compassion, minority stress, and mental health in sexual and gender minority populations: A meta-analysis and systemic review. *Clinical Psychology, 30*(1), 26–39. https://doi.org/10.1037/cps0000104

Holman, C. W., & Goldberg, J. M. (2006). Ethical, legal, and psychosocial issues in care of transgender adolescents. *International Journal of Transgenderism, 9*(3–4), 95–110. https://doi.org/10.1300/J485v09n03_05

Iacono, G., Craig, S. L., Crowder, R., Brennan, D. J., & Loveland, E. K. (2022). A qualitative study of the LGBTQ+ Youth Affirmative Mindfulness Program for sexual and gender minority youth. *Mindfulness, 13*, 222–237. https://doi.org/10.1007/s12671-021-01787-2

Israel, T., Gorcheva, R., Burnes, T. R., & Walther, W. A. (2008). Helpful and unhelpful therapy experiences of LGBT clients. *Psychotherapy Research, 18*(3), 294–305. https://doi.org/10.1080/10503300701506920

Joseph, J. M., Busa, S., & Taylor, B. (2020). Using RE-CBT with transgender and gender-expansive children and youth. In M. Bernard & M. D. Terjesen (Eds.), *Rational-emotive and cognitive-behavioral approaches to child and adolescent mental health: Theory, practice, research, applications* (pp. 351–370). Springer. https://doi.org/10.1007/978-3-030-53901-6

Juszczak, L., Melinkovich, P., & Kaplan, D. (2003). Use of health and mental health services by adolescents across multiple delivery sites. *Journal of Adolescent Health, 32*(6), 108–118. https://doi.org/10.1016/S1054-139X(03)00073-9

Keefe, J. R., Rodriguez-Seijas, C., Jackson, S. D., Bränström, R., Harkness, A., Safren, S. A., Hatzenbuehler, M. L., & Pachankis, J. E. (2023). Moderators of LGBQ-affirmative cognitive behavioral therapy: ESTEEM is especially effective among Black and Latino sexual minority men. *Journal of Consulting and Clinical psychology, 91*(3), 150–164. https://doi.org/10.1037/ccp0000799

Kosciw, J. G., Clark, C. M., & Menard, L. (2022). The 2021 National School Climate Survey: The experiences of LGBTQ+ youth in our nation's schools. New York: GLSEN. Retrieved from https://www.glsen.org/sites/default/files/2022-10/NSCS-2021-Full-Report.pdf

Kovacs, M. (1978). *Children's Depression Inventory (CDI)* [Database record]. APA PsycTests. https://doi.org/10.1037/t00788-000

Lee, R. M., & Robbins, S. B. (1995). Measuring belongingness: The social connectedness and the social assurance scales. *Journal of Counseling Psychology, 42*(2), 232.

Lucassen, M. F., Merry, S. N., Hatcher, S., & Frampton, C. M. (2015). Rainbow SPARX: A novel approach to addressing depression in sexual minority youth. *Cognitive and Behavioral Practice, 22*(2), 203–216. https://doi.org/10.1016/j.cbpra.2013.12.008

McConnell, E. A., Birkett, M. A., & Mustanski, B., (2015). Typologies of social support and associations with mental health outcomes among LGBT youth. *LGBT Health, 2*(1), 55–61. http://doi.org/10.1089/lgbt.2014.0051

Meyer, I. H., & Frost, D. M. (2013). Minority stress and the health of sexual minorities. In C. J. Patterson & A. R. D'Augelli (Eds.), *Handbook of psychology and sexual orientation* (pp. 252–266). New York: Oxford University Press.

Moradi, B., & Budge, S. L. (2018). Engaging in LGBQ+ affirmative psychotherapies with all clients: Defining themes and practices. *Journal of Clinical Psychology, 74*(11), 2028–2042. http://doi.org/10.1002/jclp.22687

Morton, M. H., Samuels, G. M., Dworsky, A., & Patel, S. (2018). *Missed opportunities: LGBTQ youth homelessness in America.* Chicago, IL: Chapin Hall at the University of Chicago. Retrieved from https://www.chapinhall.org/wp-content/uploads/VoYC-LGBTQ-Brief-FINAL.pdf

Oh, S., Kim, N., McKinzie Bennet, C., & Dillman Taylor, D. (2019). Multiculturally competent intake interview with LGBTQI+ clients. *Journal of Gay & Lesbian Mental Health, 23*(2), 186–204. https://doi.org/10.1080/19359705.2019.1568943

Onken, L. S., Carroll, K. M., Shoham, V., Cuthbert, B. N., & Riddle, M. (2014). Reenvisioning clinical science: Unifying the discipline to improve the public health. *Clinical Psychological Science*, *2*(1), 22–34. https://doi.org/10.1177/2167702613497932

Ormiston, H. E., Guttman-Lapin, D., & Shriberg, D. (2021). Social justice as a framework for addressing mental health disparities. *Communiqué, 49*(5), 14–16. Retrieved from https://www.nasponline.org/publications/periodicals/communique/issues/volume-49-issue-5/social-justice-as-a-framework-for-addressing-mental-health-disparities

O'Shaughnessy, T., & Speir, Z. (2018). The state of LGBQ affirmative therapy clinical research: A mixed-methods systematic synthesis. *Psychology of Sexual Orientation and Gender Diversity, 5*(1), 82–98. https://doi.org/10.1037/sgd0000259

Pachankis, J. E., Harkness, A., Maciejewski, K. R., Behari, K., Clark, K. A., McConocha, E., Winston, R., Adeyinka, O., Reynolds, J., Bränström, R., & Esserman, D. A. (2022). LGBQ-affirmative cognitive-behavioral therapy for young gay and bisexual men's mental and sexual health: A three-arm randomized controlled trial. *Journal of Consulting and Clinical Psychology, 90*(6), 459–477. https://doi.org/10.1037/ccp0000724

Pachankis, J. E., Hatzenbuehler, M. L., Rendina, H. J., Safren, S. A., & Parsons, J. T. (2015). LGB-affirmative cognitive-behavioral therapy for young adult gay and bisexual men: A randomized controlled trial of a transdiagnostic minority stress approach. *Journal of Consulting and Clinical Psychology, 83*(5), 875–889. http://dx.doi.org/10.1037/ccp0000037

Peter, T., Campbell, C. P., & Taylor, C. (2021). Still in every class in every school: Final report on the second climate survey on homophobia, biphobia, and transphobia in Canadian schools. Key Takeaways. Toronto, ON: Egale Canada Human Rights Trust. Retrieved from https://egale.ca/awareness/still-in-every-class/

Reynolds, W. M. (2004). The Reynolds Adolescent Depression Scale-Second Edition (RADS-2). In M. J. Hilsenroth & D. L. Segal (Eds.), *Comprehensive handbook of psychological assessment, Vol. 2. Personality assessment* (pp. 224–236). John Wiley & Sons, Inc.

Robinson, B. A., & Schmitz, R. M. (2021). Beyond resilience: Resistance in the lives of LGBTQ youth. *Sociology Compass, 15*(12), 1–15. https://doi.org/10.1111/soc4.12947

Rosenberg, M. (1965). *Society and the adolescent self-image*. Princeton, NJ: Princeton University Press.

Rowley, A. A., Roesch, S. C., Jurica, B. J., & Vaughn, A. A. (2005). Developing and validating a stress appraisal measure for minority adolescents. *Journal of Adolescence*, *28*(4), 547–557. https://doi.org/10.1016/j.adolescence.2004.10.010

Russon, J., Washington, R., Machado, A., Smithee, L., & Dellinger, J. (2022). Suicide among LGBTQIA+ youth: A review of the treatment literature. *Aggression and Violent Behavior, 64*, 1–11. https://doi.org/10.1016/j.avb.2021.101578

Ryan, C., Russell, S. T., Huebner, D., Diaz, R., & Sanchez, J. (2010). Family acceptance in adolescence and the health of LGBT young adults. *Journal of Child and Adolescent Psychiatric Nursing, 23*(4), 205–213. https://doi.org/10.1111/j.1744-6171.2010.00246.x

Ryan, C., Toomey, R. B., Diaz, R. M., & Russell, S. T. (2020). Parent-initiated sexual orientation change efforts with LGBT adolescents: Implications for young adult mental health and adjustment. *Journal of Homosexuality, 67*(2), 159–173. https://doi.org/10.1080/00918369.2018.1538407

Spence, S. H. (1998). A measure of anxiety symptoms among children. *Behaviour Research and Therapy, 36*(5), 545–566.

Spitzer, R. L., Kroenke, K., Williams, J. B., & Löwe, B. (2006). A brief measure for assessing generalized anxiety disorder: The GAD-7. *Archives of Internal Medicine, 166*(10), 1092–1097. https://doi.org/10.1001/archinte.166.10.1092

Sun, S., Nardi, W., Loucks, E. B., & Operario, D. (2021). Mindfulness-based interventions for sexual and gender minorities: A systematic review and evidence evaluation. *Mindfulness, 12*, 2439–2459. https://doi.org/10.1007/s12671-021-01710-9

The Trevor Project (2022). *2022 National survey on LGBTQ youth mental health.* West Hollywood, CA: The Trevor Project. https://www.thetrevorproject.org/survey-2022/

Wei, C., & Liu, W. (2019). Coming out in mainland China: A national survey of LGBTQ students. *Journal of LGBT Youth, 16*(2) 192–219. https://doi.org/10.1080/19361 653.2019.1565795

8

SCHOOL-WIDE POSITIVE BEHAVIORAL SUPPORT

A CBT Point of View

Jessica Glass Kendorski, Katy E. Tresco and Amanda Guld Fisher

Mental health in children and adolescents is a considerable public health concern. At least one in five children under the age of 8 has a diagnosable mental health disorder, with higher rates of children experiencing sub-clinical yet concerning symptoms (Vasileva et al., 2021). The most common mental health disorder in childhood continues to be Attention-Deficit/Hyperactivity Disorder (ADHD), with estimates ranging up to 10.2% of the population (American Psychiatric Association [APA], 2022). Anxiety and depression, however, have increased in prevalence in youth and impact a considerable proportion of the school-age population (Bitsko et al., 2022). A compilation of youth survey data from the Centers for Disease Control and Prevention indicates that 9.8% of youth ages 3–17 have been identified as having anxiety concerns by their healthcare provider and that over 4% have identified depression concerns (Bitsko et al., 2022). Rates of depression in adolescents are higher, with over 20% of youth aged 12–17 self-reporting they have experienced a major depressive episode and 18.8% of adolescents reporting seriously considering suicide in the preceding 12 months. In addition, mental health concerns, including the risk of suicide, increase during times of stress, as evidenced by elevated youth suicide rates during the COVID-19 pandemic (Bridge et al., 2023). Further, it is common for mental health concerns to co-occur; approximately one-third of young children diagnosed with a mental health disorder also meet the criteria for at least one additional diagnosis (Vasileva et al., 2021). Data also suggest that youth with depression are more likely to experience anxiety and that anxiety and ADHD often co-occur (Ghandour et al., 2019. Substance use disorders are also prevalent in adolescents (4.1%) and commonly occur with other mental health concerns (Bitsko et al., 2022).

Symptoms and impairments associated with mental health concerns have long been understood to impact attention, concentration, task initiation and persistence, motivation, and engagement in activities (APA, 2022). These challenges in youth have considerable implications for social, behavioral, and academic performance in school. Both externalizing behavior and internalizing concerns have been linked to poor academic performance, school disciplinary actions, and poor peer relationships at school. (e.g., Agnafors et al., 2021; Gubbels et al., 2019). Youth who demonstrate poor school performance have lower school completion rates and are at increased risk for antisocial behavior, difficulties with the legal system, poor social relationships, poor or inconsistent job placement and work performance, and further mental health concerns in adulthood (Gubbels et al., 2019; Lansford et al., 2016).

As such, there is a considerable need to provide both preventative and responsive services for mental health concerns directly in schools, in addition to working collaboratively across service providers.

DOI: 10.4324/9781003392439-10

Although schools have often delivered such services for students with mental health concerns under federal regulations (e.g., Individuals with Disabilities Education Improvement Act, Section 504), and evidence-based school-implemented interventions for mental health have been well established (e.g., August et al., 2018), access to such interventions has been more limited. School-based mental health services are a recognized need; however, they are not widespread nor consistently integrated, and school systems experience considerable challenges to implementation, particularly in underserved areas (Kang-Yi et al., 2023; National Center for Education Statistics [NCES], 2022).

Multi-Tiered System of Supports

Multi-Tiered System of Supports (MTSS) is a systematic framework that provides layered support with a focus on prevention, screening, evidence-based interventions, and early and accurate identification (August et al., 2018; Lewis et al., 2010). The systems approach involves a three-tiered model consisting of universal supports, which are available to all students; targeted supports, which layer additional small group interventions on top of the universal supports; and intensive supports for students that may require specially designed, individualized instruction/intervention. Embedded within the model are screening procedures designed to appropriately identify children needing support beyond the universal strategies, having the added benefit of utilizing scarce educational resources where truly needed. Research has shown the effectiveness of MTSS on academic success (e.g., Response to Intervention or RtI) and appropriate social behavior (e.g., School-Wide Positive Behavioral Interventions and Supports or SWPBIS). The core features of MTSS are (1) effective teams, (2) data-based decision-making, (3) selection of evidence-based practices, (4) early access through universal screening, (5) progress monitoring for implementation fidelity and effectiveness, and (6) systems for initial and ongoing training and coaching for staff. Of late, the research has shown how the tiers and core features could be applied to support the mental health and well-being of students in educational settings (August et al., 2018). Core evidence-based systems-level frameworks can and should be utilized to support all aspects of student success and well-being. These interventions and practices can be embedded in the same overall MTSS framework and they can be seen as a way to benefit the whole student and merged to create efficiency and efficacy. Figure 8.1 shows the standard PBIS triangle showing how resources are allocated across tiers.

Tier 1: Universal

The hallmark elements of a systems-level approach are the universal screening and evidence-based interventions that benefit the majority (at least 80%) of students. These Tier 1 supports are typically designed to promote academic and behavioral success. An evidence-based academic curriculum with frequent active student responding and scaffolding supports is key to a successful universal program. Academic screens usually involve foundational reading skills to identify students who may not be responding to the universal curriculum, as well as provide data to determine whether modifications to the universal curriculum are needed. Similarly, behavioral and emotional supports in the form of universal expectations, teaching strategies and reinforcement are employed at Tier 1. Once these universal systems are in place, a systematic data collection and analysis system can determine which students require targeted or intensive, individualized intervention. Examples of universal screening procedures to identify mental health concerns can include student self-report indicators of heightened stress or teacher direct observation of overall executive functioning and coping skills. Once these screens are completed and universal goals are established, interventions can be provided to all students, such as teaching calming strategies, developing retreat spaces, and parent collaboration initiatives.

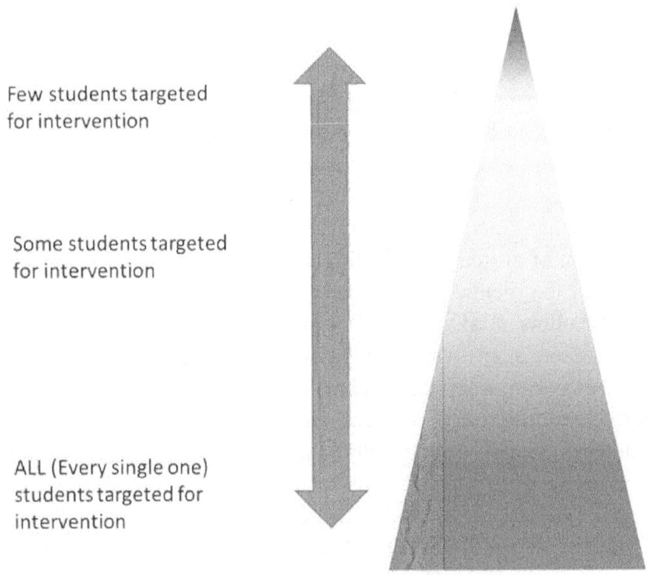

Figure 8.1 Standard PBIS Triangle

Tier 2: Targeted

When universal procedures for academic and prosocial behavior are implemented with fidelity and data collected indicate that they benefit 80% of students, then targeted interventions can be implemented for students requiring additional support (approximately 10–15%). Tier 2 (targeted) interventions are designed for students who would benefit from universal support with some additional modifications or additions. An example of Tier 2 academic support may be a 30–45 min guided reading activity with pre-correction and repeated readings conducted with a small group of target students several times per week (Lee & Yoon, 2017). The Check-In/Check-Out (CICO) intervention has been commonly used as a Tier 2 support shown to enhance the benefits of a universal positive behavior support program when implemented with small targeted groups of students. This intervention allows students to receive effective universal support with the addition of meeting with a preferred adult at the beginning of the day and the end of the day to remind students of expectations and to promote connection to the school community and self-monitoring (Drevon et al., 2019). Although CICO is often considered for externalizing behavior, research has also demonstrated the benefits of CICO for students with internalizing mental health concerns (e.g., Hunter et al., 2014; Kladis et al., 2023). The overlapping evidence-based interventions such as self-monitoring, connecting with a trusted adult, and active preparation and organization for the day could be effective for both internalizing and externalizing concerns.

Tier 3: Intensive

Intensive interventions should be utilized to support the 3–5% of students who are identified through non-response to universal interventions, possibly supplemented by additional referrals and assessment (Crone & Horner, 2003; Crone et al., 2010). These Tier 3 interventions are individualized to the student, and they can consist of specially designed instruction, individualized education plans, individualized positive behavior support plans, accommodations, or services such as individual or group counseling. It is essential in the systems-level approach to have data to confirm that at least 80% of students are responding to universal procedures so as not to burden a system's resources with too high a proportion of students requiring intensive intervention (Sugai & Horner, 2006). This approach using appropriate data-based identification of students can correctly identify students that require intensive interventions, reducing false positives and decreasing disproportionality in diagnosis and educational classification (Bradshaw et al., 2010, 2012; Gregory et al., 2017; Nelson et al., 2002; Tobin & Vincent, 2011; Vincent et al., 2011).

The logical progression of systematic identification and universal support through MTSS could be generalized to support the mental health needs of students and is known as the interconnected systems framework (ISF; Eber et al., 2019). Emotional and mental health support are intertwined with any initiative to promote academic and behavioral success. Aspects of MTSS that provide success in academic and behavioral domains, such as universal supports, data-based decision-making, screening, consultation, and utilizing a problem-solving model, can improve the mental health and identification of students in the educational setting as well (Marsh & Mathur, 2020). In line with this model, SWPBIS, perhaps the most used systems-level procedure to support prosocial behavior utilizing MTSS, also supports mental health and well-being (US Department of Education, 2021). One hallmark universal support of SWPBIS is to identify specific behavioral expectations, teach those behaviors, and provide reinforcement. However, SWPBIS is much more when it comes to providing the systems-level foundation to support the academic, social, and emotional well-being of students utilizing the five foundational elements of equity, systems, data, practices, and outcomes (Eber et al., 2019). Equity refers to the core belief that all students have a right to the interventions and strategies that will make them successful. A systems approach recognizes that a one-time change or program in intervention is not going to have as far-reaching and comprehensive effects nor maintain as well as one that targets entire systems. Practices in systems-level approaches refer to the specific strategies and interventions for addressing behavioral and mental health taught to staff, and the data collected to demonstrate positive outcomes is used to make key decisions about modifications to the system. Figure 8.2 shows the standard multi-tiered system in a visual triangle, showing how the tiers are allocated across groups of students.

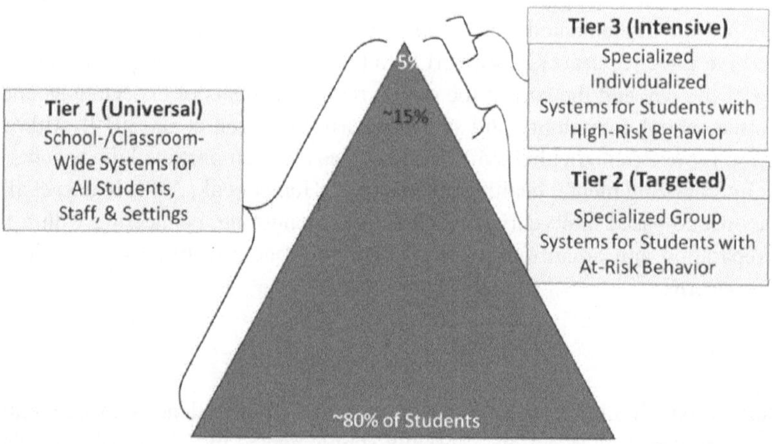

Figure 8.2 Standard Multi-tiered System Diagram

Interconnected Systems Framework and School-Wide Positive Behavior Intervention and Supports

The incorporation of mental health services into the foundation of SWPBIS to create an interconnected framework starts with the shared goal of equity. The ISF was created by experts in the field of SWPBS and School Mental Health in an effort to develop a collaborative MTSS that effectively incorporates mental health assessment and intervention into the SWPBIS model (Eber et al., 2019). ISF is based on four key messages: (1) a single system of delivery that addresses mental and behavioral health and wellness; (2) mental health strategies are useful for all; (3) access to mental health resources is not enough; and (4) the MTSS approach (see core features above) is essential to install effective school-based mental health systems. The principle of equity in an educational system ensures a natural fit into the culture and context of the specifics of the school and the outside neighborhood, as well as prioritizing the support of all students (Bradshaw et al., 2010, 2012; Gregory et al., 2017; Nelson et al., 2002; Tobin & Vincent, 2011; Vincent et al., 2011). The systems of SWPBIS have been shown to decrease disproportionality, specifically the rates of suspension and exclusionary approaches, and to increase the inclusion and availability of free and appropriate public education (FAPE) for all students (Tobin & Vincent, 2011; Vincent et al., 2011). Screening and assessing the mental health supports of students and faculty in an educational system and ensuring there is a tiered approach to address them is essential to the prevention and intervention of mental health concerns and the responsible, equitable distribution of services and FAPE.

Systems, Data, and Outcomes

Each of the foundational features/elements of MTSS and SWPBIS combine to produce a system that objectively shows a school's commitment to prioritizing prevention and providing effective and evidence-based interventions to all students while effectively identifying students in need of additional support. For example, a solid universal system of support that explicitly teaches and reinforces prosocial behavior and expectations minimizes "train and hope" approach in favor of an outcomes-based model (Sugai & Horner, 2006). The key is the identification of a school-based team, with appropriate representation, that regularly analyzes ongoing data collection to determine current global needs and allocation of resources, as well as identification of individual students for additional support. These data collection systems, created by the school teams, can include mental health screenings as well as sources of ongoing data collection used for program evaluation. A universal system of strategies that are developed by school teams, trained to competency, supported with coaching, and implemented with fidelity ensures that all adults in the building understand and are committed to the mission and philosophy of the school. Data can be collected that not only evaluate the effectiveness of interventions at all tiers but also evaluate implementation fidelity, allowing teams to problem solve to create systems that have the best ecological fit for their students and school culture.

Continually assessing acceptance and treatment fidelity through the use of systematic data collection is key to effectiveness and sustainability (Sugai et al., 2012). Systems-level initiatives typically take around three to five years to reach effectiveness and sustainability (e.g., Bradshaw et al., 2009; Kim et al., 2018). As such, it is important to incorporate both effectiveness and fidelity to monitor progress and problem-solve challenges. Treatment fidelity of a universal intervention can include direct observation of interventions, interview sampling of students and faculty, as well as objective surveys distributed to all students, faculty, and administrators. The universal mental health systems team should evaluate the data collected to determine which aspects are being implemented with fidelity and why some features are not being implemented with fidelity and then work to improve implementation.

Additionally, data collected on the effectiveness of the implementation of the universal goals should be reviewed continuously to make data-informed decisions. The analysis and collection of this data will also inform how resources should be allocated and where, as well as the overall commitment of administrators and other stakeholders. Within this framework, universal mental health supports, mental health screens, and collection of data can provide a preventive and proactive approach to mental health programming in schools.

SWPBIS Practices and Incorporation of Mental Health Initiatives

Academic, mental, and behavioral health issues are often intertwined, and therefore, interventions that are meant to target one area often result in collateral improvements in others (e.g., Bradshaw et al., 2010; Curtis et al., 2010; Lassen et al., 2006; McIntosh et al., 2008; Nelson et al., 1996). Addressing each area separately through independent initiatives is not as effective or efficient as creating a comprehensive system that incorporates and combines resources and interventions. This also aids in implementation integrity as it may be easier for staff to learn and implement one comprehensive system as opposed to various layered initiatives. Mental health initiatives can and should be systematically and thoughtfully incorporated within the identified SWPBIS practices across the three tiers. This can occur with schools that already have these practices in place at various tiers as well as schools newer to the MTSS and SWPBIS approaches in educational systems. The ISF is an example of how these two initiatives of SWPBIS and school-based mental health can be incorporated into one comprehensive multi-tiered system (Eber et al., 2019). Further, teams should inventory all systems and initiatives in the school (e.g., character education, suicide prevention, bullying prevention, SWPBIS, reading/math curricula, etc.) to allow for combinations of resources and interventions into the multi-tiered system while also determining how each fits into the missions of the school. In Figure 8.3, you can see that a siloed approach addressing all these areas in separate initiatives can be integrated into one systems approach.

To integrate mental health approaches in the educational setting, it is important to examine and establish several core aspects of systems-level structure. These include the identification of a core

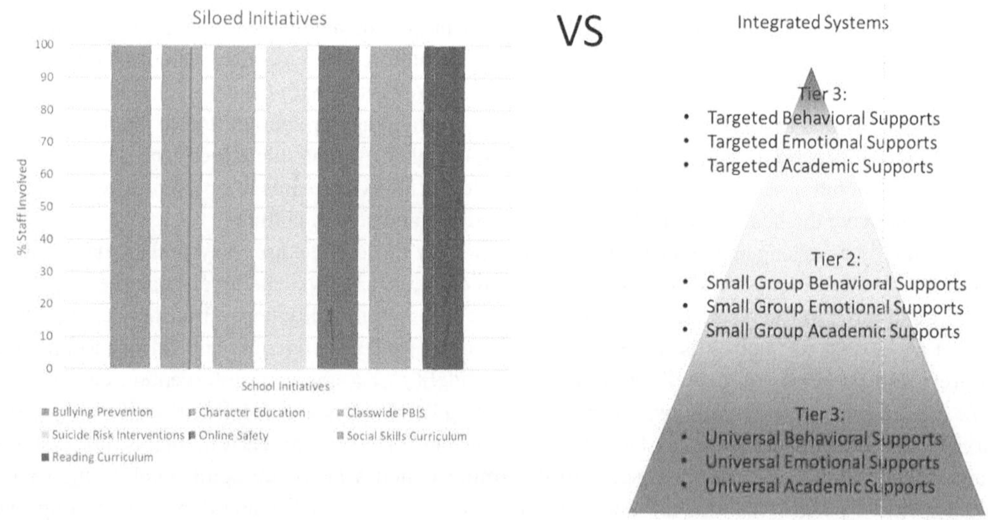

Figure 8.3 Siloed Approach

common philosophy and purpose, a committed leadership team, systematic data collection and monitoring, effective classroom practices, and effective skill, behavior, and strategy instruction and reinforcement (Eber et al., 2019). It is helpful to poll staff, take an inventory of current interventions and systems, and secure commitment before implementation. Table 8.1 shows examples of how each tier in an MTSS could include strategies for all areas of wellness: academic, mental, and behavioral health.

Table 8.1 Examples of Interventions & Strategies That May Be Found across Multi-Tiered Systems

	Academic	*Behavior*	*Mental Health*
Universal	– Evidence-based reading/ math curriculum implemented with the whole group – Active student response methods during instruction (e.g., response cards, choral responding, etc.) – Visual curriculum prompts on desks – Consistent universal screening and progress monitoring – Provide examples and non-examples – Use scaffolding and explicit instruction in teaching – Errorless teaching and error correction with immediate feedback – Small group instruction with flexible grouping – Universal curriculum-based measures (CBM) for screening	– Clear expectations presented visually and explicitly taught – Lesson plans and matrixes for expectations in different settings – Reinforcement systems – Visual cues and reminders – Proximity control – Active supervision – Progress monitoring – 4:1 ratio of praise to correction – Consistent routines – Consistent approaches to discipline across staff – Whole group practice and role plays – Noncontingent breaks (e.g., brain breaks) – Behavioral screening and progress monitoring – Pre-correction – Universal behavior screening	– Teach calming and break strategies to all students – Have a retreat space as needed – Teach conflict resolution skills – Teach emotional regulation skills – Teach coping skills – Pre-teach routines and variations in routines – Universal mental health screenings – Character education systems – Parent collaboration initiatives – Universal mental health screenings
Targeted	– Small group intensive teaching three to five times per week for 20–40 min – Reading/math specialist instruction – Increased visual cues and strategies – At-risk screening and more frequent CBM	– Small group social skills curriculum instruction – Check-in/check out – Relationship skills groups – Team collaboration – Classwide or small-group reinforcement systems – Group contingencies – Self-monitoring group programs – More frequent and detailed assessment and screening of specific skills	– Lunch bunch/guidance groups – Small group coping strategies teaching – Small group role plays and exposures – Whole group CBT workbook sessions – Self-management and self-regulation instruction – More frequent assessment and screening of specific areas (e.g., anxiety, depression scales)

(*Continued*)

Table 8.1 (Continued)

	Academic	*Behavior*	*Mental Health*
Intensive	– Research-based interventions for a specific skill such as repeated readings, corrective reading, cover, fluency drills, copy, compare, etc. – Individual specialist interventions – Individualized tutoring – Individualized progress monitoring	– Functional behavioral assessment and function-based interventions – Training and consultation with treatment integrity monitoring and progress monitoring. – Parent training and home consultation – Wraparound services and other community-based services – Individualized progress monitoring	– Individual counseling – 1:1 guided support in the classroom – Before-school/after-school sessions – 1:1 social skills instruction – Individualized treatment plan – Home counseling and wraparound services, community-based services – Individualized progress monitoring

Common Philosophy and Purpose

The first aspect of any systems approach is to identify a common philosophy and commitment to the initiative. This would entail ensuring buy-in from administrators, educational professionals, and various stakeholders that mental health and social and emotional support should be prioritized. Embedded within the common philosophy and purpose is also the commitment to the foundational aspects of SWPBIS for mental health support, such as a preventive and proactive approach to support and intervention. This common philosophy should serve as the overall approach to behavior, academic concerns, and mental health concerns. The focus should be on methods of on teaching skills, reinforcing skills, and being preventative and proactive. From a mental health support perspective, this includes a philosophy of trauma-informed practices to address student concerns, where screening for the risk of social and emotional concerns is prioritized (Hanover Research, 2019).

Leadership

Within a multi-tiered, interconnected systems of support framework, leadership commitment to and support of initiatives is an essential component (Eber et al., 2019). While leadership often includes formalized, bureaucratic leadership within the district, it can also include other stakeholders, such as leaders of teacher organizations, student organizations, and parent organizations. An essential component of establishing leadership is the development of leadership teams, which are representative of various stakeholders at varying levels of the district. A district leadership team, which consists of administrators that can make decisions regarding funding and resources, should be established to support a systems-level mental health initiative. This team will provide oversight and a way for administrators in schools within a district to collaborate on implementation within individual schools. Additionally, the district-level team can ensure that mental health supports at a systems level are funded and included in any strategic plan. Finally, this district-level team can analyze individual schools and district-level data to ensure that the initiatives and supports are effective and suggest any changes needed.

The establishment of the SWPBIS leadership teams is an essential component to providing the oversight, representation, and ongoing data evaluation of a SWPBIS initiative. When the goal of emotional and mental health support is added, the initiative could be incorporated into an already established team or created a smaller subcommittee of an existing SWPBS team. At its core, a SWPBIS leadership team that incorporates a mental health initiative would still prioritize the same overarching goals and, therefore, maintain the same or similar key players. Specifically, the leadership team should consist of a representation of grade levels and various positions within the school, an administrator, and a professional with mental health experience. This team is tasked with creating a school-wide plan to address prosocial behavior as well as emotional and mental health systems, evaluating the effectiveness of these systems and interventions, ensuring fidelity of implementation, as well as ongoing data analysis for modifications and necessary referrals.

Data Collection and Ongoing Monitoring

Core to any systems approach are data collection procedures for screening as well as active monitoring of the effectiveness of universal, targeted, and individual interventions. Prevention-oriented approaches of MTSS typically use screening tools such as DIBELS (Dynamic Indicators of Basic Early Literacy Skills) to identify students not responding to the universal language arts curriculum. Similarly, office discipline referrals may be analyzed at the school-wide level to identify students in need of additional behavioral support. From a mental health perspective, screening tools, as well as ongoing data collection procedures, can include social-emotional screening measures such as overall climate and safety surveys, as well as specific progress monitoring of social-emotional skill development and fidelity of implementation of interventions (Barrett et al., 2018).

Effective Classroom Practices

Establishing a positive, warm, predictable climate within the classroom is essential to any systems-level framework. Specifics can include active monitoring of behavior, consistent consequences, reinforcement procedures that promote prosocial behaviors, and teaching of specific prosocial behaviors (Sugai & Horner, 2006). Additionally, social, emotional, and mental health classroom practices can be implemented to ensure that there is a stable, predictable, and emotionally stable environment for students. These practices can include many of what may be common to trauma-informed practices, such as intentional relationship building with peers and teachers, which include opportunities for structured group activities and modeling and role-playing of social skills (Hanover Research, 2019). Other activities can include the identification of emotions every morning as a check-in, the identification of emotions at the end of the day, as well as time for teaching emotion regulation and coping strategies. Recently, literature related to mindfulness support and planned guided meditations has been shown to increase awareness and coping skills, as well as emotion identification and regulation (Renshaw, 2020). See Table 8.1 for examples of how effective practices can be implemented at each tier in each area of well-being (academic, mental, and behavioral health).

Teaching Skills and Behavior

It is understood that youth must be directly taught academic skills such as reading, writing, and mathematics. Similarly, identification and teaching of expected social and emotional behavior is also necessary and relevant at all tiers of intervention. These may include the prosocial behaviors identified by the system as universally important or developed more individually for students needing Tier 2 or Tier 3 support. Regardless of level, the expected behavior should be directly taught. This includes explicit instruction in the expectation, modeling of the expectation, examples of meeting the expectation, as well as non-examples. Having youth role-play meeting the expectation can also be helpful. During the initial teaching phase, expectations should be reviewed frequently. As they become learned, it may be possible to shift to a briefer and more periodic review of expectations.

Consistent with our understanding of academic and behavioral learning, youth also benefit from direct emotional instruction. The ability to identify and name how you are feeling is a recognized component of CBT interventions for youth (Kendall, 2018). Monitoring and regulating emotional expression is also a key skill. Specifically, emotion regulation typically refers to how emotions are managed and displayed and includes both the maintenance of positive emotions as well as managing responses to stressors (Gross, 1998). The use of adaptive emotion-regulation skills, those aimed at problem-solving and social support, for example, have been found to have a higher association with positive mental health (Aldao et al., 2010; Schlesier et al., 2019). It is also important to recognize developmental considerations and to teach youth how to manage emotions effectively. Emotion-regulation skills generally shift from more extrinsic adult-oriented approaches in young children, such as talking through a problem with the child or providing and modeling breathing strategies, to more intrinsically applied approaches where the youth applies strategy without guidance (Ratcliff et al., 2021; Schlesier et al., 2019). In a tiered system of support, there are opportunities for universal teaching of the identification of emotions, as well as regulation strategies to manage stress effectively. Youth at risk or in need of additional support should be taught skills more targeted toward their individual challenges. Although specific teaching strategies may vary, the general process of teaching, model, practice, and review described previously is consistent across all skills: social, emotional, behavioral, and academic. See Table 8.1 for examples of teaching strategies at each tier.

Encouraging Expected Behavior and Strategy Use

Once desired behaviors and strategies are taught, they must be supported in the natural environment to ensure they are maintained and are generalized to all settings and situations in which they are needed. Without this support it is not as likely that new skills taught will actually be displayed in non-training settings. This support and encouragement can be implemented by way of prompting and pre-correction before a desired behavior is expected to occur and reinforcement delivered after a desired behavior is to occur. For example, in a SWPBS model, the behavioral expectations are often reviewed with specific examples and non-examples across changing settings (e.g., before leaving the classroom and entering the hall to move to the cafeteria). Prompts can also be used when students are demonstrating behavior that indicates they are unsure of what to do or pausing to consider options. For example, a teacher or staff member could say, "What are some good activities to do during recess?" when a student pauses after arriving at the playground area during recess. Appropriate behaviors that are defined in the school-wide expectations can be recognized with praise and reinforced with the school reinforcement system (e.g., school store dollars, star recognition cards, weekly announcements, etc.). This will encourage the appropriate behavior to occur again in similar situations in the future.

Similarly, mental health strategies, such as identifying emotions, emotional regulation, and coping skills taught in CBT, can be encouraged in relevant triggering settings, and exposures can be contrived for practice. For example, emotional regulation strategies mentioned above can be prompted in situations that are known to trigger anxiety in children, such as changes in routines/schedules, visitors, stressful situations, and so on. This may look like a teacher prompting students to answer questions such as, "What feelings might we feel when the fire alarm rings?" and "What can we do to manage those feelings when the fire alarm rings?" prior to a fire drill. Individual students with more intensive mental health interventions can be prompted in situations that involve their individual triggers. In addition to encouraging appropriate strategy use, acknowledgment following use is also important. That is, when students display the emotional regulation strategies and coping strategies that are taught, they should be recognized and reinforced using the school reinforcement system previously described. For example, if a teacher observes a student walking to a calming corner when frustrated, asking to take a break, or using deep breathing techniques when anxious, they can deliver school store money or recognition cards and praise, including specifically stating what they were doing correctly at that moment. Students and teachers can role-play and practice these situations throughout the day and then sporadically as skills and strategies are being used more frequently.

Discouraging Unwanted Behavior

In a SWPBIS system, procedures for discouraging unwanted behavior are as important a consideration as consistent reinforcement and encouragement of expected behaviors (Sugai & Horner, 2006). A system for consistent consequences is developed and trained that typically includes defining common behavior infractions (e.g., minor and major behavioral issues) and then defining consequences for each. For example, minor behavioral issues such as classroom disruption may be responded to by the classroom teacher through verbal correction, with a brief corrective statement in a neutral tone immediately following the behavior. Teachers are then trained and coached on a consistent approach to verbal correction (e.g., a signal that an error has occurred, state-related school-wide rule/expectation, engaging in positive practice and providing positive feedback for correct positive practice). Other procedures for minor infractions may include pre-correction with role plays in problem settings, parent communications, making up lost instructional assignments, or loss of privileges. Major and more infrequent behavioral issues may be addressed by office staff and include more restrictive consequences such as office discipline referrals, parent conferences, detentions, restitution, suspension, etc. These should all be clearly defined and used with the function of the behavioral infraction in mind (e.g., staff should not issue suspensions for escape-maintained school behaviors).

The same continuum for consistent consequences can be defined and taught with ongoing coaching for issues involving mental health concerns. Redirection to the use of CBT strategies, such as relaxation/coping strategies, self-regulation techniques, access to counseling and community resources, can be defined and incorporated into a continuum of responses that indicate the specific contexts in which each should be utilized. Similarly, behavioral functions from a psychological functioning approach should be considered when determining appropriate consequences. For example, if a student has an anxiety disorder that manifests in avoidance of school activities. Special care should be taken to ensure that the consequences involve strategies such as the teaching of relaxation techniques, exposures, and coping strategies instead of reinforcing avoidance-maintained behaviors with removal from class or school.

Mental Health Professionals and Consultation

Schools have a broad range of professionals with varied expertise working to support students in all areas of well-being. Often, these professionals and their expertise are siloed, engaging in their specific expertise individually and having little consultation and collaboration with other professionals. Interprofessional collaboration is essential in the school environment, and research has shown it improves overall outcomes for students at the individual and systems levels (Borg & Drange, 2019). When building universal systems of support within an ISF, there should be identification of what expertise is available within the district, shared goals throughout professions, resources available, and what teams, assessments, and interventions are already occurring where resources could be combined. Additionally, when teams are developed and universal systems are implemented, it is essential to develop relationships within professions as well as establish buy-in for initiatives across various stakeholders in the school (Borg & Drange, 2019). Establishing this acceptance for and engagement in initiatives is achieved through surveying professionals and paraprofessionals in the school and establishing that representatives on the team use their input to develop universal interventions.

Cultivating commitment to implementing ISF involves establishing a systematic approach to collaboration and consultation. When collaborative relationships are established in an attempt to develop a systems approach to intervention, this typically entails a problem-solving approach to consultation. Problem-solving consultation is an important and often overlooked aspect of multi-tiered systems support and mental health initiatives. The steps include problem identification, problem analysis, intervention, and evaluation of intervention (Erchul & Martens, 2016; Kratochwill & Bergan, 1990). When implementing an ISF targeting mental health at a universal level, training, support, and adherence to the problem-solving model could help ensure effectiveness and sustainability. Team meetings, initiatives, universal and individual practices, and consultation should adhere to this model. The first step, problem identification, could utilize data collection specific to the school (i.e., screening data) to determine what would be an appropriate target for mental health initiatives. For example, a school identifies through screening that an elevated number of students are experiencing feelings of anxiety related to academic success. Next involves problem analysis, or an identification of why students may be feeling high levels of stress due to academic success. Examples could include a focus on high-stakes testing or over-focus in the school and community on academic success. The intervention stage would include a universal strategy that would be implemented with all students, such as mindfulness activities before exams, identification of feelings, and specific teaching of helpful versus non-helpful thoughts. Next, an evaluation of the effectiveness of the intervention, specifically measures designed to assess the same skills and competencies assessed in the problem identification, should be conducted to determine if the intervention was successful. This four-step model of collaboration can and should be used at all tiers of intervention to promote sustainability and effectiveness. In addition, the inclusion of school-based mental health professionals on problem-solving teams is key to integrating mental health expertise and services at all system levels.

Conclusion

Successful school performance is associated with mental health and well-being (e.g., Agnafors et al., 2021; Gubbels et al., 2019; Lansford, et al., 2016). As such, it is vital that educational systems provide school-based mental health services as standard practice. A systems-level model utilizing MTSS principles, such as SWPBIS, and consistent with an ISF approach, provides an ideal framework to incorporate preventive and responsive mental health programming at multiple tiers of service (Eber et al., 2019). Any school-wide system of support, whether the target is social, emotional, behavioral, or academic, follows the same principles. As such, mental health programming can be a seamless addition to standard academic and behavioral practices. Systems-level approaches include a commitment to purpose, defined and strong leadership, systematic data collection and monitoring that includes mental health indicators, and effective practices to teach and respond to behavior and strategy use at multiple levels of need (August et al., 2018; Eber et al., 2019). Universal monitoring and prevention programs to support students' understanding of emotions and use of adaptive coping strategies, as well as targeted behavioral and cognitive-behavioral approaches for students at risk and those in need of more intensive services, should be integrated into systems designed to address academic and behavioral concerns.

In addition, it is important to access and incorporate all relevant areas of expertise through interprofessional collaboration. School-based mental health professionals are integral members of problem-solving teams and have relevant input to mental health and well-being that may be impacting academic and social success in school. Shared goals and resources across professions should be established. Finally, universal systems approaches also ensure that there is fidelity of implementation, programming for generalization, equitable access, and a plan for sustainability. A structured review of data should be incorporated to allow for informed decisions regarding aspects of programming implemented with fidelity as well as overall effectiveness and acceptability. Data also inform the allocation of resources and identification of the need for additional programming.

In closing, there is a need for systematic integration of school-based mental health services, particularly in underserved areas (Kang-Yi et al., 2023; NCES, 2022). Mental health interventions within an MTSS model should be a priority in all schools, in addition to academics. Preventive and proactive interventions starting at the universal level highlight the importance of mental health as a priority for all students, and schools are a logical place for these initiatives to occur. The effectiveness of these interventions, based on the need, is best achieved within an MTSS and an ISF (Eber et al., 2019).

Reflection Questions

1. How do you perceive the role of schools in addressing the mental health needs of children and adolescents, particularly in light of the evidence presented about the prevalence of mental health disorders and their impact on academic and social success?
2. Reflect on the Multi-tiered System of Supports (MTSS) framework described in this chapter. How might implementing such a framework in schools change the way students with mental health concerns are identified and supported? Consider both the potential benefits and challenges.
3. The chapter discusses the interconnectedness of mental health with academic and behavioral outcomes. Reflect on your own experiences or observations in educational settings. How have you seen mental health concerns impact academic and social behaviors, and what interventions, if any, were effective in addressing these concerns?

References

Agnafors, S., Barmark, M., & Sydsjo (2021). Mental health and academic performance: A study on selection and causation effects from childhood to early adulthood. *Social and Psychiatry and Psychiatric Epidemiology, 56,* 857–866. https://doi.org/10.1007/s00127-020-01934-5

Aldao, A., Nolen-Hoeksema, S., & Schweizer, S. (2010). ER strategies across psychopathology: A meta-analytic review. *Clinical Psychology Review, 30,* 217–237.

American Psychiatric Association (APA) (2022). *Diagnostic and Statistical Manual of Mental Disorders, 5th Edition, Text Revision.* Washington, DC: American Psychiatric Association.

August, G. J., Piehler, T. F., & Miller, F. G. (2018). Getting "SMART" about implementing multi-tiered systems of support to promote school mental health. *Journal of School Psychology, 66,* 85–96. https://doi.org/10.1016/j.jsp.2017.10.001

Barrett, S., Eber, L., McIntosh, K., Perales, K., & Romer, N. (2018). Teaching social-emotional competencies within a PBIS framework. *PBIS.* Retrieved from https://assets-global.website files.com/5d3725188825e071f1670246/5d76ca39247bc1864c3ba932_teachingsocialemotionalcompetencieswithinapbisframework.pdf

Bitsko, R. H., Claussen, A. H., Lichtstein, J., Black, L. J., Everett Jones, S., Danielson, M. D., Hoenig, J. M., Davis Jack, S. P., Brody, D. J., Gyawali, S., Maenner, M. M., Warner, M., Holland, K. M., Perou, R., Crosby, A. E., Blumberg, S. J., Avenevoli, S., Kaminski, J. W., & Ghandour, R. M. (2022). Surveillance of Children's Mental Health – United States, 2013–2019. *Morbidity and Mortality Weekly Report, 71(Suppl-2),* 1–42. Centers for Disease Control and Prevention.

Borg, E., & Drange, I. (2019). Interprofessional collaboration in school: Effects on teaching and learning. *Improving Schools, 22,* 251–266. https://doi.org/10.1177/1365480219864812

Bradshaw, C. P., Debnam, K., Koth, C. W., & Leaf, P. (2009). Preliminary validation of the Implementation Phases Inventory for assessing fidelity of schoolwide positive behavior supports. *Journal of Positive Behavior Interventions, 11,* 145–160.

Bradshaw, C. P., Mitchell, M. M., & Leaf, P. J. (2010). Examining the effects of schoolwide positive behavioral interventions and supports on student outcomes: Results from a randomized controlled effectiveness trial in elementary schools. *Journal of Positive Behavioral Interventions, 12*, 133–148.

Bradshaw, C. P., Waasdorp, T. E., & Leaf, P. J. (2012). Effects of School-wide Positive Behavioral Intervention and Supports on child behavior problems and adjustment. *Pediatrics, 130(5*), e1136–e1145.

Bridge, J. A., Ruch, D. A., Sheftall, A., Hahm., H. C., O'Deefe, V. M., Fontanella, C. A., Brock, G., Campo, J. V., & Horowitz, L. M. (2023). *Pediatrics, 151* (3): e2022058375. https://doi.org/10.1542/peds.2022-058375

Crone, D. A., & Horner, R. H. (2003). *Building positive behavior support systems in schools: Functional behavioral assessment*. New York: Guilford Press.

Crone, D. A., Hawken, L. S., & Horner, R. H. (2010). *Responding to problem behavior in schools: The behavior education program* (2nd ed.). New York: Guilford Press.

Curtis, R., Van Horne, J., Robertson, P., & Karvonen, M. (2010). Outcomes of a school-wide positive behavior support program. *Professional School Counseling, 13*(3), 159–164.

Drevon, D. D., Hixson, M. D., Wyse, R. D., & Rigney, A. M. (2019). A meta-analytic review of the evidence for check-in check-out. *Psychology in the Schools, 56*, 293–412. https://doi.org/10.1002/pits.22195

Eber, L., Barrett, S., Perales, K., Jeffrey-Pearsall, J., Pohlman, K., Putnam, R., Splett, J., & Weist, M. D. (2019). *Advancing education effectiveness: Interconnecting school mental health and school-wide PBIS, Volume 2: An implementation guide*. Center for Positive Behavior Interventions and Supports (funded by the Office of Special Education Programs, US Department of Education). Eugene: University of Oregon Press.

Erchul, W. P., & Martens, B. K. (2016). *School consultation: Conceptual and empirical bases of practice* (3rd ed.). New York: Springer.

Ghandour, R. M., Sherman, L. J., Vladutiu, C. J., Lynch, S. E., Bitsko, R. H., & Blumber, S. J. (2019). Prevalence and treatment of depression, anxiety, and conduct problems in US children. *Journal of Pediatrics, 206*, 256–267.

Gregory, A., Skiba, R. J., & Mediratta, K. (2017). Eliminating disparities in school discipline: A framework for intervention. *Review of Research in Education, 41*, 253–278.

Gross, J. J. (1998). The emerging field of emotion regulation: An integrative review. *Review of General Psychology, 2*, 271–299.

Gubbels, C. J., van der Put, C. E., & Assink, M. (2019). Risk factors for school absenteeism and dropout: A meta-analytic review. *Journal of Youth and Adolescence, 48,* 1637–1667. https://doi.org/10.1007/s10964-019-01072-5

Hanover Research (2019). *Best practices for trauma-informed instruction.* Hanover Research. Retrieved from https://wasaoly.org/WASA/images/WASA/6.0%20Resources/Hanover/BEST%20PRACTICES%20FOR%20TRAUMA-INFORMED%20INSTRUCTION%20.pdf

Hunter, K. K., Chenier, J. S., & Gresham, F. M. (2014). Evaluation of check in/check out for students with internalizing behavior problems. *Journal of Emotional and Behavioral Disorders, 22*(3), 135–148.

Kang-Yi, C. D., Kuriyan, A., Kinkler, G., Pisciella, A. E., Williams, T., & Wolk, C. B. (2023). Generating actionable evidence for school-based mental health service delivery: Public-academic partnership based evaluations. *Community Mental Health Journal.* Retrieved from https://doi.org/10.1007/s10597-023-01147-5

Kendall, P. C. (2018). *Cognitive therapy with children and adolescents: A casebook for clinical practice* (3rd ed.). New York: The Guilford Press.

Kim, J., McIntosh, K., Mercer, S. H., & Nese, R. N. T. (2018). Longitudinal associations between SWPBIS fidelity of implementation and behavior and academic outcomes. *Behavioral Disorders, 43*(3), 357–369. https://doi.org/10.1177/0198742917747589

Kladis, K., Hawken, L. S., O'Neill, R. E., Fischer, A. J., Fuoco, K. S., O'Keeffe, B. V., & Kiuhara, S. A. (2023). Effects of check-in check-out on engagement of students demonstrating internalizing behaviors in an elementary school setting. *Behavioral Disorders, 48*, 83–96. https://doi.org/10.1177/0198742920972107

Kratochwill, T. R., & Bergan, J. R. (1990). *Behavioral consultation in applied settings: An individual guide.* New York: Plenum Press.

Lansford, J. E., Dodge, K. A., Pettit, G. S., Bates, J. E. (2016). A public health perspective on school dropout and adult outcomes: A prospective study of risk and protective factors from age 5 to 27 years. *Journal of Adolescent Health, 58*, 652–658. https://doi.org/10.1016/j.jadohealth.2016.01.014

Lassen, S., Steele, M., & Sailor, W. (2006). The relationship of school-wide positive behavior support to academic achievement in an urban middle school. *Psychology in Schools, 43*(6), 701–712.

Lee, J., & Yoon, S. Y. (2017). The effects of repeated reading on reading fluency for students with reading disabilities: A meta-analysis. *Journal of Learning Disabilities, 50*(2), 213–224. https://doi.org/10.1177/0022219415605194

Lewis, T. J., Jones, S. E. L., Horner, R. H., & Sugai, G. (2010). School-wide positive behavior support and students with emotional/behavioral disorders: Implications for prevention, identification and intervention. *Exceptionality, 18*, 82–93.

Marsh, R. J., & Mathur, S. R. (2020). Mental health in schools: An overview of multi-tiered systems of support. *Intervention in School and Clinic, 56*(2), 67–73. https://doi.org/10.1177/1053451220914896

McIntosh, K., Flannery, K. B., Sugai, G., Braun, D., & Cochrane, K. L. (2008). Relationships between academics and problem behavior in the transition from middle school to high school. *Journal of Positive Behavior Interventions, 10*(4), 243–255.

National Center for Education Statistics (NCES) (2022). Prevalence of mental health services provided by public schools and limitations in schools' efforts to provide mental health services. *Condition of Education*. US Department of Education, Institute of Education Sciences. Retrieved from https://nces.ed.gov/programs/coe/indicator/a23

Nelson, J. R., Johnson, A., & Marchand-Martella, N. (1996). Effects of direct instruction, cooperative learning, and independent learning practices on the classroom behavior of students with behavioral disorders: A comparative analysis. *Journal of Emotional and Behavioral Disorders, 4*, 53–62.

Nelson, J. R., Martella, R. M., & Marchad-Martella, N. (2002). Maximizing student learning: The effects of a comprehensive school-based program for preventing problem behaviors. *Journal of Emotional and Behavioral Disorders, 10*, 136–148.

Ratcliff, K. A., Vazquez, L. C., Lunkenheimer, E. S., & Cole, P. M. (2021). Longitudinal changes in young children's strategy use for emotion regulation. *Developmental Psychology, 27*, 1471–1489. https://doi.org/10.1037/dev0001235

Renshaw, T. L. (2020). Mindfulness-based intervention in schools. In C. Maykel & M. A. Bray (Eds.), *Promoting mind-body health in schools: Interventions for mental health professionals* (pp. 145–160). Washington, DC: American Psychological Association.

Schlesier, J., Roden, I., & Moschner, B. (2019). Emotion regulation in primary school children: A systematic review. *Children and Youth Services Review, 100*, 239–257. https://doi.org/10.1016/j.childyouth.2019.02.044

Sugai, G., & Horner, R. H. (2006). A promising approach for expanding and sustaining school-wide positive behavior support. *School Psychology Review, 35*, 245–259.

Sugai, G., O'Keefe, B. V., & Fallon, L. M. (2012). A contextual consideration of culture and school-wide positive behavior support. *Journal of Positive Behavior Interventions, 14*, 197–208.

Tobin, T. J., & Vincent, C. G. (2011). Strategies for preventing disproportionate exclusions of African American students. *Preventing School Failure, 55*, 192–201.

US Department of Education, Office of Special Education and Rehabilitative Services (2021). *Supporting child and student social, emotional, behavioral, and mental health needs*. Published by Author, Washington, DC.

Vasileva, M., Graf, R. K., Reinelt, T., Petermann, U., & Petermann, F. (2021). Research review: A meta-analysis of the international prevalence and comorbidity of mental disorders in children between 1 and 7 years. *The Journal of Child Psychology and Psychiatry, 64*, 372–381. https://doi.org/10.1111/jcpp.13261

Vincent, C. G., Swain-Bradway, J., Tobin, J. J., & Mat, S. (2011). Disciplinary referrals for culturally and linguistically diverse students with and without disabilities: Patterns resulting from school-wide positive behavior support. *Exceptionality, 19*, 175–190.

PART III

Implementing CBT Interventions for Specific Concerns

9

ANXIETY DISORDERS

Elizabeth A. Gosch, Julia Ney and Samantha Baker

Although anxiety disorders are the most prevalent mental health problems experienced by youth, it is often children with disruptive externalizing problems such as attention-deficit hyperactivity disorder (AD/HD) who come to the attention of school personnel. Children with anxiety disorders may be overlooked due to difficulty recognizing their internalizing symptoms, unfamiliarity with diagnostic criteria, and misconceptions regarding the negative consequences of these problems. Most school personnel are surprised to learn that approximately one in ten children suffers from an anxiety disorder, with epidemiological studies estimating prevalence rates between 9% and 20% in youth (Bitsko et al., 2022). Left untreated, these disorders tend to have long-term effects on social and emotional development. Negative consequences associated with anxiety disorders in youth include academic underachievement, underemployment, substance abuse, lower levels of social support, and high comorbidity with other psychiatric disorders (Wilmer et al., 2021). Moreover, evidence suggests that these disorders demonstrate a chronic course, often persisting into adulthood (Asselmann & Beesdo-Baum, 2015).

Take the example of Chris, an 11-year-old boy who is extremely shy, avoids answering questions in class, never asks his teacher for clarification when confused about assignments, accepts a failing grade rather than risk presenting in class, and does not talk much with other children. Without intervention, his grades will suffer, he will miss out on the mentorship his teacher could provide, and he will be isolated from his peers. Such a child is at risk for failing to achieve important developmental milestones. Research suggests that he is at risk for becoming depressed (Beesdo et al., 2010; Spence et al., 2018) or abusing alcohol and drugs to cope with his anxiety (Bushnell et al., 2019). However, if children like Chris could be identified early in their school years and receive appropriate interventions, this negative trajectory may be avoided. It is the purpose of this chapter to provide information to school personnel to aid them in identifying and intervening with children at risk for anxiety disorders.

Understanding Anxiety Disorders

There are eight types of anxiety disorders described in the *Diagnostic and Statistical Manual for Mental Disorders, Fifth Edition* (DSM-5; American Psychiatric Association [APA], 2022). Anxiety disorders refer to mental disorders characterized by excessive fear, anxiety, and related behavioral and cognitive disturbances, such as avoidance or anxiety-related rumination. Anxiety disorders differ by the type of situation, object, or event that elicits fear, anxiety, or leads to avoidance (APA, 2022). For this chapter, we are limiting our discussion to three of the most common anxiety

DOI: 10.4324/9781003392439-12

disorders—generalized anxiety disorder (GAD), social anxiety disorder, and separation anxiety disorder. These disorders tend to co-occur, and cognitive-behavioral treatments for these disorders follow similar protocols that are amenable to implementation in the school setting. Other childhood anxiety disorders, such as panic disorder, agoraphobia, or selective mutism, may require unique treatment components, including interoceptive exposure, social skills and language-based training, or psychopharmacological intervention (Amray et al., 2019; Bennett et al., 2016; Chhabra & Puar, 2016; Kaczkurkin & Foa, 2022).

The hallmark feature of GAD is at least six months of excessive anxiety and worry, occurring more days than not, about a number of events and activities that the child finds difficult to control (APA, 2022). The most common worries of children with GAD include worries about school performance, health, safety, and interpersonal relationships (Songco et al., 2020). GAD worries are distinct from everyday worries in that they are more pervasive, distressing, and impactful on a child's everyday functioning. Often, the worrying inherent in GAD occurs without a significant precipitant and is accompanied by physical symptoms, such as restlessness, feeling keyed up or on edge, difficulty concentrating, being easily fatigued, irritability, muscle tension, and sleep disturbance. Many children with GAD report feeling distressed by their worries or the ways their worrying impacts their ability to socialize with others, perform in school, engage in preferred activities, or interact with their family members (APA, 2022).

Social anxiety differs from GAD in that the child exhibits marked or persistent fear of specific situations—social or performance situations in which they may be negatively evaluated, leading to embarrassment or rejection (APA, 2022). Feared situations may include social interactions (e.g., having a conversation or meeting unfamiliar people), being observed (e.g., eating or drinking), or performing in front of others (e.g., public speaking, sports, or musical performances). When faced with such a situation, children with social anxiety disorder experience an intense anxiety response that may resemble a panic attack (e.g., experiencing heart pounding, sweating, and depersonalization). These children tend to avoid social or performance situations, although some may endure such situations with significant distress or discomfort. Adolescents may recognize that their fear is unreasonable, but children may not. The avoidance, fear, or anxious anticipation of these situations interferes significantly with the youth's functioning and/or causes marked distress. Due to anxiety, youth with social anxiety disorder may refuse to participate in school-related activities, such as presentations, raising their hand, writing on the board, or talking with teachers. They may also avoid eating at lunchtime, interacting with peers in and out of the school setting, or engaging in recreational performance activities, such as school band or athletic activities.

Separation anxiety disorder is characterized by at least four weeks of excessive anxiety concerning separation from the home or from major attachment figures (APA, 2022). This anxiety is beyond what is expected for the child's developmental level, occurs prior to 18 years of age, and causes significant distress or impairment. Children with this disorder may experience recurrent excessive distress when separation is anticipated or occurs, worry about harm befalling others, or worry that an untoward event will result in separation. These children are often preoccupied with the possibility of harm to themselves or attachment figures, such that they refuse to go to school, cannot sleep without attachment figures, or are unable to engage in preferred activities occurring outside the home or away from attachment figures. Many of these youth experience repeated nightmares about separation and physical symptoms (e.g., headaches, stomach aches, and nausea) when separation occurs or is anticipated (APA, 2022).

Empirical Support of School-Based CBT in Treatment of Anxiety Disorders

Cognitive-behavioral therapy (CBT) is considered an effective and 1st-line treatment for childhood anxiety disorders (Higa-McMillan et al., 2016; Levy et al., 2022; Pegg et al., 2022; Whiteside et al., 2020). Meta-analyses have concluded that approximately 60% of youth with anxiety recover following CBT treatment (Warwick et al., 2017). CBT for youth anxiety is traditionally administered individually, usually consisting of 12–20 weekly sessions, lasting up to an hour. However, it has also been found to be successfully administered in group settings, with families, and digitally. CBT incorporates a variety of cognitive and behavioral techniques to target anxiety-related cognitions and avoidance behavior. Although early efforts focused primarily on the child in treatment, more recent studies support incorporating the anxious child's social context, particularly the parents and school, into treatment. A number of treatment manuals that share many common elements have been developed for this population, perhaps best studied being the Coping Cat program (Lenz, 2015).

CBT-based prevention programs for childhood anxiety, which are delivered before the onset of a disorder, have been implemented widely in schools. In a meta-analysis examining school-based anxiety and depression prevention programs, Werner-Seidler et al. (2021) identified 33 RCTs examining anxiety-only prevention interventions which were all delivered in groups or digitally in schools. They found small but positive effects for both types of interventions (Werner-Seidler et al., 2021). An additional meta-analysis examining school-based RCTs for anxiety among school-aged children found that CBT-based programs were the most common and had significantly higher effect sizes than other types of programs (Zhang et al., 2023).

Several well-established, manualized interventions for anxiety have been successfully implemented in schools. These programs are listed in a meta-analysis by Werner-Seidler et al. (2021) and vary by the types of disorders they target (e.g., social anxiety, anxiety and depression together), whether they are targeted toward youth with anxiety symptoms or are universal prevention programs, and their use of evidence-based principles. CBT-based interventions for anxiety have several core components, outlined by Ginsburg and Smith (2023): psychoeducation, exposure, relaxation, challenging cognitions, problem-solving skills, social skills, parent psychoeducation, and relapse prevention. Here, we will highlight several well-established, CBT-based interventions delivered in schools.

The Coping Cat is a manualized CBT treatment protocol that has been proven to be effective for treating youth anxiety in a variety of large randomized controlled trials (Lenz, 2015). The Coping Cat has been adapted to school-based settings, where it has been delivered in once or twice a week groups, lasting 45 minutes each (Hajmohammadi et al., 2021). Sessions and structure are encouraged to be flexibly adapted based on school structure and provider needs. Examples of ways to flexibly adapt treatment include having 30-minute sessions twice a week, implementing the brief, eight-session Coping Cat, increasing parent involvement in treatment, and using computer-assisted lesson plans to deliver psychoeducation (Mychailyszyn et al., 2011).

The Unified Protocols for Transdiagnostic Treatment of Emotional Disorders in Children (UP-C) and Adolescents (UP-A) focus on a set of core principles and evidence-based techniques that target factors common to several disorders (e.g., anxiety, depression, obsessive-compulsive disorder, stress-related disorders), rather than anxiety alone (Kennedy et al., 2019). Treatment focuses on emotional avoidance, enhancing cognitive flexibility, and changing maladaptive actions. In a study of a nine-session, school-based UP-A group program with 28 adolescents, generalized anxiety and social anxiety symptoms (but not depressive symptoms) were significantly decreased after treatment (García-Escalera et al., 2019).

Skills for Academic and Social Success (SASS) is a CBT treatment specifically targeting social anxiety disorder that was specifically designed to be used in schools (Masia et al., 2001). A unique feature of SASS is that it is designed to be implemented by school counselors. SASS consists of 12 in-school group sessions focused on social skills, realistic thinking, and exposure. Adolescents who participated in SASS experienced significantly reduced anxiety when delivered both by counselors and by psychologists (Masia Warner et al., 2005, 2016; Mychailyszyn, 2017).

The FRIENDS program is a universal, CBT-based anxiety prevention program that is designed to be delivered in schools and provided to a whole class of children. FRIENDS has been found to be effective when delivered by psychologists, health educators, or teachers (Barrett & Turner, 2001).

The Cool Kids program is a program that is typically used with youth who are experiencing elevated anxiety, although it has been used as a universal prevention strategy as well (Ginsburg & Smith, 2023). Four studies evaluating Cool Kids, delivered in schools, found that it was associated with significant decreases in anxiety compared to both waitlist and active intervention controls (Berry & Hunt, 2009; Haugland et al., 2020; McLoone & Rapee, 2012; Mifsud & Rapee, 2005). This program has been successfully delivered in schools by researchers, school nurses, and school counselors.

Relational Considerations in the Treatment of Anxiety Disorders

Young children rely on adults in their lives to help them manage their emotions. As they age, they develop emotional regulation skills through interactions with caretakers and their environment and become more able to regulate their emotions with less help from others. When a child is anxious, it is normal and adaptive for adults to try to fix the problem and to help the children feel better as soon as possible. Adults, including school personnel, frequently help children calm down by reassuring them, soothing them, and taking them out of anxiety-provoking situations.

However, when children have anxiety disorders, these strategies may inadvertently maintain anxiety and avoidance. Over time, adults may find themselves anticipating a child's anxiety, avoiding situations that could trigger anxiety, and quickly jumping in to help the child cope with their emotions. These actions may decrease a child's upset in the short term but leave the child with fewer opportunities to learn coping strategies, thus exacerbating their anxiety and undermining their self-confidence. Lebowitz et al. (2020) describe parental accommodation of child anxiety as modifying family routines and behavior to prevent or reduce a child's anxiety in the short term. Maladaptive anxiety accommodation is different from appropriate educational accommodations required by law.

School personnel often feel pressured to engage in anxiety accommodation, including changing school routines and students' responsibilities to reduce anxiety. It is important to note that adaptive, short-term accommodations can be beneficial. For example, if a child has not been attending school due to anxiety, allowing the child to gradually increase their time in school and providing them with reinforcement for doing so may help develop positive associations with school and emotional coping strategies. However, when possible, it is recommended that school personnel work with parents, other teachers, and the child themselves to understand and decrease maladaptive anxiety accommodations.

Treatment of child anxiety proceeds best in the context of a caring, supportive relationship with a clinician who models acceptance and comfort with the child's anxiety. We have observed that the most effective clinicians demonstrate empathic attunement to the child's emotional experience while encouraging the child to face their fears gradually. Seeing a child in distress and not being able to help them can engender feelings of anxiety, helplessness, and frustration. It is most helpful to remain calm and validate the child's experience (e.g., *I am sorry you are feeling so upset*) instead of minimizing/criticizing their reactions (e.g., *There's nothing to be worried about, why are you overreacting?)* while gradually helping the child engage instead of avoiding when anxious.

Interviewing and Assessing Anxiety

Consistent with the empirical orientation of CBT, assessment occurs throughout treatment, providing information not only for case conceptualization and treatment planning but also for monitoring change over time. The CBT approach to assessment incorporates multiple methods (e.g., interviews, report inventories, and behavioral observations) and informants (e.g., child, teacher, and parent) to develop an idiographic, developmentally sensitive case conceptualization based on a comprehensive functional assessment. Drawing from Lang's tripartite model (Lang, 1968), anxiety should be assessed across cognitive, behavioral, and psychological components. Important areas to emphasize include the onset and development of anxiety symptoms as well as the historical and current socialization context (e.g., home and school) within which they developed. It is also critical to evaluate skill deficits (e.g., social skills, learning issues, emotional regulation) which can underlie anxiety issues.

Clinical interviews and functional behavioral assessment (FBA) of situations in which the child struggles yield valuable information regarding the nature of the child's anxiety symptoms as well as the conditions that trigger and maintain them. FBA helps identify the particular antecedents (i.e., what comes before) and consequences that may be associated with the child's adaptive and maladaptive responses. For example, the child may have developed classically conditioned fear responses to particular environmental triggers (e.g., fears of talking with other children after being bullied). It is not unusual for children's avoidant behaviors to be accommodated (e.g., a child with social anxiety does not have to answer questions in class), thus leading to short-term decreases in anxiety but reinforcing maladaptive anxiety, low self-efficacy, and avoidance in the long term. Similarly, FBAs help identify if the child engages in safety behaviors, actions that decrease their anxiety in the short term but perpetuate anxiety in the long run (e.g., texting a parent for reassurance while at school, only speaking in a whisper to minimize attention, hypervigilant scanning of peer's facial expressions to avoid rejection). FBAs may also reveal particular negative beliefs or thoughts children experience about themselves or situations that cue anxious arousal (e.g., *I can't do this. She thinks I'm stupid. I'm going to fail this test.*). Potential areas to assess for anxiety at school include places (e.g., cafeteria, playground, classroom), people (e.g., teachers or peers), and performance (e.g., tests, presentations, sports) (Kearney, 2008).

A clear diagnostic picture serves as a foundation for effective treatment. Semi-structured diagnostic interviews such as the Anxiety Disorders Interview for DSM-5, Parent and Child Versions (ADIS-5; Albano & Silverman, 2016) or the free Schedule for Affective Disorders and Schizophrenia for School-aged Children, Present and Lifetime Version (K-SADS-PL DSM-5; Kaufman et al., 2016) allow clinicians to do a thorough assessment of mental health disorders. The Anxiety Disorders Interview Schedule-Child/Parent, Parent Version (ADIS/ASA) can be helpful in differentiating anxiety disorders from symptoms of autism spectrum disorders (ASD) and ASD-related anxiety symptoms (Kerns et al., 2017). When time limitations in the school setting preclude administering diagnostic interviews, clinicians will still find the screening and specific diagnostic questions a good resource for targeted inquiries.

Diagnosis is only the 1st step in a meaningful assessment process. The expression of a disorder can vary widely from one youth to the next. For example, one child with anxiety in school may fear tests and experience performance anxieties, while another may experience overwhelming shyness and social concerns, and a 3rd may fear being separated from her mother. Moreover, many children meet criteria for more than one anxiety disorder. Some experts believe that an assessment along a continuum of internalizing symptoms may be more helpful for understanding and treating children's difficulties (Achenbach & Edelbrock, 1983). Many children may not meet full criteria for an anxiety disorder but still evidence difficulties with anxiety that warrant attention. Report inventories can provide information about broadband as well as specific anxiety symptoms. The Screening and Assessment Library of the School Health Assessment and Performance Evaluation System (SHAPE) developed by the National Center for School Mental Health offers an extensive list of free and low-cost measures for anxiety, depression, and other problem areas (https://www.theshapesystem.com/).

Although there are numerous report inventories, we will be limiting our discussion to a few of the most well-known, affordable, standardized measures that possess good to excellent psychometric properties (for further review, see Spence, 2018). These measures require only a short amount of time to administer, making them highly useful in school settings. Normative data for these measures enables the clinician to determine whether the child is reporting average or elevated levels of anxiety. Sensitive to change over time, they can be used to monitor treatment effects. None of these measures should be used for making a clinical diagnosis without more in-depth assessment (e.g., clinical interviews). Most of these inventories require a 2nd- or 3rd-grade reading level. For some anxious children, self-report inventories provide a less threatening means of sharing information.

Multidimensional inventories provide information about general anxiety levels and the type of anxiety symptoms experienced by youth. Three well-respected measures, the Spence Children's Anxiety Scale (SCAS; Spence, 1998), the Multidimensional Scale for Children Second Edition (MASC-2; 50 items, March, 2013), and the Screen for Anxiety-Related Emotional Disorders (SCARED; Birmaher et al., 1997) are available in numerous languages with parent and child self-report versions. An extensive research base supports their validity and reliability (for review, see Spence, 2018). These measures provide subscales that align with the DSM anxiety disorders (e.g., social, generalized, separation anxiety) and a total anxiety severity scale. A few unique aspects are noteworthy. For example, the SCAS and the SCARED are available for no cost online with some qualifications regarding use. An eight-item short form of the SCAS can be utilized to identify youth experiencing elevated levels of anxiety when evaluating larger groups of children or when time is limited (Reardon et al., 2018). Evidence supports the use of the SCAS with preschoolers and youth with ASD as well (Spence, 2018). The MASC assesses a range of anxiety symptoms while providing information about specific factors of anxiety: physical symptoms, social anxiety (humiliation/rejection, performance fears), harm avoidance (perfectionism, anxious coping), and separation/panic anxiety.

In addition to assessing anxiety in general, it may be helpful to evaluate specific aspects of anxiety through report inventories. The Severity Measure for Generalized Anxiety Disorder—Child Age 11–17 (ten items; Craske et al., 2013), the Penn State Worry Questionnaire for Children (14 items; Chorpita et al., 1997), and the Intolerance of Uncertainty Scale for Children (27 items; Comer et al., 2009; Read et al., 2013) enable clinicians to easily monitor key anxiety symptoms over time as they contain only a few items and are available online for no cost. The Revised Fear Survey Schedule for Children Child and Parent Versions (FSSC-R; Ollendick, 1983) allows clinicians to identify a child's specific fear sensitivities, providing information as to the focus of child worries. For social concerns, the Social Phobia and Anxiety Inventory for Children (Beidel et al., 1995) or the Revised Social Anxiety Scale for Children Child and Parent Versions (SASC-R; La Greca et al., 1988) may be useful. Of particular interest to school personnel, the School Refusal Assessment Scale (SRAS; Kearney & Silverman, 1993) assesses anxiety-related variables that may be involved in motivating and maintaining school refusal behavior. It is often important to assess depression as well as anxiety given the high comorbidity between these disorders. The Revised Children's Anxiety and Depression Scales (RCADS; Chorpita et al., 2000), a modification of the SCAS (Spence, 1998), includes depression and anxiety subscales (OCD, GAD, Separation anxiety, Panic and Social anxiety).

Broad assessment measures enable a more comprehensive understanding of the child's anxiety in the context of their general emotional and behavioral functioning. Frequently administered in schools, the Behavior Assessment System for Children, Third Edition (BASC-3; Reynolds et al., 2015) is a multimethod system for conducting a comprehensive assessment of behavioral and emotional functioning in youth (ages 2–25). The BASC includes teacher, parent, and youth self-report scales to gather multiple perspectives of youth behavior across settings using age-appropriate forms. Another form gathers information about the youth's course of development and family history, and a student observation form facilitates identifying and classifying directly observed classroom behavior. The BASC-3 yields clinical and adaptive behavior scales across numerous domains including an anxiety scale. Another useful system that assesses child behavior across internalizing and externalizing dimensions is the Achenbach System of Empirically Based Assessment that includes the CBCL 6–18, the Teacher Report Form (TRF), the Youth Report form (YRF), and the Caregiver-Teacher Report Form (Achenbach & Rescorla, 2000, 2001). The CBCL 6–18 provides scores on internalizing, externalizing, total problems, and DSM-IV-related scales. The TRF also includes open-ended questions which is particularly useful given that teachers have unique opportunities to observe children negotiating academic, personal, and social challenges. The CBCL 6–18 has been translated into many languages and multicultural norms are available (Achenbach & Rescorla, 2007).

A critical outcome of assessment for children with anxiety disorders is the development of a hierarchy of anxiety-provoking situations. Standardized ratings of the child's anxiety and avoidance, referred to as a subjective units of distress scale (SUDS) for each hierarchy item (e.g., 0–10 with anchor points defined), can be compared as the child progresses through treatment as another means of monitoring improvement. It often requires careful evaluation to pinpoint the exact nature of the child's fears and the optimal items to include in a hierarchy. For example, one child we treated had numerous performance concerns. Under scrutiny, it became clear that most concerns were related to his perception of his father's reaction to his performance. Thus, it was important to incorporate the father's reaction into this child's hierarchy and treatment.

CBT Conceptualization of the Problem

The cognitive-behavioral perspective views anxiety as an adaptive emotional response consisting of physiological, cognitive, and behavioral components. Anxiety can serve as a cue to signal impending danger, alerting a child to engage in adaptive behaviors to avoid stress or negative experiences, and triggering the body's "fight or flight" response (Freidl et al., 2017). An anxiety response often involves increased arousal of the autonomic nervous system, which may lead to physiological responses such as sweating, increased blood flow to the extremities, headaches, stomachaches, and tightening of muscles. The children's cognitions frequently concern estimations regarding the dangerousness of the threat and their own ability to cope. Behavioral reactions to anxiety differ from child to child but often include attempts to avoid anxiety-provoking situations or activities, crying, and expressions of irritability. Although anxiety reactions are often adaptive, some children experience maladaptive levels of anxiety in many situations that are not generally considered dangerous. These children may suffer from an anxiety disorder.

The triple vulnerability model (Barlow, 2000) views anxiety disorders as arising from three vulnerabilities: (a) a general genetic vulnerability, (b) a general psychological vulnerability concerning a sense of impending uncontrollable and unpredictable threat, and (c) a specific psychological vulnerability resulting from early learning experiences that lead a child to experience anxiety in certain situations.

Studies suggest that some individuals are more predisposed to experience increased arousal and anxiety responses to environmental triggers (Manassis et al., 2004). Kagan and colleagues (1989) identified a subset of behaviorally inhibited children who demonstrated an increased startle response, greater difficulty being soothed, and greater responsivity to novel stimuli. Family and twin studies also indicate heritability of some types of anxiety disorders (Manassis et al., 2004). Children genetically predisposed to a highly reactive arousal system, frequent negative emotional states, or difficulties understanding social interactions may experience a diminished sense of control over their emotional states, their environment, and their social world.

According to Chorpita and Barlow (1998), a sense of diminished control mediates the relationship between stressful life events and anxiety in early development and moderates this relationship in later development. Children may come to develop a sense of diminished control through experiences with their own predispositions combined with unpredictable, uncontrollable life events. Barlow (2000) hypothesized that early parenting is one avenue that affects a child's sense of control. For example, overcontrolled, unpredictable, or unresponsive family environments contribute to a sense of uncontrollability and an external locus of control. Once children have developed a diminished sense of control, they tend to perceive events as uncontrollable, even events for which the child could exhibit control. Anxious children's cognitions are characterized by overestimations of dangerousness of situations (e.g., predicting that an interaction with a teacher will frequently lead to being yelled at or humiliated) and underestimations of their ability to cope (e.g., believing that they do not know how to talk with a teacher or cannot handle it if someone is angry with them).

In terms of a specific psychological vulnerability, early socialization experiences (particularly in the family and school environments) contribute to experiencing anxiety in particular areas. As in social learning theory (Bandura & Walters, 1977), children may learn specific anxiety responses through modeling or information transmission regarding potential dangers. A child may learn to be anxious by seeing adults experiencing high levels of anxiety, underestimating their own self-efficacy, or delivering excessive warnings about potential harm. Also, children may develop heightened anxiety responses due to particular conditioning experiences that become overgeneralized. For example, a child could have a negative experience presenting in front of the class (e.g., having an anxiety attack, being harshly criticized, or being teased by peers) and then develop a conditioned, generalized anxiety response to social situations. Children may also learn that they can avoid experiencing anxiety by avoiding situations that evoke this response. Mowrer's two-factor theory (1960) posits that their avoidant responses increase in frequency as decreases in anxiety negatively reinforce them. Adults in the lives of anxious children may also come to reinforce avoidant or dependent behavior inadvertently.

Following the tripartite model, treatment could focus on multiple areas depending on the particular vulnerabilities of the child. Primarily, interventions seek to increase a child's sense of control by providing children with opportunities to exercise control over their environment, engage in mastery experiences, explore their world with age-appropriate levels of independence, develop skills, and develop coping responses (Barlow, 2000). Implementing more adaptive thinking and behavioral patterns is encouraged through teaching skills, modeling, contingency management, and exposure exercises. Interventions could occur individually or in groups within the school setting. Individual or group meetings with parents are often an important component of the treatment. Within the school and family context, treatment interventions encourage consistency, responsive teaching/parenting, adaptive modeling, and the communication of appropriate, adaptive messages regarding potential threats. Most CBT treatments recommend a combination of skill-building exercises and gradual exposure to anxiety-provoking situations to help children increase their sense of self-efficacy and decrease their perception of impending threat.

Session Structure

Although educative, the format of individual and group CBT encourages participation through questions, games, and humor. Great emphasis is placed on building group cohesion through a variety of exercises (see Flannery-Schroeder & Kendall, 2000) and making the sessions fun. Almost all sessions include time at the end to play games, such as Jenga or Nerf basketball. Children receive rewards for completing homework, called Show That I Can (STIC) tasks, between sessions to practice new skills and promote generalization of treatment effects. Each treatment session begins with a review of these tasks, which serves as a means by which the session content can be personalized to the child's current experiences. At various points in the treatment, the therapist talks with parents to gather information, update them on their child's progress, and enlist their aid in setting up therapeutic exposures to anxiety-provoking situations at home or school. Teachers also participate by providing information, monitoring in-class exposures, and praising the children for engaging in more adaptive behavior.

Component of Practice and Intervention Modules

There exists a core set of techniques found in most cognitive-behavioral treatments for anxious youth. Cognitive-behavioral treatments are based on the premise that anxious children may benefit from the internalization and subsequent use of a set of coping skills, as well as repeated and prolonged exposure to feared objects, situations, and/or events. Various CBT protocols may differ in the number, sequencing, and time devoted to the training of coping skills; however, most treatment packages include instruction in the following four domains: somatic management, cognitive restructuring, problem-solving, contingency management, and therapeutic exposure with exposure being the most underused yet impactful intervention (Whiteside et al., 2020). For a more extensive discussion of these components, see Chu and Pimentel (2023).

Somatic Management

Compared to non-anxious youth, youth with anxiety disorders have less understanding of ways in which they can modify their emotional experiences. Often, uncomfortable physical symptoms of anxiety can make a child even more nervous, leading to perceptions that a child is "out of control" of their emotional experiences. Physical symptoms of anxiety tend to exacerbate a child's already intense anxious thinking, and children may complain of intense physical discomfort in an effort to avoid feared situations.

In order to best develop skill in modifying one's own anxiety reactions, children must learn to recognize their own individualized somatic reactions to anxiety. These individual responses that are unique to each child (e.g., red ears, stomach pain, trembling voice, urge to urinate, lightheadedness, nausea, headache) serve as clues for the child to label their emotional reaction "anxious." Once labeled, children can learn various cognitive and behavioral strategies to decrease their somatic responses. Relaxation training and mindfulness techniques are powerful tools that can help children decrease their somatic arousal in a variety of situations.

Cognitive Restructuring

The use of cognitive therapy techniques in the treatment of child anxiety is based on the premise that anxiety stems from irrational or maladaptive thoughts, beliefs, or self-talk. Research has documented that anxious children demonstrate distortions in information processing, memory biases for distressing events, hypersensitivity to threat cues, and a bias toward interpreting ambiguous situations as threatening (Dudeney et al., 2015; Hadwin et al., 2006; Nikolić, 2020). Thus, the use of cognitive techniques designed to modify the maladaptive nature of anxious self-talk is compelling.

Various techniques have been developed to assist children with identifying their cognitions in anxiety-provoking situations. Kendall's use of a "thought bubble" is one example (Kendall & Hedtke, 2006). Children are shown various cartoons in which people's thoughts or statements appear in a bubble above their heads. Children are then prompted by the question, "What's in your thought bubble?" Once children are proficient at identifying self-talk, they are then instructed to undergo a rational analysis of the thoughts: Are their predictions likely to happen? Have they happened before? Would it really be so bad if they did happen? Is there another way of looking at the situation? After such an analysis, children can generate coping thoughts to counter their initial anxious thoughts. Younger children may have a more difficult time in learning to identify and modify their self-talk. They may rely on coping thoughts (e.g., *Facing my fears makes me stronger*) as opposed to cognitive restructuring to manage their anxiety reactions. Children may also benefit from externalizing their anxious thoughts through creating a character that represents their anxious thinking and behavior, such as "the worry monster." Children can then discuss what their "worry monster" is telling them and work with school clinicians to challenge or "turn down the volume" of that part of themselves.

Problem-Solving

Problem-solving interventions are intended to target the cognitive processes that mediate competence and generalize to various situations. In CBT for child anxiety, children learn to engage in problem-solving to generate and evaluate specific actions to cope more effectively with anxiety-provoking situations. Typical problem-solving steps include (1) identify situations or cues that trigger anxiety, (2) brainstorm possible coping strategies (actions and thoughts) without evaluating them, (3) evaluate the potential coping strategies, (4) select the best alternative or combination of alternatives, (5) implement the chosen coping strategies, (6) evaluate the effectiveness of the coping strategy, and (7) modify the coping strategy as needed. Implementing more effective coping strategies is posited to increase a child's self-efficacy and reduce anxiety.

The cognitive-behavioral approach to problem-solving requires that the therapist lead the anxious child sequentially through these steps under the guiding principle of collaborative empiricism. Together, the therapist and child generate numerous potential solutions without regard to their potential utility until the alternatives are exhausted. Solutions include actions and self-talk that can help children cope more effectively with anxiety-provoking situations. Once the child has identified those alternatives likely to be helpful in the resolution of the problem, he or she has developed an excellent problem-solving strategy. Children are more engaged in the problem-solving process when it is fun. Using timers, awarding prizes for generating solutions, and encouraging gentle competition can make problem-solving a game that children enjoy.

Contingency Management

One of the fundamental principles of behavior therapy is the emphasis placed on the contingencies (antecedents and consequences) of behavior. Behavior change can be achieved through the effective management of contingencies. An effective contingency management plan rests on a functional analysis of the contingencies (antecedents and consequences) maintaining maladaptive avoidant behavior and the contingencies that may support more adaptive behavior.

Children's avoidant behaviors are often negatively reinforced (leaving or avoiding a situation results in decreased feelings of anxiety in the short-term). Moreover, maladaptive responses (e.g., crying, leaving a classroom, going to the nurse) may be inadvertently positively reinforced by teachers, staff, and parents. An important component to treatment may be to discontinue reinforcement for maladaptive behavior. For example, teachers may sit a child to the side in a classroom, adopting a neutral stance, while the child calms down versus talking intently with the child in an effort to calm him. The teacher then would provide greater levels of attention when the child engages in more adaptive behavior.

In efforts to increase "brave" behavior (i.e., approach rather than avoidant strategies), anxious children are offered opportunities to earn reinforcers in many cognitive-behavioral treatment protocols. Reinforcement or "reward" systems are believed to be beneficial in reducing child anxiety by promoting engagement in treatment strategies such as homework, exposure tasks, and self-evaluation procedures. Reinforcers are used to shape and maintain behavioral improvements but are effective only to the extent that they meet with children's desires and preferences. That is, a reinforcer is only rewarding if it is desired. The successful use of contingency management procedures involves skilled selection of rewards—individualized per each child. Rewards may be material (e.g., small toys, games, sports cards) or social (e.g., playing miniature golf with a parent, seeing a movie with a friend). Often, those rewards at the start of treatment will be material, with social rewards being encouraged in the latter half of treatment. In this way, school personnel and parents will have greater success in the immediate (and less costly) provision of rewards, ultimately leading to improved maintenance of treatment effects.

Exposure

Following the skill acquisition phase of the treatment, CBT therapies use graded exposure tasks (i.e., gradual exposure to feared situations, objects, and/or events) to help children learn new, more adaptive information about the situations they fear and their own ability to cope. Exposure to feared stimuli provides the opportunity for children to learn that they can experience anxiety without truly harmful consequences and that the situations they had feared are less likely and less dangerous than they had previously believed. These new adaptive associations then compete with and inhibit previously learned associations that evoke anxiety. The experiential nature of exposures with the activation of a child's internal fear networks is critical for new learning to occur. During exposures, youth experience activation of anxiety, associated cognitions (e.g., I will look stupid and everyone will hate me, I can't handle this feeling, This feeling will never end), and behavioral responses (e.g., leave the situation, shut down, argue, ruminate, cry). Experiencing violations of their expectancies (e.g., anxiety decreasing just by staying in the situation, answering a question wrong in class does not lead to peer rejection) facilitates the learning of more realistic, adaptive associations. Exposures may be either in vivo or imaginal and can occur both in and out of the school environment.

The exposure technique can be conceived of as a gradual shaping process. It involves the use of a hierarchy of anxiety-eliciting objects and events and also often requires that the therapist address basic component skills first before moving on to more complex situations, events, or interactions. For example, while "meeting a new person" might assume a place on the hierarchy, the component skills (e.g., eye contact) would likely be addressed first. Thus, the exposure process proceeds in a gradual but incremental fashion. The fear hierarchy is created in the spirit of collaborative empiricism in which exposure tasks are conceived of as "experiments." After "experimenting," the child and therapist will examine what the child learned during the experience. Learning is facilitated by having the child predict what they think will happen prior to the exposure and comparing it to what actually happened through a process of guided discovery. The child will learn best when they discover discrepancies between their predictions and the actual outcomes versus the therapist telling them what they should think or giving them advice. For example, a child giving a talk in front of the class might predict that they will experience an anxiety level of 10 that will last for hours. The child and therapist can plot out the child's anxiety levels through SUDS scores rated before, during, and after the presentation to examine the experienced anxiety levels and compare them to the expected levels. Post-exposure processing helps solidify the child's self-efficacy, learning that they can tolerate anxiety symptoms, the anxiety-provoking situations are not actually harmful, and they can cope effectively. For further discussion of this issue and a practice-oriented description of the use of exposures in child anxiety treatment, see Chu and Pimentel (2023) and Kendall et al. (2005).

Assessment of Progress and Outcomes

Collaborative and ongoing assessment of a youth's response to treatment provides critical information. Helping youth recognize their gains through charting their anxiety levels or goals they have attained can facilitate their sense of mastery and self-efficacy. Alternatively, a lack of progress serves as a catalyst to reconsider one's case conceptualization, identify alternative maintaining factors, and adjust one's intervention strategy.

The report inventories described in the assessment section can all be utilized to measure treatment progress. Another measure sensitive to change over time, the Coping Questionnaire (CQ; parent and child versions; Kendall, 1994), assesses the child's ability to manage three anxiety-provoking situations that are identified based on interview data. The child and parent rate the child's ability to cope with each on a 7-point scale (1 = not at all able to help myself to 7 = completely able to help myself feel comfortable). Changes in coping are associated with treatment outcomes (Kendall et al., 2016; Luo & McAloon, 2021). Idiographic measures such as anxiety hierarchy SUDS ratings and tracking of operationally defined target behaviors (e.g., frequency of asking questions in class or attending school) enable one to monitor specific child-focused functional outcomes.

Several treatments for youth anxiety include measures which are intended to track treatment progress and guide clinical decision-making. This is known as measurement-based care or routine outcome monitoring (Scott & Lewis, 2015). Many of the measures that are used to assess anxiety, as mentioned earlier in this chapter, are also used to monitor treatment progress. However, the ability to compare treatments and assess their efficacy is hampered due to significant heterogeneity in outcome data reported (Patton et al., 2022). In the STARS treatment trial (Ginsburg et al., 2020), anxiety was assessed by the Clinical Global Impression—Severity and Improvement Scales (CGI- S/I; Guy, 1976), the Children's Global Assessment Scale (CGAS; Shaffer et al., 1983), and the Screen for Anxiety-Related Emotional Disorders (SCARED—P/C; Birmaher et al., 1997). In a meta-analysis assessing school-based anxiety prevention programs, the most commonly used measures used to assess anxiety symptoms were the SCAS (30% of trials; Spence, 1998), the MASC (15%; March et al., 1997), the Revised Children's Manifest Anxiety Scale (RCMAS; 12%; Reynolds & Richmond, 1978), and the DASS-Anxiety Subscale (9%; Lovibond & Lovibond, 1995).

Applications to the School Setting

School-based cognitive behavioral interventions for anxiety disorders are compelling for several reasons. First, anxiety often arises in school settings and revolves around school-related issues. It is not uncommon to see anxious children exhibiting perfectionism in homework assignments, test or performance anxiety, school refusal behavior, frequent trips to the school nurse and/or phone calls home from school, unwillingness to speak up or read aloud in school, difficulties in social interactions, and reluctance to trying new things. In CBT treatment planning, every effort is made to provide children with practice in coping with those situations which elicit anxiety. Often, it is the case that therapists working in clinics use approximations to the school situations (e.g., giving a mock test in a therapy session to a test anxious child, having a socially anxious youngster read aloud in front of the therapist); however, it is likely that these mock trials are not as potent as exposures to "real world" school events. Thus, school-based interventions are more likely to ensure that skills transfer to the natural environment.

Second, school-based interventions are amenable to group and/or classroom applications. Coping skills acquisition and practice, the focus of CBT treatments, while of relevance to anxious children, are likely to benefit non-anxious or mildly (i.e., non-clinically) anxious children as well. Classroom interventions face a captive audience, and children are accustomed to learning skills in the school setting. Just as positive health behaviors are taught in traditional health "classes," so might skills for emotional health. While CBT interventions involve standardized application in order to ensure treatment integrity, the interventions are best applied flexibly. The ease of class-wide application, potential for flexible applications, and provision of a general skill set to benefit all makes school-based prevention interventions for childhood anxiety disorders an attractive approach.

Third, educational environments are a fruitful setting in which to implement a variety of interventions because they offer the opportunity to reach a broad range of youth, including individuals who may not have otherwise had access to or been knowledgeable about needed services. Interventions in school settings can provide affordable and quality services to youth who come from under-resourced communities or to youth in lower socioeconomic brackets. Further, because youth across all demographics and with a variety of risk and resilience factors attend schools, implementing interventions in this setting can offer the 1st line of defense in addressing youth with more severe symptomatology, especially if they are initially or frequently unable to access other intervention services for a variety of reasons (e.g., income, transportation barriers, knowledge of services, etc.).

Finally, the proximity to teachers is in and of itself a compelling therapeutic feature for several reasons. Teachers often have important perspectives on children's behaviors. School settings offer teachers unique opportunities to observe children in situations that may be less likely to occur outside of school (e.g., speaking in front of a group of people). It is often the case that teachers can provide critical information about a child's anxieties that is extremely useful in treatment planning. Opportunities for training teachers about the identification and modification of anxious behaviors within the classroom should be promoted to facilitate use of such information. Teachers spend a significant proportion of time with children (approximately six to seven hours a day) and serve as very influential role models. Thus, their familiarity with key concepts in combating child anxiety (promotion of approach behaviors in the face of anxiety-eliciting events, use of positive self-talk) would be of tremendous benefit. With training of teachers as well as other key school personnel, the existing high rates of anxiety disorders may be attenuated by the effective use of proactive rather than reactive strategies. An emphasis on prevention of childhood anxiety disorders should complement the current emphasis on the successful treatment of these disorders. The following case example illustrates one way in which children's anxiety problems have been successfully treated in the school setting.

Case Example

At the beginning of this chapter, we discussed some of the difficulties experienced by Chris, a dark-haired, 11-year-old boy who was referred to the school psychologist for evaluation to determine if recent academic problems were related to a learning problem and/or fueled by Chris's anxiety. Although typically not a behavior problem at school, Chris had failed to complete several book reports that were to be accompanied by oral presentations. On several occasions, he also had "melt-downs" in the classroom when he prematurely gave up on tests or assignments, sometimes crying or trying to leave the classroom. His teacher had tried to talk with him about the problem, but he had little to offer regarding why he was not completing his work. His teacher then talked with his parents, who were surprised to learn about the uncompleted book reports but discussed how Chris's problems with perfectionism and shyness had interfered in other areas of his life, such as playing sports. For example, although Chris used to play soccer and enjoyed it, on several occasions in the past year, he left the field and refused to play after making small mistakes or during close games. In the current year, he would not play soccer at all, despite his parent's encouragement to do so. They could identify no recent stressors or changes that may have accounted for his difficulties. Given that Chris tended to perform well on other class assignments, they wondered if Chris's long-standing difficulties starting conversations with others and his tendency to avoid social situations had something to do with his current school problems.

It is important to remember that, at times, children may have an anxiety problem secondary to a learning issue. Often, these children benefit from interventions that target both learning and anxiety issues. However, an evaluation of academic achievement and cognitive skills did not reveal cognitive or learning impairments that would account for Chris's difficulties. Along with a general psychosocial interview, the school psychologist administered portions of the ADIS-5 to Chris and his parents. She found that Chris met the criteria for social anxiety disorder (severity rating 6 out of 8) and GAD (severity rating 5 out of 8). Chris did not report many symptoms but did acknowledge some social anxiety. His parents and his teacher provided the most information about the level of his avoidance. Chris appeared to feel uncomfortable in most types of social situations and avoided talking with people except his family and a few close friends he had known since kindergarten. He managed school by keeping to himself and only talking to the teacher when directly addressed. On the MASC and SASC-R, Chris scored in the clinical range and endorsed many items that he had not discussed in his interview. These measures were administered at the beginning, midpoint, and end of treatment to monitor Chris's progress. Table 9.1 provides Chris's treatment goals.

Table 9.1 Chris's Initial Treatment Goals

	The Case of Chris: Initial Treatment Goals
Goal 1	Identify and recognize somatic reactions to anxiety-provoking situations as cues to know when to use coping skills "*Am I feeling frightened?*" "*What's happening in my body?*"
Goal 2	Identify and modify anxious self-talk to decrease anxiety/avoidance and improve self-efficacy "What is my self-talk?" "Am I expecting bad things to happen?" "What else might happen?" "What is a coping thought I can have in this situation?" Examples of coping thoughts: – "It won't be as bad as I think." – "I can do hard things." – "I can help myself feel better when I get scared."
Goal 3	Develop and apply a framework of problem-solving to improve coping 1 What is the anxious situation? 2 What might someone do to make this situation less fearful? 3 Which solutions are feasible alternatives? Are there any solutions that do not make sense or are impossible? 4 What might be one of the best things to do? What is the preferred solution?
Goal 4	Engage in positive evaluation and reward oneself for engaging in challenging tasks. Examples: – Praising oneself for effort: "I did a good job today trying something new" – Playing a favorite game following a feared activity – Having a piece of candy after saying hello to a new person
Goal 5	Decrease anxiety and avoidance related to social interactions with peers, schoolwork, and playing sports while increasing coping skills and self-efficacy through therapeutic exposure Imaginal exposures examples – Imagining traveling alone to an unknown place – Picturing embarrassing oneself in front of others – Visualizing arriving late to important events In-vivo examples – going someplace new with minimal directions – making intentional errors during a sports game – arriving late to a social gathering – engaging in intentionally silly or embarrassing acts in public – making a new friend at school – making a mistake on purpose on a homework assignment – giving a speech or presentation to classmates

Course of Treatment

Chris participated in a weekly 12-session CBT group at school based on the Coping Cat Program developed by Kendall and colleagues (Flannery-Schroeder & Kendall, 2000). Table 9.2 provides an overview of the 12 sessions. The Coping Cat program teaches children to use coping strategies while

Table 9.2 Coping Cat Group Program

	Coping Cat Group Program
Session 1	Introduction to Program Build Rapport and Group Cohesion A Engage in similarities activity and I remember game B Collaboratively create group name and symbol C Share buddy list contact information D Distribute Coping Cat notebooks E Psychoeducation about anxiety; normalization of anxiety response; develop list of situations that make most people nervous F STIC assignment—write about a time when felt good and when felt anxious during the week in notebook G Participation reward
Session 2	Affective Education and Identifying Somatic Cues for Anxiety A I remember game B Review completed STIC tasks C Feelings associated with bodily cues; somatic symptoms of anxiety D Brainstorm a feelings list, role play feelings or create a feelings collage poster E Recognizing somatic anxiety cues role plays/practice F Begin FEAR plan poster—F step—feeling frightened? G Introduce Anxiety Thermometer (1–5 scale) H STIC task—record bodily reactions to anxiety over the week I Buddy assignment—contact group buddy to answer a specific question
Session 3	Relaxation training A Review STIC tasks B Feelings matching worksheet C Review STIC and buddy assignments D Complete fear-rating worksheets E Rationale for learning relaxation F Rag doll and robot exercise G Learn progressive muscle relaxation exercises or another relaxation method H Model coping with anxiety using relaxation exercise I STIC task—practice relaxation exercises three times J Buddy assignment—contact buddy to answer another closed question
Session 4	Cognitive restructuring A Review STIC task and buddy assignments B Review and practice relaxation exercises C Introduce thought-feeling connection using thought bubbles and self-talk D FEAR plan—introduce E step—expecting bad things to happen E Practice identifying self-talk with cartoons, modeling, and role plays F Practice challenging self-talk G Cohesion-building game H STIC task—record anxiety severity and thoughts in two anxious situations over the coming week I Buddy assignment—contact buddy and ask two closed questions without a script

(*Continued*)

Table 9.2 (Continued)

	Coping Cat Group Program
Session 5	Problem solving: Developing a plan to cope with anxiety A Review STIC tasks and buddy assignments B Practice identifying anxious and coping self-talk C Review FEAR plan steps F and E D Discuss strategies to cope with physiological arousal (F step) and anxious thinking (E step) E FEAR plan poster—introduce A step—actions and attitudes that help F Teach problem-solving steps G Practice problem-solving H Challenging thoughts group debate I STIC task—use FEA steps in two anxious situations J Buddy assignment—ask buddy two questions the child thinks up on their own
Session 6	Rating and rewards; review and practice FEAR plan A Review STIC tasks and buddy assignments B Practice relaxation training C FEAR plan poster—introduce R step—ratings and rewards D Teach about self-rating of one's performance and self-reinforcement E Create individualized performance barometers and rewards lists F Review FEAR plan using stories; discuss when could use FEAR plan G Make pocket-sized FEAR plan cards H Modeling/Practice how could use FEAR plan I Discuss rationale and procedure for exposures J STIC task—explain FEAR plan to another person, practice FEAR plan in one situation K Buddy assignment—contact buddy to ask open-ended and follow-up question provided by group leader
Session 7	Exposures and FEAR plan—group practice A Review STIC tasks and buddy assignments B Reinforce understanding of exposures (e.g., duration, repetition, and avoidance concepts) C Engage group in imaginal and/or in vivo exposures to low anxiety-provoking situations using FEAR plan D Collaboratively select moderate anxiety-provoking situations to practice in next session E STIC task—practice FEAR plan in one anxious situation, draw character who can help child cope with anxiety F Buddy assignment—provide information about themselves to their buddies
Session 8	Exposures and FEAR plan—group practice A Review STIC tasks and buddy assignments B Engage group in imaginal and/or in-vivo exposures to moderate anxiety-provoking situations using FEAR plan C STIC task—practice FEAR plan in two anxiety-provoking situations; create coping story for character D Buddy assignment—share stories with their buddies by phone

(*Continued*)

Table 9.2 (Continued)

	Coping Cat Group Program
Session 9	Exposures and FEAR plan—group practice A Review STIC tasks and buddy assignments B Engage group in imaginal and/or in-vivo exposures to moderate anxiety-provoking situations using FEAR plan C Video record group members practicing coping strategies during in-vivo exposures D Members re-rate performance after watching video E STIC task—Practice FEAR plan in two anxiety-provoking situations; make individual FEAR plan posters F Buddy assignment—brainstorm ideas for the end-of-program party with buddy
Session 10	Exposures and FEAR plan—individual practice A Group member leads discussion of STIC tasks B Discuss group members' feelings about the group C Engage individuals in imaginal and/or in-vivo exposures to high anxiety-provoking situations using FEAR plan D Practice relaxation in high anxiety situation E Further practice of coping strategies in vivo F STIC task—practice FEAR plan in two anxiety-provoking situations; begin planning for commercial G Buddy assignment—talk by phone with buddy
Session 11	Exposures and FEAR plan—individual practice A Group member leads discussion of STIC tasks B Discuss group members' feelings about the group C Engage individuals in imaginal and/or in-vivo exposures to high anxiety-provoking situations using FEAR plan D Plan for commercial E STIC task—practice FEAR plan in two anxiety-provoking situations; gather props for commercial F Buddy assignment—buddies discuss their feelings about the group
Final session	Termination and relapse prevention A Group members discuss STIC tasks B Videorecord the commercial C View commercial with group D Group social event E Discuss each member's accomplishments F Relapse prevention planning and exposure lifestyle G Good-bye ritual (e.g., presentation of certificate)
	Additional components
Evaluation	Pre- and post-treatment child and program assessment A Conduct pre-treatment assessment (e.g., interviews, measures) B Conduct post-treatment assessment (e.g., interviews, measures)

(*Continued*)

Table 9.2 (Continued)

	Coping Cat Group Program
Parent contact	Individualized parent phone, video, or in-person meetings and assessment May vary greatly based on need, parent interest, and school clinician's availability A Provide treatment information B Discuss child and concerns C Administer parent-report inventories before and after treatment D Educate about anxiety accommodation and FEAR plan E Hierarchy development F How parents can be involved G Prepare parents for exposure portion of program H Check-in regarding home exposures I Discuss child progress and ongoing parental concerns

engaging in activities they previously avoided due to anxiety. These coping strategies are referred to as the FEAR plan:

Step 1. The "F" Step, "Am I Feeling anxious? What does my body tell me?"
Step 2. The "E" Step, "What am I Expecting to happen? What is my self-talk?"
Step 3. The "A" Step, "What Actions and Attitudes can best help me in this situation?"
Step 4. The "R" Step, "What self-Ratings and Rewards do I receive for trying to cope?"

Chris's group consisted of three boys who shared similar concerns but also had some unique difficulties. For example, one of the group members (Jordan) had fears of separating from his mother, which led him to have difficulty attending school, resulting in missed school days, frequent trips to the school nurse, daily calls home, and crying spells in the classroom. The 3rd group member (Elijah) could be described as a "worrier." Elijah's worries involved numerous areas, including his performance in school and sports, his family's finances, his family's health, his own health, and even the health of "Bingo," his family's dog. Additionally, he exhibited a rigid insistence on punctuality and was overly concerned about looking foolish.

The focus of the 1st session was to build rapport among the group members, introduce them to the program, and encourage their participation. Chris tended to be quiet, responding with one-word answers to most questions. To facilitate group interaction, the boys played a personal facts game, decorated their program workbooks, and made lists of rewards they would like to earn in the program. Chris could only think of two possible rewards, baseball cards and Lego® bricks, so the therapist suggested he add to the list over the coming week. Children were encouraged to develop a rich, meaningful reward list that included activities (e.g., renting a movie), social events (e.g., playing a game with mom), and tangible rewards (e.g., toys). The children received information about the normal, adaptive nature of anxiety reactions and made a list of common anxieties most people experience. Chris seemed relieved to hear that one out of ten kids has some difficulties with anxiety, and all people experience anxiety in some form as a normal part of life. The therapist provided an example of a situation that made her nervous (speaking in front of other people) and how the steps in the program had helped her cope with this fear. She also talked about the ways the program had helped other children. Chris later stated that he believed the program might help him because the therapist said that the goal was to make anxiety easier to handle, not to make it completely go away, and that the program had helped other kids.

Sessions 2 and 3 focused on learning about emotions, managing somatic reactions to anxiety, and cohesion building. In Session 2, the group discussed how different feelings are associated with different physical expressions, and these physical expressions can act as clues to identify how someone is feeling. They looked at pictures of kids showing different emotions and took turns guessing what emotion the picture was demonstrating, identifying critical facial and postural clues. They played "feelings charades" and created a "feelings collage." The therapist also introduced the "feelings thermometer," a large picture of a thermometer with ratings from 0 to 8 that identify low to high levels of anxiety. The feelings thermometer helped Chris begin to identify how much anxiety he felt in different situations, giving him a means to notice differences in his levels of anxiety and language for describing his emotional experience to others. Each child then started to write down a personal hierarchy of anxiety-provoking situations, including low, mid, and high anxiety-provoking situations. Initially, Chris could only identify a few situations for his hierarchy but input from teachers and parents led to the identification of numerous anxiety-provoking situations in later sessions. The children discussed how people experience various bodily reactions when feeling anxious. For example, they talked about how a famous basketball player might experience anxiety in his body (e.g., sweaty palms, stomach ache) when having to make a free throw in the last second of the game with the score tied. They then talked about their own body's reaction to specific situations and how these reactions can serve as clues to alert the child that he is feeling anxious. Each child took a turn imagining himself in a situation that usually made him anxious to help him identify his bodily reactions. Chris imagined having the teacher call on him in class when he did not know the answer. He reported experiencing tightness in his stomach and "jittery legs." After outlining their bodies on large pieces of butcher paper placed on the floor, the children used markers to illustrate how their body responded to anxiety (e.g., butterflies in the stomach, red lines around the head for a headache, shading in the shoulders for muscle tension).

In Session 3, the group began learning relaxation exercises. The therapist discussed the idea that when someone is feeling anxious and worried, some parts of his body are likely tense. If he can relax the tense parts, he will be taking the 1st step in coping with his anxiety. The children took turns tensing their arms by making fists and noting the differences in the sensations when the arm was relaxed and when it was tense. A volunteer acted like a robot to illustrate tense muscles, and another pretended to be a wet noodle to show relaxed muscles. The boys were encouraged to lie down, close their eyes, and do a few progressive relaxation exercises. These exercises involved tensing and releasing different muscle groups to achieve a state of relaxation. See Koeppen (1974) for a young children's relaxation script and Ollendick and Cerny (2013) for an older children's script. Throughout treatment, the boys practiced the exercises by listening to audiotapes of the therapist reading portions of the relaxation script at home. In addition, relaxation was reviewed and practiced in many of the group sessions.

The goal of Session 4 was to help the children begin to identify their thoughts (particularly in anxious situations) and to understand that certain types of thoughts may increase their anxiety. The therapist began by showing cartoons with empty thought bubbles and asked the children to identify what they thought the character was thinking. They then linked what the person might feel and do if they had particular thoughts. Alternative thoughts to the same situation were proposed so the children could see that different people may have different thoughts and reactions to the same situation. Through these examples, the children learned that anxiety usually accompanied thoughts related to expecting something bad to happen. This idea led to proposing how one person may feel one way with one type of thought (e.g., expecting something bad to happen) and another way if the same person had a different type of thought (e.g., expecting something good to happen). Different cartoons and scenarios were presented while the children took turns answering questions. Chris was still very quiet in session but would occasionally answer questions and appeared to be listening when others were talking.

The therapist then told a story about a mildly anxiety-provoking situation (e.g., a boy drops a book in the hallway) and asked the group to think of a set of thoughts that would help the boy cope (reduce distress) and a set of thoughts that would lead to anxiety (more distress) as well as the behaviors that would likely follow from each set of thoughts. It was proposed that, with some practice, they could learn to change some of their anxious self-talk to coping self-talk to help themselves feel better. They were then introduced to a set of questions to ask themselves to help them begin to change their thinking and a set of "thinking traps" that often "trick" people into feeling anxious.

The group then did a few role-plays in which they began to implement the 1st two steps for coping with anxiety. The therapist had Chris imagine that he was asked a question in class. Using the FEAR plan, Chris was directed to follow the 1st step in coping with anxiety, the "F" step, and ask himself if he was feeling anxious if his body was sending him any clues (e.g., sweaty palms) that would help him tell that he was anxious. Chris said he felt "jittery" in his stomach and maybe a little anxious. Chris then was asked to engage in Step 2, the "E" step, and ask himself if he was expecting anything bad to happen. In this case, he thought he would sound stupid, other kids would laugh at him, and everyone would think he was weird. The therapist had Chris fill in a three-column table on a dry-erase board with the situation, his feelings (Step 1), and his thoughts (Step 2). Chris identified a few thinking traps characterizing his self-talk. The group then gathered evidence to support and refute Chris's negative expectations. Chris wrote down a few coping thoughts, such as "The kids in this group would not think I was stupid even if I didn't know an answer, so maybe the kids in class might not think so," "Even if they laugh at me, they might not think I'm weird because even popular kids get laughed at some times," "If they laugh at me, it will probably feel bad but only for 20 minutes or so (according to Chris's estimation); it won't feel bad forever," "Other kids might not really care so much about how I answer the question," and "Just do it."

When engaging in challenging thoughts, it was particularly critical for the therapist to adopt a posture of collaborative empiricism. Sometimes, therapists jump in too early to contradict the child's thoughts of potential harm or tell them what to think. The child then may give lip service to agreeing with the therapist's challenge but never truly question their negative assumptions. Most of these children have heard parents and teachers tell them how ridiculous or unlikely their fears are and have heard reassurances that the negative events they are predicting will not happen. Although sometimes this information is helpful to the child, they often are more open to questioning their negative assumptions when the therapist takes their concerns seriously and has the child engage in actual data gathering in order to prove or disprove his/her unrealistic thoughts. Also, children rarely just change their way of thinking completely while engaging in cognitive restructuring exercises. Rather, these exercises begin to open the door for change to occur and the children's actual experiences help solidify the adoption of new beliefs.

In Session 5, the group focused on learning an approach to problem-solving, the 3rd step in their plan for coping with anxiety. The therapist explained that in addition to knowing when you're anxious and changing your self-talk, it is often helpful to take some action or follow a plan to cope with anxiety. The therapist introduced the process of problem-solving by proposing a mildly anxiety-provoking situation (e.g., not being able to find your school sneakers when it is time to go to school). The group was instructed to brainstorm as many solutions as possible, including silly (e.g., wear my mom's shoes), unhelpful (e.g., throw a temper tantrum), and adaptive ideas (e.g., trace past steps when last wearing the shoes). At first, only one or two solutions were offered, but as the therapist added a few ideas and continued to encourage the children, more and more ideas were proposed. The children were cautioned not to judge the solutions but rather to give any ideas that came into their heads. After a long list of solutions had been developed, the group began to evaluate the solutions—looking at the pros and cons for each. Finally, the group voted and decided which solutions looked the most promising. The therapist then set up a game in which the group drew a card containing an anxiety-provoking situation, read it aloud, and each child wrote as many solutions as they could think of within one minute. The children then compared lists, receiving points for solutions that no one else had recorded. Each group member then applied the 1st three steps of their coping plan to an anxiety-provoking situation.

During Session 6, the group focused on the final step in their plan for coping with anxiety: rating and rewarding themselves for trying to cope. First, the group discussed how people tend to do things for which they receive rewards. For example, a dog will learn to shake hands to receive a biscuit; kids may do their chores for an allowance. The children then played a game in which they received a penny candy for each reward they could name, generating an impressive list of activities, toys, and snacks. The therapist pointed out that it can be fun to receive a reward and that people often feel good when they are rewarded, or they reward themselves. This point then led to discussing how people often punish and reward themselves, sometimes without even knowing it, by their self-talk. Different positive and negative scenarios were proposed (e.g., a child hits a home run in baseball or the child gets a C on a math test). The children talked about how the characters would feel, what the characters' self-talk might be, and what the characters would do in each situation. The therapist pointed out that the characters may be less likely to do some things if they punish themselves with negative self-talk (e.g., after saying hello to a classmate, a boy tells himself that he sounded stupid, so he is less likely to say hello in the future). The therapist offered slight changes to the scenarios to illustrate the importance of rewarding positive effort, not just positive results. The therapist also offered coping models from her own life in which she used reward to help motivate herself and do new things.

In this session, the group reviewed the entire four-step FEAR plan for coping with anxiety. The group practiced the steps by applying the plan to real situations encountered by group members, such as giving a class presentation or taking a test. At the close of the 1st half of the treatment, the group engaged in a social event (i.e., a pizza party) to further enhance cohesion among group members.

The 2nd half of the treatment, Sessions 7–12, consisted of applying the newly acquired skills in a variety of graduated exposures to anxiety-eliciting situations, and group cooperation was very important in this phase of treatment. The anxiety-eliciting situations were tailored to the individual fears of the children as these varied across the group. However, the therapist also strove to address concerns shared by group members by developing group exposures. The practice segments began with imaginal exposures taking place within the group, then progressed to in vivo exposures involving the group as a whole, then to in vivo exposures involving individual group members. For many groups, we find it better to move directly to in vivo exposures and only utilize imaginals when needed.

Initial exposures were designed to both target the areas of overlap among the three boys' fears as well as to provide early success experiences, which were incompatible with previous expectations. The latter was accomplished by a very gradual start. Initially, some role-play exposures involved meeting others in the group as if for the 1st time, imagining traveling to unknown destinations independently, making social and performance blunders, and arriving late to important events (e.g., school, birthday parties).

In the next phase of exposure, the group members together accomplished superordinate goals. For example, one group in vivo exposure involved a trip to a nearby park to play soccer. Jordan, the group member with separation anxiety, was responsible for leading the group to the park with minimal directions, Chris was to make intentional soccer errors during a mock game, and Elijah, the 3rd group member with concerns about punctuality, had to return the soccer ball to the school gym teacher later than requested. Thus, each child's unique anxieties were tapped into a task that could not be accomplished without the cooperation and "courageous" behaviors of each group member. For some exposures, group members with similar fears were paired to accomplish various tasks. In one exposure, both Chris and Elijah took turns engaging in very silly and potentially embarrassing behaviors to observe others' reactions. While they expected that others would laugh at them, Chris and Elijah were surprised to find that for some observers, the silliness was contagious, and the onlookers were more apt to join in than to poke fun. Other observers simply ignored the silly group mates.

The last phase of exposures involved each member tackling in vivo exposures independently. For Chris, this meant accomplishing tasks such as making a new friend at school, asking or answering a question in class, purposely making a mistake on a math test, and making numerous speeches with increasing levels of difficulty. Fellow group mates offered creative ideas/support during the pre-exposure preparation, observed during the exposures, and offered hearty congratulations upon their successful completion.

The group concluded by making a videotaped commercial about learning to cope with anxiety. The commercial was developed by the group and was intended again to promote cooperation, problem-solving, and group cohesion. In addition, the commercial served to consolidate the information learned throughout the treatment and to reinforce each child's role and participation within the group. Each group member was given a copy of the commercial to take home with them. At the end of treatment, Chris still experienced some symptoms of generalized anxiety and social anxiety but did not meet full criteria for either disorder. His scores on the MASC and the SASC-R were in the non-clinical range. He was socializing more with his classmates, talked regularly with his teacher, and was no longer afraid to ask for help when he needed it. He joined a boy scout troop and participated when the group went on a camping trip. His parents were particularly pleased that he did not seem to take his errors or mistakes as seriously and could continue to enjoy activities even when not performing perfectly.

Summary

The group treatment case discussed in this chapter serves as just one example of how a cognitive behavioral approach may be helpful in treating children's anxiety problems in a school context. Shorter treatment protocols emphasizing therapeutic exposure with select components described in this comprehensive treatment package may be adapted to the school setting for interventions with groups or individuals of diverse ages. Furthermore, great prospects exist for prevention and early intervention in the school setting with youth at risk for developing anxiety disorders. By providing information regarding the presentation, chronic course, and treatment of anxiety problems in youth, we hope to stimulate greater opportunities for these children to receive preventive and treatment services in schools.

Reflection Questions

1. In vivo and imaginal exposures are essential components of the cognitive behavioral treatment for anxiety in youth. Why does participation in exposure lead to decreased anxiety? In other words, what are the underlying mechanisms responsible for change?
2. Develop a hierarchy of anxiety-provoking situations that could be targeted in exposures for a specific child in your school. Be sure to include situations that would provoke low, moderate, and high anxiety levels.
3. Many therapists fear that exposure therapy will traumatize children, although the evidence overwhelmingly indicates that this is not the case. What can be the negative consequences of stopping exposures and facilitating child avoidance? What can you do when a child refuses to participate in an exposure or becomes upset when faced with completing an exposure?

Evidence-Based Treatment Programs for Anxiety in Youth

FRIENDS program (Barrett & Turner, 2001).
Cool Kids Program (Rapee et al., 2006). Ginsburg
Skills for Academic and Social Success (Masia et al., 1999).
Coping Cat (Kendall & Hedtke, 2006; Flannery-Schroeder & Kendall, 2000).
Building Confidence (Wood & McLeod, 2008).
Unified Protocol-Child/Adolescent Version—*For treatment of depression and anxiety* (Ehrenreich-May et al., 2018).
Baltimore Child Anxiety Treatment Study in the Schools Program (BCATSS) (Ginsburg & Drake, 2002).
Cognitive-Behavioral Intervention for Trauma in Schools (CBITS) (Stein et al., 2003).

School-Based Treatment for Anxiety Resources for Teachers and Schools

Websites

https://www.weareteachers.com/books-for-kids-with-anxiety/
http://youth.anxietybc.com
https://childmild.org/guide/a-teachers-guide-to-anxiety-in-the-classrom/
https://copingskillsforkids.com/calming-anxiety/
https://www.teachstarter.com/us/blog/classroom-mindfulness-activities-for-children-us/
https://thereachinstitute.org/reach-and-adaa-anxiety-in-children-and-teens/?gclid=Cj0KCQjw6KunBhDxARIsAKFUGs9FESj8J_5cnwXp-bYM4_T-XVd_PWbc-MH9Ciu0nEbNqiKIHNe_rSAaAsGzEALw_wcB

Books

Alber, D. (2020). *A little spot of feelings: Emotion detective*. Diane Alber Art LLC.
Dacey, J. S., Mack, M. D., & Fiore, L. B. (2016). *Your anxious child: How parents and teachers can relieve anxiety in children*. Hoboken, NJ: John Wiley & Sons.
Reilly, N. (2005). *Anxiety and depression in the classroom: A teacher's guide to fostering selfregulation in young students*. New York: W.W. Norton & Company.

References

Achenbach, T. M., & Edelbrock, C. S. (1983). Manual for the Child Behavior Checklist and Revised Child Behavior Profile. Burlington: University of Vermont, Department of Psychiatry.
Achenbach, T. M., & Rescorla, L. A. (2000). *Manual for the ASEBA preschool forms and profiles* (Vol. 30). Burlington: University of Vermont, Research Center for Children, Youth, and Families.
Achenbach, T. M., & Rescorla, L. A. (2001). *Child Behavior Checklist for ages 6–18*. Burlington: University of Vermont.
Achenbach, T. M., & Rescorla, L. A. (2007). *Multicultural understanding of child and adolescent psychopathology: Implications for mental health assessment*. New York: Guilford Press.
Albano, A. M., & Silverman, W. K. (2016). *Anxiety disorders interview schedule for DSM-5, child version*. New York: University Press.
Alber, D. (2020). *A little spot of feelings: Emotion detective*. Diane Alber Art LLC.
American Psychiatric Association (2022). Diagnostic and statistical manual of mental disorders (5th ed., text rev.). https://doi.org/10.1176/appi.books.9780890425787
Amray, A. N., Munir, K., Jahan, N., Motiwala, F. B., & Naveed, S. (2019). Psychopharmacology of pediatric anxiety disorders: A narrative review. *Cureus, 11*(8), e5487. https://doi.org/10.7759/cureus.5487
Asselmann, E., & Beesdo-Baum, K. (2015). Predictors of the course of anxiety disorders in adolescents and young adults. *Current Psychiatry Reports, 17*, 1–8.
Bandura, A., & Walters, R. H. (1977). *Social learning theory* (Vol. 1). Englewood Cliffs, NJ: Prentice Hall.
Barlow, D. H. (2000). Unraveling the mysteries of anxiety and its disorders from the perspective of emotion theory. *American Psychologist, 55*(11), 1247.

Barrett, P., & Turner, C. (2001). Prevention of anxiety symptoms in primary school children: Preliminary results from a universal school-based trial. *British Journal of Clinical Psychology, 40*(4), 399–410.

Beesdo, K., Pine, D. S., Lieb, R., & Wittchen, H.-U. (2010). Incidence and risk patterns of anxiety and depressive disorders and categorization of generalized anxiety disorder. *Archives of General Psychiatry, 67*(1), 47–57.

Beidel, D. C., Turner, S. M., & Morris, T. L. (1995). A new inventory to assess childhood social anxiety and phobia: The Social Phobia and Anxiety Inventory for Children. *Psychological Assessment, 7*(1), 73.

Bennett, K., Manassis, K., Duda, S., Bagnell, A., Bernstein, G. A., Garland, E. J., Miller, L. D., Newton, A., Thabane, L., & Wilansky, P. (2016). Treating child and adolescent anxiety effectively: Overview of systematic reviews. *Clinical Psychology Review, 50*, 80–94.

Berry, K., & Hunt, C. J. (2009). Evaluation of an intervention program for anxious adolescent boys who are bullied at school. *Journal of Adolescent Health, 45*(4), 376–382.

Birmaher, B., Khetarpal, S., Brent, D., Cully, M., Balach, L., Kaufman, J., & Neer, S. M. (1997). The Screen for Child Anxiety Related Emotional Disorders (SCARED): Scale construction and psychometric characteristics. *Journal of the American Academy of Child & Adolescent Psychiatry, 36*(4), 545–553.

Bitsko, R. H., Claussen, A. H., Lichstein, J., Black, L. I., Jones, S. E., Danielson, M. L., Hoenig, J. M., Jack, S. P. D., Brody, D. J., & Gyawali, S. (2022). Mental health surveillance among children—United States, 2013–2019. *MMWR Supplements, 71*(2), 1.

Bushnell, G. A., Gaynes, B. N., Compton, S. N., Dusetzina, S. B., Olfson, M., & Stürmer, T. (2019). Incident substance use disorder following anxiety disorder in privately insured youth. *Journal of Adolescent Health, 65*(4), 536–542.

Chhabra, T., & Puar, S. (2016). Social support in psychotherapy of panic disorder with agoraphobia in school setting. *Indian Journal of Health & Wellbeing, 7*(6), 648–650.

Chorpita, B. F., & Barlow, D. H. (1998). The development of anxiety: The role of control in the early environment. *Psychological Bulletin, 124*(1), 3.

Chorpita, B. F., Tracey, S. A., Brown, T. A., Collica, T. J., & Barlow, D. H. (1997). Assessment of worry in children and adolescents: An adaptation of the Penn State Worry Questionnaire. *Behaviour Research and Therapy, 35*(6), 569–581.

Chorpita, B. F., Yim, L., Moffitt, C., Umemoto, L. A., & Francis, S. E. (2000). Assessment of symptoms of DSM-IV anxiety and depression in children: A revised child anxiety and depression scale. *Behaviour Research and Therapy, 38*(8), 835–855.

Chu, B. C., & Pimentel, S. S. (2023). *CBT treatment plans and interventions for depression and anxiety disorders in youth.* New York: Guilford Publications.

Comer, J. S., Roy, A. K., Furr, J. M., Gotimer, K., Beidas, R. S., Dugas, M. J., & Kendall, P. C. (2009). The Intolerance of Uncertainty Scale for Children: A psychometric evaluation. *Psychological Assessment, 21*(3), 402.

Craske, M., Wittchen, U., Bogels, S., Stein, M., Andrews, G., & Lebeu, R. (2013). *Severity measure for generalized anxiety disorder—Child age 11–17* [Measurement instrument].

Dacey, J. S., Mack, M. D., & Fiore, L. B. (2016). Your anxious child: How parents and teachers can relieve anxiety in children. Hoboken, NJ: John Wiley & Sons.

Dudeney, J., Sharpe, L., & Hunt, C. (2015). Attentional bias towards threatening stimuli in children with anxiety: A meta-analysis. *Clinical Psychology Review, 40*, 66–75.

Ehrenreich-May J., Kennedy S. M., Sherman J. A., Bilek E. L., Buzzella B. A., Bennett S. M., et al. (2018). *Unified Protocols for Transdiagnostic Treatment of Emotional Disorders in Children and Adolescents: Therapist Guide.* New York: Oxford University Press.

Flannery-Schroeder, E. C., & Kendall, P. C. (2000). Group and individual cognitive-behavioral treatments for youth with anxiety disorders: A randomized clinical trial. *Cognitive Therapy and Research, 24*, 251–278.

Freidl, E. K., Stroeh, O. M., Elkins, R. M., Steinberg, E., Albano, A. M., & Rynn, M. (2017). Assessment and treatment of anxiety among children and adolescents. *Focus, 15*(2), 144–156.

García-Escalera, J., Chorot, P., Sandín, B., Ehrenreich-May, J., Prieto, A., & Valiente, R. M. (2019). An open trial applying the unified protocol for transdiagnostic treatment of emotional disorders in adolescents (UP-A) adapted as a school-based prevention program. *Child & Youth Care Forum, 48*, 29–53.

Ginsburg, G. S., & Drake, K. L. (2002). School-based treatment for anxious african-american adolescents: a controlled pilot study. *Journal of the American Academy of Child and Adolescent Psychiatry, 41*(7), 768–775. https://doi.org/10.1097/00004583-200207000-00007

Ginsburg, G. S., & Affrunti, N. W. (2013). Generalized anxiety disorder in children and adolescents. In R. A. Vasa & A. K. Roy (Eds.), *Pediatric anxiety disorders: A clinical guide* (pp. 71–90). New York: Humana Press/Springer Nature. https://doi.org/10.1007/978-1-4614-6599-7_4

Ginsburg, G. S., Pella, J. E., Pikulski, P. J., Tein, J.-Y., & Drake, K. L. (2020). School-based treatment for anxiety research study (STARS): A randomized controlled effectiveness trial. *Journal of Abnormal Child Psychology, 48*, 407–417.

Ginsburg, G. S., & Smith, I. C. (2023). School-based interventions for students with anxiety. In S. W. Evans, J. S. Owens, C. P. Bradshaw, & M. D. Weist (Eds.), *Handbook of school mental health: Innovations in science and practice* (3rd ed., pp. 21–37). Switzerland AG: Springer Nature. https://doi.org/10.1007/978-3-031-20006-9_3

Guy, W. (1976). CGI clinical global impressions. *EC-DEU Assessment Manual for Psychopharmacology,* (ADM), *76*, 338.

Hadwin, J. A., Garner, M., & Perez-Olivas, G. (2006). The development of information processing biases in childhood anxiety: A review and exploration of its origins in parenting. *Clinical Psychology Review, 26*(7), 876–894.

Hajmohammadi, Z., Haji Alizadeh, K., & Aeini, B. (2021). The effectiveness of a coping cat program on symptoms of anxiety disorders in primary schools. *International Journal of Pediatrics, 9*(11), 14801–14811.

Haugland, B. S. M., Haaland, Aa. T., Baste, V., Bjaastad, J. F., Hoffart, A., Rapee, R. M., Raknes, S., Himle, J. A., Husabø, E., & Wergeland, G. J. (2020). Effectiveness of brief and standard school-based cognitive-behavioral interventions for adolescents with anxiety: A randomized noninferiority study. *Journal of the American Academy of Child & Adolescent Psychiatry, 59*(4), 552–564.

Higa-McMillan, C. K., Francis, S. E., Rith-Najarian, L., & Chorpita, B. F. (2016). Evidence base update: 50 years of research on treatment for child and adolescent anxiety. *Journal of Clinical Child & Adolescent Psychology, 45*(2), 91–113.

Kaczkurkin, A. N., & Foa, E. B. (2022). Cognitive-behavioral therapy for anxiety disorders: An update on the empirical evidence. *Dialogues in Clinical Neuroscience. 17*(3), 337–346. https://doi.org/10.31887/DCNS.2015.17.3/akaczkurkin

Kagan, J., Reznick, J. S., & Gibbons, J. (1989). Inhibited and uninhibited types of children. *Child Development, 60*(4), 838–845.

Kaufman, J., Birmaher, B., Axelson, D., Perepletchikova, F., Brent, D., & Ryan, N. (2016). *K-SADS-PL DSM-5*. Pittsburgh, PA: Western Psychiatric Institute and Clinic.

Kearney, C. A. (2008). School absenteeism and school refusal behavior in youth: A contemporary review. *Clinical Psychology Review, 28*(3), 451–471. https://doi.org/10.1016/j.cpr.2007.07.012

Kearney, C. A., & Silverman, W. K. (1993). Measuring the function of school refusal behavior: The School Refusal Assessment Scale. *Journal of Clinical Child Psychology, 22*(1), 85–96.

Kendall, P. C., Cummings, C. M., Villabø, M. A., Narayanan, M. K., Treadwell, K., Birmaher, B., Compton, S., Piacentini, J., Sherrill, J., Walkup, J., Gosch, E., Keeton, C., Ginsburg, G., Suveg, C., & Albano, A. M. (2016). Mediators of change in the child/adolescent anxiety multimodal treatment study. *Journal of Consulting and Clinical Psychology, 84*(1), 1–14. https://doi.org/10.1037/a0039773

Kendall, P. C., & Hedtke, K. A. (2006). *Cognitive-behavioral therapy for anxious children: Therapist manual.* Ardmore, PA: Workbook Publishing.

Kendall, P. C., Robin, J. A., Hedtke, K. A., Suveg, C., Flannery-Schroeder, E., & Gosch, E. (2005). Considering CBT with anxious youth? Think exposures. *Cognitive and Behavioral Practice, 12*(1), 136–148.

Kennedy, S. M., Bilek, E. L., & Ehrenreich-May, J. (2019). A randomized controlled pilot trial of the unified protocol for transdiagnostic treatment of emotional disorders in children. *Behavior Modification, 43*(3), 330–360.

Kerns, C. M., Renno, P., Kendall, P. C., Wood, J. J., & Storch, E. A. (2017). Anxiety Disorders Interview Schedule–Autism Addendum: Reliability and validity in children with autism spectrum disorder. *Journal of Clinical Child & Adolescent Psychology, 46*(1), 88–100.

Koeppen, A. S. (1974). Relaxation training for children. *Elementary School Guidance & Counseling, 9*(1), 14–21.

La Greca, A. M., Dandes, S. K., Wick, P., Shaw, K., & Stone, W. L. (1988). Development of the Social Anxiety Scale for Children: Reliability and concurrent validity. *Journal of Clinical Child Psychology, 17*(1), 84–91.

Lang, P. J. (1968). Fear reduction and fear behavior: Problems in treating a construct. *Research in Psychotherapy Conference*, 3rd, May–June, 1966, Chicago, IL, US.

Lebowitz, E. R., Marin, C., Martino, A., Shimshoni, Y., & Silverman, W. K. (2020). Parent-based treatment as efficacious as cognitive-behavioral therapy for childhood anxiety: A randomized noninferiority study of supportive parenting for anxious childhood emotions. *Journal of the American Academy of Child and Adolescent Psychiatry, 59*(3), 362–372. https://doi.org/10.1016/j.jaac.2019.02.014

Lenz, A. S. (2015). Meta-analysis of the coping cat program for decreasing severity of anxiety symptoms among children and adolescents. *Journal of Child and Adolescent Counseling, 1*(2), 51–65. https://doi.org/10.1080/23727810.2015.1079116

Levy, H. C., Stevens, K. T., & Tolin, D. F. (2022). Research review: A meta-analysis of relapse rates in cognitive behavioral therapy for anxiety and related disorders in youth. *Journal of Child Psychology and Psychiatry, 63*(3), 252–260.

Lovibond, P. F., & Lovibond, S. H. (1995). The structure of negative emotional states: Comparison of the Depression Anxiety Stress Scales (DASS) with the Beck depression and anxiety inventories. *Behaviour Research and Therapy, 33*(3), 335–343.

Luo, A., & McAloon, J. (2021). Potential mechanisms of change in cognitive behavioral therapy for childhood anxiety: A meta-analysis. *Depression and Anxiety, 38*(2), 220–232. https://doi.org/10.1002/da.23116

Manassis, K., Hudson, J. L., Webb, A., & Albano, A. M. (2004). Beyond behavioral inhibition: Etiological factors in childhood anxiety. *Cognitive and Behavioral Practice, 11*(1), 3–12.

March, J. S. (2013). *Multidimensional Anxiety Scale for Children 2nd edition (MASC 2)*. Toronto: Multi-Health Systems Inc.

March, J. S., Parker, J. D. A., Sullivan, K., Stallings, P., & Conners, C. K. (1997). The Multidimensional Anxiety Scale for Children (MASC): Factor structure, reliability, and validity. *Journal of the American Academy of Child & Adolescent Psychiatry, 36*(4), 554–565. https://doi.org/10.1097/00004583-199704000-00019

Masia, C., Beidel, D. C., Fisher, P. H., Albano, A. M., Rapee, R. M., Turner, S. M., Morris, T. L., & Klein, R. G. (1999). Skills for academic and social success. New York: New York University School of Medicine.

Masia, C. L., Klein, R. G., Storch, E. A., & Corda, B. (2001). School-based behavioral treatment for social anxiety disorder in adolescents: Results of a pilot study. *Journal of the American Academy of Child & Adolescent Psychiatry, 40*(7), 780–786.

Masia-Warner, C., Colognori, D., Brice, C., Herzig, K., Mufson, L., Lynch, C., Reiss, P. T., Petkova, E., Fox, J., & Moceri, D. C. (2016). Can school counselors deliver cognitive-behavioral treatment for social anxiety effectively? A randomized controlled trial. *Journal of Child Psychology and Psychiatry, 57*(11), 1229–1238.

Masia-Warner, C., Klein, R. G., Dent, H. C., Fisher, P. H., Alvir, J., Albano, A. M., & Guardino, M. (2005). School-based intervention for adolescents with social anxiety disorder: Results of a controlled study. *Journal of Abnormal Child Psychology, 33*(6), 707–722. https://doi.org/10.1007/S10802-005-7649-Z

McLoone, J. K., & Rapee, R. M. (2012). Comparison of an anxiety management program for children implemented at home and school: Lessons learned. *School Mental Health, 4*, 231–242.

Mifsud, C., & Rapee, R. M. (2005). Early intervention for childhood anxiety in a school setting: Outcomes for an economically disadvantaged population. *Journal of the American Academy of Child & Adolescent Psychiatry, 44*(10), 996–1004.

Mowrer, O. (1960). Two-factor learning theory: Versions one and two. In O. H. Mowrer (Ed.), *Learning theory and behavior* (pp. 63–91). Hoboken, NJ: John Wiley & Sons Inc. https://doi.org/10.1037/10802-003

Mychailyszyn, M. P. (2017). Systematic review and meta-analysis of the Skills for Social and Academic Success (SASS) program. *Advances in School Mental Health Promotion, 10*(2), 147–160.

Mychailyszyn, M. P., Beidas, R. S., Benjamin, C. L., Edmunds, J. M., Podell, J. L., Cohen, J. S., & Kendall, P. C. (2011). Assessing and treating child anxiety in schools. *Psychology in the Schools, 48*(3), 223–232.

Nikolić, M. (2020). Disturbed social information processing as a mechanism in the development of social anxiety disorder. *Child Development Perspectives, 14*, 258–264. https://doi.org/10.1111/cdep.12390

Ollendick, T. H. (1983). Reliability and validity of the Revised Fear Survey Schedule for Children (FSSC-R). *Behaviour Research and Therapy, 21*(6), 685–692.

Ollendick, T. H., & Cerny, J. A. (2013). *Clinical behavior therapy with children*. New York: Springer Science & Business Media.

Patton, M. C., Desai, R., Noureddine, Y., Prebeg, M. J., Krause, K. R., Vohra, S., Butcher, N. J., & Monga, S. (2022). Outcomes and outcome measurement instruments reported in randomised controlled trials of anxiety disorder treatments in children and adolescents: A scoping review protocol. *BMJ Open, 12*(10), e063404.

Pegg, S., Hill, K., Argiros, A., Olatunji, B. O., & Kujawa, A. (2022). Cognitive behavioral therapy for anxiety disorders in youth: Efficacy, moderators, and new advances in predicting outcomes. *Current Psychiatry Reports, 24*(12), 853–859.

Rapee, R.M., Lyneham, H.J., Schniering, C.A., Wuthrich, V. Abbott, M.A., Hudson J.L., & Wignall, A., (2006). *The Cool Kids Child and Adolescent Anxiety Program Therapist Manual*. Sydney: Centre for Emotional Health, Macquarie University.

Read, K. L., Comer, J. S., & Kendall, P. C. (2013). The Intolerance of Uncertainty Scale for Children (IUSC): Discriminating principal anxiety diagnoses and severity. *Psychological Assessment, 25*(3), 722.

Reardon, T., Spence, S. H., Hesse, J., Shakir, A., & Creswell, C. (2018). Identifying children with anxiety disorders using brief versions of the Spence Children's Anxiety Scale for children, parents, and teachers. *Psychological Assessment, 30*(10), 1342.

Reilly, N. (2005). *Anxiety and depression in the classroom: A teacher's guide to fostering self regulation in young students.* New York: W.W. Norton & Company.

Reynolds, C. R., Kamphaus, R. W., & Vannest, K. J. (2015). *BASC3: Behavior Assessment System for Children.* Bloomington, MN: PsychCorp.

Reynolds, C. R., & Richmond, B. O. (1978). What I think and feel: A revised measure of children's manifest anxiety. *Journal of Abnormal Child Psychology, 6*, 271–280.

Scott, K., & Lewis, C. C. (2015). Using measurement-based care to enhance any treatment. *Cognitive and Behavioral Practice, 22*(1), 49–59.

Shaffer, D., Gould, M. S., Brasic, J., Ambrosini, P., Fisher, P., Bird, H., & Aluwahlia, S. (1983). A children's global assessment scale (CGAS). *Archives of General Psychiatry, 40*(11), 1228–1231.

Songco, A., Hudson, J. L., & Fox, E. (2020). A cognitive model of pathological worry in children and adolescents: A systematic review. *Clinical Child and Family Psychology Review, 23*, 229–249.

Spence, S. H. (1998). A measure of anxiety symptoms among children. *Behaviour Research and Therapy, 36*(5), 545–566.

Spence, S. H. (2018). Assessing anxiety disorders in children and adolescents. *Child and Adolescent Mental Health, 23*(3), 266–282.

Spence, S. H., Zubrick, S. R., & Lawrence, D. (2018). A profile of social, separation and generalized anxiety disorders in an Australian nationally representative sample of children and adolescents: Prevalence, comorbidity and correlates. *Australian & New Zealand Journal of Psychiatry, 52*(5), 446–460.

Stein, B., Jaycox, L., Kataoka, S., Wong, M., Tu, W., & Elliot, M. (2003). A mental health intervention for schoolchildren exposed to violence: A randomized control trial. *The Journal of the American Medical Association, 290*, 603–611.

Warwick, H., Reardon, T., Cooper, P., Murayama, K., Reynolds, S., Wilson, C., & Creswell, C. (2017). Complete recovery from anxiety disorders following cognitive behavior therapy in children and adolescents: A meta-analysis. *Clinical Psychology Review, 52*, 77–91.

Werner-Seidler, A., Spanos, S., Calear, A. L., Perry, Y., Torok, M., O'Dea, B., Christensen, H., & Newby, J. M. (2021). School-based depression and anxiety prevention programs: An updated systematic review and meta-analysis. *Clinical Psychology Review, 89*, 102079.

Whiteside, S. P. H., Sim, L. A., Morrow, A. S., Farah, W. H., Hilliker, D. R., Murad, M. H., & Wang, Z. (2020). A meta-analysis to guide the enhancement of CBT for childhood anxiety: Exposure over anxiety management. *Clinical Child and Family Psychology Review, 23*(1), 102–121.

Wilmer, M. T., Anderson, K., & Reynolds, M. (2021). Correlates of quality of life in anxiety disorders: Review of recent research. *Current Psychiatry Reports, 23*, 1–9.

Zhang, Q., Wang, J., & Neitzel, A. (2023). School-based mental health interventions targeting depression or anxiety: A meta-analysis of rigorous randomized controlled trials for school-aged children and adolescents. *Journal of Youth and Adolescence, 52*(1), 195–217.

10
SCHOOL ATTENDANCE PROBLEMS

Christopher A. Kearney, Michael Fensken and Randolph Dupont

School Attendance Problems

School attendance problems refer to a collection of issues that, for in-person educational formats, include continuous and intermittent full-day absences from school (absenteeism), skipped classes or parts of a school day, extended tardiness, morning misbehaviors designed to miss school, and substantial distress or other mental health challenges that preclude classroom attendance. School attendance problems can be extended to other educational formats as well and can include lack of participation in virtual or distance learning programs, hybrid or blended learning arrangements, or various forms of home-based instruction. School attendance problems are a key marker of deficits in multiple developmental domains for children and adolescents, including academic, behavioral, physical, and mental health, and social areas of functioning. In addition, school attendance problems typically carry particular urgency due to risk of rapid declines in academic progress, social connection, and school engagement. The problems are also a common initial treatment target for those who address youths referred to mental health and other services for a wide variety of presenting concerns.

Introduction and Overview of CBT to School Attendance Problems

Many disciplines have been involved in the study of school attendance problems over the past century and include those at a *systemic* level, with a focus on overarching contexts such as schools and broad-band variables related to policy constructs, as well as those at an *analytic* level, with a focus on specific contexts such as students and their families and narrow-band variables related to clinical constructs (Kearney, 2021). Both sets of perspectives have important contributions for defining, categorizing, conceptualizing, assessing, and treating school attendance problems, and both sets of perspectives contain nexus points that permit an integration of these viewpoints to account for the complicated ecology of school attendance problems. Two nexus points are utilized here to introduce and provide an overview of CBT for school attendance problems: systemic-oriented multi-tiered systems of support models (MTSS) and analytic-oriented treatment protocols that also have school-based applicability.

MTSS models refer to school-based service delivery models that supply different levels of resources to students with various levels of need. Most MTSS models involve a three-tier system of universal and school-wide application of primary prevention techniques and programs to bolster adaptive behavior and reduce maladaptive behavior (Tier 1); early, selective interventions involving

DOI: 10.4324/9781003392439-13

targeted and secondary prevention practices to address emerging or acute problems beyond Tier 1 (Tier 2); and extensive interventions and tertiary prevention practices to address chronic and severe problems beyond Tier 2 (Tier 3). A traditional MTSS model for an academic endeavor such as reading might involve a general curriculum for all students (Tier 1), targeted instruction for students with emerging reading difficulties (Tier 2), and special education placement for students with severe reading difficulties (Tier 3). MTSS models have been extended to various social, behavioral, and mental health problems as well, and have recently been expanded to arrange interventions for school attendance problems (Kearney & Graczyk, 2020).

Common Tier 1 interventions for school attendance and its problems include school climate interventions, safety-oriented strategies, health-based strategies, school-based mental health and social-emotional learning programs, parental involvement initiatives and culturally responsive approaches, district-wide policy review and attendance initiatives, orientation activities, summer bridge and school readiness programs, and school dropout prevention practices. Common Tier 2 interventions for school attendance problems include psychological approaches for anxiety- and non-anxiety-based absenteeism, student engagement approaches, and teacher and peer mentoring programs. Common Tier 3 interventions for school attendance problems include expanded Tier 2 interventions, alternative educational programs and schools, parent/family involvement strategies, specialized residential and inpatient programs, intensive case study and management, and 2nd chance programs designed to provide extra opportunities for high school graduation (Kumm et al., 2020). This chapter focuses primarily on Tier 2 interventions, which include those typically more clinical in nature and which are described in more detail in several sections of this chapter.

Tier 2 strategies for school attendance problems encompass the 2nd main nexus point mentioned earlier to provide an overview of CBT for this area. These strategies are more clinical in nature and have been, in many cases, applied to school settings as well, given that educational systems and their in-house support services (e.g., school-based counselors, nurses, psychologists, social workers) are often the main mental health network in many communities (Duong et al., 2021). Clinical strategies for school attendance problems rely heavily on cognitive-behavioral and family-focused techniques designed to mitigate emotional distress related to school attendance, gradually reintroduce an absent student to full-time attendance in a regular classroom setting, modify parent and other caregiver responses to absenteeism, and develop more constructive communication and problem-solving strategies for families. As such, many of these clinical techniques involve aspects of anxiety management, contingency management, and family therapy, all of which can expand as needed to address the many contextual variables often associated with this population.

Many of these clinical strategies have been adapted for school-based settings and implemented by school-based personnel (Eklund et al., 2022). Such adaptations typically involve more condensed procedures given the urgency of school attendance problems and limited time and other resources, integration with effective classroom management practices and trauma-informed practices that often also rely on key cognitive-behavioral principles, and intersection with school district policies and available alternative educational pathways (von der Embse et al., 2019). In addition, clinical strategies within a school-based setting can be included in consultation and accommodation plans for students and/or be implemented by clinicians within that setting (see also the later section on application to the school setting). Community-based clinicians often encounter Tier 2 or early Tier 3 cases of school attendance problems.

Understanding the Specific Issue

School attendance problems are characterized by substantial heterogeneity, opacity, and complexity. The *heterogeneity* of school attendance problems is evident by its many forms described earlier as well as a wide array of internalizing and externalizing behavioral symptoms that are commonly associated with the problems. Indeed, the clinical profiles of those with school attendance problems vary considerably and are often quite fluid over time. The *opacity* of school attendance problems is evident by their association with variables that make student tracking and evaluation quite difficult. Examples include close association with residential mobility, housing insecurity, transportation vulnerability, and migration patterns. The *complexity* of school attendance problems is evident by its many levels of risk variables across ecological domains. Such complexity is the main focus of this section and precedes a discussion of functional impairment for this population.

School attendance problems are associated with a plethora of risk factors at microsystem, mesosystem, exosystem, macrosystem, and chronosystem ecological domains (Childs & Scanlon, 2022). Common microsystem-level risk factors for school attendance problems, or variables involving students and their immediate environment, include problems of academic achievement and learning, substance use, psychopathology (especially emotional and disruptive behavior disorders), grade retention, risky behaviors, and poorer physical health. Common mesosystem-level risk factors for school attendance problems, or variables involving relationships among a student's microsystems, often include parent, family, and peer risk variables. Key parent risk variables include maltreatment of or inadequate attachment to a child, parental psychopathology, and less school involvement. Key family risk variables include ineffective systems such as enmeshment or conflict as well as poverty and homelessness, stressful transitions and residential movement during a school year, and transportation vulnerability. Key peer risk variables include fewer friends, less participation in extracurricular activities, proximity to absentee peers, less social competence with others, and victimization (Gubbels et al., 2019).

Common exosystem-level risk factors for school attendance problems, or variables that more distally impact a student, primarily include school-related variables. Many of these variables relate to a poor school climate, which is defined as the quality of daily school life for students (Thapa & Cohen, 2017). School-oriented risk factors for absenteeism include dangerousness, frequent teacher absences, less monitoring of absenteeism, lower quality of student-teacher relationships, reliance on punitive and exclusionary discipline practices to address absenteeism, and inadequate responsiveness to diversity issues. Regarding the latter, for example, migrant students and their parents are more often assigned pejorative labels for absenteeism and thus denied appropriate services (Rosenthal et al., 2020).

Common macrosystem-level risk factors for school attendance problems, or variables that involve broader environments, include cultural, political, and economic trends. Examples include themes related to labor distributions and markets (including economic pull factors), migration, health disparities and uneven access to care, and social injustice, among others. Macrosystem-level factors are continuing to shape education and thus the conceptualization of school attendance problems as well, including climate change, demographic shifts, school closures, technological advancements, and integration of schools with communities (see Kearney et al., 2022). Finally, school attendance problems match well with chronosystem ecological changes as students progress from preschool to elementary, middle, and high schools and encounter different challenges.

A key clinical aspect for understanding school attendance problems vis-à-vis these many contextual variables is the notion of *functional impairment*. Absenteeism severity per se is not necessarily predictive of student impairment because some youth with school attendance problems have sufficient levels of external support and thus function well. Not all absences have the same effect for each student. Clinicians should thus be aware of how certain behaviors or events interfere with performance in key domains. Kearney (2022) outlined key aspects of functional impairment related to school attendance problems that could inform decisions regarding caseness, or whether a specific instance of absenteeism should be deemed clinically problematic and in need of treatment. These aspects involve school, social, and family domains of functioning.

The *school* domain included timing of absences, interference with academic competence, and administrative or legal actions that impede future school attendance. Some absences carry greater pernicious effect depending on their timing, such as those early in the school year, during important evaluation periods, or in high-impact grades such as initial entry into elementary, middle, or high school. Absences could also interfere with academic competence for some youth, including suppressed grades and standardized testing results, less proficient academic skills, and grade retention. In addition, some cases of absenteeism trigger administrative or legal actions that impede future school attendance; examples include suspension, expulsion, arrest, court referral, and penalties that enhance barriers to attendance such as loss of driving privileges.

The *social* domain included interference with social competence, interference in interpersonal relationships, and enhanced risk of harm to others. Interference in social competence can involve erosion of social, communicative, and emotional regulation skills, among others. Interference in interpersonal relationships can involve absences that produce greater isolation from others and lack of friendships. Enhanced risk of harm to others can involve direct or indirect aggression toward others, such as in-person and cyber-bullying. The *family* domain included interference with daily functioning, maladaptive changes in family dynamics, and substantial cost to family members. Interference with daily functioning can involve distress as well as disruptions to routines and transportation and other logistical arrangements. Maladaptive changes in family dynamics can involve greater enmeshment, detachment, isolation, and conflict (Fornander & Kearney, 2019). Substantial cost to family members can involve missed school or work time as well as financial outlays for childcare and legal and health-based services. Substantial functional impairment could involve a combination of these effects or significant impairment in one to two key aspects.

Empirical Support of CBT in Treatment of School Attendance Problems

Cognitive-behavioral treatments of various sorts have been utilized for school attendance problems. One common set of strategies involves those designed for anxiety mitigation, including exposure-based practices, cognitive therapy, and somatic management techniques. Related procedures include modeling and role play, shaping, emotive imagery, and flooding (Elliott & Place, 2019). The general purposes of these strategies are to enhance school attendance on a gradual basis, to address the physiological, cognitive, and behavioral response systems relevant to school-based anxiety, and to develop skills that may have eroded during a child's absence from school. Another common set of strategies involves parent/caregiver- and/or family-oriented practices such as contingency management, contracting, and communication skills training. The general purposes of these strategies are to enhance parental/caregiver control, reinforce appropriate school attendance behavior, and improve a family's problem-solving ability, particularly with respect to school-related issues.

Large-scale empirical trials regarding cognitive-behavioral treatments for school attendance problems are sparse and are usually restricted to a narrow subset of this population, such as those with anxiety-based absenteeism. Meta-analyses reveal greater impact on attendance than anxiety (Maynard et al., 2015, 2018). The specific treatment components described above, however, have extensive empirical support with youth and their families (Kearney, 2016). In general, cognitive-behavioral treatment is better than no treatment. Readers should note as well that many interventions other than formal cognitive-behavioral treatments have also been designed for school attendance problems. Examples include mentoring, school engagement practices, and classroom behavior management (Guryan et al., 2021).

A key drawback to the use of cognitive-behavioral strategies (and treatments in general) for school attendance problems relates to the disparate nature of the field. Many professionals from various disciplines intersect with these problems and often adopt their own terminology and perspective to conceptualize and address these problems. Many therapists and caregivers are unfamiliar with school attendance problems and their treatment or view these (non-diagnostic) problems as more within the purview of the educational system than the mental health system. School-based personnel and families thus often struggle to find community-based care for this population. In addition, cognitive-behavioral and other treatments for school attendance problems have not yet been widely disseminated to therapists and schools (Kearney & Childs, 2022).

To address these issues, clinical researchers have recommended various frameworks for organizing the many interventions relevant to school attendance problems. These frameworks have various levels of adoption among therapists and other professionals and/or remain in nascent form as the field evolves. Still, each represents useful ways of thinking about how the myriad intervention options for this complex population can be contextualized. One framework was described earlier and involves MTSS models that broadly incorporate Tier 1 preventative practices, Tier 2 early and targeted intervention practices, and Tier 3 later and extensive intervention practices.

Another framework for organizing interventions for school attendance problems, and particularly cognitive-behavioral interventions, involves a functional analysis to determine the primary variables that maintain these problems on a daily basis. Kearney and colleagues have outlined four main functions with clinical profiles that often pertain to acute cases of school attendance problems: avoidance of negative affectivity associated with school-related stimuli; escape from aversive social and/or evaluative situations; pursuit of attention from significant others; and pursuit of tangible reinforcers outside of the school setting (e.g., Gonzálvez et al., 2019; Kearney & Gonzálvez, 2022). The initial two functions involve negative reinforcement, with each one generally more relevant either to younger children or to older children and adolescents. The latter two functions involve positive reinforcement, with each also generally more relevant to younger or older age groups. Each function is linked to a specific cognitive-behavioral treatment package involving an assortment of anxiety management, contingency management, and family-based practices (Kearney & Albano, 2018). A functional approach to assessing and treating school attendance problems is most relevant to emerging or acute Tier 2 cases, though some aspects can be relevant to some Tier 3 cases as well.

Other clinical researchers have organized interventions for school attendance problems by ecological level. Melvin and colleagues (2019), for example, broadly characterized interventions in this area along proximal and distal influences on school attendance problems. Proximal interventions included those that focus on student health and mental health issues, sleep problems, victimization, family functioning, economic hardship, and student/parent-teacher relationships. Distal interventions included those that focus on school climate, transportation, community services, government and school policy, and socioeconomic resources. In addition, Leduc and colleagues (2022) stated that the principles of an ecological model could guide interventions for school attendance problems. Such principles include considering a particular student within the context of their environment (interdependence); availability and distribution of resources at home and school settings (circulation of resources); ability to progress through the school system (adaptation); and the developmental impact of cumulative student experiences in their home and school settings (succession).

Relational Consideration in Treatment of School Attendance Problems

Clinicians should understand that school attendance problems are among the most disruptive, confusing, and distressing events for families. School absenteeism creates immediate challenges for caregivers with respect to child care, missed work, mandated meetings with school officials, urgent treatment-seeking, and need for altered transportation and other logistical arrangements. Many caregivers are also bewildered by these problems and are unsure whether to seek help via educational, mental health, medical, or other avenues of support. Family members are often distressed as well by school mandates to return a child to school or face administrative/legal consequences, by declining academic performance and risk of grade retention or dropout, by perceived stigma, and by concerns about sending a child back to school, particularly in anxiety-provoking situations.

Clinicians should thus understand that school absenteeism cases often require additional support compared to many other cases, particularly early in the treatment process. Empathy is helpful to understand the family's sense of distress and urgency, and a commitment to work with family members as well as with school officials is important. Family members in these cases will also be more likely to contact therapists at unusual times, such as in the early morning during the school preparation process, and so establishing boundaries in this regard is recommended. In addition, children and adolescents, and some caregivers, are highly motivated to maintain the status quo and so extended engagement on goals, timelines, treatment rationales, and potential obstacles will be necessary.

A key relational factor for the treatment of school attendance problems will be a clinician's interactions with school officials, particularly school-based counselors, social workers, nurses, and psychologists. In many school attendance problem cases, the caregiver-school official relationship has deteriorated due to friction, disagreement over strategy, and frustration with perceived refusal to help or failure to provide nuanced options for resolution. Clinicians can often serve as family advocates in these situations by communicating directly and often with school officials in a mediator-like fashion, participating in accommodation and school-based treatment plans, conducting therapy sessions at a school, working with school officials to extend treatment techniques and effects in classroom settings, and/or securing additional resources such as public assistance and legal services for families. A three-legged stool approach involving cooperation among the clinician, family members, and school officials is often crucial for resolving school attendance problems.

School attendance problems are particularly urgent and thus less amenable to wait lists and delayed treatment. As such, initial screening, consultation, and/or early assessment practices can be integrated with several generic recommendations that allow caregivers to immediately pursue some remediation as well as to establish a stronger foundation for later, more formal treatment. These recommendations include supervising a child's school attendance and daily activities closely; refraining if possible from keeping a child home from school; maintaining a regular morning routine for school preparation behaviors; improving sleep hygiene; and implementing basic rewards for attendance and disincentives for nonattendance if possible. Caregivers should also be encouraged to establish and maintain regular contact with school officials, pursue initial school reintegration if even for a short time, retrieve academic work from the school to maintain progress, and mobilize their social support network to assist with the morning routine, transportation to and from school, and homework.

Clinicians should also understand that many families encountering school attendance problems are accessing or attempting to access other systems of care as well. In addition to the educational system, many families are also interacting with medical, legal, developmental, and community systems of care. Children with medical problems and disabilities are among the most vulnerable risk groups for school attendance problems, many youths with school attendance problems are referred to truancy or family court proceedings, youth with developmental delays are often placed in special education and experience school readiness and attendance problems, and many families are preoccupied with food, housing, employment, and other survival concerns and thus have limited resources to address school attendance problems. Clinicians should interface with professionals in these other systems of care, particularly in situations requiring or involving psychiatric treatment, transitions between agencies (e.g., child protective services, court, school), psychoeducational assessment and extensive academic support needs, and public assistance and other services.

Clinicians should also understand that much intervention for school attendance problems involves interactions with family members that are outside the timeframe of formal treatment sessions. Rapport via frequent contact with caregivers and students is especially critical for these cases given their fraught nature. Emphasis should be placed on a collaborative approach, recurrent or daily interaction (especially in the 1st two weeks of formal treatment), and extensive education about the school attendance problem and relevant school policies. In addition, identifying a point person at school (e.g., school-based counselor) that family members can contact at specific times, as well as extended family members and others who can serve as strong working partners for treatment implementation, is helpful. Consider that home visits as well as school-based and other incentives for treatment participation and school attendance may be desirable in some cases.

Clinicians can also improve the relational aspects of treatment for this population by working with schools to identify nuanced avenues to resolution such as alternative schools or educational programs or modifications in course or graduation requirements. Creative and innovative options are often needed for more difficult cases, such as use of portfolio and service/experiential work in lieu of traditional classwork to demonstrate competency in a particular subject (and thus course credit). Clinicians can also ease the therapy process by focusing on gradual improvements over a short period of time (daily, weekly) as opposed to a semester or school year. In addition, some families have the wherewithal to implement only basic intervention components and so simplifying treatment may be necessary. Consider flexible and realistic end-state functioning goals as well, particularly for long-standing cases where full reintegration to a regular classroom setting is less likely.

Interviewing and Assessing School Attendance Problems

The assessment of school attendance problems is often a condensed process given the urgency of the issue. Formal structured/semi-structured interviews do have relevance for diagnostic and other important considerations related to school attendance problems, but the questions discussed next are designed to provide high-value target information amenable to a condensed assessment approach. In addition, questionnaires, observations, record reviews, and other methods are important assessment components and are covered later in this section.

Key initial questions can surround a child's current attendance status and whether they are actually enrolled in a particular school. Attendance status can include how many full days a student has missed during the current academic year in addition to partial absences that can include missed classes or sections of a school day as well as tardiness. Schools often distinguish between excused and unexcused absences, but total time missed from school, regardless of the reason, is important to consider for clinical and functional impairment purposes (Pyne et al., 2023). In related fashion, determining whether a child is still actively enrolled in a particular school is important early in the assessment process because official re-enrollment may be necessary prior to treatment procedures such as gradual reintegration to a classroom setting.

Related to current attendance status are questions surrounding a child's specific forms of absenteeism during the week and whether key patterns emerge. Some students often miss a particular day of school such as Monday or Friday, some miss specific classes that involve performance before others, some are late to school many mornings due to early misbehaviors at home or difficulty separating from caregivers or sleep problems, and others leave a school campus prematurely during the day to engage in more palatable activities. Pattern identification can be important for targeting treatment resources, such as focusing anxiety management techniques on Sunday evening and Monday morning, allowing short-term avoidance of anxiety-provoking classes prior to treatment to ensure attendance in other classes, establishing set morning routines and point of separation recommendations, and short-circuiting premature departures from school by scheduling visits to a school counselor's office at a particular time of the school day. Patterns of school attendance problems can also be informed by understanding how the problems developed over time, including key antecedents, and which prior interventions were effective or less effective.

Clinicians should also consider whether school absenteeism is actually a *more adaptive* choice for a student. Youth who feel unsafe or are victimized at school or via cyberbullying are at increased risk for school attendance problems, as are youth with particularly dangerous routes to and from home and school. Youth with recent traumatic experiences, whether in or out of school, often have subsequent difficulty navigating social and academic challenges at school. Other adolescents miss school to support family members in economic and other ways, such as via outside employment, care for siblings, and assistance for caregivers/parents with mental health or other challenges. More broadly, students of highly vulnerable groups are often subjected to biased exclusionary disciplinary policies and/or view a school setting as an oppressive, discriminating environment (Nation et al., 2020). Note as well that some caregivers deliberately keep a child home from school to conceal maltreatment, to avoid feared events such as kidnapping or deportation, or for other reasons.

Another key set of questions surrounds specific morning-based problems prior to school hours. Often, these problems involve some combination of anxiety, somatic complaints, separation concerns, oppositional behavior, or chaotic or otherwise ineffective family preparation routines. In related fashion, questions should target impairment in family functioning as a result of the school attendance problems, such as whether parents are missing work or if considerable conflict occurs. Questions should also entail how others respond to a child's school attendance problems in the morning, with a particular emphasis on ineffective responses such as acquiescing, arguing, rescuing, negotiating/bribing, threatening, lingering at school, or leaving a child at home to attend school on their own.

Another set of important questions surrounds a child's academic status, including current grades, accrued credits, ability to pass the school year, course schedule, and required make-up work. Other important topics during the interviewing process include distressing situations at school, a child's activities during school hours if not in school, eligibility for an accommodation plan, how much school attendance a child can initially tolerate (to set an early baseline and foundation for treatment), contextual factors that impact a child's absenteeism, school or district absenteeism and other policies that apply most to the case, alternative educational programs for which a student may eligible, cultural and language barriers that may influence absenteeism, and procedures, timelines, and obstacles for reintegrating a child to school.

Other important assessment techniques include questionnaires, behavioral observations, record reviews, daily ratings, and think-aloud/thought-listing procedures. Questionnaires have been developed to assess the frequency and severity of school attendance and its problems; explanations for a student's school attendance problem; impact of school attendance problems on a student academic, social, and emotional functioning; comorbid mental health conditions that may contribute to school attendance problems; and self-efficacy in school-related situations (e.g., Gonzálvez et al., 2021). Behavioral observations can be costly but can be narrowed to key situations such as the morning preparation routine, separation point at school, and classroom behaviors. Observations are commonly done in support of a functional analysis of school attendance problems to determine whether a child is primarily avoiding school or pursuing more alluring options outside of school.

Record reviews can include school attendance, health and medical status, academic progress, and psychoeducational and standardized testing results, among others. Daily ratings, such as on a 0–10 scale, may be utilized to identify patterns of anxiety and emotional distress across the morning, school day, and evening. Such ratings can help pinpoint treatment targets and gauge treatment progress. Think-aloud and thought-listing procedures are useful for recording key cognitions during and after an anxiety-provoking event such as a test to serve as fodder for cognitive therapy techniques.

Case Conceptualization

Various case conceptualization models exist for cognitive-behavioral and related interventions, some of which are quite lengthy. School attendance problems, however, generally demand a rapid case conceptualization process given their urgency and impairment. This process for this population can thus involve initial clinical presentation of the nature and severity of symptoms/problems, potential causal and maintaining factors for the symptoms/problems, current contextual factors and available support systems, treatment planning and goal setting, and identifying obstacles to treatment. Note that many case conceptualization models also emphasize hypotheses about the origin of the symptoms/problems, but the exact origins of school attendance problems are often nebulous and sometimes unnecessary for treatment purposes. However, some school attendance problems do have clearer origins with specific treatment ramifications, such as those problems that immediately follow victimization or other trauma, entry into a new school building, or classroom failure.

The case conceptualization process for school attendance problems can begin as early as the referral stage; many referrals to therapists involving primary attendance problems come from school officials and parents. School officials can inform the nature and severity of a student's attendance problems vis-à-vis immediate effects on academic achievement, risk of administrative or legal sanction, and likelihood of school reintegration. Parents can inform the nature and severity of a student's school attendance problems vis-à-vis immediate effects on social and family functioning as well as key behavioral issues. Both parties can also inform current daily functioning with respect to school preparation, degree of actual school attendance, and level of distress at home and school.

Potential causal factors for school attendance problems can involve a myriad of factors, though specific precipitants should be considered. Many school attendance problems develop gradually over time, but often some specific aspect of these problems precipitates a treatment referral. Such precipitants often involve school failure, grade retention, substantial family disruption, physical harm or bullying, school stop-out (withdrawal or unenrollment for a period of time), and school-based sanctions for absenteeism such as suspension or required parent conferences. Potential maintaining factors for school attendance problems may be more instructive for treatment development purposes and can involve the primary functions described earlier (i.e., avoidance of negative affectivity associated with school-related stimuli; escape from aversive social and/or evaluative situations; pursuit of attention from significant others; and pursuit of tangible reinforcers outside of the school setting).

Current contextual factors include those discussed earlier at various ecological levels and can inform the necessary breadth and scope of treatment. Available support systems are another important part of the case conceptualization process for this population. Recall from the earlier discussion of functional impairment that not all school absences carry the same effects. In some cases, students have substantial external support systems that potentially mitigate negative social and academic effects from absenteeism. Examples include considerable parental involvement, access to electronic equipment and tutoring, medical excusals, and school-based supports such as temporary virtual learning formats or home-based instruction. In other cases, however, few external support systems exist and therefore must be more fully developed in conjunction with the formal treatment plan.

Treatment planning and goal setting for school attendance problems are often driven by the timeline required by a school for a child to return to school. For many cases, ideally, reintegration to school should occur within four to six weeks, with additional treatment on ancillary issues for several weeks after that. For students with chronic and severe school attendance problems, treatment planning and goal setting are often driven by a student's best educational pathway toward credit accrual and/or graduation. Schools will often dictate what this pathway is, such as required summer work or an alternative educational setting, and so treatment planning and goal setting will naturally have to blend with these dictates. An essential aspect of case resolution for this population is a reintegration timeline that is agreed to by all relevant parties, and especially between school officials and parents.

Identifying obstacles to treatment is another important aspect of the case conceptualization process for school attendance problems. Treatment plans for this population often require collaboration among multiple parties as well as resolving significant logistical considerations. Common obstacles often requiring helpful collaborative efforts include transportation vulnerability, lack of supervision in the morning, and overburdened/exhausted caregivers. In many cases, efforts to mitigate obstacles must precede any attempts to resume school attendance.

Session Structure When Working with School Attendance Problems

The session structure when working with school attendance problems can be linear and stage-based but can be highly blended as well. In many urgent cases, for example, screening, assessment, and consultation processes often overlap. In addition, treatment for this population generally follows an earlier, middle, and later stage process but can also require quick recalibration and reconfiguration of strategy and goals, meaning new components must be suddenly added or subtracted. In related fashion, unforeseen goals sometimes emerge once a particular benchmark has been reached, as when a previously non-anxious student returning to school after an extended absence unexpectedly experiences substantial distress and worry about possible negative reactions from peers and teachers.

The screening process for school attendance problems should focus heavily on the current forms of absenteeism as well as the school/social/family domains of functional impairment mentioned earlier to inform the current urgency of the situation. The screening process can also include the generic recommendations mentioned earlier (relational consideration section) if formal assessment is delayed. More formal assessment can include key interview questions and behavioral assessment measures and can focus on gleaning a more complete clinical profile of possible precipitants and contextual variables. The consultation process for school attendance problems is also important and should involve ensuring that all relevant parties (especially caregivers/parents and school officials) are synchronized with respect to timeline, treatment components, and treatment rationale.

Treatment for this population generally consists of early, middle, and later stages. Early sessions focus on stabilizing school attendance, addressing immediate crises and logistical challenges, and developing communicative relationships among key stakeholders. Middle stages of treatment focus on reintegrating a student to school, implementing key support techniques such as anxiety or contingency management, and managing ancillary problems such as missed academic work. Later stages of treatment focus on consolidating treatment gains, synthesizing treatment components, finalizing full-time school attendance, and preparing for relapse prevention.

Component of Practice and Intervention Modules

Many cognitive-behavioral therapy techniques have been applied to school attendance problems, and many of these can be arranged into general categories that are discussed in this section: anxiety management, exposure and gradual reintroduction to school, contingency management, family-based procedures such as contracts, and case management approaches for chronic and severe cases. The most common primary goals of these approaches are to enhance school attendance in various forms, reduce distress associated with school, boost caregiver/parental control and ease of the school preparation process, augment a family's communication and problem-solving ability with respect to school attendance, and manage broader contextual factors that impact school attendance. Common secondary goals of these approaches are to improve general academic and family functioning, build developmental competencies that may have been delayed during absenteeism, and restore students on the path toward adult and career readiness.

Anxiety management techniques for school attendance problems are designed to address the considerable emotional distress that children and adolescents experience before and during school hours. Younger children often experience more nebulous and generalized anxiety, whereas older children and adolescents tend to experience more specific social and performance anxiety. As such, anxiety management for younger children tends to emphasize somatic management techniques such as muscle relaxation training, breathing retraining, or a menu of options (e.g., music, distraction). Anxiety management for older children and adolescents can include these techniques as well as more cognitively oriented procedures to develop more realistic thoughts in anxiety-provoking situations. Examples include examining evidence for and against certain thoughts, using dispute handles to challenge unrealistic thoughts, and decentering to enhance mindfulness, among other techniques.

Exposure-based practices are common for school attendance problems as well. Anxiety-based cases often involve extensive practice in school-related situations that tend to produce the most distress. Key examples include riding alone on a school bus, entering a classroom by oneself, being in class without one's parents, being in school without calling one's parents, engaging in transitions between classes, handling unpredictable circumstances, speaking before others, starting or maintaining conversations, attending a specialized class, eating with friends, asking or answering a question in class, taking tests, walking in hallways at school, and performing before others. In addition, anxiety- and non-anxiety-based cases can involve gradual reintroduction to a school setting, particularly following a long absence. Different methods are available for this purpose. Time in school can be gradually added (e.g., one hour or one class period per week) starting at the beginning of a school day and then forward; near the end of a school day and then backward; or at lunch and then from the middle of the day. Other gradual reintegration schedules involve starting with favorite classes or times of the school day and/or attendance in a non-classroom area of a school prior to classroom reintegration.

Contingency management techniques for this population often focus heavily on the morning school preparation routine as well as initial entry into the school building, which can be problematic especially for younger children with separation anxiety. Primary contingency management practices for school attendance problems include restructuring caregiver commands toward ones that are specific and feasible to comply with, ignoring simple inappropriate behaviors such as dawdling, designing fixed routines with ample time to complete each preparation task, establishing rewards for timely school preparation and attendance and disincentives for nonattendance, and reducing excessive reassurance-seeking behavior. Contingency management can in some cases be supplemented with aspects of forced school attendance in which two adults/caregivers physically bring a young child to school and deposit them with school officials who provide an escort into the school building. Caregivers with children with separation anxiety upon entering school are encouraged to engage in all final affection/goodbyes at home and not at school, discuss school-based problems in the evening and not the morning, and depart the separation point at school as soon as possible, ideally with school official support.

Family-based procedures for school attendance problems are generally more relevant to adolescent cases, particularly those where the student is pursuing more palatable off-campus activities during school hours. Written contracts or agreements between caregivers and the student to increase tangible incentives for school attendance and reduce tangible incentives for nonattendance are a key mechanism of this approach. Contracts should be relatively succinct, time-limited (e.g., one to two weeks), and specific and should be modified quickly as needed as school attendance improves. Communication skills training can supplement the use of contracts as well to enhance overall problem-solving ability among family members. Contracts may be supplemented as needed as well with procedures that boost the likelihood of their compliance, including escorting a youth to school and between classes, increasing supervision during school hours, improving sleep hygiene, and instructing youth on positive ways to decline offers from others to miss school.

Finally, a blend of case management practices is often needed for particularly chronic and severe cases of school attendance problems. Case management practices here involve a full understanding of the unique circumstances surrounding a particular case of severe absenteeism and providing innovative and creative workaround strategies to enhance the chances that the student will graduate from high school and/or engage in avenues that promote career and adult readiness. Examples include alternative educational pathways and 2nd chance programs available in many school districts and communities that offer flexible lanes toward school completion. Other emphases include vocational training, technical certification, and blending high school and community college work (Vargas et al., 2017). Case management practices for this population may also involve specialized, residential, or inpatient services to address severe psychopathology, family exigencies, and other substantial contextual factors and challenges.

Assessment of Progress and Outcomes

School attendance problems are highly amenable to a behavioral assessment-oriented process for gauging treatment progress and outcomes. A main outcome variable is naturally school attendance itself, which can be measured via full days, classes, and hours in school for in-person learning as well as log-ins, completed assignments, and meeting timelines for course objectives for virtual learning. Attendance for specific classes such as math or physical education that posed special difficulty for a particular student should be closely monitored as well. School attendance in general should be supervised well into the future for these cases given high potential for slips or relapse. Many school districts employ technological means to supply caregivers with immediate feedback regarding attendance, and families are encouraged to avail themselves of these measures.

Anxiety-based cases of school absenteeism can also include daily ratings of emotional distress at various times of the day to gauge progress. These would ideally occur in the morning before school, upon entry to school, midday, and after school. In addition, instances of subtle avoidance should be scrutinized as potential warning signs; examples include eating in school areas other than the cafeteria, avoiding classes with a scheduled examination, and sitting alone in the bleachers during a school event. Safety signals, or extenuating circumstances deemed necessary to perform a stressful task, should also be minimized. Examples include the need to have a family member ride a school bus or attend school with the child.

The frequency and duration of behavioral problems that were associated with a particular case of school absenteeism can be measured as well. Examples include length of dawdling or temper tantrums in the morning, time needed to separate from a caregiver at school, and number of off-campus activities during school hours. In related fashion, compliance to the school preparation morning routine, including instances of tardiness to school, can be operationalized as completing specific tasks within the scheduled timelines of the routine. Specific symptoms associated with diagnoses most relevant to school absenteeism cases, such as depression or substance use, can also be examined on a pre-post basis.

Recall as well that functional impairment domains are an important factor in determining the caseness of a particular school attendance problem. As such, assessment of progress and outcome should include the degree to which various aspects of these domains have improved. Important considerations would thus be improvements in the school domain such as grades, completed academic work, and ability to pass the school year; improvements in the social domain such as reconnection with peers and constructive interpersonal communications with teachers; and improvements in the family domain such as reduced conflict and less missed work.

Another set of important outcomes for this population includes key developmental tasks and competencies that may have eroded or become stagnant while a student was out of school for an extended period of time. Examples include handing in homework independently, visiting the school's front office to solve a problem, addressing social rejection, entering conversations with others, managing conflict, and understanding classroom and graduation requirements. Clinicians should ensure that a student is fully acclimated to their school setting and has the ability to successfully navigate challenges and novel situations. This process helps solidify treatment gains, enhance insight and self-efficacy, and reduce the chances of relapse.

Applications to the School Setting

Many of the cognitive-behavioral techniques described here for school attendance problems can interface with the school setting in various ways. One important interface of cognitive-behavioral techniques for school attendance problems with the school setting involves the use of accommodation plans. Accommodation plans typically involve a 504 plan or an individualized education plan. A 504 plan (based on Section 504 of the Rehabilitation Act of 1973) allows for supplemental services to students with physical or mental impairments that interfere with learning or other major life activities at school. An individualized education plan, or IEP (from the Individuals with Disabilities Education Act), is more stringent and usually applies most to youth formally placed in special education programs. Both accommodation plans potentially allow for inclusion of cognitive-behavioral treatment implementation recommendations at a child's school. Note that school districts vary with respect to allowing this option for school attendance problems and/or sometimes require a specific diagnosis or substantial documentation prior to plan development. Clinicians are encouraged to consult with a child's school counselor or other relevant school official in this regard.

Accommodation plans are a useful administrative mechanism to blend cognitive-behavioral treatment components into the school setting. Common components in this regard include part-time attendance schedules (to support gradual re-exposure to school), modification of test-taking times (to support interventions for performance anxiety), attendance journals and escorts into school and from class to class (to support caregiver-child separation and family-based contracts), and trauma-informed classroom practices such as cool down areas (to support somatic management techniques). Other more ancillary or supportive components in this regard include alternative educational and credit accrual pathways, modifications in class schedule and academic work, increased supervision at school, mentoring, assessment of learning and other disorders, access to school-based mental health supports, and daily feedback to caregivers regarding attendance and academic performance.

Accommodation plans should ideally be time-limited so that a regular review of its procedures can be evaluated for effectiveness and modified as needed. In addition, accommodation plans can be particularly useful in the latter half of an academic year if a student has missed many school days and is in danger of grade retention via failing courses. Plans at this stage could involve partial credit or part-time attendance for core classes (e.g., language, math), observing or auditing classes to better understand academic material in advance of a graded course, adjusting make-up work or assignments within the context of passing a course, identifying benchmarks needed to pass a class, and linking current academic progress or grades of incomplete to summer classes or other remediation avenues. Innovative strategies to demonstrate competency in a particular subject (e.g., via service/experiential work or projects) other than traditional course metrics (e.g., tests, essays) may be included as well.

Accommodation plans could also support other key interfaces of cognitive-behavioral treatments for school attendance problems and the school setting: conducting therapy sessions at the school and adapting treatment techniques for use by school officials. Common examples of the former include exposure-based practices in a classroom, cognitive restructuring immediately following an anxiety-provoking event, and assisting parents with the morning separation process on school grounds. Common examples of the latter include special in-school counseling sessions with a school-based social worker, school-based meetings with parents and school officials to implement home-based measures, and integrating youth into existing school-based mental health programs. Several resources are also available (e.g., Kearney, 2018) to modify CBT treatment techniques in line with time and resource constraints typically faced by school-based professionals.

Case Study of School Attendance Problems

The case study utilized in this section is designed as an advanced Tier 2 case, meaning that school attendance problems have likely lasted less than one calendar year but have progressed to the point where broader contextual factors and more severe functional impairment apply. As such, the case is designed to provide readers with a sense of how cognitive-behavioral treatments could be applied while at the same time demonstrating the need to work with the educational system as well as with at least one other system of care. Recall that a Tier 3 case of chronic and severe school attendance problems will likely require even greater multidisciplinary collaboration as well as more complex and flexible treatment options.

Marissa was a 12-year-old multiracial female who had entered her 1st year of middle school (6th grade in this case) in September. She attended the 1st three weeks of school but eventually became challenged by intense social and academic pressures that produced substantial anxiety and somatic complaints (fatigue, nausea). Marissa complained to her mother that she felt alienated at school and that the amount of schoolwork was confusing and overwhelming. She was also experiencing difficulty sleeping, which made the school preparation process in the morning quite difficult when Marissa could not rise on time. She missed several days of school between mid-September and the end of October, including several key days involving mid-semester examinations and class projects. The last two months of the fall semester involved a sharper decline in school attendance, parental acquiescence to the absences for fear of traumatizing their daughter, and family confusion about steps for remediation. At the end of the fall semester, the school counselor informed the family that Marissa had failed half of her classes and had surpassed the district policy limit on unexcused absences.

Marissa attended school in the 1st week of the spring semester in January but soon complained that other students were bothering her and that she felt unsafe at school. She stopped attending school completely at this point, and her family was referred by the school counselor to a community-based therapist. At the time of clinical assessment in early February, Marissa had missed about 60% of school days in the present academic year, was failing all of her current classes, was separated from her friends, and largely stayed in her room at home. The therapist and school counselor consulted on a plan to try to salvage the current academic year while at the same time addressing Marissa's psychological symptoms. The therapist referred Marissa and her family as well to a child psychiatrist for medication.

The primary initial treatment goal was to establish some form of school attendance in conjunction with a more established morning preparation routine and improved sleep hygiene. The therapist and school counselor developed a short-term accommodation plan so that Marissa could initially attend just two core classes (math, English) in the morning and be allowed to complete academic work during the other school hours at home. Transportation was arranged across several parties (extended family members, church friends) to facilitate the special schedule. In addition, a more regular sleep and waking schedule was established and linked to a more systematic school preparation routine in the morning. Tutoring was also provided for the core classes. Daily contact was conducted across the school counselor, therapist, and Marissa and her parents for two weeks, with occasional adjustments to the initial schedule, which were largely successful (Table 10.1).

The secondary treatment goal was to address Marissa's emotional distress about attending school. This involved somatic management practices, cognitive restructuring that addressed her overestimations of negative evaluation by others, and gradual exposure. A preliminary timeline was formed to complete the school reintegration process, with a goal of four weeks, adding one new class per week. This process was supplemented by a focus on re-establishing Marissa's social connections at school and addressing any school-based threats. This involved a rearrangement of Marissa's class and lunch schedule as well as greater involvement in after-school activities to boost her social support. The therapist and school counselor worked with Marissa's teachers as well to identify what work needed to be completed in the spring semester in order to merit a passing grade. The psychiatrist had also prescribed an antidepressant that appeared to help improve Marissa's energy level and mood.

Table 10.1 Initial Treatment Goals

Stabilize school attendance by establishing a baseline of minimum possible attendance.
Implement strategies such as securing academic work to help minimize functional impairment.
Ensure that all relevant stakeholders have open and frequent lines of communication.

Table 10.2 General Session Outline (Each Phase May Be Condensed, Blended, or Extended as Needed)

Session 1	Engage in consultation regarding assessment results, treatment plan, and possible obstacles; establish a baseline of attendance and a schedule for school reintegration in conjunction with input from family members and school officials and/or with an accommodation plan.
Session 2	Introduce supportive CBT techniques most specific to the case, such as those for anxiety management (e.g., somatic control exercises, cognitive techniques, mindfulness), contingency management (e.g., regular morning routine, incentives, altered caregiver commands), and/or family-based intervention (e.g., written contracts, increased supervision, communication skills training).
Sessions 3–4	Introduce the 1st step of additional school attendance (e.g., one hour or class) in conjunction with more intensive CBT techniques to support this process. Mobilize a student's social support system at school and establish external supports (e.g., tutoring, medication) as needed to ease school re-entry. Engage in daily monitoring of progress and frequent family and school contact to address problems immediately.
Sessions 5–6	Continue the gradual school reintegration process to achieve at least 50% daily attendance, continue intensive CBT, and adjust CBT techniques as needed to address unexpected problems or challenges.
Sessions 7–8	Continue the gradual school reintegration process to achieve at least 80% daily attendance, continue intensive CBT, and adjust CBT techniques as needed to address unexpected problems or challenges.
Session 9	Finalize the school reintegration process to full-time attendance and encourage family members to continue treatment procedures through the remaining sessions and to the end of the school year.
Sessions 10–11	Address key developmental competencies necessary to maintain good school attendance, such as achieving sufficient familiarity with current academic material, understanding options for seeking help at school for various issues, and engaging in new social interactions.
Session 12	Conduct relapse prevention training by focusing on future vulnerabilities such as the beginning of a new school year or during an examination period. Emphasize the need to remain vigilant about monitoring school attendance and maintaining new skills even when no school attendance problems exist.

The gradual reintegration process was uneven, as Marissa was able to initially attend a 3rd class but refused to attend a 4th class until several weeks later. She never attended her 5th and 6th classes but did attend an in-school study session in lieu of these classes; she was thus at least physically in the school building for the entire day. Treatment continued to focus on anxiety management that also eventually included family- and school-based incentives for school attendance. Marissa's accommodation plan was adjusted near the end of the academic year so that she could enroll in two modular summer classes to compensate for the subjects she missed during the regular academic year. She was eventually able to be promoted to her next grade. The therapist recommended a resumption of treatment two weeks prior to the new school year to help Marissa cope with a potentially stressful school re-entry process (Table 10.2).

Summary

Key aspects of clinical applications for school attendance problems include problem-solving and sometimes crisis-oriented approaches to resolve a highly disruptive and urgent situation. In addition, CBT components must be blended with input from relevant school-based professionals and considered within the context of school-based policies regarding attendance and absenteeism. More complex and severe cases will also likely require greater input from professionals in other systems of care. School attendance problems are often a key marker of functional impairment for youths with many different mental health and other challenges and are often an initial focus of treatment for different clinical populations. Health-based professionals are thus encouraged to familiarize themselves with key clinical strategies for school attendance problems, no matter their specialty area.

Reflection Questions

1 How might a clinician collaborate with school-based professionals to help resolve a case involving school attendance problems?
2 What contextual factors most impact school attendance problems for different student groups?
3 How can CBT practices be condensed or modified for particularly urgent school attendance problems?

Sources for Additional Treatment Detail

1 Garfi, J. (2018). *Overcoming school refusal: A practical guide for teachers, counsellors, caseworkers and parents*. Samford Valley: Australian Academic Press Group.
2 Kearney, C. A., & Albano, A. M. (2018). *When children refuse school: A cognitive-behavioral therapy approach/Therapist guide* (3rd ed.). New York: Oxford University Press.
3 Thambirajah, M. S., Grandison, K. J., & De-Hayes, L. (2008). *Understanding school refusal: A handbook for professionals in education, health and social care*. Philadelphia, PA: Jessica Kingsley Publishers.

References

Childs, J., & Scanlon, C. L. (2022). Coordinating the mesosystem: An ecological approach to addressing chronic absenteeism. *Peabody Journal of Education, 97*, 74–86. https://doi.org/10.1080/0161956X.2022.2026722

Duong, M. T., Bruns, E. J., Lee, K., Cox, S., Coifman, J., Mayworm, A., & Lyon, A. R. (2021). Rates of mental health service utilization by children and adolescents in schools and other common service settings: A systematic review and meta-analysis. *Administration and Policy in Mental Health and Mental Health Services Research, 48*, 420–439. https://doi.org/10.1007/s10488-020-01080-9

Eklund, K., Burns, M. K., Oyen, K., DeMarchena, S., & McCollom, E. M. (2022). Addressing chronic absenteeism in schools: A meta-analysis of evidence-based interventions. *School Psychology Review, 51*, 95–111. https://doi.org/10.1080/2372966X.2020.1789436

Elliott, J. G., & Place, M. (2019). Practitioner review: School refusal: Developments in conceptualisation and treatment since 2000. *Journal of Child Psychology and Psychiatry, 60*, 4–15. https://doi.org/10.1111/jcpp.12848

Fornander, M., & Kearney, C. A. (2019). Family environment variables as predictors of school absenteeism severity at multiple levels: Ensemble and classification and regression tree analysis. *Frontiers in Psychology, 10*, 2381. https://doi.org/10.3389/fpsyg.2019.02381.

Gonzálvez, C., Inglés, C. J., Kearney, C. A., Sanmartín, R., Vicent, M., & García-Fernández, J. M. (2019). Relationship between school refusal behavior and social functioning: A cluster analysis approach. *European Journal of Education and Psychology, 12*, 17–29.

Gonzálvez, C., Kearney, C. A., Vicent, M., & Sanmartín, R. (2021). Assessing school attendance problems: A critical systematic review of questionnaires. *International Journal of Educational Research, 105*, 101702. https://doi.org/10.1016/j.ijer.2020.101702

Gubbels, J., van der Put, C. E., & Assink, M. (2019). Risk factors for school absenteeism and dropout: A meta-analytic review. *Journal of Youth and Adolescence, 48*, 1637–1667. https://doi.org/10.1007/s10964-019-01072-5

Guryan, J., Christenson, S., Cureton, A., Lai, I., Ludwig, J., Schwarz, C., Shirey, E. & Turner, M. C. (2021). The effect of mentoring on school attendance and academic outcomes: A randomized evaluation of the Check & Connect Program. *Journal of Policy Analysis and Management, 40*, 841–882. https://doi.org/10.1002/pam.22264

Kearney, C. A. (2016). *Managing school absenteeism at multiple tiers: An evidence-based and practical guide for professionals*. New York: Oxford University Press.

Kearney, C. A. (2018). *Helping school refusing children and their parents: A guide for school-based professionals* (2nd ed.). New York: Oxford University Press.

Kearney, C. A. (2021). Integrating systemic and analytic approaches to school attendance problems: Synergistic frameworks for research and policy directions. *Child and Youth Care Forum, 50*, 701–742. https://doi.org/10.1007/s10566-020-09591-0

Kearney, C. A. (2022). Functional impairment guidelines for school attendance problems in youth: Recommendations for caseness in the modern era. *Professional Psychology: Research and Practice, 53*, 295–303. https://doi.org/10.1037/pro0000453

Kearney, C. A., & Albano, A. M. (2018). *When children refuse school: A cognitive-behavioral therapy approach/ Therapist guide* (3rd ed.). New York: Oxford University Press.

Kearney, C. A., Benoit, L., Gonzálvez, C., & Keppens, G. (2022). School attendance and school absenteeism: A primer for the past, present, and theory of change for the future. *Frontiers in Education, 7*, 1044608. https://doi.org/10.3389/feduc.2022.1044608.

Kearney, C. A., & Childs, J. (2022). Improving school attendance data and defining problematic and chronic school absenteeism: The next stage for educational policies and health-based practices. *Preventing School Failure: Alternative Education for Children and Youth*. https://doi.org/10.1080/1045988X.2022.2124222.

Kearney, C. A., & Gonzálvez, C. (2022). Unlearning school attendance and its problems: Moving from historical categories to postmodern dimensions. *Frontiers in Education, 7*, 977672. https://doi.org/10.3389/feduc.2022.977672.

Kearney, C. A., & Graczyk, P. A. (2020). A multidimensional, multi-tiered system of supports model to promote school attendance and address school absenteeism. *Clinical Child and Family Psychology Review, 23*, 316–337. https://doi.org/10.1007/s10567-020-00317-1

Kumm, S., Wilkinson, S., & McDaniel, S. (2020). Alternative education settings in the United States. *Intervention in School and Clinic, 56*, 123–126. https://doi.org/10.1177/1053451220914895

Leduc, K., Tougas, A. M., Robert, V., & Boulanger, C. (2022). School refusal in youth: A systematic review of ecological factors. *Child Psychiatry and Human Development*, 1–19. https://doi.org/10.1007/s10578-022-01469-7

Maynard, B. R., Brendel, K. E., Bulanda, J. J., Heyne, D., Thompson, A. M., & Pigott, T. D. (2015). Psychosocial interventions for school refusal with primary and secondary school students: A systematic review. *Campbell Systematic Reviews, 11*, 1–76. https://doi.org/10.4073/csr.2015.12

Maynard, B. R., Heyne, D., Brendel, K. E., Bulanda, J. J., Thompson, A. M., & Pigott, T. D. (2018). Treatment for school refusal among children and adolescents: A systematic review and meta-analysis. *Research on Social Work Practice, 28*, 56–67. https://doi.org/10.1177/1049731515598619

Melvin, G. A., Heyne, D., Gray, K. M., Hastings, R. P., Totsika, V., Tonge, B. J., & Freeman, M. M. (2019). The Kids and Teens at School (KiTeS) framework: An inclusive bioecological systems approach to understanding school absenteeism and school attendance problems. *Frontiers in Education, 4*. https://doi.org/10.3389/feduc.2019.00061

Nation, M., Christens, B. D., Bess, K. D., Shinn, M., Perkins, D. D., & Speer, P. W. (2020). Addressing the problems of urban education: An ecological systems perspective. *Journal of Urban Affairs, 42*, 715–730. https://doi.org/10.1080/07352166.2019.17058 47

Pyne, J., Grodsky, E., Vaade, E., McCready, B., Camburn, E., & Bradley, D. (2023). The signaling power of unexcused absence from school. *Educational Policy, 37*, 676–704. https://doi.org/10.1177/089590482110494

Rosenthal, L., Moro, M. R., & Benoit, L. (2020). Migrant parents of adolescents with school refusal: A qualitative study of parental distress and cultural barriers in access to care. *Frontiers in Psychiatry, 10*, 942. https://doi.org/10.3389/fpsyt.2019.00942

Thapa, A., & Cohen, J. (2017). School Climate Community Scale: Report on construct validity and internal consistency. *School Community Journal, 7*, 303–320.

Vargas, J., Hooker, S., & Gerwin, C. (2017). Blending high school and college can sharpen the focus of each. *Phi Delta Kappan, 99*, 13–18.

von der Embse, N., Rutherford, L., Mankin, A., & Jenkins, A. (2019). Demonstration of a trauma-informed assessment to intervention model in a large urban school district. *School Mental Health, 11*, 276–289. https://doi.org/10.1007/s12310-018-9294-z

11

REVEALING UNSPOKEN WORDS

Using CBT with Selective Mutism

Christy A. Mulligan and Ray W. Christner

Introduction

Selective Mutism (SM) is a complex and often misunderstood disorder that predominantly affects children; however, it can persist into adolescence and adulthood if not addressed early. This condition extends beyond shyness or an inhibited temperament. It presents a significant challenge to those who experience it, as it involves a consistent inability to speak in specific social situations where speech is expected. As a result, individuals with SM may remain silent in school, social gatherings, or other public contexts, hindering their ability to communicate and interact effectively. In this chapter, you will be introduced to selective mutism, how it manifests, the history of the disorder, and how it has evolved throughout the editions of the Diagnostic and Statistical Manuals III, IV, 5th, and now 5th text edition (DSM-5-TR; American Psychiatric Association, 1980, 1994, 2013, 2022) the key characteristics of subtypes of the disorder, the cognitive and behavioral strategies and techniques that are most successful, and the implication for the school environment.

What Is Selective Mutism, and How Has It Evolved?

SM is a condition where an individual is unable to speak in certain expected situations, such as school or public settings, while maintaining the ability to speak in other contexts, like at home (DSM-5-TR; American Psychiatric Association, 2022). In DSM-5-TR, it is classified under anxiety disorders, and typically, SM emerges between the ages of 3 and 6, often becoming apparent after a child enters pre-k or kindergarten. Epidemiological studies suggest a prevalence rate of approximately 1% for children with SM (Murris & Ollendick, 2015). The onset of SM during childhood can lead to significant consequences, impacting education and social interactions in the short term (Bergman et al., 2002; Kumpulainen et al., 1998).

Many clinicians have never treated a child with SM; therefore, it is important to follow the diagnostic criteria outlined by the DSM-5-TR, and it is crucial to rule out any physical disability that might hinder speech (American Psychiatric Association, 2022). Long-term outcomes reveal persistent challenges, as follow-up studies on adults who underwent various interventions for SM in childhood (average age of 8.5 years) indicate that 42%–61% continue to experience SM into adulthood (Remschmidt et al., 2001; Steinhausen et al., 2006). This suggests that SM can be an ongoing condition that hinders communication in educational, leisure, and occupational settings, often

DOI: 10.4324/9781003392439-14

accompanied by enduring dysand behavioral issues (Remschmidt et al., 2001; Steinhausen et al., 2006). Therefore, effective interventions are needed to address SM and alleviate both short-term and long-term negative effects associated with the condition.

The concept of SM has its roots in the work of Kussmaul (1822–1902), a German physician. In his groundbreaking 1877 work on speech disturbances, Kussmaul provided clinical descriptions of "absence of speech without disturbance of speech," associating it primarily with cases of "hysteria and other neuroses" (Kussmaul, 1877, p. 200). Despite this, a common misconception in subsequent literature is that Kussmaul referred to this condition as *aphasia voluntaria* (i.e., voluntary inability to speak), a misinterpretation of the term *aphrasia voluntaria* that he actually used, suggesting a more plausible meaning of "voluntary absence of speech" (Kussmaul, 1877, p. 211). Kussmaul introduced this term and positioned aphrasia voluntaria among other speech disturbances, contributing to a comprehensive frame of reference for differential diagnosis.

In 1934, another pioneer in speech disorders, Swiss child psychiatrist Tramer (1882–1963), proposed *elektiver Mutismus* (elective mutism [EM]) as a suitable term. In a detailed case report of a seven-year-old boy, Tramer suggested the name EM because the mutism was limited to contacts with a consciously chosen group of people. Tramer viewed children with this diagnosis as not aphasic but intentionally choosing to remain silent (Halpern et al., 1971; Tramer, 1934).

Although Tramer's contribution was a case report, the term *elektiver mutismus* became widely accepted. His paper's significant merit lies in its scholarly overview of the mechanisms thought to underlie the problem, covering hereditary factors, delayed phases of normal child development, psychological factors, social mechanisms, physical conditions, and major psychopathology. Therapeutically, Tramer demonstrated foresight, introducing many behavioral techniques that psychotherapists would later advocate for treating children with SM (Halpern et al., 1971; Lowenstein & Lowenstein, 1976; Wulbert et al., 1973).

EM was initially categorized in the DSM-III under Other Disorders of Infancy, Childhood, or Adolescence (American Psychiatric Association, 1980). In a departure from its "atheoretical" approach, the DSM Task Force for DSM-IV opted to replace "Elective Mutism" with "Selective Mutism" (SM). This change conveyed the idea that this type of mutism occurs in specific contexts rather than being inherently self-chosen (American Psychiatric Association, 1994). Simultaneously, researchers increasingly proposed that SM might be closely linked to anxiety (Anstendig, 1999; Black & Uhde, 1992, 1995; Dow et al., 1995; Golwyn & Weinstock, 1990), advocating for its relocation to the anxiety disorders group. Black and Uhde (1995) supported this view by finding that 97% of children with SM also met diagnostic criteria for either social phobia or avoidant personality disorder. Subsequent empirical studies consistently reported the presence of anxiety symptoms in children with SM (Carbone et al., 2010; Cohan et al., 2008; Manassis et al., 2007; Muris & Ollendick, 2015; Vecchio & Kearney, 2005), leading to the reclassification of SM as an anxiety disorder in the DSM-5 (American Psychiatric Association, 2013).

Heterogeneity of Selective Mutism

Various authors, including Muris and Ollendick (2015), have explored the relationship between SM and anxiety, noting overlap in symptomatology, etiology, and treatment approaches. However, the precise nature of this relationship remains unclear. Cohan et al.'s (2008) latent-profile analysis revealed three SM subtypes, each indicating a clinically significant presence of social anxiety. Some studies reported higher observer ratings of anxiety in children with SM compared to those with social phobia, although this finding is not consistent across all studies. Meta-analytic results also indicate that children with SM are diagnosed with an anxiety disorder in only 80% of cases (69% for social phobia) (Driessen et al., 2020). In many of these cases, unrelated diagnoses of specific phobias are common. Rozenek et al. (2020) also concluded in their review that SM was part of a heterogenic group of disorders with a multifaceted, overlapping, and complex etiology.

Notably, anxiety as a symptom is not explicitly mentioned in the DSM's diagnostic criteria for SM, despite its reclassification as an anxiety disorder. Consequently, its presence has not always been systematically assessed in empirical studies of individuals with SM. Instead, researchers often establish the link between SM and anxiety by examining the presence of comorbid anxiety disorders. While this approach has limitations, as specific phobias may not necessarily indicate a reluctance to speak in social situations, the body of literature on comorbid anxiety disorders in SM serves as a proxy for understanding the association.

Other research efforts support the notion that SM may be quite distinct from social and other anxiety disorders. Children with SM differ from those with social anxiety in key ways such as behavioral inhibition (Milic et al., 2020), endorsement of speech-demanding situations as more embarrassing (Schwenck et al., 2019), speech-based fears (Vogel et al., 2019), degree of trauma (Mulligan et al., 2015), and anxiety in school-based situations (Poole et al., 2021). Others have noted that children with SM are often rated differently by parents and teachers concerning behaviors and adaptive skills (Klein et al., 2019). Reviews additionally confirm the presence of heterogeneity among children diagnosed with SM, with several studies highlighting oppositional symptoms or coexistence of oppositional defiant disorder (ODD) that may manifest in up to 30% of youths with the disorder (Alyanak et al., 2013; Kristensen et al., 2019).

Conceptualization of Selective Mutism

Understanding SM from a cognitive-behavior therapy (CBT) framework poses challenges for clinicians due to the limited insight into the cognitive processes of children with SM. Cognitive development evolves throughout childhood and adolescence, influenced by various contextual factors such as family, peers, and school. Mennuti and Christner (2005) emphasize the need for CBT components to align with the child's developmental level. While cognitive strategies can be adapted for younger children, interventions often involve hands-on, behavioral approaches and the use of imagery rather than solely relying on verbal strategies, especially with children inhibited from speaking outside their immediate family (Drinkwater & Stewart, 2002; Mennuti et al., 2006).

In the context of a CBT framework, a popular way to conceptualize SM is to understand it along an anxiety spectrum. Treatment focuses less on compelling the child to talk and more on recognizing and addressing their anxiety effectively. Initially, behavioral interventions are crucial, given the challenges of cognitive restructuring in this population. Encouraging and reinforcing communication become key objectives alongside anxiety reduction. As treatment progresses, cognitive-based interventions gain prominence.

While cognitive aspects may be less emphasized in the direct treatment of children, they play a vital role when working with parents. Clinicians assess parental beliefs and thoughts, using cognitive restructuring to address maladaptive thinking patterns. Parents often grapple with self-blame, influenced by family history or genetic links contributing to their child's difficulties. Psychoeducational training for parents proves invaluable, offering an understanding of SM, the evaluation process, symptom treatment, and interventions for home use.

From a purely behavioral perspective, SM may be viewed as learned behavior or a response to manipulate the environment. Some researchers argue that the silent behavior of children with SM serves a specific function maintained by environmental reinforcement (Pordes, 1992). While acknowledging behavioral aspects, it's essential not to disregard the cognitive components these children experience. A behavioral or "functional" standpoint allows clinicians to explain behaviors as adaptive rather than pathological, reinforcing the need for alternative means of communication when speech is withheld. The withholding of speech often leads to secondary changes in the child, perpetuating the behavior as others accommodate or reduce demands for speech (Powell & Daily, 1995).

Conceptualization of Selective Mutism Subtypes

Researchers have identified diverse clinical symptom profiles in children with SM, reflecting the considerable heterogeneity within this population. These profiles revolve around themes of anxiety, oppositionality, communication, and other challenges. In a study by Cohan et al. (2008), caregivers of children aged 5–12 with SM were asked to assess various aspects, including communication delays, expressive and receptive language abilities, functional impairments, internalizing and externalizing symptoms, and social and behavior problems.

The study utilized latent profile analysis, revealing a three-class solution: anxious-mildly oppositional, anxious-communication delayed, and exclusively anxious. The anxious-mildly oppositional group, the largest subset (44.6%), exhibited borderline clinical scores for behavior problems and syntax, along with clinically significant social anxiety scores. Behavior problems aligned with stubborn or controlling behavior in anxiety-provoking situations. The anxious-communication delayed group, comprising 43.1%, showed poor receptive language abilities, syntax, significant social anxiety, and greater SM symptom severity compared to the exclusively anxious group. The exclusively anxious group, representing 12.3%, displayed less anxiety and better expressive and receptive language abilities than the anxious-communication delayed group. The study highlighted significant associations between oppositionality, speech, and language problems with SM (Cohan et al., 2008).

In a more recent study, five subtypes emerged with many unique characteristics (Mulligan et al., 2015): (1) Global Mutism, (2) Anxiety/Language Mutism, (3) Low Functioning Mutism, (4) Sensory/Pathology Mutism, and (5) Emotional Behavioral Mutism. Each subtype displays distinctive primary and secondary characteristics, and considering different subtypes becomes essential as it can impact the planning of appropriate treatments.

Generally, *Global Mutism* stands out as the least impaired among the various subtypes. Children classified under this subtype have typically transitioned developmentally from a subtype with more pronounced issues to the Global subtype, as their needs, particularly related to anxiety and sensory problems, are less pervasive. Notably, the children in this subtype are relatively older compared to some other subtypes, and we may hypothesize these children also experienced some degree of treatment prior to the distinction of this subtype. While children in the Global Mutism subtype may encounter challenges related to self-esteem and flexibility, they generally exhibit academic competence. Unlike some other subtypes, these children do not display significant sensory, emotional, or behavioral problems. The prevalence of the Global subtype aligns with existing literature, indicating a gender ratio of 2:1 in favor of females, cutting across all racial categories. This subtype appears to be the most prevalent, encompassing the largest percentage of children with SM. Often, children who fall into the Global Mutism do not need special education services to address academic deficits, as their academic skills are typically strong.

The *Anxiety/Language Mutism* subtype is characterized by elevated anxiety levels, often meeting the criteria for a comorbid anxiety disorder. Children within this subtype are prone to experiencing a considerable degree of environmental stress in their lives. Academically, they face challenges, and there may be delays in meeting speech and language developmental milestones on time. Consequently, these children often require speech and language services in the school setting to address their communication needs.

The *Low Functioning Mutism* subtype is marked by a general lack of academic success compared to other subtypes. These children typically do not have comorbid psychiatric conditions themselves; however, there is an increased risk of maternal psychopathology, such as depression or a history of

SM in childhood. Other relevant characteristics of this subtype include sensory and executive problems, as well as lability. These challenges are likely contributors to the academic difficulties that are a hallmark of this subtype. As a result, these children are almost invariably placed in special education to provide support for their low academic functioning.

The *Sensory/Pathology Mutism* subtype often coexists with sensory integration dysfunction. This subtype is additionally characterized by oppositional behavior and lability. Notably, the Sensory/Pathology subtype may exhibit greater racial diversity, with a higher prevalence of bilingual children. Children with SM in this subtype may also show signs of separation anxiety problems and delays in motor skills. Overall, this subtype is likely to be the most impaired when compared to the other subtypes. It is common to observe comorbid diagnoses of learning disabilities, ADHD, ODD, and depression within this subtype.

Lastly, the *Emotional/Behavioral Mutism* subtype, unique with a 10:1 gender ratio favoring females, exhibits difficulties in executive control, emotional lability, and oppositional behavior. Surprisingly, these children do not face significant academic issues despite executive functioning difficulties. Recognizing these subtype distinctions allows clinicians to conceptualize SM better and differentiate between students needing special education services, those requiring a 504 service agreement, or regular education. With these findings, it is hoped that clinicians will gain deeper insights and develop evidence-based treatments tailored to each subtype (Mulligan et al., 2015).

With the identification of these subtypes, clinicians now have a clearer framework to conceptualize children with SM. This distinction also aids in understanding why some students require special education services while others may need services under a 504 service agreement or can be serviced in a regular education setting. The hope is that these new findings from Mulligan et al. (2015) will not only provide clinicians with greater insight and the ability to conceptualize this complex disorder but will also pave the way for the development of new evidence-based treatments tailored to the specific needs of each subtype. In the next section, we will highlight some strategies and interventions that may be useful to use for each subtype, including service delivery and placement options.

Treatment Strategies for Selective Mutism Subtypes

Currently, the predominant effective treatments for SM involve behavioral elements, such as reinforcement, stimulus fading, token procedures, shaping procedures, contingency management, self-modeling, or response-initiation procedures (Gidden et al., 1997; Kehle et al., 1998). Successful approaches to treating selectively mute children should encompass a thorough analysis of the child and their environment (Anstendig, 1999). One advantage of these strategies is their applicability in various settings, including home, school, and the community.

Looking at the subtypes of SM and considering cognitive and behavioral strategies, it is recommended to think about the following interventions to incorporate into treatment. It is recognized that each child who suffers from SM is unique, and the disorder is more heterogeneous; therefore, Table 11.1 provides a recommended guide or starting point to help make gains in functionality in school.

The above strategies are not exhaustive, and tailoring interventions to the specific needs of the individual child with SM is critical in successful progress and maintenance toward verbal communication. One caution for any subtype or any form of treatment is to deemphasize speech or verbal communication. For example, if you encourage verbal communication for a child whose primary issue is anxiety, this, in turn, could stifle progress by focusing on speech. Similarly, for those youth with SM who are experiencing oppositional tendencies, if the therapist's goal is speaking, this may spark an internal battle between the youth and those who encourage verbal communication.

Table 11.1 Recommended Intervention Options and Supports

Subtype	*Treatment Intervention*	*Placement Consideration/Related Services*
Global mutism	• Build rapport • Benefit from psychoeducation • Cognitive strategies can be employed, e.g., graded exposure, feelings thermometer, moving toward Socratic questioning and cognitive restructuring • Activity scheduling • Therapeutic journaling • Small group social skills training, with typical peers included • Promote and build self-efficacy • Interviews with those closest to the student, e.g., parents/teachers	• Regular education or • 504 for psychological services
Anxiety/language mutism	• Build rapport • Ecological evaluation to better understand the youth's environment • Build in verbal intermediaries • Relaxation training, imaginal exposure • Build confidence and self-efficacy • Psychoeducation for those working with the child not to pressure speech • Provide acceptable non-verbal alternatives to verbal communication, e.g., red card/green card • Parent-guided exposure • Small group work • Mindfulness	• Special education services, e.g., speech and language services • In-school psychological services • May consider outside counseling
Low functioning mutism	• Build rapport • Assess for deficits in executive functioning • Sensory diet may be appropriate • Behavioral interventions, such as reinforcement, shaping, contingency management • Behavioral experiments • Video modeling • Verbal praise • Ecological evaluation to better understand the youth's environment	• Special education • In-school psychological services
Sensory/pathology mutism	• Build rapport • Sensory diet • Psychoeducation • Help the youth to understand triggers • Provide choices for communication • Teach social skills, self-monitoring • Interviews with those closest to the student, e.g., parents/teachers	• Special education • 504 • OT • PT • FBA/BIP • Psychological services • Behavior specialist • Possible outside counseling

(*Continued*)

Table 11.1 (Continued)

Subtype	*Treatment Intervention*	*Placement Consideration/Related Services*
Emotional/ behavioral mutism	• Build rapport • Psychoeducation • Assess for deficits in executive functioning • Teach connection between thoughts/feelings/ behaviors • Providing choices of acceptable alternative forms of communication • Teach the youth how to communicate a break if overwhelmed • Cognitive strategies, e.g., graded exposure, stimulus fading, shaping, therapeutic journaling, moving toward cognitive restructuring, Socratic questioning	• Special education • 504 • FBA/BIP • Psychological services • Behavior specialist • Possible outside counseling

The diversity within SM is also reflected in the various multimodal treatment approaches that researchers and practitioners have employed to address the distinct characteristics of this population (Østergaard, 2018). Recent efforts in multimodal treatment have expanded toward intensive and group-oriented interventions. Lorenzo et al. (2020) utilized a combination of parent-child interaction therapy, live parent coaching and child-directed interaction, and cognitive-behavioral techniques like stimulus fading in a multi-day, all-day group setting, supplemented by videoconferencing and school outreach, to address young children with SM. Similarly, Cornacchio et al. (2019) employed a comparable strategy, and they found that intensive group therapy led to significant remissions of SM, reductions in social anxiety, and long-term improvements in functional outcomes compared to a wait-list control. Skedgell et al. (2017) employed personalized individual and group therapy, integrating exposure-based and contingency management procedures to bring about change in young children with SM. Indeed, involving multiple stakeholders is now recognized as a crucial aspect of SM treatment (Catchpole et al., 2019).

CBT stands out as a prominent approach in aiding children with SM. CBT interventions aim to help children recognize and acknowledge their SM through psychoeducation while guiding them in altering their thoughts and behaviors to alleviate anxieties and enhance self-assurance in social contexts. CBT interventions need to highlight the child's positive attributes alongside addressing areas of concern. While traditional CBT techniques may emphasize verbalization, adaptations can be made to accommodate children with SM. Knell (1993) has introduced cognitive-behavioral play therapy, blending cognitive-behavioral interventions with elements of play therapy, which proves promising, especially for younger children and those with SM.

It may not be easy to monitor progress, as often the child may whisper, almost inaudibly, as they begin to make progress. Therefore, one potential solution to this issue is the adoption of an objective measure for assessing speaking behavior. A notable example stemming from recent advancements in wearable technology is passive audio vocal measurement. This technology demonstrates the ability to quantitatively assess child vocalizations, vocal volume, and other conversational metrics (Xu et al., 2018). Although wearable technology is still undergoing refinement and development, its potential to enhance the quality of SM research in the future is significant.

Implications and Applications to the School Setting

SM often becomes apparent when a child enters school, underscoring the crucial role of school support in treatment. Framing SM as an anxiety disorder within the school setting can yield more effective support compared to relying solely on standard special education and remedial services (Shipon-Blum, 2007). Students with SM may benefit from in-school accommodations, many of which can be formalized through a 504 Service Agreement rather than opting for special education services. To adequately address the individual needs of each child, schools should allocate resources to conduct a thorough evaluation. This comprehensive approach ensures tailored support and accommodations to facilitate the child's academic and social progress.

The significance of the relationship between students and teachers greatly influences children's development, especially during their initial years of schooling. It's during this time that children solidify essential skills for academic success and form precise cognitive perceptions of themselves as learners (Entwisle & Hayduk, 1988; Pianta & Walsh, 1996). This influence becomes even more pronounced for students with atypical development (Robertson et al., 2003). Therefore, classroom teachers can implement several strategies to create a more comfortable and supportive environment for students with SM. Firstly, conducting a home visit can help the child become familiar with the teacher in a relaxed setting. If possible, allowing the child to witness positive interactions between the teacher and parent during drop-off can also ease anxiety. We cannot underscore the importance of a strong home/school relationship with consistent communication.

Within the classroom, pairing students with SM with a buddy during breaks, recess, and lunch can encourage socialization. Initially, teachers can facilitate nonverbal forms of communication, such as using index cards with greetings like "Good morning" or "Goodbye." Acknowledging and rewarding these attempts at communication are essential components of any classroom behavior plan. All efforts toward communication should be rewarded, albeit not overly praised (Shipon-Blum, 2007), as teachers should be sensitive to the fact that children with SM may feel easily embarrassed by effusive verbal reinforcement. To mitigate discomfort, teachers should avoid drawing unnecessary attention to the child and minimize direct eye contact when speaking to them.

Lastly, teachers should serve as a point of contact for professionals working with the child outside of school, including physicians, psychologists, or other therapists (Shipon-Blum, 2007). Collaboration between school and external professionals is vital for coordinating support and interventions to meet the child's needs best.

If a child with SM qualifies for special education services, several accommodations and interventions can support their educational experience. Recommendations from Shipon-Blum (2007) include:

1 **Small Group or Buddy Work**: Allowing the child to work in small groups or with a designated "buddy" can provide a supportive environment for social interaction and academic participation.
2 **Parental Involvement**: Encouraging parental involvement in the school helps create a collaborative support network and ensures consistency between home and school environments.
3 **Alone Time with a Friend**: Providing opportunities for the child to spend alone time with a trusted friend can foster social connections and reduce anxiety.
4 **Extended Time and Alternative Assessments**: Offering extended time for assignments or tests, as well as providing alternative assessment formats such as taped or written verbal reports, accommodates the child's needs and allows for varied modes of expression.
5 **Nonverbal Communication**: Supporting nonverbal communication methods and preparing the child for changes in routine helps alleviate anxiety and promotes participation.
6 **One-on-One Time with the Teacher**: Providing dedicated one-on-one time with the teacher allows for personalized support and guidance tailored to the child's needs.

7 **Creative Learning Environments**: Incorporating visual and spatial activities into the curriculum creates engaging and accessible learning experiences for children with SM.
8 Efforts toward both nonverbal and verbal communication should be recognized and rewarded to reinforce positive behaviors and efforts.
9 In addition to accommodations and interventions, related services may be considered as part of the child's programming. These services, which may include speech and language therapy, occupational therapy, or psychological counseling, can address specific needs and support the child's overall development within the school setting. The necessity of related services should be assessed on a case-by-case basis to ensure comprehensive and individualized support for children with SM.

As a child with SM progress through treatment, school professionals often observe improvements in their behaviors. These improvements may include increased verbalization and social interaction with peers, as well as a noticeable reduction in anxiety levels, if present. Observable signs of decreased anxiety might include more frequent smiling, increased eye contact, relaxed body posture, spontaneous initiation of verbal or nonverbal communication, and quicker responses to questions.

For the treatment team working with a child with SM, the most rewarding outcome is hearing the child's voice being communicated to others. Witnessing the child's progress and seeing them engage more confidently in social interactions represents a significant achievement and underscores the effectiveness of the intervention efforts. This tangible improvement not only reflects the child's growth but also validates the collaborative efforts of the treatment team in supporting the child's development and well-being.

Conclusions and Future Directions

Several factors should be considered for the future understanding of SM. One such factor is using assessments extending beyond anxiety symptoms to understand better the complexities of the disorder, such as associated cognitive and behavioral patterns, temperament, environment, and physiological influences. Objective measures, such as psychophysiological assessments, are preferable to subjective evaluations by parents, teachers, or clinicians, especially when children with SM are unable to confirm their experiences (Driessen et al., 2020) verbally. It may also be beneficial to extend the research to treatment-resistant SM and the adult population, as research in this area is scant (Dreissen et al., 2019).

Research on treating children with SM remains mixed in the review of what interventions work to increase verbal communication. However, implementing current CBT strategies for anxious children and children who demonstrate varying degrees of oppositional behavior, as well as executive deficits and sensory sensitivities, offers practical strategies for developing goals and approaches to reduce negative symptomatology for youth with SM. School-based professionals should employ creativity in adapting these interventions to minimize reliance on verbal interactions during treatment sessions. This approach acknowledges the diverse needs of children with SM, the heterogeneity of the disorder, and the communication styles of children with SM, ensuring interventions are tailored to their individual needs.

Further research needs to be conducted on subtyping and evidence-based treatments to truly determine which strategies have the greatest effect size for each subtype. However, the hope is by providing suggestions on where to begin, school-based clinicians will be able to develop an initial treatment plan. By recognizing the variability within SM presentations and utilizing adaptable treatment strategies informed by CBT principles, professionals can better support children with SM in navigating social and educational settings more effectively. This proactive and flexible approach enhances the prospects for positive outcomes and improved quality of life and communication for children with SM in schools and their community settings.

Reflection Questions

1 How do the evolving diagnostic criteria and understanding of SM across different editions of the DSM influence the approach to identifying and treating individuals with SM?
2 Reflect on the heterogeneity within SM. How does recognizing these subtypes enhance the effectiveness of treatment plans, and what challenges might clinicians face in accurately identifying and addressing the specific needs of each subtype?
3 Considering a child you have worked with who experiences SM, reflect on the role of schools in supporting the student. What are the key components of a successful school-based intervention, and how can educators, psychologists, and parents collaborate to create a supportive environment that facilitates communication and reduces anxiety for students with SM?

References

Alyanak, B., Kilincaslan, A., Harmanci, H. S., Demirkaya, S. K., Yurtbay, T., & Vehid, H. E. (2013). Parental adjustment, parenting attitudes and emotional and behavioral problems in children with selective mutism. *Journal of Anxiety Disorders, 27*, 9–15. https://doi.org/10.1016/j.janxdis.2012.10.001

American Psychiatric Association (1980). *Diagnostic and statistical manual of mental disorders* (3rd ed.). Washington, DC: American Psychiatric Association.

American Psychiatric Association (1994). *Diagnostic and statistical manual of mental disorders* (4th ed.). Washington, DC: American Psychiatric Association.

American Psychiatric Association (2013). *Diagnostic and statistical manual of mental disorders* (5th ed.). Washington, DC: American Psychiatric Association.

American Psychiatric Association (2022). *Diagnostic and statistical manual of mental disorders* (5th ed., text rev.). https://doi.org/10.1176/appi.books.9780890425787

Anstendig, K. D. (1999). Is selective mutism an anxiety disorder? Rethinking its DSM-IV classification. *Journal of Anxiety Disorders, 13*(4), 417–434.

Bergman, R. L., Piacentini, J., & McKracken, J. T. (2002). Prevalence and description of selective mutism in a school-based sample. *Journal of American Academy of Child and Adolescent Psychiatry, 41*, 938–946.

Black, B., & Uhde, T. W. (1992). Case study: Elective mutism as a variant of social phobia. *Journal of the American Academy of Child & Adolescent Psychiatry, 31*(6), 1090–1094.

Black, B. B., & Uhde, T. W. (1995). Psychiatric characteristics of children with selective mutism: A pilot study. *Journal of the American Academy of Child and Adolescent Psychiatry, 34*, 847–855.

Carbone, D., Schmidt, L. A., Cunningham, C. C., McHolm, A. E., Edison, S., St. Pierre, J. et al. (2010). Behavioral and socio-emotional functioning in children with selective mutism: A comparison with anxious and typically developing children across multiple informants. *Journal of Abnormal Child Psychology, 38*, 1057–1067.

Catchpole, R., Young, A., Baer, S., & Salih, T. (2019). Examining a novel, parent child interaction therapy-informed, behavioral treatment of selective mutism. *Journal of Anxiety Disorders, 66*, 102112. https://doi.org/10.1016/j.janxdis.2019.102112

Cohan, S. L., Chavira, D. A., Shipon-Blum, E., Hitchcock, C., Roesch, S. C., & Stein, M. B. (2008). Refining the classification of children with selective mutism: A latent profile analysis. *Journal of Clinical Child and Adolescent Psychology*, 37, 770–784. https://doi.org/10.1080/15374410802359759

Cornacchio, D., Furr, J. M., Sanchez, A. L., Hong, N., Feinberg, L. K., Tenenbaum, R., et al. (2019). Intensive group behavioral treatment (IGBT) for children with selective mutism: A preliminary randomized clinical trial. *Journal of Consulting and Clinical Psychology, 87*, 720–733. https://doi.org/10.1037/ccp0000422

Driessen, J., Blom, J. D., Muris, P., Blashfield, R. K., & Molendijk, M. L. (2020). Anxiety in children with selective mutism: a meta-analysis. *Child Psychiatry & Human Development, 51*(2), 330–341.

Dow, S. P., Sonies, B. C., Scheib, D., Moss, S. E., & Leonard, H. L. (1995). Practical guidelines for the assessment and treatment of selective mutism. *Journal of the American Academy of Child and Adolescent Psychiatry, 34*, 836–845.

Driessen, J., Blom, J. D., Muris, P., Blashfield, R. K., Molendijk, M. L. (2020). Anxiety in children with selective mutism: A meta-analysis. *Child Psychiatry & Human Development, 51*, 330–341.

Drinkwater, J., & Stewart, A. (2002). Cognitive behaviour therapy for young people. *Current Opinions in Psychiatry, 15*, 377–381.

Entwisle, D. R., & Hayduk, L. A. (1988). Lasting effect of elementary school. *Sociology of Education, 61*, 147–159.

Gidden, J. J., Ross, G. J., Sechler, L. L., & Becker, B. R. (1997). Selective mutism in elementary school: Multidisciplinary interventions. *Language, Speech and Hearing Services in Schools, 28*, 127–133. https://doi.org/10.1044/0161-1461.2802.127

Golwyn, D. H., & Weinstock, R. C. (1990). Phenelzine treatment of elective mutism: A case report. *The Journal of Clinical Psychiatry, 51*, 384–385.

Halpern, W. I., Hammond, J., & Cohen, R. (1971). A therapeutic approach to speech phobia: Elective mutism reexamined. *Journal of the American Academy of Child Psychiatry, 10*, 94–107.

Kehle, T. J., Madaus, M. R., Baratta, V. S., & Bray, M. A. (1998). Augmented self-modeling as a treatment for children with selective mutism. *Journal of Psychology, 36*, 247–260.

Klein, E. R., Ruiz, C. E., Morales, K., & Stanley, P. (2019). Variations in parent and teacher ratings of internalizing, externalizing, adaptive skills, and behavioral symptoms in children with selective mutism. *Journal of Environmental Research and Public Health, 16*, 4070. https://doi.org/10.3390/ijerph16214070

Knell, S. M. (1993). *Cognitive-behavioral play therapy*. New York: Guilford Press.

Kristensen, H., Oerbeck, B., & Manassis, K. (2019). Selective mutism. In S. N. Compton, M. A. Villabø & H. Kristensen (Eds.), *Pediatric anxiety disorders* (pp. 225–250). New York: Academic Press.

Kumpulainen, K., Rasanen, E., Raaska, H., & Somppi, V. (1998). Selective mutism among second graders in elementary school. *European Child and Adolescent Psychiatry*, 11, 71–78.

Kussmaul, A. (1877). *Die Störungen der sprache: Versuch einer pathologie der sprache*. Leipzig: Verlag von F.C.W Vogel.

Lorenzo, N. E., Cornacchio, D., Chou, T., Kurtz, S. M., Furr, J. M., & Comer, J. S. (2020). Expanding treatment options for children with selective mutism: Rationale, principles, and procedures for an intensive group behavioral treatment. *Cognitive Behavior Practice*. https://doi.org/10.1016/j.cbpra.2020.06.002

Lowenstein, L. F., & Lowenstein, K. (1976). The treatment and follow-up of a number of cases of elective mutism. *Behavioural and Cognitive Psychotherapy, 4*(3), 41–46.

Manassis, K., Tannock, R., Garland, E. J., Minde, K., Mcinnes, A., & Clark, S. (2007). The sounds of silence: Language, cognition, and anxiety in selective mutism. *Journal of the American Academy of Child and Adolescent Psychiatry, 46*(9), 1187–1195. https://doi.org/10.1097/CHI.0b013e318076b7ab

Mennuti, R. B., & Christner, R. W. (2005). School-based cognitive behavioral therapy (CBT). In A. Freeman (Ed.), *International encyclopedia of cognitive behavior therapy* (pp. 343–347). New York: Klewer/Springer.

Mennuti, R. B., Christner, R. W., & Freeman, R. (Eds.) (2006). *Cognitive behavioral interventions in educational settings: A handbook for practice*. New York: Guilford.

Milic, M. I., Carl, T., & Rapee, R. M. (2020). Similarities and differences between young children with selective mutism and social anxiety disorder. *Behaviour Research and Therapy, 133*, 103696. https://doi.org/10.1016/j.brat.2020.103696

Mulligan, C. A., Hale, J. B., & Shipon-Blum, E. (2015). Selective mutism: Identification of subtypes and implications for treatment. *Journal of Education and Human Development, 4*, 79–96. https://doi.org/10.15640/jehd.v4n1a9

Murris, P., & Ollendick, H. T. (2015). Children who are anxious in silence: A review on selective mutism, the new anxiety disorder in DSM-5. *Clinical Child and Family Psychology Review, 18*, 151–169. https://doi.org/10.1007/s10567-015-0181-y

Østergaard, K. R. (2018). Treatment of selective mutism based on cognitive behavioural therapy, psychopharmacology and combination therapy – A systematic review. *Nordic Journal of Psychiatry, 72*, 240–250. https://doi.org/10.1080/08039488.2018.1439530

Pianta, R. C., & Walsh, D. J. (1996). *High-risk children in schools: Constructing sustaining relationships*. New York: Routledge.

Poole, K. L., Cunningham, C. E., McHolm, A. E., & Schmidt, L. A. (2021). Distinguishing selective mutism and social anxiety in children: A multi-method study. *European Child & Adolescent Psychiatry, 30*(7), 1059–1069. https://doi.org/10.1007/s00787-020-01588-3

Pordes, M. D. (1992). Intervention with the selectively mute child. *Psychology in the Schools, 29*, 367–376.

Powell, S., & Dailey, M. (1995). When to intervene in selective mutism: The multimodal treatment of a case of persistent selective mutism. *Psychology in Schools, 32*, 114–123.

Remschmidt, H., Poller, M., Herpertz-Dahlmann, B., Hennighausen, K., & Gutenbrunner, C. (2001). A follow-up study of 45 patients with elective mutism. *European Archives of Psychiatry and Clinical Neuroscience, 251*, 284–296. https://doi.org/10.1007/pl00007547

Robertson, K., Chamberlain, B., & Kasari, C. (2003). General education teachers' relationship with included students with autism. *Journal of Autism and Developmental Disorders, 33*, 123–130.

Rozenek, E. B., Orlof, W., Nowicka, Z. M., Wilczyn ́ska, K., & Waszkiewicz, N. (2020). Selective mutism-an overview of the condition and etiology: Is the absence of speech just the tip of the iceberg? *Psychiatria Polska, 54*, 333–349. https://doi.org/10.12740/PP/OnlineFirst/108503

Schwenck, C., Gensthaler, A., & Vogel, F. (2019). Anxiety levels in children with selective mutism and social anxiety disorder. *Current Psychology, 40*, 1–8. https://doi.org/10.1007/s12144-019-00546w

Shipon-Blum, E. (2007). When the words just won't come out: Understanding selective mutism. Retrieved https://www.yumpu.com/en/document/read/12133154/when-the-words-just-wont-come-out-selective-mutism-group

Skedgell, K. K., Fornander, M., & Kearney, C. A. (2017). Personalized individual and group therapy for multifaceted selective mutism. *Clinical Case Studies, 16*, 166–181. https://doi.org/10.1177/1534650116685619

Steinhausen, H., Wachter, M., Laimbock, K., & Winkler Metzke, C. (2006). A long-term outcome study of selective mutism in childhood. *Journal of Child Psychology and Psychiatry, 47*, 751–756. https://doi.org/10.1111/j.1469-7610.2005.01560.x

Tramer, M. (1934). Elktiver Mutism bie Kindern. *Z Kindrpsychiat, 1*, 30–35.

Vecchio, J. L., & Kearney, C. A. (2005). Selective mutism in children: Comparison to youths with and without anxiety disorders. *Journal of Psychopathology and Behavior Assessment, 27*, 31–37. https://doi.org/10.1007/s10862-005-3263-1

Vogel, F., Gensthaler, A., Stahl, J., & Schwenck, C. (2019). Fears and fear-related cognitions in children with selective mutism. *European Journal of Child and Adolescent Psychiatry, 28*, 1169–1181. https://doi.org/10.1007/s00787-019-01281-0

Wulbert, M., Nyman, B. A., Snow, D., & Owen, Y. (1973). The efficacy of stimulus fading and contingency management in the treatment of elective mutism: A case study. *Journal of Applied Behavioral Analysis, 6*, 435–441.

Xu, H. Y., Stroud, J., Jozanovic, R. K., Clucas, J., Son, J. J., Koo, B., … & Milham, M. P. (2018). Clinical perspective on passive audio vocal measurement in the evaluation of selective mutism. *Frontiers in Psychiatry, 443*, 1–7. https://doi.org/10.3389/fpsyt.2018.00443

12

CBT FOR TRAUMA AND POSTTRAUMATIC STRESS DISORDER

Dana Milakovic

CBT for Trauma and Posttraumatic Stress Disorder

Pre-pandemic statistics on the rates of exposure of youth to traumatic events suggested that up to 61% of youth were exposed to at least one traumatic event in their life prior to age 18 (CDC, 2023). The most current data from the Youth Risk Behavior Survey (YRBS) and a variety of other mental health surveys indicate that up to 80% of students have been exposed to at least one type of traumatic event, two-thirds have been exposed to more than two or more types of traumatic events (CDC, 2023; Conners-Edge et al., 2022; Forkey et al., 2021). Exposure to traumatic events has been widely shown to have detrimental effects on developing brains, resulting in developmental, social, emotional, behavioral, and academic difficulties in the school setting. The American Academy of Pediatrics (Forkey et al., 2021) provides guidance to pediatricians regarding engaging in trauma-informed practices and how this supports children and adolescents. The range of support includes the development of relationships through referral for specialized care. This same referral process is made possible in trauma-informed school settings.

According to the National Child Traumatic Stress Network (2016), a trauma-informed school is one in which all members of a school community are provided the necessary support and training to recognize and respond to the impact of trauma on students and other school community members with an overall goal of maximizing physical and psychological safety, facilitating the recovery or adjustment of the child and family, and supporting their ability to thrive. This focus is best described as a tiered framework to prevent traumatization and support students when they experience trauma. Trauma-informed school systems promote a safe, supportive, and welcoming climate and seek to create a structured and predictable learning environment that avoids re-traumatization and reduces trauma reminders, proactively builds positive peer-to-peer and student-to-teacher relationships, has balanced disciplinary and restorative practices, and has suicide prevention and bullying prevention in place (The National Child Traumatic Stress Network, Schools Committee, 2017). When this tiered approach is present, school staff are able to recognize and appropriately refer students who are experiencing behavioral, emotional, or academic concerns that are likely to be the result of a traumatic experience. In other cases, the close relationships present between the school and community support family involvement and the safe disclosure of families to school mental health (SMH) staff when a traumatic event occurs. This can facilitate the provision of services in the school setting to reduce the neurocognitive and developmental effects of trauma as well as provide opportunities for support

DOI: 10.4324/9781003392439-15

rather than re-traumatization through discipline procedures (Conners-Edge et al., 2022; Guarino & Chagnon, 2018).

With the wide range of negative impacts of trauma on academic, behavioral, and social performance in the school setting, providing services to students who have experienced trauma and are showing signs in the school setting is vital in optimizing educational opportunities and growth. The best evidence-based treatments for trauma and posttraumatic stress disorder (PTSD) are individualized trauma-focused cognitive-behavior therapy (TF-CBT) (Conners-Eduge et al., 2022; Davis et al., 2023; Lindebo Knutsen et al., 2019; Lyon et al., 2021); however, current staffing shortages and high demand for mental health providers have resulted in a large number of youth who are not able to access services. With students spending a large portion of their day in the school setting and immediate staff access to students when they are in school, the provision of school-based services can help reduce the gap between treatment needs and the provision of services. School-based mental health (SBMH) services currently account for 50%–80% of all youth mental health services in the United States; however, TF-CBT has not been scaled up into the educational setting and often therapy modalities that have not shown evidence-based effectiveness for trauma and PTSD are utilized (Davis et al., 2023; Lyon et al., 2021). While barriers can be present and will be reviewed, along with opportunities to address them, TF-CBT continues to be shown as an effective group or individual treatment option for youth who have experienced trauma, regardless of the nature of the traumatic event (Conners-Eduge et al., 2022; Davis et al., 2023; Lindebo Knutsen et al., 2019; Lyon et al., 2021).

Understanding Trauma and PTSD

Trauma has been defined in many ways; however, a unifying theme across all definitions is exposure and long-lasting effects. According to the Substance Abuse and Mental Health Services Administration (SAMHSA, 2014), trauma results from an event, series of events, or set of circumstances that is experienced as physically or emotionally harmful or life-threatening and that results in lasting effects on functioning or well-being (mental, physical, social, emotional, or spiritual). Trauma impacts every school system across the United States. Current data on exposure to trauma and the immediate and intergenerational effects revolve around studying adverse childhood experiences (ACEs).

While exposure to a traumatic event does not immediately result in a psychological diagnosis, there are several trauma and stressor-related disorders that require exposure to a traumatic event in the Diagnostic Statistical Manual-5-TR (American Psychiatric Association [APA], 2022). These include reactive attachment disorder, disinhibited social engagement disorder, PTSD, acute stress disorder, adjustment disorder, and other specified trauma- and stressor-related disorders. For this work, a focus will remain on exposure to trauma, without requirements of a trauma- or stress-related disorder, including PTSD.

Adverse Childhood Experiences

When seeking to understand trauma, conversations must begin with exposure. ACEs are potentially traumatic events that occur during childhood and adolescence. While the original study on ACEs focused on abuse, neglect, witnessing violence, and specific household dysfunction (e.g., having a parent incarcerated, divorce/separation, or mental illness and substance abuse) (Felitti et al., 1998), current research on ACEs have expanded the definition to include systemic and environmental exposure to potentially traumatic events as well (Forkey et al., 2021; Research & Evaluation Group, 2013; Sacks & Murphey, 2018). It is important to note that these systemic factors and the resulting exposures of some families can put youth at increased risk of experiencing trauma. Children who are in foster care remain at home following a child protective services investigation or are moved to kinship care following investigation have higher levels of reported abuse and neglect. Additional populations with higher risk for exposure to ACEs include immigrant and refugee children, children living in poverty, and underrepresented racial, ethnic, and religious groups (Forkey et al., 2021; Guarino & Chagnon, 2018). In addition to systemic factors that increase the risk of exposure to ACEs, individual characteristics of youth can increase their rates of bullying and community violence. Lesbian, gay, bisexual, transgender, and queer youth, children of color, American Indian and Alaskan native children, immigrant children, neurodiverse youth, and youth who are overweight are at higher risk for exposure to ACEs in their homes and community (Forkey et al., 2021; Guarino & Chagnon, 2018; Trevor Project, 2023).

ACEs have been found to impact individuals differently, and similar to other aspects of trauma, it has been found that the level of exposure, acuteness vs. chronicity of exposure, and severity of exposure have been associated with a higher level of negative outcomes (McRae et al., 2021). When looking at a youth or adolescent in the school setting that experiences a traumatic event but has not yet reached criteria for PTSD, it is important to be aware of their history of adverse experiences, as these can serve as an enduring risk factor that predisposes them to increased determinantal effects when exposed to trauma, as well as reduce their level of natural resiliency (Conners-Edge et al., 2022; Forkey et al., 2021; Tsehay et al., 2020).

Cultural Considerations

In addition to assessing the youth in our school setting, when examining trauma exposure and resiliency, a family perspective is also highly relevant. Research focusing on epigenetics provides insights into how a familial history of trauma can impact youth. Epigenetics involve the study of how environmental experiences can impact gene expression in individuals and future generations, including physiological and psychological expression of genetics (Dubois & Guaspare, 2020; Kealohi Sato Conching & Thayer, 2019; Thumfart et al., 2022). Research on epigenetics has been focused on communities who have experienced known cultural trauma and began with studying the outcomes of offspring of Holocaust survivors and has expanded to health outcomes of groups who have traumatic exposure to war and populations that have been historically and systematically subjugated (Dubois & Guaspare, 2020; Kealohi Sato Conching & Tahyer, 2019). Epigenetics has provided a research base that supports historical and cultural trauma (also referred to as transgenerational or intergenerational trauma) as preexisting ACEs for students whose families have experienced trauma, as well as for populations that experience ongoing racism (Phipps & Thorne, 2019; Thumfart et al., 2022).

Cultural considerations and knowledge of transgenerational or intergenerational trauma are vital to providing support to students and families. The establishment of a therapeutic relationship that is rooted in psychological safety is key to being able to meet the core needs of students prior to beginning therapy and will be reviewed in depth; however, this begins with the acknowledgment and validation of individual and family experiences. TF-CBT has been documented to be effective in students who have experienced significant trauma, including cultural and historical trauma, but modifications may need to be made to address cultural needs (Chipalo, 2021; Kim et al., 2023; Phipps & Thorne, 2019).

Intersection of Trauma and PTSD

PTSD requires exposure to one or more traumatic events. Criteria for a diagnosis of PTSD vary depending on age, and the DSM-5-TR (APA, 2022) differentiates criteria for individuals older than six and individuals six and under. Eligibility for PTSD requires an exposure to a traumatic event, as discussed previously, and requires that that exposure was an actual or threatened death, serious injury, or sexual violence. The exposure can occur through either directly experiencing the event, witnessing it occurring to others in person, learning that the event occurred to a close family member or friend, or experiencing reoccurring trauma or adversity (APA, 2022). Intrusive symptoms mark PTSD, avoidance of trauma-related thoughts or environmental triggers, alterations in mood and cognitions (e.g., distorted beliefs), altered arousal and reactivity (e.g., hypervigilance, sleep problems, concentration difficulties), and increases in aggression in youth (APA, 2022).

PTSD prevalence estimates for criteria based on the DSM-5 are estimated to be 6.1%–8.3% (APA, 2022). Emerging research focusing on the intersection of trauma and PTSD suggests that child maltreatment is more strongly associated with negative outcomes, aggression in young males, and the development of PTSD (McRae et al., 2021). With current CDC estimates including one in seven children experiencing child abuse or neglect in a given year, 14 youth dying daily from homicide, and more than 1,300 youth receiving treatment in an emergency room for violence-related injuries (CDC, 2023), SMH professionals will likely see multiple youth per year with traumatic stress or PTSD.

Empirical Support of CBT Treatment with Trauma and PTSD

CBT has a well-established research base for usage with anxiety and depression in children and adolescents (Christ et al., 2020; Whiteside et al., 2022), and the development of TF-CBT was developed based on traditional CBT. TF-CBT includes both individual and joint parent and child sessions to address the developmental, behavioral, and cognitive impacts of trauma on youth. TF-CBT utilizes the acronym of P.R.A.C.T.I.C.E. to summarize the main components of TF:CBT: Psychoeducation, Parenting skills, Relaxation skills, Affective modulation skills, Cognitive coping skills, Trauma narrative, and Cognitive processing of traumatic events (Chipalo, 2021).

TF-CBT has been documented to be an evidence-based treatment for children and adolescents who have a memory of the trauma event. TF-CBT has been found to be effective in individual and group settings (Conners-Eduge et al., 2022; Davis et al., 2023; Lindebo Knutsen et al., 2019; Lyon et al., 2021). Lewey et al. (2018) conducted a meta-analysis of TF-CBT, and they found that modifications for young children, including acting out trauma with puppets, creating a scrapbook with pictures and words, songwriting, and drawing, were all effective ways to process traumatic events when done within a TF-CBT structure. Syros et al. (2022) conducted an extensive review of TF-CBT studies and reported the efficacy of utilization across multiracial populations, as well as usage in schools and community settings. Furthermore, in their review of studies with randomized trials, Syros et al. (2022) reported clinically significant improvements that sustained for six months, one year, and two years following treatment.

Davis et al. (2023) conducted a meta-analysis of group-based interventions for treating PTSD symptoms in youth, and they found that manualized TF-CBT training provided effective treatments for symptoms regardless of the population or complexity of trauma exposure. TF-CBT has been found to be effective across a range of traumas, regardless of the timing of the incident or severity. This includes refugee populations (Chipalo, 2021) and cultural trauma in African American youth (Phipps & Thorne, 2019).

Relational Consideration in Treatment of Trauma and PTSD

Exposure to traumatic events can have significant impacts on a youth's emotional, behavioral, relational, cognitive, and developmental functioning. When addressing trauma exposure and possible traumatic impact, it is important to ensure that the clinician is engaging from a trauma-informed lens.

Trauma-Informed Care Values

SAMHSA (2014) provides guidance for a trauma-informed approach with the goal of developing a shared understanding of trauma and trauma-informed care. SAMHSA acknowledges the impact of trauma on youth and families, as well as promoting the healing journey that is possible with interventions rooted in trauma-informed care. SAMHSA (2014) provides a set of six key principles of a trauma-informed approach: safety; trustworthiness and transparency; peer support; collaboration and mutuality; empowerment, choice, and voice; and cultural, historical, and gender issues.

Students and families who have experienced trauma are particularly vulnerable to traumatization. Often, trust has been lost through the trauma experience, and by focusing initially on the development of emotional, social, behavioral, physical, and psychological safety, SMH professionals can begin to develop a relationship rooted in trust. Providing opportunities for students to voice their experiences without judgment begins to build a therapeutic alliance and support healing.

The Importance of Safety in the Therapeutic Relationship

The success of any therapy, including TF-CBT, requires the development of a therapeutic alliance that supports client growth. Recognizing the disproportionality of trauma exposure for populations that have been historically marginalized requires clinicians to be aware of their own biases and ensure cultural humility while working with students and their families. Recognizing the intersection of individual trauma with societal factors is a key factor in supporting youth and families who have experienced trauma. While understanding the individual ACE for the child and family is important, taking a step back and assessing the possibility of an Adverse Community Environment is also an important step for SMH professionals. Ellis et al. (2022) review structural racism and how this adversity fosters ACE, including food insecurity, parental unemployment, housing instability and homelessness, domestic violence, maternal depression, parental incarceration, household substance abuse, neglect, and physical or emotional abuse.

Providing support through a trauma-informed approach moves beyond the understanding of trauma and transitions to a focus on promoting resiliency and healing. When developing a therapeutic alliance, ensuring physical and psychological safety through the lens of trauma-informed care values allows SMH professionals to respond by integrating their knowledge of trauma into treatment planning and session design, as well as actively resisting re-traumatizing youth so healing can occur.

Assessing for Trauma

Assessing trauma in the educational setting can be a challenging task. When a widespread traumatic event occurs in a community, there can be a tendency of school staff and mental health providers to assign the label of "trauma" to every student affected. This approach does not account for the research showing healing is the norm following a traumatic event. Research has suggested that some anxiety is normal following a traumatic event and is a healthy response to a stressful situation (Brock & Louvar-Reeves, 2019). Referrals for trauma screening following a traumatic event should not generally occur until at least one week out to allow for adaptive coping to begin to occur. However, monitoring of students should begin immediately, and for students with prior trauma histories, referrals may need to be made sooner.

The National Association of School Psychologists (NASP) provides one possible model to assist school and community mental health providers in assessing trauma responses, identifying and prioritizing crisis problems, and evaluating and concluding treatment. School crisis prevention and intervention: the PREPaRE model, 2nd Edition (Brock & Louvar-Reeves, 2019) provides a framework that can assist schools with triaging students based on their proximity to the event, preexisting vulnerabilities, immediate reactions during the crisis, and current or ongoing reactions and coping. Schools are encouraged to have a set trauma response model that includes prevention, early detection, and triaging of students based on exposure to traumatic events in their school and community. SBMH staff should be a part of that plan to assist in triaging students, managing referrals, and helping staff understand trauma processing.

Not all trauma reactions are the result of a known traumatic event occurring in the school or community. When students are living in an environment of chronic stress, especially in the absence of a stable adult, they can experience toxic stress or trauma reactions. Additionally, current data from the Center for Disease Control (CDC, 2023) indicates that 61% of adults reported experiencing one or more traumatic events prior to the age of 18. The most recent data from the Youth Risk Behavior Survey (YRBS, 2023) indicates that trends for violence in youth's lives are increasing. The data reported by youth continues to show that they are experiencing traumatic events that may be unknown to adults in their lives at an elevated rate. For this reason, one of the most important ways to address trauma in educational settings is to educate staff on behaviors that are often seen in students who are experiencing trauma.

Referral

A primary way to identify trauma is education of school staff, as referrals are likely to come from educational staff or parents. To improve referral processes, it is important for SBMH professionals to educate staff and parents on the signs and symptoms of trauma. This includes differentiating what trauma responses look like in varying developmental stages. As part of every referral for behavioral concerns, a screening and/or interview should occur to ensure that the referral reason is valid and not related to trauma.

Clinical Interview

Clinical interviews should be conducted with both the student and family. When addressing trauma in the school setting, SMH professionals should use a structured or semi-structured interview to allow for complete interviews without additional probing for trauma details. Trauma details are explored more in-depth during treatment, and probing prior to establishing safety and coping skills can exacerbate symptoms and negatively impact the therapeutic alliance. Interviews should serve to inform treatment and planning. Due to the sensitive nature of interviewing for trauma, it can be helpful to practice interviews in a peer clinical setting to increase clinician comfortability with interviews. Choi et al. (2019) provide two different examples of structured interviews for parents and children to assess exposure to traumatic events.

Following the identification of exposure to traumatic events, SMH professionals can conduct a behavioral interview. The goal of a behavioral interview is to determine potential antecedents and consequences for the behaviors of concern. As part of the behavioral interview, SMH professionals should be aware of themes that can provide insight into trauma triggers. If known, trauma triggers should be documented as part of the interview process. Questions around trauma triggers should include directly asking the student and family if they know what increases behaviors.

Other Assessment Data

Incorporating behavioral rating scales into the comprehensive assessment can provide additional data on the impact of trauma symptoms on the individual and their social and learning environment.

The Child Behavior Assessment System for Children, 3rd Edition (BASC-3; Reynolds & Kamphaus, 2015) is a paper-and-pencil or electronic measure that provides the opportunity for multiple responders and comparison across settings. Individual scores on the BASC-3 can inform the necessity for additional rating scales to address specific internalizing or externalizing behaviors. Treatment planning for behavioral needs may be supported by conducting a functional behavior assessment.

Through the usage of a comprehensive assessment, school teams can support treatment planning and intervention across the school setting. Screening and interview data support treatment planning and session planning, while a full assessment supports collaboration with other educational staff. Trauma behaviors in the school are likely to impact all areas of the student's functioning, and providing a comprehensive plan can increase feelings of safety in the school, resulting in fewer trauma reminders and subsequent behaviors. For a comprehensive list of research-based screenings and interviews, readers are encouraged to access the School Health Assessment and Performance Evaluation System's (SHAPE) screening and assessment library (National Center for School Mental Health, 2019).

Application of CBT for Students with Trauma or PTSD

Case Conceptualization

Understanding the behaviors and emotions of individuals with trauma relies on the acceptance that when an individual is experiencing trauma reactions, the emotional reactivity of their brain is in overdrive and behaviors and cognitions are secondary to the emotional reactions. CBT serves to align emotions with what is occurring in the environment and assist youth with making cognitive decisions regarding their behaviors rather than relying on emotional reactions. TF-CBT provides a structured method of providing support through phases with increased exposure to trauma reminders while building skills to develop new cognitions (Cohen & Mannarino, 2015). Cohen and Mannarino (2015) summarize the overarching goals of TF-CBT of addressing and re-regulating the child's trauma impact domains, which can include affective, behavioral, biological, cognitive/perceptual, and social/school.

Treatment goals and session structure should be guided by the comprehensive assessment completed to document trauma behaviors, trauma exposure(s), impact on the academic environment, impact on socialization in school, and behavioral presentation. Initial planning with the family to determine how often they can participate, how participation can be supported, and optimal outcomes assist with sustained engagement of the family throughout the sessions.

Session Structure

Balancing treatment goals and educational goals for a student is an important consideration for students receiving services in the school setting. Planning how the student will balance missed work instruction and when sessions can be scheduled to ensure the same educational material is not missed weekly will be important considerations.

Regardless of the age of the student, psychoeducation with the youth and family should be a primary goal in TF-CBT. Flexibility, no matter how the psychoeducational is provided to family members, can assist mental health staff and families with time management, as well as the establishment of a positive, supportive relationship. Providing opportunities for virtual participation in sessions, especially for sessions that involve psychoeducation, can increase parental involvement and participation.

TF-CBT involves phases of stabilization, trauma narrative and processing, and integration and consolidation and is provided in sessions of 60–90 minutes in length. Exposure has been verified through decades of research to be a vital part of CBT and is also a key component of TF-CBT (Cohen & Mannarina, 2015). Gradual exposure should be included throughout all TF-CBT sessions and increased as youth are able to process and gain control over trauma reminders.

Component of Practice and Intervention Modules

TF-CBT is a family approach that requires fidelity of implementation to achieve desired outcomes. When implementing this approach in a school setting, staff training should be considered, as well as the capacity of staff to implement the programming with fidelity. Due to the difficulties in a school setting with access to time and resources, many mental health professionals have been asked to implement individual and group services. While most CBT research for trauma has been focused on individual outcomes, studies have shown that manualized TF-CBT, Cognitive-Behavioral Intervention for Trauma in Schools (CBITS), Teaching Recovery Techniques (TrT), and Bounce Back have shown efficacy in a group and individual settings (Davis et al., 2023). When utilized in a group setting, research suggests that peers may provide support that a client's family typically does and parental involvement may not be as detrimental if not able to be provided (Davis et al., 2023). Training for each program is required and can be done in an online setting; however, supervision should be provided by previously trained and experienced clinicians. Addressing implementation barriers is best done with consideration for school climates and should involve decision makers to allow for the reduction in barriers (Lyon et al., 2021).

Trauma-Focused Cognitive-Behavior Therapy

TF-CBT consists of 12–20 sessions and has been shown to be appropriate for ages 3–18 years. The TF-CBIT model requires specialized training, which can be provided in person or virtually. TF-CBT Web is a web-based training for learning TF-CBT provided by the Medical University of South Carolina (2017) and has been endorsed by SAMHSA.

TF-CBT includes nine components that utilize the acronym PRACTICE. Psychoeducation (P) includes educating the child/adolescent about clinical and neurobiological aspects of trauma and therapeutic options. The development of a therapeutic alliance is part of psychoeducation. A secondary component of psychoeducation is supporting parenting skills and the management of trauma symptoms and parenting skill development to reinforce learned skills. Relaxation (R) includes teaching specific skills such as breathing exercises and progressive muscle relaxation to reduce the physiological signs of traumatic stress. Affective modulation involves emotional education and regulation skills, including utilization of positive self-talk and thought interruption. Cognitive coping (C) is designed to repair cognitive distortions that are identified through the processing and narration of trauma (T). The development of a trauma narrative is a core component of TF-CBT. While not always required, in-vivo (I) control over childhood trauma reminders uses exposure principles of CBT to increase exposure and reduce fearful reactions to trauma reminders. This is necessary when specific fears are identified through the therapeutic process. Child-parent sessions are conducted (C) to support the child in telling their family about the trauma event, as well as providing psychoeducational information to families. Enhancement (E) of future safety and development of the child is the final stage of TF-CBT and is designed to assist the child with addressing safety concerns to return them to a typical developmental trajectory (Medical University of South Carolina, 2017; Syros, 2022).

Cognitive-Behavioral Intervention for Trauma in Schools

CBITS has extensive research supporting usage in a group setting, especially for children with PTSD (Syros et al., 2022). Jaycox et al. (2018) provide the CBITS-2nd Edition through the Rand Corporation. CBITS was originally published in 2003, and the 2nd Edition includes updates based on lessons learned through research. Jaycox et al. (2018) report that CBITS is designed for groups of students who are experiencing relational or behavioral problems following exposure to significant traumatic experiences. CBITS has been designed for students who are in 4th grade or above and was initially developed for trauma-impacted, recently immigrated students from Latino, Korean, Armenian, and Russian backgrounds (Syros et al., 2022). It has been widely used in both rural and urban school settings following natural disasters and following significant community violence (Jaycox et al., 2018; Syros et al., 2022). CBITS is not recommended for students in crisis, students with significant behavioral needs that prohibit group engagement, or students with severe intellectual delays (Jaycox et al., 2018). CBITS consists of ten group sessions, one to three individual student sessions, two caregiver meetings, and an optional school staff informational session (Jaycox et al., 2018).

Teaching Recovery Techniques

TrT is a manualized group intervention developed by the Children and War Foundation (Smith et al., 1999) in Norway and is based on TF-CBT. TrT was designed to meet the needs of low-resource settings where large numbers of children needed intervention following trauma exposure (Sarkadi et al., 2018). TrT was designed for youth eight and above and consists of seven sessions for youth and two sessions for parents and is delivered by TrT trained staff. The session length is between 90 and 120 minutes and includes skill training and skill rehearsal. Homework is provided to be completed between sessions and reviewed at the subsequent session. Sessions are designed to build a therapeutic alliance (Session 1), intrusions and normalizing experiences (Sessions 2 and 3), relaxation and coping self-statements (Session 4), exposure and traumatic reminders (Sessions 5 and 6), and a follow-up session (Session 7). Parents' sessions are done without youth present and are conducted prior to the intervention beginning and between the 2nd and 4th youth group sessions. TrT has been used effectively worldwide, and research supports usage in the school setting for groups of students who have experienced traumatic events (Davis et al., 2023; Durbeej et al., 2021; Sarkadi et al., 2018).

Bounce Back

Bounce Back is an adaptation of the CBITS program and is designed for students in kindergarten through 5th grade. Similar to CBITS, Bounce Back is a group intervention that occurs over ten group sessions. Activities are designed for a younger developmental age and teach coping skills and healing from trauma through games and activities. Bounce Back develops a trauma narrative with students through individual sessions. Trauma narratives are then shared with parents through parent sessions. Parent training is included in the protocols to assist with psychoeducation and skill development (Syros et al., 2022). Bounce Back is available through the Center for Safe and Resilient Schools and Workplaces (2023).

Eye Movement Desensitization and Reprocessing

Eye Movement Desensitization and Reprocessing (EMDR) is a manualized treatment that was initially designed to treat trauma in a short period, with as little as one session (Lewey et al., 2018; Shapiro, 1989). EMDR was designed to use saccadic eye movements in a rhythmic pattern while cognitively focusing on the prominent aspects of the traumatic memory (Shapiro, 1989). EMDR has been widely studied as a treatment for PTSD and trauma and has been shown to have positive effects on behaviors and cognitions associated with trauma. Ongoing research on EMDR has suggested developmental changes for youth and adolescents, and a change in view to suggest that EMDR is more closely associated with exposure therapy and cognitive restructuring (Lewey et al., 2018).

EMDR has an underlying assumption that traumatic memories are stored inappropriately in memory, resulting in problem behaviors and reactions to trauma reminders (Teke & Avsaroglu, 2022). By reprocessing these memories while engaged in rapid and rhythmic eye movements, clients are able to increase their adaptive functioning and decrease trauma responses (Shapiro, 1989; Teke & Avsaroglu, 2022). EMDR has been shown to be a relatively quick, effective intervention for youth who have experienced trauma. Training for EMDR is not included in most clinical programs, and specific training and supervision are necessary to effectively utilize EMDR in mental health practices (Teke & Avsaroglu, 2022).

Assessment of Progress and Monitoring

Monitoring for progress should be primarily based on the referral and presenting behavioral and emotional presentation. Progress should be monitored consistently over the treatment sessions. While this is a key component of all CBT programs, providing CBT in an educational setting increases the need for progress monitoring and documentation of effectiveness and impact (Orminston et al., 2020). Readers are encouraged to view the screening and assessment library found in the SHAPE resources (National Center for School Mental Health, 2019) or the National Traumatic Stress Network's (NTSN) trauma screening and assessment resource for up-to-date, validated scales. Monitoring of progress should include a validated measure prior to the initiation of services and a measure following the conclusion of services. SMH professionals should consider utilizing a screening measure during the comprehensive assessment that can be repeated post-treatment. A review of research on treatment outcomes indicates a wide range of child-report or parent/child-report measures of PTSD or anxiety symptoms checklists.

Daily monitoring of symptoms can be done through using anxiety or symptom check-ins, Sudden Units of Distress (SUD) ratings, or virtual reporting of moods. Both low-tech and high-tech options are available for monitoring, and readers are encouraged to discuss monitoring with students and engage in shared decision-making to support compliance and utilization of monitoring tools.

Application to School Setting

SBMH services are in-person or telehealth services provided to students in the school setting. This can include services to promote skill development, create supportive learning environments, and provide intensive support for signs of mental illness. While SMHs are often individuals not employed by the school setting but providing services in the school setting, for this writing, all employees providing mental health services in a school will be broadly categorized as SMHs. This includes school-employed mental health providers such as school counselors, school psychologists, and social workers. Services provided can be categorized as assessment, prevention, and implementation services designed to support learning through the creation of supportive learning environments (Kern et al., 2022; Ormiston et al., 2021). SBMH services are widely used in the United States, and a recent poll indicated that 96% of public schools offer at least one type of mental health service to their student, with 84% of those services being individual-based interventions (Panchal et al., 2022).

Multi-Tiered System of Support

Implementation of individual services to address a student who has experienced trauma should ideally be provided in a framework including a multi-tiered system of support (MTSS). MTSS can address student mental health concerns through a tiered model that promotes systemic changes and a needed foundation of safety and trustworthiness in the school setting. Trauma-informed systems that highlight the need for the development of a safe and supportive environment as a core component of their everyday functioning provide the infrastructure necessary to implement TF-CBT for students who have experienced trauma. Providing a safe, supportive environment promotes feelings of physical as a core feature. Additionally, the focus on staff awareness and understanding of trauma signs and symptoms allows for a transition between the clinical setting and the classroom setting with fewer undesirable behavioral and discipline outcomes (Conners-Edge et al., 2022; Guarino & Chagnon, 2018).

In Tier 1, also referred to as universal, schools provide support through a program delivered to all students that is designed to introduce a common language and communicate the expectations and skills needed to be successful. This tier supports resiliency building for students through positive reinforcement, skill building, and cognitive-behavioral elements (e.g., modeling, cognitive mediation techniques) with a goal of developing appropriate social skills and problem-solving skills (Kern et al., 2022; Orminston et al., 2021). Tier 1 supports also provide support for educational staff by providing universal training for school staff on mental health and trauma signs/symptoms. This allows for faster referrals for behaviors of concern and promotes collaboration and consultation across disciplines.

Tier 2 services are often referred to as targeted prevention or early intervention and are provided to students who are unresponsive or minimally responsive to universal support. This level of support typically involves group work and skill development to address reported or observed skill deficits. With youth who have experienced trauma, this could involve psychoeducational groups or skill-building groups based on a common experience (e.g., grief groups, divorce groups). In a school setting, TF-CBT has also been shown to be an effective group intervention when groups of students are homogeneous in terms of either trauma exposure or behavioral expression and services are provided by an experienced mental health clinician (Davis et al., 2023; Phipps & Thorne, 2019).

A mental health professional typically provides Tier 3 services in a SMH model. This level of service is intensive and individual intervention. This level of support should be determined to be necessary following a comprehensive assessment and determination of a level of need (Kern et al., 2022; Ormiston et al., 2021). For students who have experienced trauma or have been diagnosed with PTSD, this level of support may be necessary for some time to assist them in accessing educational opportunities in the least restrictive environment. Support at this level should be individualized and comprehensive to ensure the support being provided is designed to achieve a specific goal(s).

Logistical Considerations

Treatment in a school setting has several advantages, including having the student readily available, ease of collaboration with educational staff, ready access to behavioral and attendance data, and ease of monitoring treatment outcomes. While these advantages can serve to enhance treatment outcomes, staff should be aware of barriers that exist and plan for those barriers prior to implementing services. Prior consideration and planning for individual school climate, policy and procedures, school leadership support, and flexibility of scheduling can support the implementation of TF-CBT with fidelity and lead to more effective outcomes for students.

When developing treatment goals and objectives for services in the school setting, consideration should be given to the duration of each session, how long you can maintain a student in treatment, and how family engagement will be structured. Sessions may differ depending on age, with younger students being generally easier to schedule and the duration of treatment becoming more critical as you begin to treat middle school and high school students. Consultation with educational staff to address how missed academics will be addressed should be done prior to beginning services to promote collaboration and reduce the stress on youth. Psychoeducation on trauma and how it impacts academics can be helpful in supporting educational staff in understanding why services are being implemented. Addressing the time limit of the services can also reduce barriers and increase staff buy-in for problem-solving. Behaviors of concern and consequences can be framed in a fight/flight/freeze view to determine how to address them through the therapeutic process. Behaviors that involve safety (e.g., harm to self/others, elopement) should be addressed through behavioral planning as well as during individual sessions.

Trauma Case Study

This case study is being presented from an elementary school perspective as presented to a SMH professional. The case presentation will be presented through the stages of referral, assessment, and treatment planning.

Referral

Mark is a 4th grade student who was referred due to behaviors in the classroom setting. The school administration referred him following a physical altercation between him and two other 4th grade boys. Behaviors of concern included inattention, arguing with peers, disrespect toward adults, and crying. His teacher reported that he is often tired, and she must wake him up at least once during the week. He has been asking to visit the bathroom more often than normal and has been going to the nurse complaining of stomach aches two to three times per week. Prior to referring him, his teacher attempted to speak with his parents but was unable to reach his mother. His father has been removed from the contact information in the educational information system.

Screening and Clinical Interview

The initial assessment of the student involved reviewing his cumulative educational records. Mark's educational history is non-significant through the 3rd grade. No behavioral referrals were documented, and his academics were within the average to high-average range. Attendance records indicate no concerns through the 3rd grade. A review of his previous report cards shows positive teacher comments and no socialization concerns.

Initial contact with Mark's mother, Mrs. Smith, was inconclusive, and she presented as angry and withdrawn. Following an initial conversation with the administration regarding his behaviors of concern, Mrs. Smith was asked to stop at the mental health professional's office. She was upset about the behaviors and became frustrated when discussing his school behaviors. She was initially reluctant to discuss home behaviors but following rapport being built, she was willing to discuss how additional support could be helpful. Mrs. Smith reported that she was struggling with feelings of sadness and anxiety following the death of her husband in a car accident eight months ago. The family was together in the car when the accident occurred. Mark was treated and released; his mother was hospitalized for a week following the accident, and his father died following an extended hospital stay. She reports that Mark has been playing video games more often, is less likely to talk, and wants to be with her all the time. He had been having problems sleeping but seems to be doing better and is now able to sleep in his own room. He was initially involved in a community grief group and was doing well. While she has been seeing a therapist, he has not wanted to engage in therapy, so she has been monitoring his behaviors. Mrs. Smith gave permission for Mark to have a formal screening and for the mental health professional to meet with Mark.

Mark's initial interview was conducted with his mother present to assist in rapport development and increase his feelings of physical and psychological safety. Following an initial low-level conversation focused on his favorite video games and peer relationships, the interviewer began to discuss recent behaviors in the school setting. Mark reported that he is often angry, or his stomach hurts, and he can't seem to control what he's feeling. He reported that he was doing okay and was able to stop thinking about his dad dying during school until the class started talking about family history in social studies, and he was asked to do a family tree. He stated that he tried telling his teacher he didn't want to do the project, but she told him projects were not up for discussion. Mark reported he doesn't trust his teacher now, and when he's upset, he doesn't think he can ask for help.

Mark was administered the Penn State Worry Questionnaire for Children (Meyer et al., 1990). Following elevated scores, Mark and his mother completed, respectively, self and parent versions of the Screen for Child Anxiety-Related Emotional Disorders (SCARED; Birmaher et al., 1999). Results of the individual anxiety screening indicated elevated scores for separation anxiety disorder (self and parent) and significant somatic symptoms (self).

Other Assessment Data

Following a conversation with Mrs. Smith, it was determined that a school-based referral for short-term services would be the initial step. This was decided due to the majority of the behaviors occurring in the school setting and as a way to reduce the demand on Mark's mother to find additional support outside of school, which would add stress due to her work schedule. In addition to the clinical interview and screening, data was collected to determine his anxiety level throughout the day. Data was collected through Closegap (2022) to allow for parent and school data sharing and trend analysis. His teacher took additional data to track any behaviors for a week to help identify triggers. Table 12.1 provides an example of initial treatment goals, and Table 12.2 offers a sample session outline.

Table 12.1 Initial Treatment Goals and Objectives for Case Study

Goal	*Objectives*
Mark and his mother will learn accurate information about trauma, trauma reminders, common responses to trauma reminders, and the grief process.	a Mark will learn accurate information about his neurological trauma responses, common physical reactions, and the grief process. b Mark's mother will be provided with accurate information on developmental reactions to trauma, trauma reminders, and warning signs for increased pathology.
Mark will understand how to help himself return to a feeling of psychological safety.	a Mark will identify how his body feels when a trauma reminder is present. b Mark will identify trauma reminders that decrease his psychological safety.
Mark will increase his relaxation skills and emotional coping by developing skills to reduce levels of psychological arousal when faced with stressful experiences or trauma reminders.	a Mark will learn controlled breathing. b Mark will learn progressive muscle relaxation. c Mark will learn grounding techniques. d Mark will teach grounding, breathing, and progressive muscle relaxation to his mother and teacher.

Table 12.2 Session Outline Example

Goal	*Methods*
Session 1: Psychoeducation	
• Goal setting • Establish goals and norms for sessions revolving around blame and affective statements. • Provide education around TF-CBT, including homework, what sessions will look like, and how it has helped other youth and families. • Provide an initial introduction to the cognitive triangle to promote understanding of how emotions, thoughts, and behaviors are linked.	Descriptions should be brief and developmentally appropriate. Regardless of the age of the student, making sure the explanation is simple will help with understanding and processing. One way of introducing TF-CBT is: "TF-CBT is an approach that has been shown to help children/teens understand their trauma and learn coping skills. You will also learn ways to keep yourself physically and emotionally safe. I would like to work on setting our goals together. How does that sound?" Follow-up questions can include: • What questions do you have? • What do you want to accomplish in our time together? • How often do you think we should have your mom in? Are you okay if your mom participates over the computer sometimes? (providing a virtual option can increase availability and decrease demand on staff and family). • What could I do that would help the most (and least)? The session should include a "getting to know you" portion. This can include asking about favorite hobbies, doing art activities, or playing a game while you talk.
Session 2: Psychoeducation	
• Normalize exposure to trauma. • Explain and normalize symptoms and avoidance. • Introduce trauma information, including signs, symptoms, and physiological reactions to trauma reminders. • Explain trauma, traumatic grief, and trauma reminders. *Parenting goal:* • Normalize trauma responses and link behaviors to trauma. • Teach/Review basic behavioral modification strategies and provide guidance based on parent needs.	• Resources that can be sent home and reviewed are helpful for the family to have after the session to reference. The National Child Traumatic Stress Network maintains up-to-date childhood traumatic grief and trauma resources for families and schools. • After reviewing video(s) and/or providing information, consider questions such as: o Which trauma reactions do you think you show? o Tell me about some trauma reminders. o What does your grief feel like? o How do you think your grief is different than your trauma reminders? • Consider using videos to provide information in a developmentally appropriate manner. One example is All Connected: A Place for Belonging (Connect our Kids, 2022) on YouTube. Ensure all examples used are from reputable sources. • Additional methods include: o Games o Discussion o Worksheets o Using creative ideas based on their areas of interest or hobbies (e.g., podcast, private TikTok)

(*Continued*)

Table 12.2 (Continued)

Goal	*Methods*
Session 3: Relaxation	
• Relaxation skills are designed to address the physiological aspects of stress and anxiety by reducing muscle tension, slowing down breathing, and calming the mind. • The goal of teaching relaxation skills is to teach what it feels like when the body is anxious and tense to promote the identification of changes in the physiological state. • Skills must be taught prior to trauma narrative.	• Identify what skills are being used now (hobbies, sports, crafts, music, activities). • Teach progressive muscle relaxation. • Practice controlled breathing. • Listen to relaxation activities online. • Identification of soothing activities (sounds, smells, nature). • Body awareness exercises. • Slow-paced diaphragmatic breathing. *Consider additional activities based on developmental age:* • Dancing • Blowing bubbles • Songs • Crafts *Homework consideration:* • Calendar with a check for each day practiced. The goal is to practice at least once per day in school and/or at home. • Writing down activities in a relaxation plan can provide reminders for practice and communication. This can be simple and a separate plan or listed out in the header/footer of the calendar.
Session 4: Affect modulation	
• Increase emotional identification and provide emotion words to internal feelings. • Rate feelings at different intensities. • Normalize emotional avoidance and conflicting feelings. • Learn strategies to regulate emotions.	• Problem-solve a "toolkit" that can be used when youth is upset. This should include a wide range of activities. • Develop a five-point scale for younger students to provide visual reminders of how to use a toolkit. • Feelings games • Watching a movie clip or video clip with sound turned off to help identify emotions based on behaviors
Session 5: Cognitive processing skills	
• Teach the connection between thoughts, feelings, and behaviors (cognitive triangle). • Help students learn to identify automatic or inaccurate thoughts that are maladaptive. Gain agreement that thoughts drive feelings and thoughts can be changed.	***Student:*** A variety of techniques can be used, including: • Progressive logical questioning (Socratic questioning): ask about the belief, sum up their belief, ask for evidence, challenge the assumption, and repeat until challenging is no longer necessary. • Responsibility pie: use a pie chart to develop initial belief, identify causal factors, and revise the pie chart to revised belief statement. • Best friend role play ***Parent:*** • Introduce the cognitive triangle and begin by processing parent maladaptive cognitions. For many parents of youth with trauma, this will include cognitions related to blame, inability to protect, the child never being able to heal, and/or feelings they should have known about the trauma sooner.

(*Continued*)

Table 12.2 (Continued)

Goal	*Methods*
	Homework consideration: • Have the student and parent complete the Challenging Belief Worksheet (cpt.musc.edu) following an example of completion during the session.
Session 6: Coping skills	
• Review previous sessions and continue development of coping skills and affect regulation prior to beginning trauma narrative. • Provide youth and parents with a discrete coping skill for bringing awareness into the moment.	• Review usage of coping skills and effectiveness for trauma reminders. Continue with coping skills if effective. • Grounding exercise. • Teach parent grounding technique. • Role play.
Sessions 7 and 8: Trauma narrative	
Writing a trauma narrative can help youth learn to experience, process, and reduce the negative thoughts and feelings associated with traumatic events. When done intentionally, with family support, this can help them resolve feelings and incorporate coping skills into their life. It is important to carefully schedule this with a supportive family member present and at a time when the youth will be able to leave the school following the session. Adequate time for these sessions should be given. If you are not able to schedule this at a time when the youth will not have to return to class and with family support, these sessions are not recommended. Goals: • Help youth face traumatic events in a supportive environment. • Identify inaccurate or maladaptive trauma-related cognitions. • Identify more helpful thought patterns about traumatic exposure, the world, family, and self.	1 Start with the facts. Have the student retell the trauma story with only facts. Encourage factual information over feelings by asking who, what, where, and when questions. 2 After the facts are recorded, ask the child to read the narrative slowly (or read aloud to them) and add feelings and thoughts they experienced during their trauma experience. Avoid challenging thoughts and feelings during this step and use open-ended questions to facilitate sharing of feelings. 3 Dig deeper into the traumatic event. Once the student is comfortable sharing, ask them what the worst part or about their trauma or what the worst memory was. Revise what has been written and add more detail gradually. 4 Once the student's narrative has been read and re-read and detail has been added, utilize cognitive skills. Review the story and challenge any irrational thoughts. Allow revisions based on those challenges. 5 Add a final paragraph asking the student what they've learned, how now is different, and/or how they have grown. Ask them to conclude by giving advice to someone who has experienced a similar traumatic event.
Session 9: Enhancing safety	
• Re-establishing feelings of power and control in self. • Teach safety skills for future potentially traumatic events. • Identify where to get help if needed and whom youth can go to for support. • Have a discrete safety plan in case of suicidal thoughts.	• Develop a formal safety plan. • List of people to reach out to in the school setting if trauma reminder occurs and coping skills are overwhelming. • Programming crisis text number in their phone. • Identify risks/warning signs and provide them to parents. • Role play help-seeking skills.

Summary

Trauma exposure and diagnoses of PTSD are continuing to rise in children and adolescents. Current pre-pandemic estimates suggest that two out of three students have been exposed to at least one traumatic event. With increasing exposure to traumatic events being linked to detrimental neurobiological effects that result in developmental, social, emotional, behavioral, and academic difficulties in the school, providing services to students who have experienced trauma and are showing signs in the school setting is necessary for optimizing educational opportunities and growth. Assessing for trauma exposure was reviewed as a necessary component of all comprehensive behavioral evaluations, as the connection between maladaptive behaviors and neurocognitive disruptions related to trauma has been explicitly linked.

Evidence for the usage of CBT was presented with a focus on how evidence-based treatment programs for trauma have been adapted successfully for usage with traumatized youth. A review of relevant research throughout this chapter provided validation of TF-CBT as an individual and group treatment for trauma and PTSD, regardless of the source of the trauma exposure. Trauma cannot be adequately understood or addressed without understanding the cultural and societal influences that lead historically marginalized children and adolescents to have an increased likelihood of exposure to trauma. These factors were addressed through research indicating TF-CBT has been shown to be effective in usage with many of the most vulnerable youth, including those experiencing racism, refugees, children of incarcerated parents, and survivors of mass casualty events and war.

While specialized training is required to provide evidence-based approaches for addressing trauma and PTSD, training programs endorsed by SAMHSA have been developed and are provided online through the Medical University of South Carolina at a minimal cost. Training programs advance the concepts of traditional CBT to include psychoeducation on trauma and the development of a trauma narrative. Utilizing the PRACTICE components of TF-CBT, a case conceptualization was provided through a case study demonstrating the process from assessment through the development of sessions. For readers who are new to CBT and trauma, manualized evidence-based programs, including CBITS, Bounce Back, and TrT, were also reviewed.

Reflection Questions

1 What supports, resources, and policies will you need to ensure are in place prior to providing TF-CBT in your school setting (e.g., supervision, permissions, space, time, and caseload limits)?
2 Reflecting on what you have learned about trauma, why would trauma narratives be inappropriate if the student is required to return to the classroom setting immediately?
3 What trauma reminders or anxiety triggers do you need to address prior to providing TF-CBT to ensure a psychologically safe environment?

Evidence-Based Treatment Programs for Trauma and PTSD

- Trauma-Focused Cognitive-Behavioral Therapy (TF-CBT).
- Cognitive Behavior Intervention for Trauma in Schools (CBITS).
- Bounce Back.
- Support for Students Exposed to Trauma (SSET).
- Eye Movement Desensitization and Reprocessing (EMDR).
- Teaching Recovery Techniques (TrT).

References

American Psychiatric Association (APA) (2022). *Diagnostic and statistical manual of mental disorders, fifth edition, text revision*. Washington, DC: American Psychiatric Association.

Birmaher, B., Brent, D. A., Chiappetta, L., Bridge, J., Monga, S., & Baugher, M. (1999). Psychometric properties of the Screen for Child Anxiety Related Emotional Disorders (SCARED): A replication study. *Journal of the American Academy of Child and Adolescent Psychiatry, 38*(10), 1230–1236.

Brock, S. E., & Louvar-Reeves, M. A. (2019). *Mental health crisis intervention: Responding to an acute traumatic stressor in schools*. Bethesda, MD: National Association of School Psychologists.

Broekhof, R., Nordahl, H., Bjornelv, S., & Selvik, S. (2022). Prevalence of adverse childhood experiences and their co-occurrence in a large population of adolescents: A young HUNT 3 study. *Social Psychiatry and Psychiatric Epidemiology, 57*, 2359–2366. https://doi.org/10.1007/s00127-022-02277-z

Brown, D., Anda, R., Tiemeier, H., Felitti, V., Edwards, V., Croft, J., & Giles, W. (2009). Adverse childhood experiences and the risk of premature mortality. *American Journal of Prevention Medicine, 37*(5), 389–396. https://doi.org/10.1016.j.amepre.2009.06.021

Center for Disease Control and Prevention: National Center for HIV, Viral Hepatitis, STD, and TB Prevention, Division of Adolescent and School Health (2023). Youth risk behavior survey: Data summary and trends report. Meyer TJ, Miller ML, Metzger RL, Borkovec TD: Development and Validation of the Penn State Worry Questionnaire. *Behavior Research and Therapy, 28*, 487–495, 1990.

Center for Safe and Resilient Schools and Workplaces (2023). *Bounce back*. Retrieved from https://traumaawaresch.wpengine.com/index.php/learn-more-bounce-back/

Chipalo, E. (2021). Is trauma focused-cognitive behavioral therapy (TF-CBT) effective in reducing trauma symptoms among traumatized refugee children? A systemic review. *Journal of Child and Adolescent Trauma, 14*(4), 545–558. https://doi.org/10.1007/s40653-021-00370-0

Choi, K. R., McCreary, M., Ford, J. D., Rahmanian Koushkaki, S., Kenan, K. N., & Zima, B. T. (2019). Validation of the traumatic events screening inventory for ACEs. *Pediatrics, 143*(4). https://doi.org/10.1542/peds.2018-2546

Christ, C., Schouten, M., Blanderrs, M., van Schaik, D., Beekman, A., Wisman, M., Stikkelbroek, Y., & Dekker, J. (2020). Internet and computer-based cognitive behavioral therapy for anxiety and depression in adolescents and youth adults: Systematic review and meta-analysis. *Journal of Medical Internet Research, 22*(9). https://doi.org/10.2096/17831

Cohen, J., & Mannarino, A. (2015). Trauma-focused cognitive behavioral therapy for traumatized children and youth. *Child and Adolescent Psychiatry Clinics of North America, 24*(3), 557–570. https://doi.org/10.1016/j.chc.2015.02.005

Connect our Kids (2022, November 17). All Connected: A Place for Belonging *Season 1: How trauma affects your brain*. [Video]. Retrieved from https://youtube.com/playlist?list=PLsLWimD2L4FvUHe3eh5MlMRFKxrfe8prO

Conners Edge, N., Holmes, K., Wilburn, E., & Sutton, M. (2022). Fostering informed and responsive systems for trauma in early care and education (FIRST:ECE): A preliminary evaluation. *Early Childhood Education Journal*. https://doi.org/10.1007/s10643-022-01390-7

Closegap. (2022). *School toolkit*. Retrieved from https://www.closegap.org/educator-toolkit

Davis, R., Meiser-Stedman, R., Afzal, M., Devaney, J., Halligan, S., Lofthouse, K., Smith, P., Stallard, P., Ye, S., & Hiller, R. (2023). Meta-analytic review: Group-based interventions for treating posttraumatic stress symptoms in children and adolescents. *Journal of the American Academy of Child & Adolescent Psychiatry*. https://doi.org/10.1016/j.jaac.2023.02.013

Dubois, M., & Guaspare, C. (2020). From cellular memory to the memory of trauma: Social epigenetics and its public circulation. *Social Science Information, 59*(1), 144–183. https://doi.org/10.1177/053901841987600

Durbeej, N., McDiarmid, S., Sarkadi, A., Feldman, I., Punamaki, R., Kankaanpaa, R., Anderson, A., Hilden, P., Verelst, A., Derluyn, I., & Osman, F. (2021). Evaluation of a school-based intervention to promote mental health of refugee youth in Sweden (TheRefugeesWellSchool Trial): Study protocol for a cluster randomized controlled trial. *Trials, 22*. https://doi.org/10.1186/s13063-020-04995-8

Ellis, W., Dietz, W., & Chen, K. (2022). Community resilience: A dynamic model for public health 3.0. *Journal of Public Health Management and Practice, 28*(1), 18–26. https://doi.org/10.1072/PHH.0000000000001413

Felitti, V., Anda, R., Norndenberg, D., Williamson, D., Spitz, A., Edwards, V., Koss, M., & Marks, J. (1998). Relationship of childhood abuse and household dysfunction to many of the leading causes of death in adults. The Adverse Childhood Experiences (ACE) study. *American Journal of Prevention Medicine, 14*(4), 245–258. https://doi.org/10.1016/s0749-3797(98)00017-8

Ford, J., Racusin, R., Rogers, K., Schiffman, J., Ribbe, D., & Edwards, J. (2002). *Traumatic events screening inventory of children (TESI-C) version 8.4*. National Center for PTSD and Dartmouth Child Psychiatry Research Group. Retrieved from https://www.ptsd.va.gov/professional/assessment/documents/TESI-C.pdf

Forkey, H., Szilagyi, M., Kelly, E., & Duffee, J. (2021). Trauma-informed care. *Pediatrics, 148*(2). https://doi.org/10.1542/peds.2021-052580

Guarino, K., & Chagnon, E. (2018). *Trauma-sensitive schools training package*. National Center on Safe Supportive Learning Environments. Retrieved from https://safesupportivelearning.ed.gov/trauma-sensitive-schools-training-package

Herrenkohl, T., Hong, S., & Verbrugge, B. (2019). Trauma-informed programs based in schools: Linking concepts to practices and assessing the evidence. *American Journal of Community Psychology, 64*, 373–388. https://doi.org/10.1002/ajcp.12362

Jaycox, L. H., Audra, K. L., & Sharon, A. H. (2018). *Cognitive behavioral intervention for trauma in schools (CBITS)* (2nd ed.). Santa Monica, CA: RAND Corporation. Retrieved from https://www.rand.org/pubs/tools/TL272.html. Also available in print form.

Kealohi Sato Conching, A., & Thayer, Z. (2019). Biological pathways for historical trauma to affect health: A conceptual model focusing on epigenetic modifications. *Social Science and Medicine, 230*, 74–82. https://doi.org/10.1016/j.socscimed.2019.04.001

Kern, L., Weist, M., Mathur, S., & Barber, B. (2022). Empowering school staff to implement effective school mental health services. *Behavioral Disorders, 47*(3), 207–219. https://doi.org/0.1177/01987429211030860

Kim, I., Kim, N., & Jang, H. (2023). Adverse childhood experiences and intersectionality of sex, race, and poverty in adolescents: A descriptive analysis. *Journal of Asia Pacific Counseling, 13*(1), 79–94. https://doi.org/10.18401/2023.13.1.6

Kliethermes, M., Goodman, R. F., Epstein, C., Cohen, J. A., The Philadelphia Alliance for Child Trauma Services (PACTS), & the Child Traumatic Grief and Traumatic Separation Collaborative Group (2020). *Childhood traumatic grief: Youth information sheet*. Los Angeles, CA, and Durham, NC: National Center for Child Traumatic Stress. Retrieved from https://www.nctsn.org/sites/default/ files/resources/fact- sheet/childhood_traumatic_grief youth_information_sheet.pdf

Lewey, J., Smith, C., Burcham, B., Saunders, N., Elfallal, D., & O'Toole, S. (2018). Comparing the effectiveness of EMDR and TF-CBT for children and adolescents: A meta-analysis. *Journal of Child and Adolescent Trauma, 11*, 457–472. https://doi.org/10.1007/s40653-018-0212-1

Lindebo Knutsen, M., Sachser, C., Holt, T., Goldbeck, L., & Jensen, T. (2019). Trajectories and possible predictors of treatment outcome for youth receiving trauma-focused cognitive behavioral therapy. *Psychological Trauma: Theory, Research, Practice, and Policy*. https://doi.org/10.1037/tra0000482

Lyon, A., Pullmann, M., Dorsey, S., Levin, C., Gaias, L., Brewer, S., Larson, M., Corbin, C., Davis, C., Muse, I., Joshi, M., Reyes, R., Jungbluth, J., Barrett, R., Hong, D., Bomez, M., & Cook, C. (2021). Protocol for a hybrid type 2 cluster randomized trial of trauma-focused cognitive behavioral therapy and a pragmatic individual-level implementation strategy. *Implementation Science, 16*(3). https://doi.org/10.1186/s13012-020-01064-1

McRae, E. M., Stoppelbein, L., O'Kelley, S. E., Fite, Pl, & Smith, S. B. (2021). An examination of posttraumatic stress symptoms and aggression among children with a history of adverse childhood experiences. *Journal of Psychopathology and Behavioral Assessment, 43*, 657–670. https://doi.org/10.1007/s10862-021-09884-1

Medical University of South Carolina (2017). *TF-CBT Web: A course for trauma-focused cognitive behavioral therapy*. Retrieved from https://tfcbt2.musc.edu/

Metzger, I., Anderson, R., Are, F., & Ritchwood, T. (2021). Healing interpersonal and racial trauma: Integrating racial socialization into trauma-focused cognitive behavioral therapy for African American youth. *Child Maltreatment, 26*(1), 17–27. https://doi.org/10.1177/1077559520921457

Meyer, T., Miller, M., Metzger, R., & Borkovec, T. (1990). Development and validation of the Penn State worry questionnaire. *Behavior Research and Therapy, 28*(6), 487–495. https://doi.org/10.1016/0005-7967(90)90135-6

Minne, E., & Gorelik, G. (2022). The protective role of trauma informed attitudes on perceived stress among teachers and school staff. *Journal of Child and Adolescent Trauma, 15*, 275–283. https://doi.org/10.1007/s40653-021-00389-3

National Center for School Mental Health (2019). *School Health Assessment and Performance Evaluation System (SHAPE)*. Retrieved from https://www.theshapesystem.com/

Ormiston, H. E., Nygaard, M. A., & Heck, O. C. (2020). The role of school psychologists in the implementation of trauma-informed multi-tiered systems of support in schools. Journal of Applied School Psychology, *37*(4), 319–351. https://doi.org/10.1080/15377903.2020.1848955

Orminson, H., Nygaard, M., Heck, O., Wood, M., Rodriguez, N., Maze, M., Asomani-Adem, A., Ingmire, K., Burgess, B., & Shriberg, D. (2021). Educator perspectives on mental health resources and practices in their school. *Psychology in Schools, 58,* 2148–2174. https://doi.org/10.1002/pits.22582

Panchal, N., Cox, C., & Rudowits, R. (Sept. 6, 2022). The landscape of school-based mental health services. KFF. Retrieved from https://www.kff.org/other/issue-brief/the-landscape-of-school-based-mental-health-services/

Phipps, R., & Thorne, S. (2019). Utilizing trauma-focused cognitive behavioral therapy as a framework for addressing cultural trauma in African American children and adolescents: A proposal. *The Professional Counselor, 9*(1), 35–50. https://doi.org/10.15241/rp.9.1.35

Research and Evaluation Group at Public Health Management Corporation (2013). *Findings from the Philadelphia urban ACE survey*. Retrieved from https://simplebooklet.com/findingsfrom philadelphiaacesurveyand comparedacequestions#page=1

Reynolds, C. R., & Kamphaus, R. W. (2015). *Behavior assessment for children: Third edition (BASC-3)*. Bloomington, MN: Pearson.

Ross, S., Sharma-Patel, K., Brown, E., Huntt, J., & Chaplin, W. (2021). Complex trauma and trauma-focused cognitive behavioral therapy: How do trauma chronicity and PTSD presentation affect treatment outcome? *Child Abuse and Neglect, 111*. https://doi.org/10.1016/j.chiabu.2020.104734

Rucci, P. (2000). Instrument development in the Italy-USA collaborative spectrum project. *Epidemiologia e Psichiatria Sociale, 9*, 249–256. https://doi.org/10.1017/s1121189x00008381

Sacks, V., & Murphey, D. (2018). The prevalence of adverse childhood experiences, nationally, by state, and by race or ethnicity. *Child Trends*. Retrieved from https://www.childtrends.org/publications/prevalence-adverse-childhood-experiences-nationally-state-race-ethnicity

Sarkadi, A., Adahl, K., Stenvall, E., Ssegonja, R., Batti, H., Gavra, P., Kangstrom, K., & Salari, R. (2018). Teaching recovery techniques: Evaluation of a group intervention for unaccompanied refugee minors with symptoms of PTSD in Sweden. *European Child and Adolescent Psychiatry, 27*, 467–479. https://doi.org/10.1007/s00787-017-1093-9

Shapiro, F. (1989). Efficacy of the eye movement desensitization procedure in the treatment of traumatic memories. *Journal of Traumatic Stress, 2*(2), 199–223. https://doi.org/10.1002/jts.2490020207

Smith, P., Dyregrov, A., Yule, W., Perrin, S., Gupta, L., & Gjestad, R. (1999). *Teaching recovery techniques manual: A manual for teaching survival techniques to child survivors of war and major disasters*. Foundation for Children and War. Retrieved from https://www.childrenandwar.org

Substance Abuse and Mental Health Services Administration (2014). *SAMHSA's concept of trauma and guidance for a trauma-informed approach. HHS publication No. (SMA) 14–4884*. Substance Abuse and Mental Health Services Administration.

Syros, I., Karantzali, A., & Anastassiou-Hadjicharalambous, X. (2022). Trauma-focused cognitive behavior therapy (TF-CBT), cognitive behavioral intervention on trauma in schools (CBITS), and other promising practices in the treatment of posttraumatic stress disorder in children and adolescents: Evidence evaluation. *OMB Neurobiology, 6*(4). https://doi.org/10.21926/obm.neurobiol.2204146

Teke, E., & Avsaroglu, S. (2022). Efficacy of eye movement desensitization and reprocessing (EMDR) therapy for children and adolescents with posttraumatic stress disorder. *Journal of School and Educational Psychology, 2*(1), 1–12. https://doi.org/10.47602/josep.v2i1.1

The National Child Traumatic Stress Network, Schools Committee (2017). Creating, supporting, and sustaining trauma-informed schools: A System Framework. National Center for child Traumatic Stress. Retrieved from https://www.nctsn.org/sites/default/files/resources//creating_supporting_sustaining_trauma_informed_schools_a_systems_framework.pdf

Thumfart, K., Jawaid, A., Bright, K., Flashmann, M., & Mansuy, I. (2022). Epigenetics of childhood trauma: Long term sequelae and potential for treatment. *Neuroscience & Behavioral Reviews, 132*, 1049–1066. https://doi.org/10.1016/j.neubiorev.2021.10.042

Trevor Project (2023). *2023 U.S. national survey on the mental health of LGBTQ young people*. Retrieved from https://www.thetrevorproject.org/survey-2023/assets/static/05_TREVOR05_2023survey.pdf

Tsehay, M., Necho, M., & Mekonnen, W. (2020). The role of adverse childhood experience on depression symptom, prevalence, and severity among school going adolescents. *Depression Research and Treatment, 2020*(5951792), 1–9. Published by Hindawi Research. https://doi.org/10.1155/2020/5951792

Whiteside, S., Sim, L., Morrow, A., Farah, W., Hilliker, D., Hassan Murad, M., & Wang, Z. (2022). A meta-analysis to guide the enhancement of CBT for childhood anxiety: Exposure of anxiety management. *Clinical Child and Family Psychology Review, 23*(1), 102–121. https://doi.org/10.1007/s10567-019-00303-2

13

CULTURALLY RESPONSIVE CBT INTERVENTIONS FOR REFUGEE AND MIGRANT STUDENTS

Bridging the Gap to Well-Being

Diana M. Diaków

Understanding the Terminology and Heterogeneity of Refugee and Migrant Children and Families)

Forcibly displaced persons (FDPs) represent a complex and diverse population, encompassing individuals forced to leave their homelands due to life-threatening circumstances. The terminology surrounding this population includes distinct categories such as refugees, asylum seekers, stateless persons, internally displaced persons (IDPs), and migrants, each characterized by unique legal statuses and circumstances. This section aims to elucidate these terms, provide relevant statistics, and emphasize the heterogeneity within the refugee population.

Refugees constitute a subset of FDPs who have fled their homeland due to imminent threats such as war, political oppression, or persecution. The term "refugee" originated during the First and Second World Wars, with the Universal Declaration of Human Rights ([UDHR], 1948) delineating specific criteria for obtaining refugee status. According to the UDHR, individuals seeking refugee status must demonstrate a "well-founded fear of being persecuted for reasons of race, religion, nationality, membership of a particular social group, or political opinion" (UDHR, 1948, p. 14). The non-refoulement principle of international law, outlined in the UDHR (1948), ensures that a person granted refugee status should not be forcibly returned to their home country due to hazardous living conditions. It is important to note, however, that apart from the impetus of war, climate change also drives global displacement, especially in the Global South (Koehn et al., 2023). Asylum seekers are individuals who have left their country of origin and formally applied for asylum in another nation, awaiting a conclusive decision on their application.

In addition to those who seek safety abroad, a significant proportion of FDPs comprises IDPs. IDPs are individuals who have left their homes due to life-threatening circumstances but remain within the borders of their home country, relocating to safer regions. Their journey may evolve, with an individual starting as an IDP and later becoming a migrant, asylum seeker, or refugee. The experiences of IDPs underscore the multifaceted nature of forced displacement, highlighting the intricate web of challenges faced by individuals who navigate the complex terrain within their own national boundaries.

Stateless persons lack citizenship in any nation or state, often resulting from fleeing their country of former habitual residence due to persecution or life-threatening events. Their legal status raises

DOI: 10.4324/9781003392439-16

unique challenges concerning economic, employment, and housing conditions, distinguishing them from other displaced groups.

The term "migrant" encompasses individuals who leave their homes, either voluntarily or forcibly, for reasons such as economic hardship or a desire to live and work in another country. It is crucial to note that migrants may experience psychological challenges similar to refugees, emphasizing the common thread of relocation among forcibly displaced individuals.

As of mid-2023, the global forcibly displaced population reached an estimated 110 million, with over one-third identified as refugees (The United Nations Higher Commissioner for Refugees [UNHCR], 2023). Notably, 43.3 million, or over 40%, were minors under 18 years old, and 1.9 million children were born as refugees (UNHCR, 2023). The top countries of origin for refugees included Syria, Afghanistan, and Ukraine, with significant numbers seeking refuge in countries like The Islamic Republic of Iran and Turkey.

In conclusion, understanding the nuances of terminology and the heterogeneity within the forcibly displaced population is crucial for clinicians working with refugee and migrant children and families. The legal status, reasons for displacement, and diverse adversities experienced by these individuals underscore the need for a nuanced and culturally sensitive approach to providing cognitive-behavioral therapy (CBT) to this heterogeneous group.

Displacement Stages

Pre-Flight Stage

The pre-flight stage, marking the commencement of a refugee's journey, unfolds in their homeland, rendered unsafe by various life-threatening events such as natural disasters or armed conflicts (Sullivan & Simonson, 2016). This phase exposes refugee youth to a myriad of stressors, including physical, sexual, and emotional abuse, exploitation, famine, and recruitment by armed groups (Betancourt et al., 2012). Premigration adversities, especially violence and loss of family members, significantly elevate the risk of psychopathology among youth.

Flight Stage

As refugees embark on the migration stage, transitioning from their homes to safer locations, they encounter challenges in meeting basic needs, including access to food, water, sanitation, shelter, and electricity (The Royal Institute of International Affairs [RIOIA], 2016). Exposure to violence persists during this flight stage, with humanitarian workers reporting witnessing acts of aggression and gender-based assaults in poorly lit and unsafe refugee camps (Diaków, 2021). Limited mental health services in temporary shelters contribute to heightened risks of mental health disorders among refugees, including incidents of deliberate self-harm and suicides (Diaków, 2021; Tyrer & Fazel, 2014).

Resettlement Stage

The post-migration or resettlement stage, culminating in forcibly displaced children and families reaching their destination country, introduces new challenges despite the prospect of safety and support from resettlement agencies (Hodes et al., 2008). Refugees, particularly youth fleeing life-threatening circumstances, grapple with uncertainty, fear of return, grief, and changes in socioeconomic status (Durà-Vila et al., 2012; Tyrer & Fazel, 2014). Throughout resettlement, refugee children and families confront economic hardships, cultural adjustments, social isolation, and racism. Exposure to stressors like bullying, generational differences, and deteriorating family relationships unfold in the host countries (Hodes et al., 2008. Refugee parents' postmigration difficulties and mental health problems are linked with harsh parenting and, further, with externalizing and internalizing symptoms among children (Bryant et al., 2018). Limited access to specialized mental health care compounds the challenges faced by refugee children and families, attributed to factors such as age, high internalizing symptoms frequency, and racial/ethnic minority status (Durà-Vila et al., 2012; Sullivan & Simonson, 2016).

In the host community, language barriers contribute to social and school difficulties, with refugees viewed as an outer group perceived as threatening to the local community's cultural and political backgrounds (Borrell et al., 2015). For example, Muslim immigrant youth face rejection due to religious heritage. Syrian refugee boys experience bullying, physical attacks, and humiliation, and refugee women face social stigmatization due to cultural differences related to polygamous marriages (Phalet et al., 2018; Yaylaci, 2018). Discrimination and stigmatization based on ethnic or religious backgrounds, alongside the challenges of navigating cultural differences, language acquisition, and educational adjustments, further contribute to psychological challenges (Durà-Vila et al., 2012).

Resilience

Despite these challenges, the resettlement process offers opportunities for the accumulation of socioecological protective factors spanning across individual, familial, and environmental attributes, including language proficiency, access to community services (e.g., church, mosque), employment, expanded social support, and formal and informal educational opportunities (Kuru & Ungar, 2020). As the refugee journey progresses, the balance between risk and protective factors evolves, influencing the mental health and well-being of children and families. Understanding these dynamics is essential for clinicians to tailor interventions that promote resilience and support the intricate psychological needs of this diverse and vulnerable population.

Psychopathology among Refugee and Migrant Children: A Comprehensive Exploration

The trajectory of trauma experienced by FDPs, spanning from pre-flight to resettlement, manifests in a complex interplay of risk and protective factors, ultimately influencing their mental health and well-being (Betancourt et al., 2012). The varied forms of trauma, refugee children, and families are vulnerable to psychological maltreatment, sexual abuse, and physical abuse, as well as exploitation, famine, murder, torture, and recruitment by armed groups, creating a multifaceted backdrop for the mental health challenges faced by these vulnerable populations (Betancourt et al., 2012; Spinazzola et al., 2014).

The enduring exposure to trauma among refugee youth leaves an indelible mark on their neurobiological development. Early trauma, reflected in altered cortisol levels, may lead to persistent functional impairments in neurobiological structures such as the amygdala and hippocampus (De Bellis & Zisk, 2014). Furthermore, trauma is associated with structural changes in the limbic system, presenting as hippocampal atrophy and an enlarged amygdala, with implications for memory, concentration, anxiety, stress, fear, aggression, and the onset of depressive symptoms (Carrion et al., 2007; De Bellis & Zisk, 2014).

Continuous exposure to trauma during early development correlates with poorer cognitive functions and academic achievement in youth, affecting domains such as visual attention, verbal memory, learning, inhibitory control, problem-solving, reading, mathematics, and speeded naming (Jaffee & Maikovich-Fong, 2010; Malarbi et al., 2017; Pollak et al., 2010).

Trauma, Internalizing, and Externalizing Symptoms

The consequences of trauma extend to the heightened risk of mental health disorders, including internalizing (i.e., anxiety, depression) and externalizing symptoms (e.g., aggression, hyperactivity, inattention, relational insecurity, and negative self-perceptions; Rizkalla et al., 2020). Speidel et al. (2021) found that male refugee children were rated higher in externalizing symptoms than female children. Importantly, familial pre-migration adversities are consistently associated with higher levels of refugee children's internalizing and externalizing symptoms (Speidel et al., 2021).

Among refugee youth, gender-based differences manifest, with varying rates of PTSD and depressive symptoms. A subgroup of refugee youth, child soldiers, faces heightened risks of depression, anxiety, suicidal ideation, and substance abuse due to their direct involvement in violence (de Silva, 2001). Psychopathological challenges observed in refugee youth also extend to the classroom, impacting attention, behavior, and withdrawal, underscoring the importance of recognizing trauma-related issues in educational settings (Rousseau et al.,1996).

Empirical Support of CBT in Treatment of the Trauma-Related Symptoms in Refugee and Migrant Children and Families)

CBT emerges as a cornerstone in psychological interventions, exhibiting consistent efficacy across diverse mental health challenges such as depression, PTSD, and anxiety. As articulated by The Royal College of Psychiatrists (2022), CBT is a verbal therapeutic modality that delves into an individual's cognitive appraisals, emotional responses, and subsequent behavioral patterns in response to various situations. The collaborative nature of CBT involves both therapist and client actively working together to reshape maladaptive thoughts and behaviors, breaking free from cycles of negativity and acquiring practical skills for positive progression. Notably, CBT often employs clinical strategies that are aimed at fostering clients' healing across various domains of their functioning, including protective factors such as optimism and emotional regulation skills (Speidel et al., 2021).

Trauma-Focused CBT: Nurturing Resilience in Trauma Survivors

Within the broader landscape of CBT, trauma-focused CBT (TF-CBT) stands out as a specialized framework explicitly designed to address posttraumatic stress disorder (PTSD). TF-CBT adopts a comprehensive approach, incorporating elements such as psychoeducation, parent training, relaxation techniques, affective modulation, cognitive coping, trauma narrative development, exposure to trauma-related stimuli, and safety-focused interventions (Cohen & Mannarino, 2015).

The acronym P.R.A.C.T.I.C.E. succinctly encapsulates the key components of TF-CBT, emphasizing Psychoeducation, Parenting Skills, Relaxation skills, Affective modulation skills, Cognitive coping skills, Trauma narrative, Cognitive processing of traumatic events, In vivo mastery of trauma reminders, Conjoint child-parent sessions, and Enhancing safety and future development trajectory (Cohen & Mannarino, 2015). This approach, renowned for its cultural sensitivity, has gained international recognition and is recommended as a 1st-line treatment for traumatized children and youth (Cohen et al., 2006).

While TF-CBT has shown promise in studies with non-refugee populations, its effectiveness in the context of refugee children and displaced individuals from non-Western countries requires further exploration (Cohen et al., 2006). The systematic review conducted by Chipalo (2021) supports TF-CBT's efficacy, particularly in sessions lasting between 12 and 28 weeks, as observed in studies involving culturally diverse refugee children and families in the United States and Germany.

The integration of TF-CBT into the broader spectrum of CBT aligns seamlessly with the adaptability required when working with refugee and migrant families. As clinicians engage with these populations, the structured and evidence-based nature of TF-CBT proves invaluable.

The success of CBT interventions, as demonstrated by Ehntholt et al. (2005), is marked by a significant reduction in overall PTSD symptom severity and intrusive PTSD symptoms among participating children. However, the application of trauma-informed and evidence-based treatments for refugee youth necessitates careful consideration of cultural variations.

Western cultural frameworks, predominantly rooted in individualism, may not fully address the mental health needs of refugee youth socialized in collectivist cultures (Hutchinson & Dorsett, 2012). For example, grief is a culturally universal condition; however, the expression of mourning is culture-bound (Cohen et al., 2006).

To overcome these challenges, culturally responsive adaptations to therapeutic approaches are essential. Chowdhary et al. (2014) stress the significance of understanding cultural determinants of health advocating for the inclusion of local remedies, health practices, stories, parables, and symbols. For instance, interventions for Vietnamese and Cambodian refugees in the United States incorporated culturally relevant symbols, such as a lotus bloom spinning in the wind, as part of a relaxation technique (Roemer & Orsillo, 2002). Storytelling and expressive techniques, including painting, music, and poetry, can supplement the CBT techniques to facilitate the healing of refugee children and families who come from Middle Eastern and African backgrounds (Diaków, 2021; Moore, 2017).

Adapting CBT to specific populations involves focusing on family relations before delving into personal aspects (Dwairy, 2009), recognizing the preference of Malaysian of Malay and Chinese ethnicity patients to describe health through physical rather than psychological problems (Khaiyom et al., 2015), and incorporating the recitation of verses of the Qur'an addressing concerns like worry or using Islamic prayer for Muslim clients (Subhas et al., 2021).

Beyond cultural considerations, empirical evidence from CBT randomized controlled trials conducted on war-traumatized non-displaced children showcases the success of CBT in reducing PTSD, anxiety, and depression symptoms, with effect sizes ranging from medium to large (Barron et al., 2013). This robust body of research underscores the potential of CBT, including specialized approaches like TF-CBT, as valuable therapeutic tools in addressing trauma-related disorders in refugee children and youth.

Relational Consideration in Treatment of Problem Area (Connecting)

Navigating mental health services can be a formidable challenge for refugee children and families, who may perceive such services as stigmatizing and harbor trust issues stemming from prior adversities (Majumder et al., 2014). Fear of stigmatization and a distinct conceptualization of mental health problems pose significant barriers to accessing specialized mental health treatment for this population (Unterhitzenberger et al., 2019). To surmount these challenges, clinicians must prioritize the establishment of a robust rapport with their refugee and migrant clients. This involves dedicating time to elucidate the therapist's role and the treatment modality.

Refugee children and families may encounter challenges in establishing trust with clinicians, given their past encounters with authority figures (Majumder et al., 2014). Moreover, these families have undergone diverse forms of interrogation throughout their journey, including interviews integral to their asylum applications. Consequently, clinicians must ensure a transparent data-gathering process, clearly articulating its purpose and delineating how sensitive information will be handled. It is imperative to reassure clients that the narratives shared will not adversely affect their migration status. This assurance holds particular significance for individuals contending with various stressors in the host country, such as domestic or community violence.

Cultural nuances play a pivotal role in shaping interactions, with many non-Western communities endorsing the value of "Saving Face" by refraining from questioning authority figures as a sign of respect (Unterhitzenberger et al., 2019). Recognizing this, clinicians can employ strategic communication techniques, such as asking clients to articulate their understanding in their own words after introducing concepts or methods instead of using potentially anxiety-provoking inquiries like "Do you have any questions?"

Chipalo (2021) advocates for the involvement of professional interpreters trained in TF-CBT to mitigate communication barriers arising from technical terms or culturally specific emotional responses. While leveraging interpreters, clinicians need to be mindful of potential distortions in interpretation, ranging from linguistic deficiencies to interpreter attitudes toward either the client or the clinicians (Marcos, 1979).

The language barrier, a significant stressor for refugee and migrant families in a host country, should be addressed with sensitivity. Clinicians can openly acknowledge their own language limitations and emphasize the importance of understanding the client's experiences and perspectives, fostering a collaborative approach. Instead of stating, "I will invite an interpreter because your English is not enough for us to work," clinicians can convey acceptance and non-judgment by saying, "Unfortunately, I do not speak your language, and I really would like to make sure I can understand your experiences and perspectives."

Trust issues, rooted in past experiences of persecution and political violence, may affect the willingness of refugee families to work with interpreters and authority figures (Majumder et al., 2014). Clinicians must explore these views before assuming readiness for collaboration. Additionally, considering the preferences of clients, especially regarding the gender or ethnicity of interpreters, is crucial, particularly for Muslim and Middle Eastern clients with potential cultural and ideological tensions (Diaków, 2021).

To cater to the cultural norms of Muslim Arab clients, Dwairy (2009) suggests an initial focus on family relations rather than personality traits, intrapsychic feelings, attitudes, and thoughts. Encouraging refugee youth to describe their family well-being and relationships with specific family members aligns with this approach. Psychotherapies can further benefit from psychosocial interventions that include creative arts, proven to enhance the well-being of refugee youth while addressing emotional and relational challenges (Ager et al., 2011).

Interviewing and Assessing Problem Area (Assessing)

In the realm of assessing mental health in refugee youth, challenges arise from the scarcity of culturally responsive tools specifically normed for this population (Gadeberg et al., 2017). While trauma-related assessments exist for survivors in clinical settings, limited attention has been given to culturally relevant assessments for refugee youth (Gadeberg et al., 2017). Gadeberg and colleagues (2017) underscored the gap in validated tools for children below six years old, emphasizing the need for early screening to prevent adverse outcomes from early trauma.

Most assessments deployed thus far have been normed on Western adult populations, lacking child-specific considerations (Hollifield et al., 2002). Gadeberg et al. (2017) stressed the importance of using culturally sensitive screening tools that incorporate child-specific methods, such as doll-plays, to capture youth's internalized reactions effectively.

Considering the diverse linguistic backgrounds of refugee youth, translated tools become imperative (Gadeberg et al., 2017). For instance, translations of the Child Behavior Checklist (CBCL) and the Child Posttraumatic Stress Disorder Symptom Scale Interview (CPSS-I) into Somali have proven beneficial (Hall et al., 2014). Similarly, culturally adjusted screeners like the Reaction of Adolescents to Traumatic Stress Questionnaire (RATS) cater to bilingual needs, addressing the linguistic diversity within refugee communities (Bean et al., 2006).

To account for literacy skills, innovative adaptations like pairing Likert scales with coloring, as seen in RATS, enhance comprehension for refugee youth (Bean et al., 2006). Despite the heterogeneity among refugees, their shared experience of fleeing life-threatening circumstances justifies the need for cross-culturally valid screening tools (Gadeberg et al., 2017).

Somatic complaints, often prevalent in this population, can be measured using the Diagnostic Predictive Scales (DPS; Lucas et al., 2001). Anxiety symptoms find assessment through the Screen for Child Anxiety Related Emotional Disorders (SCARED; Birmaher et al., 1997). These tools contribute to a comprehensive evaluation of mental health in refugee children and youth, addressing the nuanced challenges they may present. See Table 13.1 for a comprehensive list of assessment tools suitable for refugee children and youth.

Acknowledging the diverse cultural backgrounds of refugee children and families underscores the importance of employing comprehensive assessment strategies, particularly during interviews with caregivers. Embracing relational interviewing proves to be a valuable clinical tool, aligning with the prevalent orientation toward relationships within many refugee families (Hydén, 2014). The dynamics of relationships, especially the hierarchy embedded within them, require thoughtful consideration during these interviews. For instance, in cultures where children are expected to moderate eye contact when addressing adults, understanding this nuance becomes crucial, as it is a significant clinical data point. Recommendations by Piña-Watson et al. (2013) further emphasize the significance of considering cultural values like *familismo*, emphasizing obligation and connectedness to the family, when working with Latinx families. This highlights the need to extend interviews beyond parents to gain a more holistic understanding of family dynamics.

Within the framework of relational interviewing with children and their families, careful attention must be given to the introduction and prompts for questions. These prompts should be designed to elicit narratives, recognizing the cultural relevance of storytelling, a prevalent practice in, for example, Middle Eastern cultures. The inclusion of culturally sensitive prompts ensures that the interview process is not only clinically effective but also responsive to the diverse cultural norms of the families being assessed. Clinical interviewing should attempt to mimic storytelling by, e.g., inviting caregivers to share stories about their child or narrate their recent journey to the community. These prompts align with cultural practices and encourage a more nuanced exploration of the child's experiences and challenges within their cultural context.

- Tell me your story about your child's journey to this community. What were the significant moments or challenges along the way?
- In your family, are there any traditions or cultural practices that hold particular significance? Could you share a story related to one of these practices?
- Could you please share with me a story about your child's strengths?
- Tell me the story about what has been troubling your child lately. Are there any specific events or challenges that seem to have impacted them?
- I am curious about how your child copes with challenges. Can you share a story that highlights their coping mechanisms or strategies during difficult times?

Case Conceptualization (Understanding)

Samir, a ten-year-old Muslim Syrian boy, and his family's journey reflect the profound impact of forced displacement on their lives. Arriving in Germany with his biological mother and younger sibling, Samir's experiences are rooted in the traumatic loss of his father during a bombing incident in Syria. Witnessing his father's death while fleeing their home profoundly affected Samir, prompting his mother to prioritize immediate escape, leaving his father behind due to collapsing structures.

Samir's educational journey has been disrupted by civil unrest and military violence in Syria, depriving him of structured schooling. The family's arduous transition, from escaping to Turkey and enduring a hazardous sea crossing to Greece, marked by stays in refugee camps, exposed Samir to community violence and instances of physical and sexual abuse. Despite participating in psychosocial and educational programs in Greek refugee camps, his engagement was repeatedly interrupted by environmental hazards. Amidst these challenges, Samir's medical history remains incomplete due to lost documents during migration.

In Germany, Samir's mother grapples with her own mental health challenges, undergoing outpatient treatment for PTSD and depression while navigating the complexities of adjusting to a new environment. Samir, exhibiting trauma-related symptoms, displays strong startle responses, daily nightmares, bedwetting, aggressive behaviors (i.e., biting his mother, throwing objects), and self-harming (i.e., banging his head on the wall) tendencies. His limited verbal communication, preference for drawing disturbing imagery, and heightened distress when separated from his mother further illustrate the depth of his psychological struggles. Samir tends to express a sense of guilt for his father's death. He tends to say, "Baba would be still with us if I was a good boy."

Despite the adversities, Samir maintains a connection with close family members still in Greek refugee camps, often inquiring about his cousins. His interests include playing with blocks, drawing, and finding comfort in his mother's lullabies. While adapting to the German language, Samir's ability to express simple words and phrases reflects a glimpse of resilience in the face of adversity.

Treatment Goal 1: Establishing Emotional Regulation

Objective: Over the next 12 sessions, Samir will demonstrate improved emotional regulation by reducing the frequency and intensity of aggressive behaviors (e.g., throwing objects, biting) and self-harming tendencies (e.g., head-banging) in response to distressing stimuli.

Intervention plan: Implement relaxation techniques and stress management strategies tailored to Samir's age and cultural background. Utilize play therapy and creative expression to provide alternative outlets for emotional expression, fostering a sense of safety and self-soothing.

Treatment Goal 2: Addressing Trauma-Related Nightmares and Sleep Disturbances

Objective: Within 12 sessions, Samir will experience a decrease in the occurrence of daily nightmares and achieve at least a 50% reduction in bedwetting incidents.

Intervention plan: Introduce narrative exposure techniques to process and integrate traumatic memories gradually. Implement a consistent bedtime routine incorporating calming activities and validating Samir's emotional experiences. Collaborate with Samir's mother to create a secure sleep environment that promotes a sense of safety.

Treatment Goal 3: Empowering the Mother in Supporting Samir's Emotional Regulation

Objective: Within 12 sessions, Samir's mother will develop effective strategies to support Samir's emotional regulation and manage his distress, contributing to a more stable family environment.

Intervention plan: Provide psychoeducation on trauma-informed parenting, focusing on Samir's unique needs and triggers. Collaboratively create a personalized toolkit of coping mechanisms for Samir, incorporating culturally relevant calming techniques. Offer guidance on recognizing Samir's cues for distress and responding empathetically.

Session Structure: Building Rapport and Establishing Emotional Regulation

A sample session structure can involve a warm-up, mood/distress check-in, guided relaxation, Psychoeducation, and wrap-up. Embarking on the therapeutic journey with Samir, the 1st session is meticulously crafted to establish a secure and inviting space. This initial encounter sets the tone for a nurturing environment, crucial for Samir to feel at ease and engaged in the forthcoming therapeutic process. We begin by initiating an open dialogue, allowing Samir to share at his own pace, preferably through plan (e.g., blocks, drawing).

In the segment addressing *Stress in My Body* (see a sample bundle of forms for this segment in Form 3 in the Appendix of this book), the session delves into Samir's emotional and physiological symptoms. Here, we engage Samir in articulating his mood and somatic symptoms, providing a valuable snapshot of his current level of distress. This exploration is pivotal in establishing a comprehensive understanding of how stress manifests physically, creating a foundation for future emotional expression.

Recognizing Samir's distress, a guided relaxation exercise precedes the main focus of the session. This strategic step is designed to ease Samir into a state of emotional receptivity, ensuring an optimal environment for engaging with the therapeutic goals. Post-relaxation, another mood, and somatic symptoms rating is obtained, offering tangible insights into the impact of relaxation techniques on Samir's emotional well-being.

Seamlessly integrating psychoeducation, the session imparts age-appropriate insights into trauma-related symptoms (e.g., tension in the body). This knowledge empowers Samir with a sense of understanding, laying the groundwork for emotional regulation. As the session gracefully concludes, a thoughtful wrapping-up process ensures Samir departs with emotional stability, setting the stage for continued exploration and healing in subsequent sessions. Homework can be assigned to promote Samir's ability to utilize newly acquired skills across various settings.

Component of Practice and Intervention Modules (Intervening)

Attuning to Somatic Distress: A Culturally Responsive Coloring Exercise

In the multifaceted realm of TF-CBT for refugee children, the incorporation of culturally sensitive interventions is paramount. Tailored to foster rapport and enhance therapeutic outcomes, *Stress in My Body* (see a sample bundle of forms for this segment in Form 3 in the Appendix of this book) endeavors to guide children in attuning to somatic symptoms of distress within a visual and expressive modality. As explained earlier, for many migrant and refugee children, exploring somatic symptoms may feel more familiar than discussing their thoughts or feelings. Navigating the complexities of trauma with refugee populations requires a nuanced approach that respects and integrates cultural variations in emotional expression. *Stress in My Body* was developed by Dr. Diaków and used in group sessions with Middle Eastern female teens in a refugee camp in Greece.

The primary goal of this exercise is to provide refugee children with a tangible and culturally responsive method to articulate their bodily sensations. Commencing with a comprehensive introduction and psychoeducation, the clinician emphasizes the interconnectedness of emotions and bodily experiences, acknowledging diverse cultural expressions of distress. Collaboration with caregivers is integral, with a pre-exercise consultation to gather insights into potential medical considerations that may influence the child's bodily experiences. As the child engages in the coloring activity, using a culturally responsive body outline, they are encouraged to mark areas of tension or discomfort with a range of colors. Clinicians can ask a follow-up scaling question to assess the intensity of distress/ discomfort by asking, e.g., "How big or small is this feeling?" These questions can further foster therapeutic alliance by creating a cooperative atmosphere. This visual representation serves as a personalized reference for tracking changes over sessions or interventions. Utilizing this exercise at the outset and conclusion of sessions, or before and after specific interventions, creates a visual narrative of the child's emotional journey, aligning with the principles of TF-CBT within a culturally sensitive framework.

Culturally Responsive Guided Relaxation Exercises

The following guided relaxation script is designed for ten-year-old Samir, attuning to his cultural background. Dr. Diaków originally developed this script for group sessions with four- to seven-year-old Muslim Arab refugee children in a refugee camp in Greece. The intention is to offer a template that clinicians can adapt and modify to align with the cultural nuances and individual needs of each child. This intervention underscores the importance of avoiding potentially triggering elements in guided relaxation (e.g., sea or ocean waves imaginary or sounds), particularly for those, like Samir, who have undergone traumatic experiences, such as sea crossings. Customization ensures that the therapeutic journey remains safe, culturally responsive, and attuned to the specific needs of refugee children.

<u>Introduction</u>

Find a cozy spot, maybe sit or lie down alone or next to your parents, whatever feels comfy for you. This time is just for you to feel calm and safe.

<u>Breathing</u>

Let's start with some easy breathing. Inhale through your nose, like you're sniffing a flower, and exhale through your mouth, like you're blowing that flower. Smell the sweet scent? That's your favorite flower, making each breath cozy and nice.

<u>Engaging the Senses: Magical Garden</u>

Imagine a magical garden with all the colors you love. There's a cool fountain there, and when you dip your fingers in, it feels like a warm hug from the person that you love. Can you hear the leaves rustling?

<u>Soothing Imagery</u>

Picture a golden light above, just like the warm sun in your hometown. Feel it coming down, wrapping you up like a big, comfy blanket. Any tightness you feel?

<u>Connection to Culture</u>

Imagine the call to prayer humming softly. It's like a familiar tune, giving you strength and hope. Imagine it in the background, making you feel all peaceful inside.

<u>Progressive Relaxation</u>

Time to say goodbye to any wiggles or jiggles. Imagine each part of you—toes, legs, tummy, and all—getting super relaxed. Like warm wind, washing over you, making everything feel gooey and comfy.

<u>Closing</u>

Guess what? You can visit this cozy place whenever you want. When you're ready, wiggle your fingers and toes, and you're back feeling calm. Remember you're strong and can handle anything that comes your way. Ready?

Culturally Responsive Trauma Narrative That Also Spotlights Client's Strengths: My Mountain

To gain insight into client's experiences and their perceptions of their problems, clinicians can use Exploratory Graphics (e.g., *My Mountain*; see Figure 13.1). They are child-friendly and language-free tools that help to understand a client's background better. Dr. Diaków has developed *My Mountain* to work with Uzbeki and Kazakh teen students who migrated to Poland and who presented with trauma-related symptoms. Before incorporating *My Mountain* into a session, clinicians need to make sure that the client is familiar with this particular landscape and has not experienced trauma associated with the mountains to reduce potential triggers. Clinicians are encouraged to create their own graphics that may feel familiar to their clients, depending on their cultural background and personal experiences. By incorporating elements of creative expression and storytelling which may be familiar to Middle Eastern and African refugee children and families (Diaków, 2021; Moore, 2017), this intervention can be not only a great culturally responsive segway to a trauma narrative but also a part of resilience building sessions.

Follow these steps:

1 Present the *My Mountain* to the client and explain to them that

Each of us is climbing a mountain. Sometimes, we are surrounded by beautiful flowers and chirping birds, and sometimes, we are exposed to harsh weather, and we feel lonely summiting the peak. It is a journey and we face a number of obstacles on the way. The higher we are, the

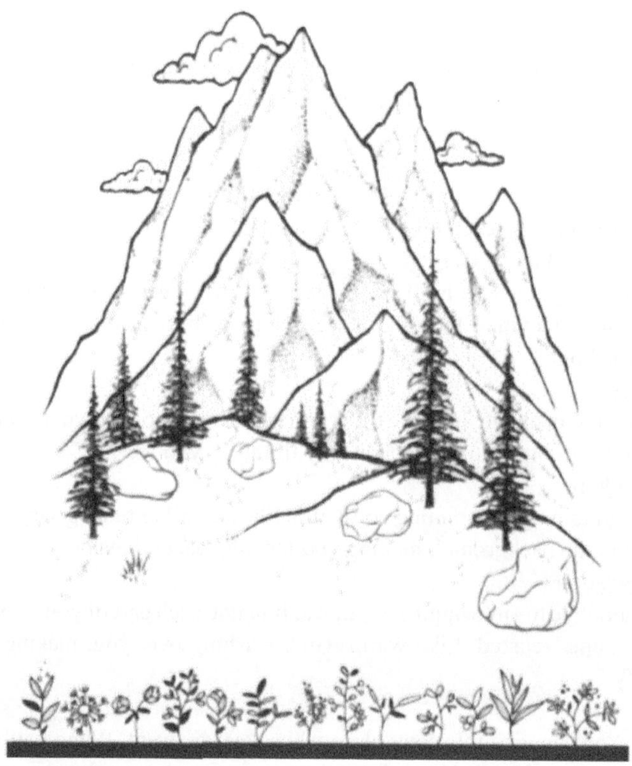

Figure 13.1 Exploratory Graphic: *My Mountain*

more dangerous it gets. Sometimes, there are rocks falling down, and we may be very scared. I want you to think about your life experiences, both those that are positive and those that are negative. These positive experiences, things that have made you happy, are like flowers that blossom in beautiful colors, and those negative experiences, your fears, and worries are like falling rocks—you are afraid of them.

2 Give crayons to your client and allow them to draft their experiences on the paper.
3 Facilitate the discussion by asking these questions: *Tell me about your flowers. Why do they make you happy? How often are you in their presence? How is that for you to be around these flowers (ask about emotions, thoughts, and physical sensations)? Tell me about these falling rocks. What does it look like when you are afraid of them (ask about emotions, thoughts, and physical sensations)?*
4 Comment on your client's resilience and endurance. Empower them.

Assessment of Progress and Outcomes (Monitoring)

A robust tool for assessing the progress and outcomes of therapeutic interventions with refugee and migrant children is the Strengths and Difficulties Questionnaire (SDQ), developed by Goodman (1997). This widely utilized questionnaire comprises 25 items distributed across 5 subscales, each encompassing five items. These subscales assess emotional symptoms, conduct problems, hyperactivity-inattention, peer problems, and personal strengths. Available in parent, teacher, and self-rating formats, the SDQ caters to children and youth aged 3–16. It boasts translation into over 70 languages and dialects, although normative data are accessible for only ten countries.

A notable strength of the SDQ lies in its versatility, enabling a comprehensive evaluation of both psychopathological symptoms and individual strengths. The questionnaire's reliability in capturing difficulties is well-established, with recommendations favoring the use of total scores over subscale scores due to higher reliability (Hoofs et al., 2015). The SDQ's applicability extends across diverse cultural settings, aligning with the varied backgrounds of refugee children. To enhance the sensitivity and accuracy of psychopathological assessments, it is advisable to adopt a multimethod, multiscore approach.

Despite its strengths, the SDQ confronts challenges in the absence of appropriate norms for immigrant populations. This limitation restricts the validity and generalizability of obtained scores, particularly concerning the lack of norms for refugee and migrant children's home countries. Consequently, assessments are confined to measures with established validity evidence (Sullivan & Simonson, 2016).

The SDQ stands out as one of the most researched measures in cross-cultural contexts, providing a comprehensive overview of not only psychopathological symptoms but also individual strengths. Its availability in parent and teacher formats enhances the richness of data points, enabling a more nuanced analysis of progress and outcomes in therapeutic interventions. In addition to the comprehensive assessment provided by the SDQ, monitoring progress in therapeutic interventions necessitates a nuanced evaluation of specific presenting concerns.

An uncomplicated yet universally applicable tool for monitoring progress is the Subjective Units of Distress Scale (SUDS). This versatile scale can be tailored to accommodate younger children or individuals with limited literacy skills by adopting visual representations. It's crucial to acknowledge that, due to disrupted education, some refugee and migrant individuals might not be familiar with metric systems or thermometers. Therefore, adopting culturally responsive scales becomes imperative. Clinicians are encouraged to bring creativity into this aspect, utilizing culturally relevant symbols such as warmth, temperature, or visual depictions of size. Through the implementation of SUDS, clinicians can effectively assess a child's distress levels. Ratings can be collected both before

Table 13.1 Assessment and Progress Monitoring Tools

Category	*Tool Name*
PTSD symptoms	The University of California at Los Angeles (UCLA-PTSD)
	Posttraumatic stress disorder reaction index for DSM-5
	Children's Revised Impact of Event Scale 8/13 (CRIES-8/13)
	Child Posttraumatic Stress Reaction Index (CPTS-RI)
	Posttraumatic Diagnosis Scale (PDS)
	Parent Report of Posttraumatic Stress Symptoms (PROPS)
	Clinician administered PTSD scale—Child/Adolescent version (CAPS-CA)
	Child and Adolescent Trauma Scale (CATS)
Anxiety	The Spence Children's Anxiety Scale (SCAS)
	Revised Children's Manifest Anxiety Scale (RCMAS)
	Screen for Child Anxiety Related Disorders (SCARED)
Depression	Depression Self Rating Scale for Children (DSRS)
	Patient Health Questionnaire Depression Scale (PHQ-8)
	Children's Depression Inventory (CDI)
	Montgomery-Asberg Depression Rating Scale Self-report (MADRS-S)
Broad measures	Strengths and Difficulties Questionnaire (SDQ)
Resilience	Child And Youth Resilience Measure (CYRM)

and after specific interventions, like relaxation exercises or trauma narratives, as well as at the commencement and conclusion of counseling sessions. This approach ensures a nuanced understanding of the child's emotional state and facilitates a dynamic assessment of progress throughout therapeutic engagement.

A range of outcome measures tailored to address the multifaceted nature of refugee and migrant children's mental health concerns enhances the precision of treatment evaluation. Table 13.1 presents a diverse array of measures designed to assess progress across various domains, including PTSD symptoms, anxiety, depression, and broader measures of mental health. Each instrument is selected for its relevance and effectiveness in capturing the unique challenges and strengths within this population.

Applications to the School Setting

Refugee services within schools have become a pressing international concern, particularly considering that a significant percentage of individuals of concern and refugees are under 18 years old (UNHCR, 2023). Leveraging the school setting for interventions holds promise as it offers a non-stigmatizing and easily accessible avenue for mental health care for a large cohort of refugee children. Schools, for many refugee and migrant children, serve as a vital and sometimes sole connection to the wider community (Sullivan & Simonson, 2016).

School-based interventions are categorized into two types: targeted interventions, directed at selected symptomatic children (e.g., TF-CBT, the UCLA Trauma/Grief Program, the Children and War: Teaching Recovery Techniques), and universal interventions, which focus on building resilience and strengthening students' access to resources without requiring specific clinical intervention (Ehntholt et al., 2005). Programs like Healing after Trauma Skills (HATS; Gurwitch & Messenbaugh, 2001), The Building Resilience Project (BRP; Baum, 2005), and The Threat of Terrorism, incorporating elements of CBT, art therapy, body-oriented strategies, and narrative approaches (Berger et al., 2007), exemplify the diverse strategies employed. The Classroom-Based Intervention Program

(CBI; Macy et al., 2003), grounded in CBT and incorporating expressive therapy techniques, showcases another effective approach.

Collaborative efforts between teachers and mental health professionals, as demonstrated by Ehntholt et al. (2005) and O'Shea et al. (2000), underscore the efficacy of school-based services in reaching a population of children who may not readily access traditional mental health facilities. Schools, being a primary providers of mental health services for children and youth, play a crucial role in ensuring that these young refugees receive the necessary support, considering the interconnectedness of mental health, academic performance, and general well-being.

Recognizing that anxiety disorders, including PTSD, may not always manifest visibly in classroom settings, creative approaches are essential. Techniques such as writing, drawing, and creative expression workshops, proven to decrease externalizing and internalizing symptoms and increase self-reported popularity (Kalantari et al., 2012; Rousseau et al., 2005), can be invaluable. Drama workshops and storytelling, fostering exploration of identities and backgrounds, further contribute to supporting students' resilience (Rousseau et al., 2014). The incorporation of CBT programs, such as the one developed by Fox et al. (2005) for Southeast Asian refugees, which integrates discussions on ethnic traditions and resettlement experiences, adds a comprehensive dimension to coping skill development.

Critical considerations from the research conducted by Layne et al. (2001) on school-based post-war intervention with traumatized Bosnian adolescents emphasize the need for educators to evaluate the appropriateness of interventions for the specific population and available resources. Additionally, teacher training in the psychological techniques required for faithful intervention implementation in classroom settings is essential, as highlighted by Ehntholt et al. (2005). The extended time children spend in schools makes school-based mental health interventions a practical avenue for practicing coping skills in vivo.

Group Intervention

The clustering of refugees during resettlement makes group treatments a pragmatic and cost-effective choice (Ehntholt et al., 2005). Therapeutic groups offer additional benefits by alleviating children's feelings of hopelessness and loneliness while also normalizing their reactions (Ehntholt et al., 2005). An example of group intervention is found in the "Children and War: Teaching Recovery Techniques" manual (Yule et al., 2013), specifically designed for non-mental health professionals like teachers. This manual equips them with cognitive-behavioral tools to effectively address PTSD in children.

Ensuring appropriateness for group inclusion is crucial, considering not all refugee children may exhibit PTSD symptoms. If the group's criteria are met by only a small number of refugee children, sessions may need to include children from various ethnic backgrounds and ages who have encountered diverse traumatic experiences (Ehntholt et al., 2005).

The psycho-social-educational program within the intervention aims to educate children about PTSD symptoms and impart developmentally appropriate coping strategies. The six manual-based sessions, addressing intrusion, arousal, and avoidance symptoms, have been successfully implemented in Turkey, Greece, and the UK (Ehntholt et al., 2005). Non-mental health professionals, under supervision, such as licensed school psychologists, can effectively deliver this CBT manualized program.

Incorporating "pull-out" sessions for individualized attention is a viable approach, allowing clinicians to address specific issues with each child. For instance, introducing graded exposure individually can be beneficial for certain children reporting PTSD symptoms of avoidance (Ehntholt et al., 2005).

Adapting the program for specific populations requires careful consideration of cultural factors. Ehntholt et al. (2005) noted that teen Kosovan Albanian boys refrained from group participation, viewing discussions about emotions as a sign of weakness. It is suggested that their involvement might be facilitated if a male teacher, known and respected by them, led the sessions.

Group homogeneity, with children from the same country, ethnic background, or those with similar traumatic experiences and a shared 1st language, is recommended. Larger groups, especially those with older children, benefit from having a group co-leader, and with younger children, it is considered essential (Ehntholt et al., 2005).

However, this group intervention might not be suitable for newly arrived refugee children, as they need time to adjust to the host country's culture and language. While organizing parallel sessions for parents poses time challenges, it is highly recommended.

Table 13.2 Treatment Plan for Samir and His Mother

Session	*Description and Practice*
1	Psychoeducation, Parenting skills: Psychoeducation about trauma, trauma-related symptoms, and the rationale of TF-CBT; normalizing the symptoms; teaching positive parenting skills (e.g., praise, active ignoring, contingency management strategies); psychoeducation about sleep hygiene.
2	Relaxation: Information about the rationale of relaxation; demonstration and practicing relaxation techniques (e.g., play-based emotional regulation exercises, controlled breathing). Some culturally responsive relaxation practices can involve lullabies, or reading/telling stories, psychoeducation regarding stress reactions.
3	Affective modulation: Explanation of rationale; identification of feelings; expression of feelings; rating the intensity level of emotions; positive self-instructions; coping with difficult/unpleasant emotions. It is important to refer to distress in the body and help Samir understand the physiological component of his big feelings; Psychoeducation regarding stress reactions.
4	Cognitive processing, I: Outline the cognitive triangle; identify dysfunctional thoughts in daily life (i.e., "I'm a bad boy"); help Samir to generate more accurate and helpful thoughts; it may be helpful to refer to the verses from the Qur'an to help Samir find positive affirmations about himself. Other resilience-building activities may be used here (e.g., *Petals of Resilience*).
5–8	Trauma narrative: Decide on a format for the narrative; describe the perception of the event, including the worst moment; read the narrative and thoughts and feelings. It may be helpful to let Samir draw his story to bridge the language gap. He may also want to use blocks to depict the events that occurred. Exploratory Graphics, e.g., *My Mountain*, can be used to help Samir tell his story.
9	Cognitive processing II: Exploring and correcting cognitive errors concerning the traumatic experience (e.g., cognitions of guilt for the father's death); dual attention tasks (EMDR techniques)
10	In-vivo exposure: Explaining the rationale; development of a "plan" (if necessary, instruct the mother for co-therapeutic exposure); "Safe Place Coping Technique."
11	Conjoint child/caregiver session: Explaining the rationale; Prepare child and parent for a conjoint session; sharing the trauma narrative; answering questions; fostering child-parent communication.
12	Enhancing safety and future skills: Developing a feeling of safety; a safety plan; teaching safety skills.

Cultural and Linguistic Considerations

Considering linguistic and cultural diversity, potential conflicts arising for political reasons, and differing gender roles, group interventions with more than one interpreter become impractical. Access to competent interpreters is essential, and clinicians must acquire the skills to effectively collaborate with them. In line with the National Association of School Psychologists (NASP, 2019) guidelines, employing interpreters in therapeutic activities and translating deliverables into the native languages of refugee students is crucial for effective communication. Furthermore, school psychologists must refrain from involving refugee youth's siblings or friends as interpreters, given the age-inappropriate roles often taken on by refugee youth in their families during displacement (NASP, 2019).

Case Study of Problem Area

Treatment Goal 1: Establishing Emotional Regulation

Treatment Goal 2: Addressing Trauma-Related Nightmares and Sleep Disturbances

Treatment Goal 3: Empowering the Mother in Supporting Samir's Emotional Regulation

TF-CBT P.R.A.C.T.I.C.E. Sessions according to Cohen et al. (2006) (Adapted from Cohen et al., 2006) (Table 13.2)

Summary

The existing research landscape in refugee mental health interventions remains limited, necessitating a pragmatic evaluation strategy focused on understanding the intervention recipients, their backgrounds, and nuanced interactions between the treatment program itself and the targeted group (Bonell et al., 2013). Examining the applicability and social validity of interventions applied to refugee populations is a critical step, considering the need to understand their effectiveness in context, even when assumptions about their relevance based on similarities with other traumatized youth groups exist. Moreover, the shortage of longitudinal studies, coupled with small sample sizes and cultural insensitivity in tools, poses limitations to understanding refugee youth's mental health (Gadeberg et al., 2017). Advancements in research methodologies are crucial to meeting the mental health needs of refugee youth, regardless of their migration status.

To advance our understanding, the development of practice-based evidence from real-world contexts is essential. This involves utilizing diverse research methodologies, such as single-case designs, mixed methods, quasi-experimental group designs, or regression discontinuity designs when experimental designs are not feasible (Kratochwill et al., 2012).

Given the diverse challenges faced by refugee children, mental health services must offer a comprehensive range of interventions. This inclusivity is crucial for addressing various issues, including disruptive behavior disorders, anxiety symptoms, and PTSD. Given that forced displacement is a global issue, clinicians and practitioners across emergency and non-emergency settings, including schools and community-based facilities, should strive to provide refugee mental health services that are culturally responsive and geared not only toward adults but also children.

Reflection Questions

1 How might building rapport and initial assessments foster or hinder your refugee or migrant client's resilience and also the overall success of TF-CBT?
2 Suppose you have no interpreters available and you are working with a child with whom you do not have a commonly spoken language. What steps could you take to ensure that you deliver

clinical support ethically, given that access to specialized mental health services is very scarce for refugees?

3 How may your sociocultural background manifest in your clinical relationship with a refugee family? How can you mitigate potential biases that you bring to this relationship? What can you do when a conflict of values arises, for example, when you observe a parenting style that does not align with your worldview?

References

Ager, A., Akesson, B., Stark, L., Flouri, E., Okot, B., McCollister, F., & Boothby, N. (2011). The impact of the school-based Psychosocial Structured Activities (PSSA) program on conflict-affected children in northern Uganda. *Journal of Child Psychology and Psychiatry, 52*(11), 1124–1133. https://doi.org/10.1111/j.1469-7610.2011.02407.x

Barron, I. G., Abdallah, G., & Smith, P. (2013). Randomized control trial of a CBT trauma recovery program in Palestinian schools. *Journal of Loss and Trauma, 18*(4), 306–321. https://doi.org/10.1080/15325024.2012.688712

Baum, N. L. (2005). Building resilience. *Journal of Aggression, Maltreatment & Trauma, 10*(1–2), 487–498. https://doi.org/10.1300/j146v10n01_08

Bean, T., Derluyn, I., Elisabeth H. M., Eurelings-Bontekoe, Broekaert, E., & Spinhoven, P. (2006). Reactions of adolescents to traumatic stress questionnaire–multiple language versions. *PsycTESTS Dataset*. https://doi.org/10.1037/t69684-000

Berger, R., Pat-Horenczyk, R., & Gelkopf, M. (2007). School-based intervention for prevention and treatment of elementary-students' terror-related distress in Israel: A quasi-randomized controlled trial. *Journal of Traumatic Stress, 20*(4), 541–551. https://doi.org/10.1002/jts.20225

Betancourt, T. S., Newnham, E. A., Layne, C. M., Kim, S., Steinberg, A. M., Ellis, H., & Birman, D. (2012). Trauma history and psychopathology in war-affected refugee children referred for trauma-related mental health services in the United States. *Journal of Traumatic Stress, 25*(6), 682–690. https://doi.org/10.1002/jts.21749

Birmaher, B., Khetarpal, S., Brent, D., Cully, M., Balach, L., Kaufman, J., & Neer, S. M. (1997). The Screen for Child Anxiety Related Emotional Disorders (SCARED): Scale construction and psychometric characteristics. *Journal of the American Academy of Child & Adolescent Psychiatry, 36*(4), 545–553. https://doi.org/10 1097/00004583-199704000-00018

Bonell, C., Fletcher, A., Morton, M., Lorenc, T., & Moore, L. (2013). Methods don't make assumptions, researchers do: A response to Marchal et al. *Social Science & Medicine, 94*, 81–82. https://doi.org/10.1016/j.socscimed.2013.06.026

Borrell, C., Palència, L., Bartoll, X., Ikram, U., & Malmusi, D. (2015). Perceived discrimination and health among immigrants in Europe according to national integration policies. *International Journal of Environmental Research and Public Health, 12*(9), 10687–10699. https://doi.org/10.3390/ijerph120910687

Bryant, R. A., Edwards, B., Creamer, M., O'Donnell, M., Forbes, D., Felmingham, K. L., Silove, D., Steel, Z., Nickerson, A., McFarlane, A. C., Van Hooff, M., & Hadzi-Pavlovic, D. (2018). The effect of posttraumatic stress disorder on refugees' parenting and their children's mental health: A cohort study. *The Lancet Public Health, 3*(5), e249–e258. https://doi.org/10.1016/s2468-2667(18)30051-3

Carrion, V. G., Weems, C. F., & Reiss, A. L. (2007). Stress predicts brain changes in children: A pilot longitudinal study on youth stress, posttraumatic stress disorder, and the hippocampus. *Pediatrics, 119*(3), 509–516. https://doi.org/10.1542/peds.2006-2028

Chipalo, E. (2021). Is Trauma Focused-Cognitive Behavioral Therapy (TF-CBT) effective in reducing trauma symptoms among traumatized refugee children? A systematic review. *Journal of Child & Adolescent Trauma, 14*(4). https://doi.org/10.1007/s40653-021-00370-0

Chowdhary, N., Jotheeswaran, A. T., Nadkarni, A., Hollon, S. D., King, M., Jordans, M. J. D., Rahman, A., Verdeli, H., Araya, R., & Patel, V. (2014). The methods and outcomes of cultural adaptations of psychological treatments for depressive disorders: A systematic review. *Psychological Medicine, 44*(6), 1131–1146. https://doi.org/10.1017/S0033291713001785

Cohen, J. A., & Mannarino, A. P. (2015). Trauma-focused cognitive behavior therapy for traumatized children and families. *Child and Adolescent Psychiatric Clinics of North America, 24*(3), 557–570. https://doi.org/10.1016/j.chc.2015.02.005

Cohen, J. A., Mannarino, A. P., & Deblinger, E. (2006). *Treating trauma and traumatic grief in children and adolescents*. New York: Guilford Press.

De Bellis, M. D., & Zisk, A. (2014). The biological effects of childhood trauma. *Child and Adolescent Psychiatric Clinics of North America, 23*(2), 185–222. https://doi.org/10.1016/j.chc.2014.01.002

de Silva, D. G. H. (2001). Conscription of children in armed conflict. *BMJ, 322*(7298), 1372–1372. https://doi.org/10.1136/bmj.322.7298.1372

Diaków, D. M. (2021). *Humanitarian workers' perspectives on mental health and resilience of refugee youth: Implications for school psychology* [Doctoral Dissertation, University of Montana]. ScholarWorks University of Montana.

Durà-Vilà, G., Klasen, H., Makatini, Z., Rahimi, Z., & Hodes, M. (2012). Mental health problems of young refugees: Duration of settlement, risk factors and community-based interventions. *Clinical Child Psychology and Psychiatry, 18*(4), 604–623. https://doi.org/10.1177/1359104512462549

Dwairy, M. (2009). Culture analysis and metaphor psychotherapy with Arab-Muslim clients. *Journal of Clinical Psychology, 65*(2), 199–209. https://doi.org/10.1002/jclp.20568

Ehntholt, K. A., Smith, P. A., & Yule, W. (2005). School-based cognitive-behavioural therapy group intervention for refugee children who have experienced war-related trauma. *Clinical Child Psychology and Psychiatry, 10*(2), 235–250. https://doi.org/10.1177/1359104505051214

Fox, P. G., Rossetti, J., Burns, K. R., & Popovich, J. M. (2005). Southeast Asian refugee children: A school-based mental health intervention. *The International Journal of Psychiatric Nursing Research, 11*(1), 1227–1236.

Gadeberg, A. K., Montgomery, E., Frederiksen, H. W., & Norredam, M. (2017). Assessing trauma and mental health in refugee children and youth: A systematic review of validated screening and measurement tools. *European Journal of Public Health, 27*(3), 439–446. https://doi.org/10.1093/eurpub/ckx034

Goodman, R. (1997). The strengths and difficulties questionnaire: A research note. *Journal of Child Psychology and Psychiatry, 38*(5), 581–586. https://doi.org/10.1111/j.1469-7610.1997.tb01545.x

Gurwitch, R. H., & Messenbaugh, A. (2001). *Healing after trauma skills: A manual for professionals, teachers and families working with children after trauma/disaster*. Oklahoma City, OK: Children's Medical Research Foundation.

Hall, B. J., Puffer, E., Murray, L. K., Ismael, A., Bass, J. K., Sim, A., & Bolton, P. A. (2014). The importance of establishing reliability and validity of assessment instruments for mental health problems: An example from Somali children and adolescents living in three refugee camps in Ethiopia. *Psychological Injury and Law, 7*(2), 153–164. https://doi.org/10.1007/s12207-014-9188-9

Hodes, M., Jagdev, D., Chandra, N., & Cunniff, A. (2008). Risk and resilience for psychological distress amongst unaccompanied asylum seeking adolescents. *Journal of Child Psychology and Psychiatry, 49*(7), 723–732. https://doi.org/10.1111/j.1469-7610.2008.01912.x

Hollifield, M., Warner, T. D., Lian, N., Krakow, B., Jenkins, J. H., Kesler, J., Stevenson, J., & Westermeyer, J. (2002). Measuring trauma and health status in refugees. *JAMA, 288*(5), 611. https://doi.org/10.1001/jama.288.5.611

Hoofs, H., Jansen, N., Danielle, Jansen, M., & Kant, Ij. (2015). The context dependency of the self-report version of the Strength and Difficulties Questionnaire (SDQ): A cross-sectional study between two administration settings. *PLoS One*, *10*(4), e0120930–e0120930. https://doi.org/10.1371/journal.pone.0120930

Hutchinson, M., & Dorsett, P. (2012). What does the literature say about resilience in refugee people? Implications for practice. *Journal of Social Inclusion, 3*(2), 55–78.

Hydén, M. (2014). The teller-focused interview: Interviewing as a relational practice. *Qualitative Social Work: Research and Practice, 13*(6), 795–812. https://doi.org/10.1177/1473325013506247

Jaffee, S. R., & Maikovich-Fong, A. K. (2010). Effects of chronic maltreatment and maltreatment timing on children's behavior and cognitive abilities. *Journal of Child Psychology and Psychiatry*, *52*(2), 184–194. https://doi.org/10.1111/j.1469-7610.2010.02304.x

Kalantari, M., Yule, W., Dyregrov, A., Neshatdoost, H., & Ahmadi, S. J. (2012). Efficacy of writing for recovery on traumatic grief symptoms of Afghani refugee bereaved adolescents: A randomized control trial. *OMEGA – Journal of Death and Dying, 65*(2), 139–150. https://doi.org/10.2190/om.65.2.d

Khaiyom, J. H., Mukhtar, F., Ibrahim, N., Mohd Sidik, S., & Oei, T. P. S. (2015). Psychometric properties of the Catastrophic Cognitions Questionnaire-Modified (CCQ-Modified) among community samples in Malaysia. *Stress and Health, 32*(5), 543–550. https://doi.org/10.1002/smi.2660

Koehn, P. H., Bo-Yuen Ngai, P., Uitto, J. I., & Diaków, D. M. (2023). *Migrant health and resilience: Transnational competence in conflict and climate displacement situations*. New York: Routledge.

Kratochwill, T. R., Hoagwood, K. E., Kazak, A. E., Weisz, J. R., Hood, K., Vargas, L. A., & Banez, G. A. (2012). Practice-based evidence for children and adolescents: Advancing the research agenda in schools. *School Psychology Review, 41*(2), 215–235. https://doi.org/10.1080/02796015.2012.12087521

Kuru, N., & Ungar, M. (2020). Refugee children's resilience: A qualitative social ecological study of life in a camp. *Journal of Refugee Studies*. https://doi.org/10.1093/jrs/feaa092

Layne, C. M., Pynoos, R. S., Saltzman, W. R., Arslanagić, B., Black, M., Savjak, N., Popović, T., Duraković, E., Mušić, M., Ćampara, N., Djapo, N., & Houston, R. (2001). Trauma/grief-focused group psychotherapy: School-based postwar intervention with traumatized Bosnian adolescents. *Group Dynamics: Theory, Research, and Practice, 5*(4), 277–290. https://doi.org/10.1037/1089-2699.5.4.277

Lucas, C. P., Zhang, H., Fisher, P. W., Shaffer, D., Regier, D. A., Narrow, W. E., Bourdon, K., Dulcan, M. K., Canino, G., Rubio-Stipec, M., Lahey, B. B., & Friman, P. (2001). The DISC Predictive Scales (DPS): Efficiently screening for diagnoses. *Journal of the American Academy of Child & Adolescent Psychiatry, 40*(4), 443–449. https://doi.org/10.1097/00004583-200104000-00013

Macy, R. D., Johnson Macy, D., Gross, S. I., & Brighton, P. (2003). Healing in familiar settings: Support for children and youth in the classroom and community. *New Directions for Youth Development, 2003*(98), 51–79. https://doi.org/10.1002/yd.44

Majumder, P., O'Reilly, M., Karim, K., & Vostanis, P. (2014). "This doctor, I do not trust him, I'm not safe": The perceptions of mental health and services by unaccompanied refugee adolescents. *International Journal of Social Psychiatry, 61*(2), 129–136. https://doi.org/10.1177/0020764014537236

Malarbi, S., Abu-Rayya, H. M., Muscara, F., & Stargatt, R. (2017). Neuropsychological functioning of childhood trauma and posttraumatic stress disorder: A meta-analysis. *Neuroscience & Biobehavioral Reviews, 72*, 68–86. https://doi.org/10.1016/j.neubiorev.2016.11.004

Marcos, L. (1979). Effects of interpreters on the evaluation of psychopathology in non-English-speaking patients. *American Journal of Psychiatry, 136*(2), 171–174. https://doi.org/10.1176/ajp.136.2.171

Moore, T. (2017). Strengths-based narrative storytelling as therapeutic intervention for refugees in Greece. *World Federation of Occupational Therapists Bulletin, 73*(1), 45–51. https://doi.org/10.1080/14473828.2017.1298557

National Association of School Psychologists (NASP) (2019). *Students who are displaced persons, refugees, or asylum-seekers* [Position statement practice recommendations]. Bethesda, MD: Author.

O'shea, B., Hodes, M., Down, G., & Bramley, J. (2000). A school-based mental health service for refugee children. *Clinical Child Psychology and Psychiatry, 5*(2), 189–201. https://doi.org/10.1177/1359104500005002004

Phalet, K., Fleischmann, F., & Hillekens, J. (2018). Religious identity and acculturation of immigrant minority youth. *European Psychologist, 23*(1), 32–43. https://doi.org/10.1027/1016-9040/a000309

Piña-Watson, B., Ojeda, L., Castellon, N. E., & Dornhecker, M. (2013). Familismo, ethnic identity, and bicultural stress as predictors of Mexican American adolescents' positive psychological functioning. *Journal of Latina/O Psychology, 1*(4), 204–217. https://doi.org/10.1037/lat0000006

Pollak, S. D., Schlaak, M. F., Roeber, B. J., Nelson, C. A., Wewerka, S. S., Wiik, K. L., Frenn, K. A., Loman, M. M., & Gunnar, M. R. (2010). Neurodevelopmental effects of early deprivation in postinstitutionalized children. *Child Development, 81*(1), 224–236. https://www.jstor.org/stable/40598975

Rizkalla, N., Mallat, N. K., Arafa, R., Adi, S., Soudi, L., & Segal, S. P. (2020). "Children are not children anymore; They are a lost generation": Adverse physical and mental health consequences on syrian refugee children. *International Journal of Environmental Research and Public Health, 17*(22), 8378. https://doi.org/10.3390/ijerph17228378

Roemer, L., & Orsillo, S. M. (2002). Expanding our conceptualization of and treatment for Generalized Anxiety Disorder: Integrating mindfulness/acceptance-based approaches with existing cognitive-behavioral models. *Clinical Psychology: Science and Practice, 9*(1), 54–68. https://doi.org/10.1093/clipsy.9.1.54

Rousseau, C., Beauregard, C., Daignault, K., Petrakos, H., Thombs, B. D., Steele, R., Vasiliadis, H.-M., & Hechtman, L. (2014). A cluster randomized-controlled trial of a classroom-based drama workshop program to improve mental health outcomes among immigrant and refugee youth in special classes. *PLoS One, 9*(8), e104704. https://doi.org/10.1371/journal.pone.0104704

Rousseau, C., Drapeau, A., & Corin, E. (1996). School performance and emotional problems in refugee children. *American Journal of Orthopsychiatry, 66*(2), 239–251. https://doi.org/10.1037/h0080175

Rousseau, C., Drapeau, A., Lacroix, L., Bagilishya, D., & Heusch, N. (2005). Evaluation of a classroom program of creative expression workshops for refugee and immigrant children. *Journal of Child Psychology and Psychiatry, 46*(2), 180–185. https://doi.org/10.1111/j.1469-7610.2004.00344.x

Royal College of Psychiatrists (2022). *Cognitive behavioural therapy (CBT)*. Royal College of Psychiatrists. Retrieved from https://www.rcpsych.ac.uk/mental-health/treatments-and-wellbeing/cognitive-behavioural-therapy-(cbt)

Speidel, R., Galarneau, E., Elsayed, D., Mahhouk, S., Filippelli, J., Colasante, T., & Malti, T. (2021). Refugee children's social-emotional capacities: Links to mental health upon resettlement and buffering effects on pre-migratory adversity. *International Journal of Environmental Research and Public Health, 18*(22), 12180. https://doi.org/10.3390/ijerph182212180

Spinazzola, J., Hodgdon, H., Liang, L-J., Ford, J. D., Layne, C. M., Pynoo, S. R., Briggs, E. C., Stolbach, B., & Kisiel, C. (2014). Unseen wounds: The contribution of psychological maltreatment to child and adolescent mental health and risk outcomes. *Psychological Trauma: Theory, Research, Practice, and Policy, 6*(1), 18–28. https://doi.org/10.1037/a0037766

Subhas, N., Mukhtar, F., & Munawar, K. (2021). Adapting cognitive-behavioral therapy for a Malaysian Muslim. *Medical Journal of the Islamic Republic of Iran*. https://doi.org/10.47176/mjiri.35.28

Sullivan, A. L., & Simonson, G. R. (2016). A systematic review of school-based social-emotional interventions for refugee and war-traumatized youth. *Review of Educational Research, 86*(2), 503–530. https://doi.org/10.3102/0034654315609419

The Royal Institute of International Affairs (RIOIA) (2016). Service delivery in the refugee camps of Greece: Improving coordination and strengthening resilience. Retrieved from https://www.chathamhouse.org/sites/default/files/publications/research/Meeting%20Summary%20-%20Service%20Delivery%20in%20the%20Refugee%20Camps%20of%20Greece.pdf

The United Nations (UDHR) (1948). Universal declaration of human rights. Retrieved from https://www.un.org/en/udhrbook/pdf/udhr_booklet_en_web.pdf

The United Nations Higher Commissioner for Refugees (UNHCR) (2023). *Refugee statistics*. UNHCR. Retrieved from https://www.unhcr.org/refugee-statistics/

Tyrer, R. A., & Fazel, M. (2014). School and community-based interventions for refugee and Asylum seeking children: A systematic review. *PLoS One, 9*(2), e89359. https://doi.org/10.1371/journal.pone.0089359

Unterhitzenberger J., Wintersohl S., Lang M., König J., & Rosner R. (2019). Providing manualized individual trauma-focused CBT to unaccompanied refugee minors with uncertain residence status: a pilot study. *Child Adolesc Psychiatry Ment Health, 13*, 22. https://doi.org/10.1186/s13034-019-0282-3

Yaylaci, F. T. (2018). Trauma and resilient functioning among Syrian refugee children. *Development and Psychopathology, 30*(5), 1923–1936. https://doi.org/10.1017/s0954579418001293

Yule, W., Dyregrov, A., Raundalen, M., & Smith, P. (2013). Children and war: The work of the children and war foundation. *European Journal of Psychotraumatology, 4*(1), 18424. https://doi.org/10.3402/ejpt.v4i0.18424

14

ANGER AND AGGRESSION

John E. Lochman, Caroline L. Boxmeyer, Nicole P. Powell, Salma Siddiqui, Sara L. Stromeyer and Meghann Sallee

In educational settings, students who display problems with anger and aggression have become an increasing concern. Not only do these problems present challenges to safety and order, they can also interfere with the educational process. Aggressors, their victims, and school personnel all stand to bear negative effects from displays of anger in the school setting. Children who display aggressive behavior and those who are on the receiving end of aggressive acts are both at risk for academic problems (e.g., Ma et al., 2009) and poor school attendance (e.g., Gubbels et al., 2019; Kokko et al., 2006). Further, even the learning of non-aggressive students may be compromised when they attend classrooms with high overall levels of aggression (Blank & Shavit, 2016). For teachers, the challenges associated with managing students' aggressive behavior can lead to increased levels of work-related stress and burnout (Winding et al., 2022).

Students who demonstrate problems with anger and aggression are at risk for difficulties in several other important areas of functioning. These students are at elevated risk for mental health disorders, including those involving externalizing behaviors (e.g., Oppositional Defiant Disorder, Conduct Disorder), as well as internalizing disorders such as depression and anxiety (American Psychiatric Association, 2013; Evans et al., 2017). Aggression can lead to disruptions in peer relationships, and aggressive students are frequently rejected by their peers. Academically, aggression directed to peers and to teachers is associated with problems with reading (e.g., Kremer et al., 2017) and mathematics (e.g., Pagani et al., 2010), as well as with skills important for academic success such as motivation, academic engagement, and on-task behavior. Aggressive students are more frequently retained and are also more likely to prematurely drop out of school (Jaafar et al., 2013; Risi et al., 2003) . In the long-term, students whose problems with anger and aggression go unchecked are at risk for serious consequences including delinquency, violent behavior, and substance abuse (e.g., Fite et al., 2008; Kassing et al., 2019).

Concerns about the implications of students' anger and aggression have spurred the development of intervention programs designed to target these problems. Given students' near universal attendance at schools and the availability of qualified professionals in the school setting, school-based programs have been developed to address students' aggressive behavior problems. Increasingly, school systems are turning to empirically supported intervention programs to address student emotional and behavioral needs, many of which incorporate cognitive-behavior therapy (CBT) principles, as evident in the What Works Clearinghouse website maintained by the Institute for Education Sciences. Following a review of empirical evidence supporting the effectiveness of CBT in the treatment of

DOI: 10.4324/9781003392439-17

problems with anger and aggression in youth, this chapter will provide a conceptualization of these problems from a CBT perspective. Assessment and treatment planning will also be discussed, followed by a review of effective programs incorporating CBT techniques and their application in the school setting, and illustrative case examples.

Empirical Support for CBT Targeting Anger and Aggression in Youth

Although problems with anger and aggression in youth can be persistent and difficult to treat, CBT strategies have been shown to effect positive changes in children and adolescents with externalizing behavior problems. Treatment addresses both the experience (i.e., the inner feeling) and expression of anger (i.e., aggression), with the goal of moving from maladaptive strategies to adaptive coping and control skills. CBT approaches target emotion regulation, reducing arousal and social problem-solving skills that are associated with aggressive behavior. Common components include recognizing and regulating emotions, identifying antecedents and consequences of aggression, cognitive restructuring of hostile attributions, and problem-solving, along with modeling and rehearsal of socially appropriate behaviors (Sukhodolsky et al., 2016). Several meta-analytic studies have provided support for CBT interventions in the prevention and treatment of conduct problems in youth.

A particularly relevant review targeted CBT for anger management interventions in students with special education needs (Ho et al., 2010). Eighteen treatment outcome studies were included, the majority of which involved delivery of anger-focused CBT to high school-aged students in the school setting. A total of 408 students were included, the majority of whom were receiving special education services for emotional or behavioral issues. The authors concluded that CBT techniques were moderately effective in reducing displays of anger and aggression, improving anger control skills, and addressing deficiencies related to social cognitive abilities and affect.

Similar conclusions were drawn from a broader meta-analytic study which focused on the delivery of CBT to typically developing children and adolescents with externalizing behavior problems. Sukhodolsky et al. (2004) examined the effectiveness of 40 treatment outcome studies, 21 published and 19 unpublished studies, of CBT programs for youth aged 6–18 years. Treatment was mainly delivered in a group format, and treatment length was short term, ranging from 8 to 18 hours. The authors reported a moderate effect size (0.67) across all studies, consistent with prior outcome studies of psychotherapy with children. Youth whose problems were categorized in the moderate range appeared to benefit most (effect size of 0.80), compared to children with severe (0.59) or mild (0.57) problems with anger and aggression.

Sukhodolsky and colleagues also analyzed different components of CBT, finding the largest effect sizes for skills development (0.79) and multimodal treatment (0.74), followed by problem-solving (0.67) and affective education (0.36). In order to evaluate specific therapeutic mechanisms, treatment techniques were coded as follows: instruction, discussion, modeling, role-play, feedback, emotion identification, relaxation, self-instruction, exposure, homework, and reinforcement. Feedback, modeling, and homework emerged as being significantly related to the magnitude of the overall effect size. That is, the effectiveness of treatment increases as the amount of modeling and feedback increases. It was found that improvement in anger experience domain was twice as great for problem-solving treatments ($d = 1.05$) than for affective education treatments ($d = 0.52$). Problem-solving treatments included learning how to think about causes, consequences, and solutions for anger-provoking situations while affective education treatments included relaxation, positive imagery, and education on emotions. Interestingly, no differences were observed based on duration of treatment and delivery format (e.g., group versus individual).

Three other meta-analytic studies have also supported the effectiveness of CBT interventions for anger and aggression in youth. Robinson et al. (1999) reported a mean effect size of 0.64, in the moderate range, in their meta-analysis of 23 studies investigating CBT effects on externalizing behavior symptoms. Bennett and Gibbons (2000) reviewed 30 studies targeting antisocial behavior in children and adolescents, finding support for both short-term (mean post-treatment effect size = 0.23) and long-term (mean follow-up effect size = 0.51) effects. Results further suggested that CBT tended to be more effective for adolescents and older elementary school-aged youth than for younger children, but that factors such as treatment components, number of treatment sessions, and session length were unrelated to outcomes. McCart et al. (2006) found stronger effects for adolescents than for younger children in their examination of 71 CBT outcome studies and suggested that the effectiveness of CBT interventions may increase with advances in cognitive development.

Studies investigating the Coping Power Program delineated several factors to consider in effectively disseminating and implementing CBT treatment for anger and aggression in youth. In addition to exploring the intensity of training provided to practitioners (Lochman, Boxmeyer, et al., 2009), several studies have sought to address a barrier to care involving participants and practitioners finding evidence-based CBT programs too demanding and too lengthy. An abbreviated version of Coping Power was implemented, with findings suggesting similar long-term (i.e., three year) positive effects on children's externalizing behaviors. Additionally, it was found that booster sessions following the abbreviated preventative intervention did not add to the intervention effects across time, lending further evidence to the sufficiency of the briefer version of the intervention (Lochman, Baden, et al., 2014). Extending this effort to reduce the length of intervention, a hybrid version of Coping Power involved an even briefer form of the intervention (less than half the number of in-person sessions in the original program) in combination with an internet component, was effective in producing a lower level of post-intervention conduct problems, in comparison to a treatment-as-usual condition (Lochman, Boxmeyer, et al., 2017).

In sum, there is a large body of evidence supporting the effectiveness of CBT interventions for youth who display problems with anger and aggression. CBT techniques appear to alter targeted processes, such as affect regulation, anger control, and social cognitive skills, leading to reductions in problem behaviors. Older children and adolescents may benefit most, and treatment can be effective when delivered in schools, in a group setting, and over a relatively short time period. Notably, data suggest direct feedback to those providing and receiving treatment for anger and aggression produces improved outcomes in treatment targets.

Assessment Techniques for Anger and Aggression in Schools

Accurate assessment of anger and aggression is an important 1st step to intervening with children in schools. School-based assessment of these problems should focus on identifying functional impairment, specific problem behaviors and symptoms, and skill deficits, as well as the child's strengths. A variety of assessment tools can be used in schools as part of a multi-source, comprehensive assessment. Additionally, identification and resolution of major discrepancies across sources will help to better conceptualize each child's case (Sattler, 2022).

Assessment should 1st consider the child's impairment in functioning, which provides a quality-of-life perspective that goes beyond simple symptom counting (Goldstein & Naglieri, 2016a). Research has indicated that long-term outcomes are better predicted by functional impairment than by diagnostic symptoms (Pelham & Burrows-Maclean, 2005). The Children's Impairment Rating Scale (CIRS; Fabiano et al., 2006) assesses impairment in areas such as peer relations, academic functioning, and classroom behavior, and can be easily used for progress monitoring, due to its quick, efficient administration. Another instrument which can be used by parents and teachers, and which has strong psychometric qualities and provides useful information about treatment planning with children, is the Rating Scale of Impairment (Goldstein & Naglieri, 2016b).

In planning the assessment, it is important to also assess for comorbid problems, such as attentional difficulties, social skills deficits, and depressive symptoms, because children with anger and aggression problems are more likely to have other mental health issues, which can result in more functional impairment and can impact interventions (McMahon & Frick, 2007). Assessment of internalizing as well as externalizing problems is important, because research suggests that the initiation and maintenance of internalizing and externalizing behavior problems can be influenced by a common set of risk factors (e.g., irritable temperament, harsh parental discipline, psychological stress, social-cognitive deficiencies), and that intervention can have transdiagnostic outcomes by addressing these mechanisms (Lochman, Powell, et al., 2014). Additionally, intellectual and achievement testing are not only useful to identify the child's current level of functioning but also can help to rule out a possible learning disability or low cognitive functioning, which may be impacting the child's anger or aggression.

Additionally, it is helpful to gather information from both parents and teachers, in order to determine the consistency of the child's behaviors across settings (Takeda et al., 2016). However, it should be noted that these reports can be subjective to the rater's perspective and so have the potential for bias. Children over the age of about eight years can also provide valid ratings of their own symptoms (Kamphaus & Frick, 2001), and several rating systems include a child self-report measure. Several valid and reliable behavior rating scales exist for measuring a variety of behavioral, social, and emotional competencies. The Behavior Assessment System for Children-3 (BASC-3; Reynolds et al., 2015), Revised Behavior Problem Checklist (RBPC; Quay & Peterson, 1996), and the Conners' Rating Scales-Revised (CRS-R; Conners, 1997) can be used to compare and integrate information from multiple informants. Additionally, the Student Behavior Survey (SBS; Lachar et al., 2000) and the Child Behavior Checklist (CBCL; Achenbach, 1991) and its teacher (TRF) and child counterparts (YSR) can be used for screening of behavior problems.

Clinical interviews can also be conducted with parents or teachers, to gain more in-depth and detailed information about the child's behavior. Structured interviews, such as the Diagnostic Interview Schedule for Children Adolescents and Parents (DISCAP-5; Tissue et al., 2022), may also be useful because they are norm-referenced and provide diagnostic information about Conduct Disorder and Oppositional Defiant Disorder, as well as comorbid diagnoses. If children with Oppositional Defiant Disorder have the subgroup of angry-irritable symptoms, they can be particularly at-risk for having co-morbid depression symptoms (Evans et al., 2017). The weakness of this assessment method is that interviews can be time-consuming, which may present a problem in busy schools.

Direct behavioral observation of the child in the classroom is also useful for more objective measurement of the child's behavior (Sattler, 2022). Standardized observation systems which can be used by the clinician include the BASC-3 Student Observation System (Reynolds et al., 2015) and the CBCL Direct Observation Form (CBCL DOF; Achenbach & Rescorla, 2001). See Nock and Kurtz (2005) for a complete review of school observational procedures. These measures can be used as part of a functional behavior assessment, in which antecedents to and consequences of the child's behavior are identified, which are then used as targets for interventions.

It is also helpful to gather information about the child's social functioning, which may impact anger and aggression. Teachers can rate children's social skills using the Social Skills Rating System (SSRS; Gresham & Elliott, 1990). Even though teachers may be able to provide some insight about children's peer relationships, it is important to attempt to gather information from the child's peers, as they are likely to be more accurate reporters of social relationships and behavior. Other children in the child's class can provide data about how well-liked or not well-liked a child is, or how often they start fights, tease others, or get into trouble.

Finally, it is important to understand the child's social-cognitive skills, as they are an important target for intervention in children with anger and aggression problems and can play a large role in the child's problems. Vignettes and hypothetical situations, in which children identify how they perceive the situation and indicate how likely they would be to perform certain actions, can be used to assess these social-cognitive processes. Examples of clinically useful social-cognitive measures include the Selman and Byrne test (1974), the Means-End Problem Solving Inventory (MEPS; Platt & Spivack, 1989), the Social Cognitive Skills Test (SCST; Van Manen et al., 2001), and a web-based measure of social information processing using videotaped vignettes (Kupersmidt et al., 2011).

Cognitive-Behavioral Conceptualization of Anger

It has been observed that cognitive and behavioral deficits contribute to angry affect and aggressive behavior (e.g., Crick & Dodge, 1994). Given these deficits, it follows that any strategy to help manage anger and other associated problems must focus on the restructuring of cognitions and teaching adaptive behavior. Most anger management interventions are based on CBT which includes a focus on both behavior modification (Dodge, 1993) and also how a person construes reality.

The central premise of CBT is that thoughts influence the way individuals feel and act. There are many important elements in this assumption: the perception of an event, how we encode, process, and interpret the information, emote, and then react defines the behavior in question. CBT draws heavily from principles of social learning and social information processing theory. The social learning model dates back to Rotter (1954) who stressed that an individual's expectations of reinforcement have an impact on behavior. This perspective was further expanded to the impact of observing someone else being rewarded on subjective reward contingencies and decision-making processes (Miller & Dollard, 1941). The Cognitive Social Learning Model further elaborated this by incorporating variables such as encoding aspects of a situation, expectancies consequent upon behavior, affective responses, goals and values one wants to achieve, and the capacity to engage in goal-directed behaviors (Mischel, 1973). This led to an understanding that behavior is a product of both person and situation variables. Ineffective problem solving is also considered part of problem behavior. Incorporating problem solving as a component of treatment has resulted in improvement, sustained even after a year (Shure & Spivack, 1980).

The Social Information Processing model (Crick & Dodge, 1994) attempts to explain behavior as a product of cognitive processes (i.e., encoding of selected information from the event one is experiencing, its specific representation in memory, and accessing one or more possible responses from the memory). This is followed by deciding in favor of and then initiating a behavioral response which is determined by the linguistic and motor repertoire available to a person (Dodge, 1986). The literature documents that aggressive children tend to encode and interpret information differently than do non-aggressive children. Aggressive children may recall fewer nonhostile cues about a social event (Lochman & Dodge, 1994), and reactively aggressive children may display a hostile attribution bias; that is, they may inaccurately attribute negative intentions to others' motivations in social situations (Dodge et al., 1997; Yaros et al., 2014).

Aggressive children also display cognitive deficiencies in the later stages of social information processing. Specifically, their goals in social situations tend to be characterized by dominance and revenge (Lochman et al., 1993; McDonald & Lochman, 2012), and the responses they generate for problem situations are often inappropriately action-oriented and nonverbal rather than incorporating more effective skills such as verbal assertion and compromise (Dunn et al., 1997; Lochman & Dodge, 1994). Further, aggressive children tend to evaluate aggressive behavior in a positive way (Crick & Werner, 1998) and expect that it will lead to positive outcomes for them (Lochman & Dodge, 1994).

Two additional constructs are important regarding social information processing; one is the role of schema and the other is the heightened level of negative affective and emotional arousal. Schemas, which are regarded as our underlying beliefs consistent across situations, can determine the quality of attention one gives to an aspect of a situation and can influence our perception of social cues in managing social and emotional conflict. A dysfunctional schema can result in emotional and behavioral problems by negatively influencing each social information step (Lochman & Dodge, 1998). Information processing in a social situation is influenced by, and impacts upon, negative affect and level of emotional arousal as emotions tend to mediate the relation between attribution and behavior (Weiner, 1990; Williams et al., 2003). Physiological arousal is influenced by autonomic nervous system functioning (Kassing et al., 2018) and temperamental predispositions, as well as by an individual's interpretations of a given event. At heightened levels of arousal, aggressive children are likely to generate and enact less competent solutions to social problems. This conceptualization holds ground in other cultural contexts as well; anger appears to mediate the relationship between automatic thoughts and aggressive behaviors, as automatic thoughts result in anger which is expressed through physical aggression (Yavuzer & Karataş, 2013). Anger is also seen to determine how children construe the viability of relationship with peers when they face provocation as revenge goals appear to be related to aggression similarly across groups belonging to two different cultures (McDonald et al., 2022).

Treatment Planning and Intervention Strategies

Strategies for Individual Cases

This section summarizes seven common areas for strategies that can be included in treatment plans for children with problems with aggressive behavior and anger dysregulation.

Goal Setting

A common initial element of CBT approaches for aggressive children is to have them identify long-term and short-term goals for themselves in their home and school settings. Children identify personally meaningful long-term goals to work on for the current school year (e.g., to raise C's to B's; to be promoted to the next grade). Using input from teachers, clinicians assist children in breaking the long-term goals into manageable steps or short-term goals. Short-term goals are typically "prosocial opposites" of problem behaviors, and the short-term behavioral goals are entered onto behavioral goal sheets, monitored daily by teachers or parents, and lead to points that children can exchange for agreed-upon rewards. Research has indicated that a goal-setting component in a CBT program can help to generalize children's behavioral change into school and home settings. Goal setting likely leads children to focus more on the consequences of their daily behaviors.

Organization and Study Skills

Given the frequency with which externalizing problems co-occur with behavioral difficulties in the school setting, CBT programs often include activities that directly address the importance of organizational skills and students' study habits. To address aggressive children's concomitant academic problems, children identify useful and not-useful study habits and then create a plan to use the useful ones when completing homework and long-term projects at school. Children and parents also can jointly create a homework contract which specifies when and where homework will be done, and how parents will monitor homework completion and provide contingent rewards for homework completion.

Emotion Awareness

As a precursor to anger management training, children can participate in activities designed to normalize the experience of various emotions and to help them accurately recognize and label their feelings and the triggers for their feelings. Students describe various emotions in terms of associated physiological sensations, behaviors, and cognitions. Children increase their accuracy in identifying emotions in others as well as in themselves. There is typically an initial focus on a wide range of emotions children experience, including emotions that they perceive as making them vulnerable (sadness, anxiety), and which they may not recognize in themselves. Then, there is focused attention on the cognitive (ruminative "angry thoughts") and physiological correlates of anger. Students can use a thermometer analogy to help them recognize the range of intensity with which emotions occur. Labels are given to emotions at varying levels on the thermometer (e.g., "annoyed" at the bottom, "mad" in the middle, and "furious" at the top). These activities are helpful to students who might experience their feelings in an "on-off" manner, failing to recognize the range in intensity of their experience and then missing early opportunities to manage their angry feelings. Children then learn to identify "triggers" that lead to each level of anger.

Emotion Regulation

Children's increased awareness of their anger arousal leads to a variety of anger management activities that help children better manage their arousal in situations that they perceive to be threatening. Students learn several active strategies for self-control, including the use of distraction, relaxation (e.g., abdominal breathing, progressive relaxation, guided imagery), and coping self-statements. Students can implement anger management skills both before they become flooded with emotion, while their anger is still at a manageable level, and also after becoming anger aroused to aid them to recover more quickly from their aroused state. To help them manage their levels of anger and related physiological arousal, students participate in exercises in which they practice directing their focus away from an annoying or stressful situation. Typically, a series of graded exposure activities are used to assist children in practicing their self-regulation skills 1st in indirect ways (e.g., through puppet role-plays) and then, after demonstrating proficiency in using skills in the puppet role-play, in direct person-to-person role-plays. The clinician monitors children's arousal and serves as a coach to the child during the role-plays.

Perspective-Taking

Children with externalizing behavior problems often have problems with perspective-taking, and this can be especially evident in their hostile attribution biases. Before aggressive children can accurately perceive the problem situations they face, and begin the social problem-solving procedures, they must develop an ability to accurately perceive others' perspectives and intentions. After a set of fun game-like tasks that illustrate how a single stimulus can be perceived in quite different ways, children can engage in role-play tasks, where different people's different perceptions of events and of others' intentions are explored. Although the focus is primarily often on children's perceptions of their peer interactions, clinicians can also focus on teacher-child and parent-child interactions if warranted. The primary focus in perspective-taking training with aggressive children is on retraining the hostile attribution bias evident in reactive aggressive children, encouraging them to consider that it is sometimes hard to tell what others intend in problematic situations (rather than erroneously assuming hostile intentions in ambiguous situations).

Social Problem-Solving

Along with anger management training, problem-solving skill training is the most common CBT technique used with aggressive children. Children learn a step-wise approach to thinking about problem resolution, typically including steps for problem identification, generation of choices or solutions to resolve the problem, consideration of consequences for each solution, and a method for making a decision about which choice to enact. Problem-solving can be more successful when the experienced problem can be reframed into a positive goal to be achieved and when the child initially tries to resolve problems that trigger low-to-moderate levels of anger. When generating solutions to a problem, students are encouraged to brainstorm broadly about choices and clinicians accept even "bad" choices as discussion points for the next step that involves considering consequences. Brainstorming about the consequences (perceived as positive and negative; short and long term) for each choice being considered is likely one of the most important aspects of the problem-solving process. A series of activities are used to progressively develop and refine social problem-solving skills, ranging from discussion activities, to game-like tasks, to role-playing, to video or audio recording an enactment of the problem-solving process. Use of video or audio recording provides an engaging way for students to solidify their understanding of problem-solving and allows them to view and critique their skills in enacting various options.

Handling Peer Pressure

As children enter adolescence, there is often a focus in CBT on helping children handle developmentally sensitive risks, such as peer pressure to engage in antisocial behavior. Students participate in role-plays to practice using strategies to resist peer pressure and discuss how peer pressure can operate in students' neighborhoods. Students discuss their involvement in groups or cliques, and they consider the implications of associating with various types of peer groups. Students consider their personal strengths and leadership qualities and discuss how they can use their abilities to become involved with less deviant and more prosocial peer groups.

Manualized Evidence-Based CBT Programs

There are a variety of CBT programs for school-age aggressive children that can be used either for universal prevention by targeting whole classrooms or whole schools or for children screened and targeted for their aggressive behavior. In the latter case, programs can either serve as targeted prevention programs for at-risk children or for treatment with children diagnosed with disruptive behavior disorders (DBD). This section provides example programs; a more complete list can be found elsewhere (e.g., Matthys & Lochman, 2017; Powell et al., 2011).

During the preschool and early elementary school years, an effective universal prevention program is Promoting Alternative Thinking Strategies (PATHS). PATHS is delivered by trained classroom teachers and promotes children's emotion awareness, emotional regulation, and social-problem-solving. Overall, results at one- and two-year follow-ups have indicated that children receiving the PATHS intervention were better at understanding emotions, better at problem-solving, and had reported decreases in conduct problems and impulsivity compared to children in a control group (Greenberg et al., 2001, 2006).

A well-researched program for targeted prevention or treatment during the preschool and early elementary school years is The Incredible Years program, which includes parent training, a child training program (Dinosaur School), and a teacher component for young children with DBD (Webster-Stratton, 2005; Webster-Stratton & Reid, 2010). Research findings regarding the effectiveness of the Incredible Years child, parent, and teacher training interventions alone and in combination have been impressively replicated across multiple samples. The Incredible Years child intervention has also been shown to produce significant reductions in the amount of conduct problems children exhibit at home and school and to produce increases in social problem-solving skills in comparison to waitlist control conditions (Webster-Stratton & Hammond, 1997; Webster-Stratton et al., 2004).

During later childhood, The Seattle Social Development Project (SSDP) is a universal prevention program designed to reduce aggression by creating a positive school environment. Teachers are trained to use nonpunitive classroom behavioral management strategies such as positive reinforcement, and more recent versions of the intervention have also included parent training and child problem-solving and social skills training (Hawkins et al., 1999). Longitudinal research conducted with the SSDP has found stronger commitment to school and improved academic achievement (Hawkins et al., 1999), significant prevention of alcohol use (Hawkins et al., 1999; Lonczak et al., 2001), reductions in delinquency, and decreased reports of pregnancy for females and causing pregnancy for males (Hawkins et al., 1999).

Two evidence-based targeted prevention and treatment programs during the preadolescent years are the Problem Solving Skills Training plus Parent Management Training (PSST + PMT) program and Coping Power. PSST + PMT is targeted for school-aged children with disruptive behavior who are between 7 and 13 years old and includes 25 weekly sessions (Kazdin et al., 1992). The combination of PSST with the PMT parent-focused intervention was found to have greater improvements in reducing adult reports of children's aggression and delinquency, as compared to PSST or parent-focused interventions alone (Kazdin et al., 1992).

The Coping Power Program was derived from earlier research on an Anger Coping Program (Lochman, 1992). Coping Power has cognitive-behavioral child and parent components (Lochman et al., 2008; Wells et al., 2008). Coping Power was originally designed to be implemented with 4th–6th grade children in school or clinic settings but has been successfully adapted for younger and older children. In comparison to randomly assigned control groups in two separate samples, the Coping Power Program has produced decreases in self-reported delinquency, substance use, and aggressive behavior at school at one-year and three-year follow-ups (Lochman & Wells, 2003, 2004; Lochman et al., 2013). Mediation analyses, using path analytic techniques, indicate that the Coping Power intervention effect on the outcomes at the one-year follow-up was mediated by intervention-produced improvements in parental consistency and in children's internal locus of control, attributional biases, person perception, and children's expectations that aggression would not work for them (Lochman & Wells, 2002). These positive effects of Coping Power have been replicated in a variety of settings (e.g., Eiraldi et al., 2018; Ludmer et al., 2018; Mushtaq et al., 2017). For example, Mushtaq and colleagues (2017) found that preadolescent boys in Pakistan who had been screened for having high levels of aggressive behaviors had greater reductions in externalizing and internalizing behaviors, and reactive and proactive aggression if they had received the Coping Power program. Research has also examined whether the Coping Power program could be optimized for children with high levels of reactive aggressive behaviors by integrating aspects of mindfulness training into the program, and results have indicated that children have greater improvements in emotional regulation with Mindful Coping Power in comparison to usual Coping Power (Boxmeyer et al., 2021, 2023). In a clinical sample, Coping Power reduced the overt aggression of children with ODD or CD in Dutch outpatient clinics in comparison to care-as-usual children (van de Wiel et al., 2007) and had preventive effects by reducing adolescent marijuana and cigarette use of CP children in comparison to the care-as-usual children (Zonnevylle-Bender et al., 2007). In randomized control studies, Coping Power and its adaptations have also demonstrated positive long-term follow-up effects on externalizing behavior problems with clinically diagnosed ODD and CD youth in Italy (Muratori, Milone et al., 2019), with children with attention deficit/hyperactivity disorder (Vanzin et al., 2018), with children with borderline intellectual disability (Schuiringa et al., 2017), and the Coping Power child component has added to the effects of behavioral parent training for children with high levels of ODD symptoms (Helander et al., 2018).

A manualized treatment developed specifically for female juvenile offenders, Juvenile Justice Anger Management (JJAM), is a cognitive-behavioral intervention adapted from the Coping Power

Program to address the unique needs of adolescent girls in residential juvenile justice settings. Research has supported gender differences in the expression and development of anger and aggression, including females being more likely to be angered by someone they love, to act aggressively in the home, and to engage in physical and relational aggression. JJAM includes gender-specific considerations, including additional instruction on relational aggression (e.g., spreading rumors, excluding someone from a group, giving the silent treatment) along with skill-building specifically related to developing, strengthening, and repairing relationships (Goldstein et al., 2013). In an efficacy study of 57 female youth aged 14–20 years, Goldstein and colleagues (2018) found JJAM led to greater reductions in anger, reactive physical aggression, and reactive relational aggression when compared to a treatment as usual control condition.

During the adolescent years, the Life Skills Training Program is an example of a universal prevention program designed to prevent substance abuse (Botvin & Griffin, 2004). The program was developed for middle school students. Cognitive-behavioral skills-training techniques are used to teach students' personal self-management skills, social skills, and drug resistance skills. The program has been shown to be highly effective in reducing alcohol, tobacco, marijuana, and polydrug use in a series of randomized controlled efficacy trials and in two effectiveness studies.

Multisystemic therapy (MST) is a well-researched treatment program for adolescents. MST is an intensive family and community-based treatment program that has been implemented with chronic and violent juvenile offenders, substance-abusing juvenile offenders, adolescent sexual offenders, youths in psychiatric crisis (i.e., homicidal, suicidal, psychotic), and maltreating families (Henggeler & Lee, 2003). Clinicians are guided by a set of nine MST principles which include concepts like focusing on systems strengths, delivering developmentally appropriate treatment, and improving effective family functioning. Evaluations of the effectiveness of MST with chronic and violent juvenile offenders have produced promising results. Several investigations have shown that families who receive MST report lower levels of adolescent behavior problems and improvements in family functioning at post-treatment and lower recidivism in a four-year follow-up in comparison to alternative treatment conditions (Borduin et al., 1995; Henggeler et al., 1992).

The Modular Approach to Therapy for Children with Anxiety, Depression, Trauma, or Conduct Problems (MATCH; Chorpita & Weisz, 2009) is a CBT and BPT (behavior parent training) manualized treatment comprised of 33 modules that can be flexibly chosen to provide a bespoke arrangement of content, order, and dose of treatment. Two randomized effectiveness studies in typical practice settings have found MATCH to outperform usual clinical care across diagnostic concerns, including externalizing behaviors (Chorpita et al., 2017). Notably, Evans and colleagues (2020) found in comparison to usual care and standard manualized treatments, MATCH participants showed faster rates of improvement, possibly due to the more adaptable and personalized implementation of the empirically supported interventions.

Implications and Applications to the School Setting

Problems with anger and aggression often interfere with school success (Larson & Lochman, 2011). Children who exhibit anger and aggression cause distractions within the classroom, negatively impacting upon the learning environment (Powell et al., 2011). Due to their engagement in antisocial behaviors, aggressive children are more likely to experience angry, punitive, and avoidant reactions from their teachers and peers. This can exacerbate the problem, as peer rejection has been shown to have a bidirectional relationship with aggression. That is, while antisocial behaviors may lead to peer rejection, the experience of being rejected can also be a trigger for further aggression (Powers et al., 2013), and the combination of rejection from peers and engagement in aggressive behavior compounds the children's risk for serious later behavioral problems (Coie et al., 1992). Children exhibiting aggressive, disruptive behaviors in school are likely to have reductions in their academic achievement (Chow & Wehby, 2018; Pas et al., 2010) and increased rates of school drop-out (Fabelo et al., 2011). Negative consequences of aggression within the classroom do not only affect aggressors, but also their peers, teachers, and school administrators. Research suggests that both aggressors and victims are at risk for lower levels of academic competence (Ma et al., 2009).

Disciplinary approaches aimed at reducing anger and aggression often include stern lectures, phone calls home, and detention. Not only do these practices take up a significant amount of teachers' and administrators' time, most importantly, they do not address the child's needs. The punitive response from teachers and administrators assumes that the child knows how to behave appropriately. Conversely, the problem behaviors are sometimes due to a lack of skill rather than a lack of motivation. Children who have problems with anger and aggression are often in need of an intervention focusing on skills such as anger regulation, impulse control, and problem solving (Larson & Lochman, 2011; Lochman & Wells, 2002).

Because of contextual factors maintaining children's aggressive behavior in the school environment, and the children's negative effect on the school environment, the school setting has long been recognized as an optimal setting for multilevel intervention focusing on universal and targeted prevention (Allen et al., 1976). This is particularly important given the reliance on school systems to address the mental health needs of students (Rones & Hoagwood, 2000). The school environment provides an opportunity (1) to assess need and monitor progress, (2) to reinforce skills in the classroom through positive behavior supports and effective consequences, (3) for students to observe and engage in prosocial behavior, and (4) for educational professionals to consult and collaborate (Larson & Lochman, 2011).

Tier 1 universal prevention approaches for all children (Lochman, Boxmeyer, et al., 2019), such as codes of conduct, classroom rules, and social-emotional education, will address the behavioral needs of most students. For example, Universal Coping Power is a classroom-wide adaptation of the Coping Power program which has been found to reduce students' behavioral and emotional problems in elementary and middle school settings (Muratori et al., 2017, 2020). These universal interventions can in turn lead to improvements in pre-mathematics and language abilities in the preschool years (Muratori, Lochman, et al., 2019) and to academic achievement and school retention in later school years (Bradshaw et al., 2009). However, there is a small subset of children in need of greater individualized support in developing the necessary behavioral skills to be successful in school and can be screened for Tier II interventions (Lochman, Boxmeyer, et al., 2019; McDaniel et al., 2018). For these students, CBT interventions, such as those described earlier (e.g., Lochman & Wells, 2003, 2004), can be effectively applied in the school setting to improve children's behavior as well as their academic outcomes (Lochman et al., 2012; McDaniel et al., 2018).

While there are empirically supported treatments that have been shown to be efficacious, implementation in a real-world setting can have a significant effect on treatment outcome. Effective and efficient dissemination of CBT as a Tier II intervention is a significant challenge, and three prominent concerns are (1) child engagement and therapeutic alliance, (2) child and clinician issues with group-based interventions with this population of children, and (3) the nature and intensity needed for effective training of clinicians.

Because of their oppositional and disruptive behaviors, children with externalizing problems can be especially difficult to engage in targeted Tier II interventions. However, intervention engagement is an important predictor of good outcomes. Children who display higher levels of negative affect in early sessions are more likely to have poor and sharply declining attendance of Coping Power sessions (Pas et al., 2020). Conversely, children who have displayed greater engagement midway through Coping Power intervention, evident in greater accomplishment of weekly behavioral goals and positive behavior in sessions, have been found to have lower levels of externalizing behavior one year after intervention (Lindsey et al., 2019) and to simulate greater parent attendance in co-occurring parent meetings (Ellis et al., 2013). In a related vein, children who establish stronger emotional and relationship bonds with their clinician in early Coping Power sessions have greater reductions in externalizing behavior through a follow-up period (Mitchell et al., 2021). Thus, it is important for clinicians to monitor children's therapeutic alliance in early sessions and to tailor the session to maximize their engagement.

A 2nd concern to address is that, although there are evident unique strengths for using a group format with angry and aggressive youth (e.g., opportunities for peer reinforcement, role-playing, group rewards), there are a set of potential obstacles (e.g., disruptive behavior, noncompliance, reinforcement of deviant behavior by peers) that can interfere with the optimal functioning of the group and which can detract from the effectiveness of the intervention. In a study of the delivery of the Coping Power program in group versus individual format, teacher-rated externalizing problems declined significantly for both intervention conditions, but the reductions were significantly greater for children receiving Coping Power in an individual format (Lochman, Dishion, et al., 2015). Children who had extreme levels of behavioral disinhibition, emotional dysregulation, and need for social bonding were found to have better outcomes if seen individually (Glenn et al., 2018, 2019; Lochman, Dishion et al., 2015). Clinician factors also affect how well children with aggressive behavior problems profit from participation in group-based intervention. Clinicians who have more conscientious and agreeable personality traits implement the program with greater intervention fidelity and quality and are more likely to sustain their use of the program in later years (Lochman, Powell, et al., 2009, 2015). Conversely, counselors with high levels of cynicism working in schools where there was little staff autonomy and a focus on managerial control had difficulty successfully implementing the program (Lochman, Powell, et al., 2009). In addition, clinicians who conduct group sessions with greater warmth and less irritability have children who have greater reductions in externalizing behavior problems through later follow-ups up to four years after intervention (Lochman, Dishion, et al. 2017; Lochman, Glenn, et al., 2019). Thus, children's and clinicians' characteristics can affect group delivery of CBT and should be addressed in the training of clinicians.

Third, intensity of training of clinicians plays a role in effective dissemination (Lochman, Boxmeyer, et al., 2009). A controlled dissemination study of the Coping Power program found that the intensity of training provided to school counselors impacted child outcomes. Providing counselors with the standard training workshop, monthly meetings, and immediate supervisory feedback based on recorded sessions led to significant reductions in child externalizing behavior and improvements in social and academic skills. These positive child outcomes did not emerge for counselors who had only participated in the standard training workshop (Lochman, Boxmeyer, et al., 2009).

These findings suggest that empirically supported interventions for anger and aggression can be successfully implemented in the school setting. However, intensive training using performance feedback and counselor screening should be included to ensure effective dissemination. School-based interventions afford opportunities to children in need, their peers, teachers, and administrators; resulting decreases in anger and aggression can have a positive impact on the entire school community.

Case Example—Group-Based Implementation of Coping Power

Dr. Bitner is a school psychologist at Norwood Elementary School, a neighborhood school in a large urban city. She is responsible for providing behavioral intervention for students who need Tier II or Tier III behavioral intervention. Dr. Bitner has several 5th and 6th grade students in need of behavioral intervention for disruptive and aggressive behavior problems. She is required to deliver interventions that have research support for their effectiveness, thus she selected the Coping Power program from a list of evidence-based interventions.

Because a group size of five to six students is recommended for Coping Power, Dr. Bitner identified six students with disruptive and aggressive behavior to take part in a Coping Power group. She asked the social work intern, Ms. Erikson, to co-lead the group with her. Before starting the group, Dr. Bitner and Ms. Erikson met individually with each of the students and their parents/guardians to describe the purpose of the group and to determine their willingness to participate. The group consisted of Jarrod, a 5th grade boy who tended to lash out at anyone who seemed to have it out for him; Jayla, a 6th grade girl who was very eager to please but was often rejected by her peers due to her overbearing nature and emotional lability; Mark, a 6th grade boy whose disruptive behavior seemed to primarily reflect untreated hyperactivity/impulsivity; Xavier, a 5th grade boy who had numerous suspensions for fighting, stealing, and threatening others; Isabel, a 5th grade girl who was described as a bully by her teacher and classmates; and Anthony, a 6th grade boy who often appeared sullen and had trouble getting along with others.

During the 1st session, Dr. Bitner described the purpose of the group and led the students in a get-acquainted activity. She then had the students generate a list of group rules (e.g., take turns talking; treat each other with respect; what we say here stays here). Once the rules were established, Dr. Bitner indicated that each student would earn one point for following the rules during each Coping Power session. If they broke a rule, they would earn a warning "strike." If they earned three strikes, they would not earn their point for following the rules. After hearing this, Isabel shouted out, "This is a group for bad kids, isn't it?" Dr. Bitner responded that none of the group members were bad kids, rather they were invited to be in the group because they could use some extra help with their behavior. Mark whispered to Jarrod, "isn't that the same as saying we are bad kids?" which led Jarrod to laugh and roll his eyes. Ms. Erikson observed this exchange and gestured to Mark and Jarrod to listen to Dr. Bitner. Sensing that Mark and Jarrod might continue to be disruptive, Ms. Erikson moved her seat between them. In the meantime, she noticed that Anthony had his head down on his desk, so she gently tapped his shoulder and encouraged him to sit up and participate.

Dr. Bitner led the group in a discussion about why the group was called Coping Power and how the program would help the group members learn new ways of coping with, or handling, strong feelings and difficult situations. She indicated that learning to cope effectively is a skill and can help you meet the goals you have for yourself and get along well with others. Dr. Bitner asked the group members if they knew what a personal goal is. Jayla raised her hand excitedly and said, "It is something you want to do." "That's right," said Dr. Bitner, "a goal is something that you want to accomplish or reach. Long-term goals are objectives that you want to accomplish in the future, and short-terms goals are things you can do each day, or each week, that will help you reach your long-term goal." Dr. Bitner informed the group that they were going to be talking more about goal-setting during their next few meetings and asked the group members to think of some goals they might like to accomplish (or behaviors they could improve on). She let the students know that she was planning to talk to their parents and teachers to obtain their ideas about possible behavior goals for each group member as well.

At the end of the 1st session, Dr. Bitner complimented the group members for being willing to give Coping Power a try and for their good participation in the 1st session. She gave everyone a point for positive participation, except for Anthony, who had put his head on his desk and been disengaged for at least half of the session. Dr. Bitner let Anthony know that he could earn his point at the next group session if he kept his head off his desk and contributed to the discussion. Dr. Bitner also awarded a point for following the rules to five of the group members. Xavier had not earned his point because he had gotten three strikes for kicking another group member and for talking back to the leader. Ms. Erikson modeled how they would end each Coping Power session by giving each group member a turn to share what he or she had learned and to provide compliments to other group members for positive behavior. Dr. Bitner and Ms. Erikson also gave the group time to look through the

Prize Box, which contained school supplies, coupons for incentives such as free homework passes, and small games and toys, which the group members could purchase with their points earned in Coping Power sessions.

As the group continued in Coping Power, the group members began to set weekly behavior goals for themselves and were responsible for taking their goal sheet to their teacher to obtain daily feedback. By Session 8, Jarrod was working on a goal of "keeping his anger at medium or lower on his anger thermometer." Jayla was working on a goal of "giving others appropriate personal space." Mark had set a goal of "keeping his eyes on the teacher during lessons." Isabel's goal was to "treat others nicely." Finally, Anthony's goal was to "make at least two contributions during each classroom discussion." Despite his participation in the 1st five Coping Power sessions, Xavier had continued to show problematic behavior at school and had been sent to alternative school after stealing a teacher's cell phone. Because Dr. Bitner also provided behavioral intervention to students at the alternative school, she met with Xavier individually there, and they continued to discuss and practice the same skills the group was learning in Coping Power.

By Session 11, the group had practiced setting long-term and short-term goals and learned academic skills such as keeping track of their assignments, keeping their backpacks organized, and utilizing positive study habits. They had also begun a unit on emotional awareness in which they had learned to accurately label and measure specific emotions and to recognize the early physical signs of anger (e.g., heart racing, face feeling hot, hands in a fist). They had also become more aware of their own thoughts and the link between what they say to themselves and how they feel (e.g., "I hate my sister," "school is stupid," "my teacher has it out for me," "nobody likes me," "I'll show him who is the boss"). They had completed several homework assignments in which they made note of at least one situation in which they felt angry each day and described what had happened, the level of anger they experienced, what thoughts they had when they were angry, and how they tried to cope with their anger.

Isabel came to Session 11 wanting to talk about a problem she had had at school. She was angry that she had been sent to the principal's office for yelling at a classmate. Isabel felt that it wasn't fair because the classmate had been rude to her 1st and wouldn't stop bugging her even though she had told her to leave her alone. Isabel thought that the classmate should have been the one to get in trouble. Dr. Bitner thanked Isabel for being willing to share this real-life problem with the group. She asked Isabel if it would be okay if the group used her example for the lesson that day. Isabel indicated that it would be fine to do so.

During the group review, the group members recalled that they had been practicing ways to cope with anger, in particular, using coping self-statements to reduce angry thoughts and feelings following teasing by peers. They had learned that anger is a normal feeling that can alert us to something important that is bothering us, such as teaching. They had also learned that we tend to make better decisions about the best way to handle situations in which we feel angry, if we take time to calm down first and think things through. They knew they were just practicing the 1st step, of noticing and calming their anger first, so they could then make a wise choice about how to handle the situation.

Dr. Bitner asked Isabel to recall what she was thinking when the classmate started taunting her. Isabel said she was thinking that the other girl "was a loser and had better watch her back because she had it coming to her." Dr. Bitner asked Isabel whether thinking these things made her feel more angry or less angry. "Well, these things are true but thinking about them probably made me more angry." "What do you think you could have said to yourself instead that might have made you less angry?" asked Dr. Bitner.

> I guess I could have told myself that I don't like how she is talking to me … but I also don't want to get into a fight. I could try to tell myself to 'not be a fool, just keep my cool,' then figure out how to deal with the other girl later.

Isabel said. Dr. Bitner asked Isabel how she might have felt if she had thought these thoughts instead. Isabel indicated that her anger probably would have gone down. "Then you have given us a good example of a coping statement," said Dr. Bitner. "Would it be okay if I pretend to be the girl who was bugging you? While I say some mean things, you can practice saying coping statements to keep your cool." Isabel indicated that would be fine. With some coaching from Ms. Erikson, Isabel was able to keep her anger low by reciting coping statements while Dr. Bitner pretended to taunt her. After discussing how this went for Isabel, Dr. Bitner let each of the group members have a turn practicing using coping statements to control their anger. Dr. Bitner reminded them that the purpose of this activity was to practice keeping their cool long enough to make a wise choice about how to handle the situation, and that they would practice wise problem-solving next.

By Session 22, Xavier had returned to Norwood Elementary and was interested in re-joining the Coping Power group. In the meantime, Anthony had been hospitalized following a violent emotional outburst and was likely to remain in a day treatment classroom. Dr. Bitner helped the group welcome Xavier back and process the fact that Anthony was not likely to return to Coping Power. The group caught Xavier up on the new approach they had been learning to solve interpersonal problems. They were preparing to make a video to teach other students how to use P-I-C-C (Problem Identification, Choices and Consequences) to stop and brainstorm choices and think ahead about consequences before deciding how to solve a problem. The group had decided to act out a problem scene in which a teacher yells at a student for talking in class. After identifying the problem from each person's perspective, they acted out three different choices for solving the problem. For the 1st choice, the student talked back to the teacher in a rude voice and got written up in the disciplinary book. For the 2nd choice, the student blamed the person next to him for talking. The teacher said, "be quiet and worry about yourself." For the 3rd choice, the student apologized and remained quiet during the rest of the lesson. Later, when the teacher was not busy, the student went to her desk and politely explained that he had been trying to help his classmate find the right page. The consequence of the 3rd choice was that the teacher was understanding and seemed to appreciate his explanation, especially that he had waited to give it at a more appropriate time. The group members enjoyed making the video and were eager for their parents to see it at the end of the Coping Power parent group that was taking place simultaneously.

The Coping Power child group met several more times, with the remaining sessions focusing on fostering relationships with positive peers, resisting deviant peer influences, and celebrating the group members' positive qualities and gains made while in Coping Power. Dr. Bitner and the other group members praised Jarrod for learning to stop and see things from other people's perspectives and pointed out that this change seemed to help him reduce his arguments with others. The group gave Jayla positive feedback for staying calm rather than reacting with anger in provocation situations and for learning to give others more personal space. Ms. Erikson praised Isabel for making a big improvement in how nicely she treated others and for learning to use coping statements to control her anger. The group members told Xavier they were glad he had returned to the group and complimented him for being more positively engaged and trustworthy since he returned. Finally, the group members praised Mark for always being willing help others and for being calmer and more organized with his belongings and schoolwork. The group celebrated the end of Coping Power with a pizza party that they had earned by working as a team and obtaining 70% of the total points possible. After the group ended, Dr. Bitner described each student's behavior gains to their parents and IEP team and, when needed, provided recommendations for additional intervention.

Case Example—Individual Implementation of Coping Power

While Xavier was attending alternative school, Dr. Bitner met with him individually and continued to use Coping Power to address his behavior. Given his history of antisocial behavior, Dr. Bitner spent extra time trying to develop rapport with Xavier and helping him see how his behavior interfered with his personal goals. One of the challenges Dr. Bitner faced was that Xavier did not see much of a future for himself. He said he disliked school and spent most of his time after school hanging out with his high-school age cousins while his mother worked two jobs to provide for the family. Xavier said the only things he liked about school were P.E. and getting to spend time on the computer. He said he wanted to play on the school basketball team but was not eligible because he had been suspended.

Xavier and Dr. Bitner worked together to develop a long-term goal for Xavier to be able to join the basketball team next semester. They established short term goals for improving Xavier's behavior at school to reduce his suspensions so that he would be eligible to play (e.g., resolve problems without fighting; catch my anger early and use a coping statement to stay calm; ask for permission before borrowing things from others). Dr. Bitner also worked with Xavier's teacher to set up a classroom incentive system such that for every day that Xavier met his goal of "resolving problems without fighting," he earned ten extra minutes of computer time. In addition, every time Xavier earned 25 Coping Power points, he was able to serve as a peer teacher for the 1st grade P.E. class for the day.

Once these goals and incentives were established, Xavier showed notable effort to improve his behavior. Dr. Bitner felt that the problem-solving unit of Coping Power was most helpful for Xavier, in helping him recognize that aggressive solutions did not help him reach his goals as well as he thought. Xavier began to generate more socially skilled solutions (such as verbal assertion, bargaining, and compromise solutions) and to enact them more effectively, 1st by practicing them with Dr. Bitner and then by trying to apply them in real-life problem situations. By the time Xavier returned to Norwood Elementary and the Coping Power group, he had 30% fewer aggressive interactions and showed more interest in getting along with others. Xavier enjoyed the times he earned the opportunity to serve as the peer teacher for P.E. and this helped him begin to enjoy going to school again. The P.E. teacher took Xavier under his wing, made sure he completed his homework on days Xavier went to the aftercare program, then gave him basketball pointers to help him get ready to make the team next year. Figure 14.1 provides a sample treatment plan. Table 14.1 offers an outline of Coping Power sessions.

Summary

Angry and aggressive behaviors present significant challenges within the educational environment. Addressing these problems is particularly important given that their effects are likely to extend beyond short-term disruptions, with aggressive youth at heightened risk for serious, negative long-term consequences. Schools have responded to student problems with anger and aggression by implementing evidence-based CBT interventions, which are available for students from preschool through high school age. By targeting cognitive deficiencies and distortions common to youth with aggressive behavior problems, and by addressing social skills deficits, problems with emotion regulation, and difficulties with social problem-solving, these interventions have been shown to reduce disruptive behaviors and improve students' social functioning. Recent research has investigated factors involved in effectively disseminating these programs, and continued efforts in this domain will help to ensure that troubled students' difficulties with anger and aggression are effectively addressed.

Reflection Questions

1 You are a school psychologist who has been asked to evaluate a 5th grade student who is defiant in the classroom and is frequently aggressive to peers. Describe your approach to assessment, including information gathering strategies and informants to be consulted.

Description of the Problem: Student displays frequent anger outbursts and initiates physical fights with other students. He is disrespectful to the teacher and acts out when the teacher enforces classroom rules. He has threatened other students physically and verbally. Student puts little effort into school work and disrupts the class during instructional time.

Treatment Goal 1: To increase the student's school bonding and motivation to learn

Treatment strategies to meet Goal 1: To utilize the goal-setting portion of the Coping Power child curriculum to help the student identify personal short-term and long-term goals and to help the student make linkages between his academic work and attainment of current and future personal goals. To develop school-based incentives for rewarding increased effort toward schoolwork, including incentives likely to increase school-bonding. To utilize the Coping Power parent curriculum to increase home-school communication and increase parental support of student's academic work and behavior at school.

Treatment strategies to meet Goal 1: Progress will be assessed based on student's school attendance; student's completion of class work and homework assignments; student's attainment of daily behavior goals related to class participation on Coping Power goal sheet; and on structured and unstructured assessments of the student's classroom behavior

Treatment Goal 2: To increase the student's emotional coping skills

Treatment strategies to meet Goal 2: To utilize the emotional awareness and anger coping portions of the Coping Power child curriculum to help the student recognize thoughts, feelings, and physiological cues associated with early signs of anger and to utilize a range of coping strategies (e.g., distraction, relaxation, deep breathing, and self-instruction via coping self-statements) to keep anger at low to medium levels. To help the student's teacher and parents encourage his use of these skills throughout the day at school and at home.

Method of assessing progress toward Goal 2: Progress will be assessed based on student, parent, and teacher feedback using structured and unstructured methods; through the student's attainment of daily behavior goals related to emotional coping on Coping Power goal sheet; and via a reduction in disciplinary actions.

Treatment Goal 3: To increase the student's use of non-aggressive solutions to problems

Treatment strategies to meet Goal 3: To utilize the problem-solving portion of the Coping Power child curriculum to help the student learn to use alternate solutions to interpersonal problems and to anticipate the consequences of his actions. To help the student's teacher and parents encourage his use of effective, non-aggressive solutions to interpersonal problems.

Method of assessing progress toward Goal 3: Progress will be assessed based on student, parent, and teacher feedback; through attainment of daily behavior goals related to effective problem-solving on Coping Power goal sheet; and via a reduction in disciplinary actions.

Figure 14.1 Sample Treatment Plan

2 Imagine that your assessment of the student described above reveals a child who has little difficulty with anger control but uses aggression to meet social and instrumental needs. Which of the CBT strategies described would be important to include in a treatment plan for this student? How might you put these strategies into practice?
3 Imagine that you are running a school-based group for adolescents with aggressive behavior problems. How might you address hostile attribution biases that member might display? Develop ideas for several activities that might encourage members to consider other (non-hostile) reasons for others' actions.

Table 14.1 Overview of Coping Power Intervention Objectives by Session

Child Component		*Parent Component*	
Session	*Content and Main Objectives*	*Session*	*Content and Main Objectives*
1	Introduce program purpose and structure; build rapport; foster group cohesion	1	Provide overview of program structure and content; introduce parent academic support in the home
2 and 3	Introduce concept of goal-setting; assist students in identifying long-term and short-term personal goals; discuss barriers to achieving goals	2	Discuss homework monitoring and develop structure for parent-teacher interaction
4	Discuss importance of organization and effective study habits for academic success	3	Introduce topic of stress management for parents; discuss effects of stress; practice relaxation for stress management
5 and 6	Identify behavioral, physiological, and cognitive cues for emotions, especially anger	4	Introduce time management strategies for stress management; introduce and practice using cognitive model for stress management
7	Practice use of distraction to cope with anger	5	Present social learning theory, including the role of antecedents and consequences on shaping behavior; discuss and model use of praise
8–10	Practice use of coping self-statements to manage anger	6	Discuss and role-play ignoring to manage minor disruptive behaviors
11	Practice using relaxation to manage anger	7	Present features of effective instructions
12–14	Introduce concept of perspective-taking; encourage students to consider non-hostile motivations for others' actions	8	Discuss the importance of rules and expectations in the home
15	Introduce PICC problem-solving model; discuss 1st step: Problem Identification	9	Discuss discipline and punishment; present steps for using time-out effectively
16	Introduce Choices step of PICC model; practice identifying potential solutions to social problems	10	Discuss and role-play use of privilege removal and work chores as consequences for inappropriate behaviors and rule violations
17–18	Introduce Consequences step of PICC model; practice identifying consequences to various solutions; practice evaluating consequences	11	Help parents prepare and plan for summer breaks
19	Identify obstacles to problem-solving and practice persistence in overcoming them	12	Review information on academic support in the home
20	Begin planning for PICC video-making activity	13	Identify activities that promote family cohesiveness
21	Videotape students describing PICC model and role-playing problem situation, choices, and consequences	14	Discuss application of PICC to problems that may occur within the home
22	Complete videotape production; review and discuss video; review content	15	Assist parents in setting up structures to facilitate family communication

(Continued)

Table 14.1 (Continued)

Child Component		*Parent Component*	
Session	*Content and Main Objectives*	*Session*	*Content and Main Objectives*
23	Review group purpose and structure	16	Review and summarize key concepts; identify community resources for families
24	Review organization and study skills		
25	Use PICC model to practice solving social problems involving teachers		
26	Practice social skills for joining positive peer groups and making friends		
27	Use PICC model to practice solving social problems related to group entry and negotiation with peers		
28	Use PICC model to practice solving social problems involving siblings		
29	Identify skills to resist peer pressure		
30	Practice skills to resist peer pressure using a variety of role-played situations		
31	Use PICC model to practice solving social problems that may occur in students' neighborhoods; assist students in identifying their group memberships and status within social groups		
32	Create a poster illustrating skills to resist peer pressure		
33	Discuss ways to affiliate with positive peer groups		
34	Review and summarize key concepts; help students experience a sense of closure as the program ends		

Suggested Readings

Kendall, P. C. (2011). *Child and adolescent therapy: Cognitive behavioral procedures* (4th ed.). New York: Guilford Press.

Matthys, W., & Lochman, J. E. (2017). *Oppositional defiant disorder and conduct disorder in childhood* (2nd ed.). Oxford: Wiley-Blackwell.

Nelson, W. M. III, Finch, A. J., & Hart, K. J. (2006). *Comparative treatment of conduct disorder.* New York: Springer.

References

Achenbach, T. M. (1991). *Manual for the child behavior checklist and 1991 profile.* Burlington, VT: University Associates in Psychiatry.

Achenbach, T. M., & Rescorla, L. A. (2001). *Manual for ASEBA school-age forms & profiles.* Burlington: University of Vermont, Research Center for Children, Youth, & Families.

Allen, G. J., Chinsky, J. M., Larcen, S. W., Lochman, J. E., & Selinger, H. V. (1976). *Community psychology in the schools: A behaviorally oriented multilevel preventive approach.* Hillsdale, NJ: Erlbaum (Re-issued by Routledge Publishing in 2018).

American Psychiatric Association. (2013). *Diagnostic and statistical manual of mental disorders* (5th ed.) (DSM-5). Washington, DC: American Psychiatric Association.

Bennett, D. S., & Gibbons, T. A. (2000). Efficacy of child cognitive-behavioral interventions for antisocial behavior: A meta-analysis. *Child & Family Behavior Therapy, 22*(1), 1–15.

Blank, C., & Shavit, Y. (2016). The association between student reports of classmates' disruptive behavior and student achievement. *AERA Open, 2*(3), 1–17. https://doi.org/10.177/2332858416653921

Borduin, C. M., Mann, B. J., Cone, L. T., Henggeler, S. W., Fucci, B. R., Blaske, D. M., & Williams, R. A. (1995). Multisystemic treatment of serious juvenile offenders: Long-term prevention of criminality and violence. *Journal of Consulting and Clinical Psychology, 63,* 569–578.

Botvin, G. J., & Griffin, K. W. (2004). Life skills training: Empirical findings and future directions. *Journal of Primary Prevention, 25*(2), 211–232.

Boxmeyer, C. L., Miller, S., Romero, D. E., Powell, N. P., Jones, S. B., Qu, L., Tueller, S., & Lochman, J. E. (2021). Mindful Coping Power: Comparative effects on children's reactive aggression and self-regulation. *Brain Sciences, 11,* 1119. https://doi.org/10.3390/brainsci11091119

Boxmeyer, C. L., Stager, C. G., Miller, S., Lochman, J. E., Romero, D. E., Powell, N. P., Bui, C., & Qu, L. (2023). Mindful Coping Power effects on children's autonomic nervous system functioning and long-term behavioral outcomes. *Journal of Clinical Medicine.* https://doi.org/10.3390/jcm12113621

Bradshaw, C. P., Zmuda, J. H., Kellam, S. G., & Ialongo, N. S. (2009). Longitudinal impact of two universal preventive interventions in first grade on educational outcomes in high school. *Journal of Educational Psychology, 101*(4), 926–937. https://doi.org/10.1037/a0016586

Chorpita, B. F., Daleiden, E. L., Park, A. L., Ward, A. M., Levy, M. C., Cromley, T., Chiu, A. W., Letamendi, A. M., Tsai, K. H., & Krull, J. L. (2017). Child STEPs in California: A cluster randomized effectiveness trial comparing modular treatment with community implemented treatment for youth with anxiety, depression, conduct problems, or traumatic stress. *Journal of Consulting and Clinical Psychology, 85*(1), 13–25.

Chorpita, B. F., & Weisz, J. R. (2009). *MATCH-ADTC: Modular approach to therapy for children with anxiety, depression, trauma, or conduct problems.* Satellite Beach, FL: PracticeWise.

Chow, J. C., & Wehby, J. H. (2018). Associations between language and problem behavior: A systematic review and correlational meta-analysis. *Educational Psychology Review, 30*(1), 61–82. https://doi.org/10.1007/s10648-016-9385-z

Coie, J. D., Lochman, J. E., Terry, R., & Hyman, C. (1992). Predicting early adolescent disorders from childhood aggression and peer rejection. *Journal of Consulting and Clinical Psychology, 60,* 783–792.

Conners, C. K. (1997). *Conners' Rating Scales-Revised: Technical manual.* North Tonawanda, NY: Multi-Health Systems.

Crick, N. R., & Dodge, K. A. (1994). A review and reformulation of social information processing mechanisms in children's social adjustment. *Psychological Bulletin, 115,* 74–101.

Crick, N. R., & Werner, N. E. (1998). Response decision processes in relational and overt aggression. *Child Development, 69,* 1630–1639.

Dodge, K. A. (1986). A social information processing model of social competence in children. In M. Perlmutter (Ed.), *The Minnesota symposia on child psychology: Vol.18. Cognitive perspectives on children's social and behavioral development* (pp. 77–125). Hillsdale, NJ: Erlbaum.

Dodge, K. A. (1993). Social cognitive mechanisms in the development of conduct disorder and depression. *Annual Review of Psychology, 44,* 559–584.

Dodge, K. A., Lochman, J. E., Harnish, J. D., Bates, J. E., & Pettit, G. S. (1997). Reactive and proactive aggression in school children and psychiatrically impaired chronically assaultive youth. *Journal of Abnormal Psychology, 106,* 37–51.

Dunn, S. E., Lochman, J. E., & Colder, C. R. (1997). Social problem-solving skills in boys with Conduct and Oppositional Defiant Disorders. *Aggressive Behavior, 23,* 457–469.

Eiraldi, R., Mautone, J. A., Khanna, M. S., Power, T. J., Orapallo, A., Cacia, J., Schwartz, B. S., McCurdy, B., Keiffer, J., Paidipati, C., Kanine, R., Abraham, M., Tulio, S., Swift, L., Bressler, S. N., Cabello, B., & Jawad, A. F. (2018). Group CBT for externalizing disorders in urban schools: Effect of training strategy on treatment fidelity and child outcomes. *Behavior Therapy, 49,* 538–550.

Ellis, M. L., Lindsey, M., Barker, E. D., Boxmeyer, C. L., & Lochman, J. E. (2013). Predictors of engagement in a school-based family preventive intervention for youth experiencing behavioral difficulties. *Prevention Science, 14,* 457–467.

Evans, S. C., Burke, J. D., Roberts, M. C., Fite, P. J., Lochman, J. E., de la Pena, F. R., & Reed, G. M. (2017). Irritability in child and adolescent psychopathology: An integrative review for ICD-11. *Clinical Psychology Review, 53*, 29–45.

Evans, S. C., Weisz, J. R., Carvalho, A. C., Garibaldi, P. M., Bearman, S. K., Chorpita, B. F. (2020). Effects of standard and modular psychotherapies in the treatment of youth with severe irritability. *Journal of Consulting and Clinical Psychology, 88*(3), 255–268.

Fabelo, T., Thompson, M. D., Plotkin, M., Carmichael, D., Marchbanks, M. P., III, & Booth, E. A. (2011). *Breaking schools' rules: A statewide study of how school discipline relates to students' success and juvenile justice involvement.* New York: Council of State Governments Justice Center.

Fabiano, G. A., Pelham, W. E., Jr., Waschbusch, D. A., Gnagy, E. M., Lahey, B. B., Chronis, A. M., … & Burrows-MacLean, L. (2006). A practical measure of impairment: Psychometric properties of the Impairment Rating Scale in samples of children with Attention Deficit Hyperactivity Disorder and two school-based samples. *Journal of Clinical Child and Adolescent Psychology, 35*, 369–385.

Fite, P. J., Colder, C. R., Lochman, J. E., & Wells, K. C. (2008). The relation between childhood proactive and reactive aggression and substance use initiation. *Journal of Abnormal Child Psychology, 36*, 261–271.

Glenn, A. L., Lochman, J. E., Dishion, T., Powell, N. P., Boxmeyer, C., Kassing, F., Qu, L., & Romero, D. (2019). Toward tailored interventions: Sympathetic and parasympathetic functioning predicts responses to an intervention for conduct problems delivered in two formats. *Prevention Science, 20*, 30–40.

Glenn, A. L., Lochman, J. E., Dishion, T., Powell, N. P., Boxmeyer, C., & Qu, L. (2018). Oxytocin receptor gene variant interacts with intervention delivery format in predicting intervention outcomes for youth with conduct problems. *Prevention Science, 19*, 38–48.

Goldstein, N. E. S., Giallella, C. L., Haney-Caron, E., Peterson, L., Serico, J., Kemp, K., Romaine, C. R., Zelechoski, A. D., Holliday, S. B., Kalbeitzer, R., Kelley, S. M., Hinz, H., Sallee, M., Pennacchia, D., Prelic, A., Burkard, C., Grisso, T., Heilbrun, K., Núñez, A., … & Lochman, J. (2018). Juvenile Justice Anger Management (JJAM) treatment for girls: Results of a randomized controlled trial. *Psychological Services, 15*(4), 386–397.

Goldstein, N. E. S., Serico, J. M., Riggs Romaine, C., Zelechoski, A. D., Kalbeitzer, R., Kemp, K., & Lane, C. (2013). Development of the juvenile justice anger management treatment for girls. *Cognitive and Behavioral Practice, 20*, 171–188.

Goldstein, S., & Naglieri, J. A. (Eds.) (2016a). *Assessing impairment: From theory to practice* (2nd ed.). New York: Springer.

Goldstein, S., & Naglieri, J. A. (2016b). Measuring impairment with the Rating Scale of Impairment. In S. Goldstein & J. A. Naglieri (Eds.), *Assessing impairment: From theory to practice* (2nd ed.) (pp. 247–255). New York: Springer.

Greenberg, M. T., Domitrovich, C., & Bumbarger, B. (2001). The prevention of mental disorders in school-aged children: Current state of the field. *Prevention and Treatment, 4*. Available on the World Wide Web: Retrieved from http://journals.apa.org/prevention/volume4/pre0040001c.html.

Greenberg, M. T., & Kusche, C. A. (2006). Building social and emotional competence: The PATHS curriculum. In S. R. Jimerson & M. Furlong (Eds.), *Handbook of school violence and school safety: From research to practice* (pp. 395–412). Mahwah, NJ: Lawrence Erlbaum Associates.

Gresham, F. M., & Elliott, S. N. (1990). *Social skills rating system: Manual.* Circle Pines, MN: American Guidance Service.

Gubbels, J., van der Put, C. E., & Assink, M. (2019). Risk factors for school absenteeism and dropout: A meta-analytic review. *Journal of Youth and Adolescence, 48*, 1637–1667. https://doi.org/10.1007/s10964-019-01072-5

Hawkins, J. D., Catalano, R. F., Kosterman, R., Abbott, R. D., & Hill, K. G. (1999). Preventing adolescent health-risk behaviors by strengthening protection during childhood. *Archives of Pediatrics and Adolescent Medicine, 153*, 226–234.

Helander, M., Lochman, J., Högström, J., Ljòtsson, B., Hellner, C., & Enebrink, P. (2018). The effect of adding Coping Power Program-Sweden to Parent Management Training-Effects and moderators in a randomized controlled trial. *Behavior Research and Therapy, 103*, 43–52.

Henggeler, S. W., & Lee, T. (2003). Multisystemic treatment of serious clinical problems. In A. E. Kazdin & J. R. Weisz (Eds.), *Evidence-based psychotherapies for children and adolescents* (pp. 301–322). New York: Guilford.

Henggeler, S. W., Melton, G. B., & Smith, L. A. (1992). Family preservation using multisystemic therapy: An effective alternative to incarcerating serious juvenile offenders. *Journal of Consulting and Clinical Psychology, 60*, 953–961.

Ho, B. P. V., Carter, M., & Stephenson, J. (2010). Anger management using a cognitive-behavioral approach for children with special education needs: A literature review and meta-analysis. *International Journal of Disability, Development, and Education, 57*(3), 245–265.

Jaafar, N. R. N., Iryani, M. D. T., Salwina, W. I. W., Nazri, A. R. F., Kamal, N. A., Prakash, R. J., & Shah, S. A. (2013). Externalizing and internalizing syndromes in relation to school truancy among adolescents in high-risk urban schools. *Asia-Pacific Psychiatry, 5*, 27–34.

Kamphaus, R. W., & Frick, P. J. (2001). *Clinical assessment of child and adolescent personality and behavior* (2nd ed.). Needham Heights, MA: Allyn & Bacon.

Kassing, F., Godwin, J., Lochman, J. E., Coie, J. D., & Conduct Problems Prevention Research Group (2019). Using early childhood behavior problems to predict adult convictions. *Journal of Abnormal Child Psychology, 47*, 765–778.

Kassing, F., Lochman, J. E., & Glenn, A. (2018). Autonomic functioning in reactive versus proactive aggression: The influential role of inconsistent parenting. *Aggressive Behavior, 44*, 524–536.

Kazdin, A. E., Siegal, T. C., & Bass, D. (1992). Cognitive problem-solving skills training and parent management training in the treatment of antisocial behavior in children. *Journal of Consulting and Clinical Psychology, 60*, 733–747.

Kokko, K., Tremblay, R. E., Lacourse, E., Nagin, D. S., & Vitaro, F. (2006). Trajectories of prosocial behavior and physical aggression in middle childhood: Links to adolescent school dropout and physical violence. *Journal of Research on Adolescence, 16*(3), 403–428.

Kremer, K. P., Flower, A., Huang, J., & Vaughn, M. G. (2017). Behavior problems and children's academic achievement: A test of growth-curve models with gender and racial differences. *Children Youth Services Review, 67*, 95–104. https://doi.org/10.1016/j.childyouth.2016.06.003

Kupersmidt, J. B., Stelter, B., & Dodge, K. A. (2011). Development and validation of the Social Information Processing Application: A web-based measure of social information processing patterns in elementary school-age boys. *Psychological Assessment, 23*(4), 834–847.

Lachar, D., Wingenfeld, S. A., Kline, R. B., & Gruber, C. P. (2000). *Student behavior survey.* Los Angeles, CA: Western Psychological Services.

Larson, J., & Lochman, J. E. (2011). Helping schoolchildren cope with anger: A cognitive-behavioral intervention (2nd ed.). New York: Guilford Press.

Lindsey, M. A., Romanelli, M., Ellis, M. L., Barker, E. D., Boxmeyer, C. L., & Lochman, J. E. (2019). The influence of treatment engagement on positive outcomes in the context of a school-based intervention for students with externalizing behavior problems. *Journal of Abnormal Child Psychology, 47*, 1437–1454.

Lochman, J. E. (1992). Cognitive-behavioral intervention with aggressive boys: Three year follow-up and preventive effects. *Journal of Consulting and Clinical Psychology, 60*, 426–432.

Lochman, J. E., Baden, R. E., Boxmeyer, C. L., Powell, N. P., Qu, L., Salekin, K. L., & Windle, M. (2014). Does a booster intervention augment the preventative effects of an abbreviated version of the coping power program for aggressive children? *Journal of Abnormal Psychology, 42*(3), 367–381.

Lochman, J. E., Boxmeyer, C. L., Ialongo, N. S., McDaniel, S. C., Pas, E. T., & Powell, N. P. (2019). Tier II family-school partnership programs. In A. Garbacz (Ed.), *Implementing family-school partnerships: Student success in school psychology research and practice* (pp. 88–110). New York: Routledge.

Lochman, J. E., Boxmeyer, C. L., Jones, S., Qu, L., Ewoldsen, D., & Nelson, W. M. III (2017). Testing the feasibility of a briefer school-based preventive intervention with aggressive children: A hybrid intervention with face-to-face and internet components. *Journal of School Psychology, 62*, 33–50. https://doi.org/10.1016/j.jsp.2017.03.010

Lochman, J. E., Boxmeyer, C. L., Powell, N. P., Qu, L., Wells, K., & Windle, M. (2009). Dissemination of the coping power program: Importance of intensity of counselor training. *Journal of Consulting and Clinical Psychology, 77*, 397–409.

Lochman, J. E., Boxmeyer, C. L., Powell, N. P., Qu, L., Wells, K., & Windle, M. (2012). Coping power dissemination study: Intervention and special education effects on academic outcomes. *Behavioral Disorders, 37*, 192–205.

Lochman, J. E., Dishion, T. J., Boxmeyer, C. L., Powell, N. P., & Qu, L. (2017). Variations in response to evidence-based group preventive intervention for disruptive behavior problems: A view from 938 Coping Power sessions. *Journal of Abnormal Child Psychology, 45*, 1271–1284. https://doi.org/10.1007/s10802-016-0252-7

Lochman, J. E., Dishion, T. J., Powell, N. P., Boxmeyer, C. L., Qu, L., & Sallee, M. (2015). Evidence-based preventive intervention for preadolescent aggressive children: One-year outcomes following randomization to group versus individual delivery. *Journal of Consulting and Clinical Psychology, 83*, 728–735.

Lochman, J. E., & Dodge, K. A. (1994). Social-cognitive processes of severely violent, moderately aggressive and nonaggressive boys. *Journal of Consulting and Clinical Psychology, 62*, 366–374.

Lochman, J. E., & Dodge, K. A. (1998). Distorted perceptions in dyadic interactions of aggressive and nonaggressive boys: Effects of prior expectations, context, and boys' age. *Development and Psychopathology, 10*, 495–512.

Lochman, J. E., Glenn, A. L., Powell, N. P., Boxmeyer, C. L., Bui, C., Kassing, F., Qu, L., Romero, D., & Dishion, T. (2019). Group versus individual format of intervention for aggressive children: Moderators and predictors of outcomes through four years after intervention. *Development and Psychopathology, 31*(5), 1757–1775.

Lochman, J. E., Powell, N. P., Boxmeyer, C. L., Ford, H. L., & Minney, J. A. (2014). Beyond disruptive behaviors: Applications of the Coping Power program. In J. Ehrenreich-May & B. Chu (Eds.), *Transdiagnostic mechanisms and treatment for youth psychopathology* (pp. 293–312). New York: Guilford Press.

Lochman, J. E., Powell, N. P., Boxmeyer, C. L., Qu, L., Sallee, M., Wells, K. C., & Windle, M. (2015). Counselor-level predictors of sustained use of an indicated preventive intervention for aggressive children. *Prevention Science, 16*, 1075–1085. https://doi.org/10.1007/s11121-014-0511-1

Lochman, J. E., Powell, N. P., Boxmeyer, C. L., Qu, L., Wells, K. C., & Windle, M. (2009). Implementation of a school-based prevention program: Effects of counselor and school characteristics. *Professional Psychology: Research and Practice, 40*, 476–482.

Lochman, J. E., Wayland, K. K., & White, K. J. (1993). Social goals: Relationship to adolescent adjustment and to social problem solving. *Journal of Abnormal Child Psychology, 21*, 135–151.

Lochman, J. E., & Wells, K. C. (2002). Contextual social-cognitive mediators and child outcome: A test of the theoretical model in the Coping Power Program. *Development and Psychopathology, 14*, 971–993.

Lochman, J. E., & Wells, K. C. (2003). Effectiveness study of Coping Power and classroom intervention with aggressive children: Outcomes at a one-year follow-up. *Behavior Therapy, 34*, 493–515.

Lochman, J. E., & Wells, K. C. (2004). The Coping Power program for preadolescent aggressive boys and their parents: Outcome effects at the one-year follow-up. *Journal of Consulting and Clinical Psychology, 72*, 571–578.

Lochman, J. E., Wells, K. C., & Lenhart, L. A. (2008). *Coping Power child group program: Facilitator guide.* New York: Oxford.

Lochman, J. E., Wells, K. C., Qu, L., & Chen, L. (2013). Three year follow-up of Coping Power intervention effects: Evidence of neighborhood moderation? *Prevention Science, 14*, 364–376.

Lonczak, H. S., Huang, B., Catalano, R. F., Hawkins, J. D., Hill, K. G., Abbott, R. D., Ryan, J. A. M., & Kosterman, R. (2001). The social predictors of adolescent alcohol misuse: A test of the Social Development Model. *Journal of Studies on Alcohol, 62*, 179–189.

Ludmer, J. A., Sanches, M., Propp, L., & Andrade, B. F. (2018). Comparing multicomponent Coping Power Program to individualized parent-child treatment for improving parenting efficacy and satisfaction of parents of children with conduct problems. *Child Psychiatry and Human Development, 49*, 100–108.

Ma, L., Phelps, E., Lerner, J. V., & Lerner, R. M. (2009). Academic competence for adolescents who bully and who are bullied: Findings from the 4-H Study of Positive Youth Development. *The Journal of Early Adolescence, 29*(6), 862–897.

Matthys, W., & Lochman, J. E. (2017). *Oppositional defiant disorder and conduct disorder in childhood* (2nd ed.). Oxford: Wiley-Blackwell.

McCart, M. R., Priester, P. E., Davies, W. H., & Azen, R. (2006). Differential effectivenss of behavioral parent-training and cognitve-beahviroal therapy for antisocial youth: A meta-analysis. *Journal of Abnormal Child Psychology, 34*(4), 527–525.

McDaniel, S. C., Lochman, J. E., Tomek, S., Powell, N., Irwin, A., & Kerr, S. (2018). Reducing levels of behavioral risk in late elementary school: A comparison of two targeted interventions. *Behavioral Disorders, 43*, 370–382.

McDonald, K. L., & Lochman, J. E. (2012). Predictors and outcomes associated with trajectories of revenge goals from fourth grade through seventh grade. *Journal of Abnormal Child Psychology, 40*, 225–236.

McDonald, K. L., Siddiqui, S., Seo, S., & Gibson, C. E. (2022). Interpretations and revenge goals in response to peer provocations: Comparing adolescents in the United States and Pakistan. *International Journal of Behavioral Development, 46*(6), 555–561. https://doi.org/10.1177/01650254221121840.

McMahon, R. J., & Frick, P. J. (2007). Conduct and oppositional disorders. In E. J. Mash & R. A. Barkley (Eds.), *Assessment of childhood disorders* (4th ed.) (pp. 132–183). New York: Guilford.

Miller, N. E., & Dollard, J. (1941). *Social learning and imitation.* New Haven, CT: Yale University Press.

Mischel, W. (1973). Toward a cognitive social learning conceptualization of personality. *Psychological Review, 80*, 252–283.

Mitchell, Q. P., Younginer, S. T., Lochman, J. E., Vernberg, E. M., Powell, N. P., & Qu, L. (2021). Examining for the protective effects of therapeutic engagement on child aggression. *Journal of Emotional and Behavioral Disorders, 29*(3), 162–174. https://doi.org/10.1177/1063426620980701

Muratori, P., Bertacchi, I., Catone, G., Mannucci, F., Nocentini, A., Pisano, S., & Lochman, J. E. (2020). Coping Power Universal for middle school students: The first efficacy study. *Journal of Adolescence, 79*, 49–58.

Muratori, P., Bertacchi, I., Giuli, C., Nocentini, A., & Lochman, J. E. (2017). Implementing Coping Power adapted as a universal prevention program in Italian primary schools: A randomized control trial. *Prevention Science, 18*, 754–761. https://doi.org/10.1007/s11121-016-0715-7

Muratori, P., Lochman, J., Bertacchi, I., Giuli, C., Guarguagli, E., Pisano, S., Gallani, A., & Mammarella, I. C. (2019). Universal Coping Power for pre-schoolers: Effects on children's behavioral difficulties and pre-academic skills. *School Psychology International, 40*(2), 128–144.

Muratori, P., Milone, A., Levantini, V., Ruglioni, R., Lambruschi, F., Pisano, S., Masi, G., & Lochman, J. E. (2019). Six-year outcome for children with ODD or CD treated with Coping Power Program. *Psychiatry Research, 271*, 454–458.

Mushtaq, A., Lochman, J. E., Tariq, P. N., & Sabih, F. (2017). Preliminary effectiveness study of Coping Power program for aggressive children in Pakistan. *Prevention Science, 18*, 762–771. https://doi.org/10.1007/s11121-016-0721-9

Nock, M. K., & Kurtz, S. M. S. (2005). Direct behavioral observation in school settings: Bringing science to practice. *Cognitive and Behavioral Practice, 12*(3), 359–370.

Pagani, L. S., Fitzpatrick, C., Archambault, I., & Janosz, M. (2010). School readiness and later achievement: A French Canadian replication and extension. *Developmental Psychology, 46*(5), 984–994.

Pas, E. T., Bradshaw, C. P., Hershfeldt, P. A., & Leaf, P. J. (2010). A multilevel exploration of the influence of teacher efficacy and burnout on response to student problem behavior and school-based service use. *School Psychology Quarterly, 25*(1), 13–27.

Pas, E. T., Kaiser, L., Rabinowitz, J., Lochman, J. E., & Bradshaw, C. P. (2020). Identifying factors associated with patterns of student attendance and participation in a group Tier 2 preventive intervention: Implications for adaptation. *Journal of Applied School Psychology, 29*, 198–226.

Pelham, W. E. Jr., & Burrows-Maclean, L. (2005). Mental mealth intervetions: Evidence-based approaches. In L. Osborn, T. Dewitt, L. First & J. Zenel (Eds.), *Pediatrics* (pp. 1940–1948). Philadelphia, PA: Elsevier Mosby.

Platt, J., & Spivack, G. (1989). *The MEPS procedure manual.* Philadelphia, PA: Hahnemann University, Department of Mental Health Sciences.

Powell, N. P., Boxmeyer, C. L., Baden, R., Stromeyer, S., Minney, J. A., Mushtaq, A., & Lochman, J. E. (2011). Assessing and treating aggression and conduct problems in schools. *Psychology in the Schools, 48*, 233–242.

Powers, C. J., Bierman, K. L., & Conduct Problems Prevention Research Group (2013). The multifaceted impact of peer relations on aggressive-disruptive behavior in early elementary school. *Developmental Psychology, 49*, 1174–1186.

Quay, H. C., & Peterson, D. R. (1996). *Revised behavior problem checklist, PAR Edition.* Odessa, TX: Psychological Assessment Resources.

Reynolds, C. R., Kamphaus, R. W., & Vannest, K. (2015). *Behavior Assessment System for Children—3 (BASC-3)*. Bloomington, MN: Pearson Assessments.

Risi, S., Gerhardstein, R., & Kistner, J. (2003). Children's classroom peer relationships and subsequent educational outcomes. *Journal of Clinical Child & Adolescent Psychology, 32*(3), 351–361.

Robinson, T. R., Smith, S. W., Miller, M. D., & Brownell, M. T. (1999). Cognitive behavior modification of hyperactivity–impulsivity and aggression: A meta-analysis of school-based studies. *Journal of Educational Psychology, 91*(2), 195–203.

Rones, M., & Hoagwood, K. (2000). School-based mental health services: A research review. *Clinical Child and Family Psychology Review, 3*, 223–241.

Rotter, J. B. (1954). *Social learning and clinical psychology*. New York: Prentice Hall.

Sattler, J. M. (2022). *Foundations of behavioral, social, and clinical assessment of children* (7th ed.). La Mesa, CA: Jerome M. Sattler, Publisher, Inc.

Schuiringa, H., van Nieuwenhuijzen, M., Orobio de Castro, B., Lochman, J. E., & Matthys, W. (2017). Effectiveness of an intervention for children with externalizing behavior and mild to borderline intellectual disabilities: A randomized trial. *Cognitive Therapy and Research, 41*, 237–251. https://doi.org/10.1007/s10608-016-9815-8

Selman, R. L., & Byrne, D. F. (1974). A structural-developmental analysis of levels of role taking in middle childhood. *Child Development, 45,* 803–806.

Shure, M. B., & Spivack, G. (1980). Interpersonal problem solving as a mediator of behavioral adjustment in preschool and kindergarten children. *Journal of Applied Developmental Psychology, 1*, 29–44.

Sukhodolsky, D. G., Kassinove, H., & Gorman, B. S. (2004). Cognitive-behavioral therapy for anger in children and adolescents: A meta-analysis. *Aggression and Violent Behavior, 9*(3), 247–269.

Sukhodolsky, D. G., Smith, S. D., McCauley, S. A., Ibrahim, K., & Piasecka, J. (2016). Behavioral interventions for anger, irritability, and aggression in children and adolescents. *Journal of Child and Adolescent Psychopharmacology, 26*(1), 58–64.

Takeda, T., Nissley-Tsiopinis, J., Nanda, S., & Eiraldi, R. (2016). Factors associated with discrepancy in parent-teacher reporting of symptoms of ADHD in a large clinic-referred sample of children. *Journal of Attention Disorders, 24*, 1605–1615.

Tissue, A. D., Hawes, D. J., Lechowicz, M. E., & Dadds, M. R. (2022). Reliability and validity of the DSM-5 Diagnostic Interview Schedule for Children, Adolescents, and Parents-5 in externalizing disorders and common comorbidities. *Clinical Child Psychology and Psychiatry, 27*(3), 870–881.

Van de Wiel, N. M. H., Matthys, W., Cohen-Kettenis, P. T., Maassen, G. H., Lochman, J. E., & van Engeland, H. (2007). The effectiveness of an experimental treatment when compared with care as usual depends on the type of care as usual. *Behavior Modification, 31*, 298–312.

Van Manen, T. G., Prins, P. J. M., & Emmelkamp, P. M. G. (2001). Assessing social cognitive skills in aggressive children from a developmental perspective: The social cognitive skills test. *Clinical Psychology and Psychotherapy, 8*, 341–351.

Vanzin, L., Colombo, P., Valli, A., Mauri, V., Ceccarelli, S. B., Pozzi, M., Molteni, M., & Nobile, M. (2018). The effectiveness of Coping Power Program for ADHD: An observational outcome study. *Journal of Child and Family Studies, 27*(4), 3554–3563.

Webster-Stratton, C. (2005). The incredible years: A training series for the prevention and treatment of conduct problems in young children. In E. D. Hibbs & P. S. Jensen (Eds.), *Psychosocial treatments for child and adolescent disorders: Empirically based strategies for clinical practice* (2nd ed.) (pp. 507–555). Washington, DC: American Psychological Association.

Webster-Stratton, C., & Hammond, M. (1997). Treating children with early-onset conduct problems: A comparison of child and parent training interventions. *Journal of Consulting and Clinical Psychology, 65*, 93–109.

Webster-Stratton, C., & Reid, M. J. (2010). The incredible years parents, teachers, and children training series: A multifaceted treatment approach for young children with conduct disorders. In J. R. Weisz & A. E. Kazdin (Eds.), *Evidence-based psychotherapies for children and adolescents* (pp. 117–138). New York: Guilford.

Webster-Stratton, C., Reid, M. J., & Hammond, M. (2004). Treating children with early-onset conduct problems: Intervention outcomes for parent, child, and teacher training. *Journal of Clinical Child and Adolescent Psychology, 33*, 105–124.

Weiner, B. (1990). Attributions in personality psychology. In L. Pervin (Ed.), *Handbook of personality: Theory and research* (pp. 609–637). New York: Guilford.

Wells, K. C., Lochman, J. E., & Lenhart, L. A. (2008). *Coping Power parent group program: Facilitator guide*. New York: Oxford.

Williams, S. C., Lochman, J. E., Phllips, N. C., & Barry, T. (2003). Aggressive and nonaggressive boys' physiological and cognitive processes in response to peer provocations. *Journal of Clinical Child and Adolescent Psychology, 32*, 568–576.

Winding, T. N., Aust, B., & Andersen, L. P. S. (2022). The association between pupils' aggressive behaviour and burnout among Danish school teachers – The role of stress and social support at work. *BMC Public Health, 22*, 316. https://doi.org/10.1186/s12889-022-12606-1

Yaros, A., Lochman, J. E., Rosenbaum, J., & Jimenez-Camargo, L. A. (2014). Real-time hostile attribution measurement and aggression in children. *Aggressive Behavior, 40*, 409–420.

Yavuzer, Y., & Karataş, Z. (2013). Ergenlerde otomatik düşünceler ile fiziksel saldırganlık arasındaki ilişkide öfkenin aracı rolü [The mediating role of anger in the relationship between automatic thoughts and physical aggression in adolescents]. *Turk Psikiyatri Derg, 24*(2), 117–123. Turkish. PMID: 23754265.

Zonnevylle-Bender, M. J. S., Matthys, W., van de Wiel, N. M. H., & Lochman, J. (2007). Preventive effects of treatment of DBD in middle childhood on substance use and delinquent behavior. *Journal of the American Academy of Child and Adolescent Psychiatry, 46*, 33–39.

15
DEPRESSIVE DISORDERS

Courtney L. Leone and Hannah Brimkov

Introduction

Depression is a prevalent mental health condition that affects individuals of all ages, including children and adolescents. Data collected by the Substance Abuse and Mental Health Services Administration showed that in the United States, an estimated 4.1 million, or 17%, of adolescents aged 12–17 years old had at least one major depressive episode in their lives (SAMHSA, 2021). Among this statistic, the rates were consistently higher among adolescent females compared to males (Flanagan et al., 2015; National Institute of Mental Health [NIMH], 2022; Wijnhoven et al., 2014). The impact of depression on young individuals extends beyond their emotional well-being and can significantly disrupt their academic performance, social interactions, and overall quality of life. Adolescents between 12 and 17 years old who reported they received mental health services in an educational setting "felt depressed" (SAMHSA, 2021). Therefore, it is crucial to explore effective treatment approaches that address depression specifically within the unique context of educational settings.

Cognitive-behavioral therapy (CBT) has emerged as a leading evidence-based treatment modality for prevention and treatment of depression in children and adolescents. CBT offers a structured, goal-oriented, and collaborative approach that targets maladaptive thoughts, behaviors, and emotions associated with depression. By equipping young individuals with essential cognitive and behavioral skills, CBT aims to alleviate depressive symptoms and foster resilience, leading to improved academic functioning and overall psychological well-being.

This chapter explores the theoretical foundations of CBT and its adaptation for the unique developmental needs and challenges faced by young individuals.

This chapter is written to provide a comprehensive guide for mental health professionals working in schools, educators who are leading the development of mental health systems in schools, and researchers interested in exploring the use of CBT for prevention and treatment of depression in children and adolescents within educational settings. In the next several pages, a comprehensive overview of the application of CBT techniques, strategies, and interventions in educational settings to effectively address depressive symptoms in the school setting is discussed. Throughout, current empirical research, evidence, and practical insights are highlighted within the context of the applicability of CBT in educational settings. By examining the current literature and emerging trends,

DOI: 10.4324/9781003392439-18

this chapter empathizes how the status of the literature can be integrated into educational environments to support the mental health and well-being of children and adolescents with depression.

Overview of CBT and Depressive Disorders

As already stated, depressive disorders are a significant concern among children and adolescents, and their impact on educational settings is well recognized. Since the mid- to late 1900s, CBT emerged to treat adult individuals with depressive disorders. For several decades now, CBT has been used and adapted as an evidence-based treatment for children and adolescents with depression (Chand et al., 2022). Dr. Aaron T. Beck, widely recognized as the father of cognitive therapy, played a pivotal role in laying the foundation for CBT. His early work focused on working with adults with depressive symptoms and formed the basis for CBT interventions. Although Beck's early research was mainly with adults, his groundbreaking research and theoretical insights paved the way for adaptation of CBT for younger populations. Building upon Beck's work, Drs. Donald Meichenbaum, Philip C. Kendall, and Alan E. Kazdin made substantial contributions in adapting CBT for children and adolescents with various disorders, including anxiety and oppositional defiance disorder. Their research and clinical innovations helped to refine and expand the application of CBT techniques specifically tailored to the unique needs of younger individuals. Additionally, Dr. Judy S. Beck has played an influential role in guiding clinicians to adapt CBT for more challenging cases, especially in children and adolescents. Collectively, these pioneers have shaped the field of CBT through their theoretical contributions, extensive research efforts, and clinical work. Their research has solidified CBT as an effective therapeutic approach for addressing a wide range of psychological difficulties in children and adolescents.

In educational settings, CBT can be a valuable intervention for depressive symptoms. CBT offers structure and is very much goal-oriented, allowing adaptations to meet the unique needs of individual children and adolescents. Incorporating CBT into educational settings can help students to develop adaptive thinking patterns and effective coping skills to manage any depressive symptoms they might be experiencing. CBT goes beyond just working within counseling settings and requires collaboration between different professionals within the school. CBT focuses on the connection between thoughts, feelings, and behaviors. The goal is to focus on and identify negative thought patterns and modify them to develop healthy coping skills. The key components of CBT for depressive disorders in children and adolescents include psychoeducation, cognitive restructuring, behavioral activation, problem-solving skills, and social skills training.

Psychoeducation

Provides age-appropriate information about depression, its causes, and the role of thoughts, emotions, and behaviors in maintaining depressive symptoms to help students understand their experiences and reduce stigma associated with mental health challenges. This can be incorporated into health and physical education classes, daily classroom routine, as well as weekly mental health challenges for students. Providing psychoeducation can act as a proactive and preventative process, but it can also bring awareness to school personnel, staff, and peers.

Cognitive Restructuring

Helps students identify and challenge negative and distorted thinking patterns that contribute to depressive symptoms. By replacing negative thoughts with more realistic and positive ones, students can reframe their perceptions and improve their emotional well-being. In an educational setting, this can be done during group sessions or by allowing students opportunities to identify thoughts by using interventions such as journal writing or active discussion.

Behavioral Activation

Encourages engagement in pleasurable and meaningful activities to counteract the withdrawal isolation often associated with depression. By increasing participation in positive experiences, students can enhance their mood and regain a sense of enjoyment. This can be achieved by collaborating with the child or adolescent to create structured activities and tasks throughout each day to reach individual goals that they set. To ensure the individual participates in positive experiences, the professional helping the student can collaborate with him/her on pleasant events scheduling. This may involve incorporating breaks for relaxation, scheduling in their hobbies or interest regularly, or participating in social interactions with peers. Additionally, establishing behavioral contracts between students, teachers, and parents to maintain specific behavioral goals and rewards can motivate students to engage in positive behaviors (e.g., completing assignments, participating in class, or attending school events).

Problem-Solving Skills

Teaches students effective problem-solving techniques to address challenges and setbacks they may encounter. These skills empower students to find constructive solutions and build resilience when faced with difficult situations. Even offering collaboration to solve problems fosters a more positive school experience.

Social Skills Training

Assist students in developing and improving their social skills, including communication, assertiveness, and conflict resolution. By working on social skills, social competence can strengthen relationships and support networks, both of which are vital protective factors against depression. There are currently several popular, evidence-based social skills training programs for educational settings. Some include The Social Skills Improvement System (SSIS; Gresham & Elliot, 2017), Promoting Alternative Thinking Strategies (PATHS; Domitrovich & Greenber, 2017), FRIENDS for Life (Barret et al., 2006), and Skillstreaming (McGinnis & Goldstein, 2019).

Understanding Depressive Disorders

In children and adolescents, depressive symptoms can appear similarly to symptoms in adults. Some symptoms can manifest as anxiety for a child. A child or adolescent can appear as sad or hopeless, or they can begin to lose interest in their favorite activities. This is similar to what an adult may experience, but a child or adolescent may have inconsistencies with their emotions and can also show irritability or crankiness, behavioral outbursts, physical complaints (e.g., headaches, stomachaches, fatigue), sleep disturbances, and separation anxiety. In a school setting, symptoms can interfere with academic performance. Depressive symptoms may not allow a child to concentrate on the tasks at hand due to lack of sleep, low energy, or lack of motivation and productivity.

The Diagnostic and Statistical Manual of Mental Disorders, 5th edition (DSM 5-TR) plays a significant role in guiding assessment, diagnosis, and treatment planning for treating depression in children and adolescents in educational settings. The DSM 5-TR offers a range of depressive disorders that may be relevant to children and adolescents, including Major Depressive Disorder (MDD),

Table 15.1 DSM 5-TR Criteria for Specific Depressive Disorders

Depressive Disorder	*DSM 5-TR Criteria*
Major Depressive Disorder (MDD)	According to the DSM 5-TR, to receive a diagnosis of MDD, five or more of the following symptoms must be present during the same two-week period and represent a change from previous functioning. The symptoms are (1) depressed mood most of the day, nearly every day, or irritability in children; (2) markedly diminished interest or pleasure in all, or almost all, activities most of the day nearly every day; (3) in a child, the failure to make their expected weight gain; (4) insomnia or hypersomnia nearly every day; (5) observed restlessness or being slowed down; (6) fatigue or loss of energy nearly every day; (7) feelings of worthlessness or excessive or inappropriate guilt nearly every day; (8) diminished ability to think or concentrate, or indecisiveness, nearly every day; or (9) recurrent thoughts of death, recurrent suicidal ideation without a specific plan, or a suicide attempt or a specific plan for committing suicide. In addition, at least one of the symptoms must be either depressed mood or loss of interest or pleasure. Diagnosis also requires that the symptoms cause clinically significant distress or impairment in social, occupational, or other important areas of functioning. The depressive episode may not be attributable to the physiological effects of a substance or to another medical condition. At least one major depressive episode may not be better explained by other psychotic disorders. There also should never have been a manic episode or hypomanic episode (American Psychiatric Association [APA], 2022)
Disruptive Mood Dysregulation Disorder (DMDD)	The DSM-5-TR defines DMDD by the following symptoms: (1) severe recurrent temper outbursts manifested verbally (e.g., verbal rages) and/or behaviorally (e.g., physical aggression toward people or property) that are grossly out of proportion in intensity or duration to the situation or provocation; (2) temper outbursts are inconsistent with developmental level; (3) temper outbursts occur, on average, three or more times per week; (4) all the former criteria have been present for 12 or more months with no period lasting 3 or more consecutive months without any symptoms; (5) all the former criteria are present in at least two of three settings (e.g., at home, at school, with peers) and are severe in at least one of these; (6) diagnosis is made for the 1st time between the ages of 6 and 18 years old; (7) there has never been a distinct period lasting more than one day during which the full symptom criteria, except duration, for a manic or hypomanic episode have been met (when developmentally inappropriate); (8) the behaviors do not occur exclusively during an episode of MDD and are not better explained by another mental disorder; and (9) the symptoms are not attributable to the physiological effects of a substance or to another medical or neurological condition. Note that this diagnosis cannot coexist with oppositional defiant disorder, intermittent explosive disorder, or bipolar disorder. It can, however, coexist with MDD, attention-deficit hyperactivity disorder, conduct disorder, and substance use disorders. There should not have been a manic or hypomanic episode (APA, 2022)

(*Continued*)

Table 15.1 (Continued)

Depressive Disorder	*DSM 5-TR Criteria*
Persistent Depressive Disorder (PDD)	In the DSM 5-TR, a diagnosis for dysthymia includes the following symptoms: (1) depressed mood for most of the day, for more days than not, and in children this can show as irritability for at least a year; (2) presence of two or more of poor appetite or overeating, insomnia or hypersomnia, low energy or fatigue, low self-esteem, poor concentration or difficulty making decisions, or feelings of hopelessness; (3) during the one year period of the disturbance the child has never been without the previously stated symptoms for more than two months at a time; (4) criteria for an MDD may be continuously present for two years; (5) there has never been a manic episode or a hypomanic episode, and criteria have never been met for cyclothymic disorder; (6) the disturbance is not better explained by another psychotic disorder; (7) the symptoms are not attributable to the physiological effects of a substance or other medical condition; and (8) the symptoms cause clinically significant distress or impairment in social, occupational, or other important areas of functioning (APA, 2022)

Disruptive Mood Dysregulation (DMDD), Persistent Depressive Disorder (PDD), and Other Specified and Unspecified Depressive Disorders. Each of these disorders has specific criteria that need to be met for a diagnosis to be made which are outlined in Table 15.1.

Individuals with Disabilities Education Act

Although the DSM 5-TR guides assessment and treatment planning, in an educational setting, the Individuals with Disabilities Education Act (IDEA) (2004) ensures students with disabilities have access to a free appropriate public education (FAPE). Under IDEA, depression can be considered a disabling condition that may impact a student's ability to access and benefit from his/her education. IDEA recognizes that students with mental health conditions, including depression, may require special education and related services to meet their unique needs. According to the disability categories included in IDEA, two are most relevant to children and adolescents struggling with symptoms associated with depression—Emotional Disturbance and Other Health Impairment (OHI). If a student qualifies due to a disability category and has educational need, the student is determined to be eligible for special education and an Individualized Education Program (IEP) is then developed by an educational team.

Emotional Disturbance

Under IDEA, an emotional disturbance (ED) qualifies as a condition exhibiting one or more of the following characteristics over a long period of time and to a marked degree that adversely affects a child's educational performance: (1) an inability to learn that cannot be explained by intellectual, sensory, or health factors; (2) an inability to build or maintain satisfactory interpersonal relationships with peers and teachers; (3) inappropriate types of behavior or feelings under normal circumstances; (4) a general pervasive mood of unhappiness or depression; and (5) a tendency to develop physical symptoms or fears associated with personal or school problems (U.S. Department of Education, 2004).

Other Health Impairment

According to IDEA, the definition of an OHI is a person who has limited strength, vitality, or alertness (including to environmental stimuli) which impacts the individual's ability to function in an educational environment. This condition is due to chronic or acute health problems, and it impacts the child's educational performance (U.S. Department of Education, 2004).

Individualized Education Program

If a student's depressive symptoms significantly impact his/her educational performance, he/she may be eligible for special education services. The student's educational team, including parents, educators, and other professionals, collaborate to develop an IEP. The IEP outlines the student's educational goals, accommodations, modifications, related services, and supports necessary to address the depression and ensure access to a FAPE. Examples of supports and services include individual or group counseling services from a qualified mental health professional, adjustments to the educational environment (e.g., extended time for tests, modified homework, preferential seating), social skills training, peer support programs, or transition planning if the student is older.

Section 504 of the Rehabilitation Act of 1973

A 504 plan is based on Section 504 of the Rehabilitation Act of 1973 and is intended to provide accommodations and support to students who have a physical or mental impairment that substantially limits one or more major life activities, including learning (U.S. Department of Education, 2010). Therefore, if a student is not suspected as having a disability that requires special education services, but rather has a disability that impacts his/her ability to access public education, accommodations may be more appropriate, and a 504 evaluation and subsequent accommodation plan may be implemented. Examples of accommodations for a student with a 504 plan tailored to depressive symptoms might include flexible deadlines, frequent breaks, self-care activities, preferential seating, note-taking support, reduced workload (e.g., providing alternative assignments, modifying existing assignments, providing options for homework), emotional support, communication plan, individual or group counseling, or social skills supports.

Empirical Support of CBT in Treatment of Depressive Disorders

In the last several decades, CBT has been considered the "Gold Standard" or the "best standard" in the field of psychology for treatment of depressive disorders. CBT is the most researched, is systematically sound, and aligns with the processes of one's mind more than many other psychotherapies (David et al., 2018). The reason CBT is researched more is because the treatment can be easily operationally defined and measured compared to other therapies. For researchers, this is an important component when determining the efficacy of any treatment. CBT has shown that it can work in many different settings and has an ability to be tailored to these settings and remain effective.

As previously stated, CBT is the most researched psychotherapy treatment. There is a considerable body of empirical evidence supporting the efficacy of CBT for the treatment of depression in children and adolescents. There are several meta-analytic reviews of randomized controlled trials (RCTs) that have consistently demonstrated that CBT is an effective intervention for reducing depressive symptoms in this population. For example, a meta-analysis conducted by Weisz and colleagues (2017) included 38 RCTs of psychological treatments for youth depression, including CBT. The authors found that CBT was significantly more effective than control conditions in reducing depressive symptoms, with a moderate effect size ($d = 0.58$). Moreover, the effects of CBT were comparable to those of other evidence-based treatments for depression, such as antidepressant medication and interpersonal psychotherapy. Another meta-analysis by Hetrick and colleagues (2016) included 28 RCTs of psychological treatments for depression. The authors found that CBT was significantly more effective than control conditions in reducing depressive symptoms, with a moderate effect size ($d = 0.38$). The effects of CBT in this study were also found to be comparable to those of other evidence-based treatments for adolescent depression. In both cases, CBT was found to be just as effective as pharmacological interventions and other psychotherapies.

In addition to these meta-analyses, other studies have shown the effectiveness that CBT offers. In 2004, the Treatment for Adolescents with Depression Study (TADS) published an RCT with 439 patients between the ages of 12 and 17 years old to evaluate the effectiveness of four treatments: Fluoxetine, CBT with Fluoxetine, CBT alone, or placebo (March et al., 2004). The results of this study showed that the use of CBT in combination with the drug was superior to just the drug alone, but that the drug alone was a better treatment than CBT alone. This was the case during the 1st 12 weeks that the study was initially checked. By week 18, however, CBT alone was found to be just as effective as the drug alone. The more time that was invested with CBT, the more effective it was (March et al., 2004). The TADS team also published an RCT in 2009 that revisited this topic but focused on length of time with a naturalistic follow-up. This study further emphasized that combined treatment was superior compared to solely one or the other. Furthermore, it showed that CBT was best used over a longer time period much like the previous study proved (March et al., 2009).

More specifically, a well-known cognitive-behavioral treatment that has been widely used and studied is the Coping With Depression (CWD) course. CWD focuses on psychoeducation in which a standardized protocol is followed independently by the patient through several modalities (e.g., laptop, CD, or TV). CWD can also be used in individual or group settings; however, it is more often used in groups. In the last decade or so, it has also been modified for use on the internet as well. CWD also focuses on providing a "toolbox" of skills that the patient can refer to later in life. Lastly, CWD can be administered by healthcare professionals, in addition to psychologists and mental health professionals (Clarke & Lewinsohn, 1989). CWD is also known for its adaptability and flexibility for target populations. When modifying an evidence-based intervention, such as CWD, Clarke and colleagues (2022) research suggested following the three pillars of evidence-based practice in psychology. One can do this by integrating the best available research with clinical expertise in the context of the patient's characteristics, culture, and preferences. A 30-year review of the CWD showed that in the RCT trials observed, it is one of the best cognitive-behavioral treatments that is adaptable for prevention, treatment, and relapse of depression (Cuijpers et al., 2009).

Overall, these meta-analytic reviews and additional studies provide strong empirical support for the efficacy of CBT in the treatment of depression in children and adolescents. Continually with time, CBT has been shown to be an effective and durable intervention for reducing depressive symptoms in this population, and its effects are comparable to those of other evidence-based treatments. There are several programs that have been created using CBT approaches and have shown tremendous results in treating depression in adolescents. These programs will be discussed later in this chapter.

Relational Consideration in Treatment of Depressive Disorders

One of the key symptoms associated with depression is withdrawal. When a child or adolescent is withdrawn from people that they used to find connection with, it can be difficult to find ways to draw them back in and find joy in those interactions again. In an educational setting, withdrawal can look like limited peer interaction, reduced participation, decreased eye contact, increased absenteeism, and avoidance of tasks or interactions with peers. In the treatment of depression in children and adolescents within educational settings, relational considerations play a significant role in promoting positive outcomes. Recognizing and addressing the relational dynamics and connections that students have with their teachers, peers, and family members can contribute to a more comprehensive and effective treatment approach. There are several key points to consider regarding relationships in the treatment of depression. Some include building a therapeutic alliance, school-home collaboration, peer support, teacher-student relationships, emotional regulation skills, communication skills, positive reinforcement, and culturally responsive approaches to treatment. It is important to recognize that each student is unique, to tailor interventions to the student's specific needs, and to understand these needs by having personalized discussions to consider strengths and areas of improvement.

Building a Therapeutic Alliance

Building a strong alliance between the student and the mental health professional is crucial. It involves establishing trust, empathy, and a supportive relationship, all of which can enhance treatment engagement and collaboration (Campbell & Simmonds, 2011). There are several ways that building an alliance can be achieved in an educational setting: (1) take the time to create a safe and welcoming environment where the student feels comfortable sharing thoughts and feelings and (2) establish trust and build rapport by showing empathy, actively listening, and validating their experiences (Murphy & Hutton, 2018). CBT in educational settings is generally manualized and can lack time to build an alliance with the child or adolescent (Fernandes, 2022). Because of this, it is also important to involve the student in the treatment process as much as possible and to ensure the student has time to connect with the people he/she is working with in the educational setting. This can be done by setting goals together, which ensures that the student's input and preferences are considered. Moreover, it empowers the student to take ownership of his/her mental health journey.

School-Home Collaboration

Collaborating with parents/guardians and teachers is essential to understanding each student's unique context, gathering valuable insights, and implementing consistent strategies across various settings. This collaboration promotes a holistic approach to treatment. Keeping open lines of communication with the student, their parents, and relevant staff is key to having effective treatment. Open lines of communication may include regularly updating progress, providing feedback, addressing any concerns or questions, and using various methods to communicate (e.g., emails, phone calls, or in-person meetings) to discuss interventions being used and any challenges the student may be facing. It is important to actively involve parents/guardians in the student's educational journey by (1) seeking their input, perspectives, and insights regarding any needs; (2) encouraging the family to participate in school activities, meetings, and decision-making processes; (3) providing resources, workshops, or training sessions for parents/guardians on understanding depression and supporting their child's mental health; and (4) offering information on community resources, support groups, and counseling services that exist outside of the school.

Peer Support

Encouraging positive peer relationships and fostering a supportive social environment can contribute to the student's emotional well-being. Activities that promote social interaction, empathy, and inclusivity can help reduce feelings of isolation and enhance the student's sense of belonging. One example is the use of peer mentoring programs. This is where older students or trained peer mentors provide support and guidance to students with depressive disorders. The mentor can offer a listening ear, share coping strategies, and help navigate the school environment. Using psychoeducational projects to educate peers on depression is also a way to empower students dealing with depressive symptoms (i.e., Peer-to-Peer Depression Awareness Program; Parikh et al., 2018). Encourage students to talk with peers and share experiences through presentations, workshops (e.g., sensitivity training, social skills training), or awareness campaigns. In doing this, students are promoting understanding and reducing the stigma (Lapshina et al., 2019).

Teacher-Student Relationships

Nurturing positive relationships between teachers and students can create a supportive and validating educational environment. Teachers who demonstrate understanding, patience, and flexibility can positively influence the student's motivation, engagement, and overall well-being. A teacher who establishes a warm and inclusive classroom environment allows students to feel safe, valued, and respected (Cook et al., 2018; Martin & Collie, 2019). It is imperative to take the time to understand each student's unique challenges and experiences and offer support, encouragement, and reassurance when needed. The teacher can also schedule regular one-on-one check-ins with students to offer guidance or address emotional needs (i.e., The Adolescent Goal-Setting Intervention; Lind et al., 2017). Professional development and training can provide teachers opportunities to learn active listening skills and effective strategies for supporting students (Krane et al., 2017).

Emotional Regulation Skills

Teaching children and adolescents effective emotional regulation skills can empower them to cope with depressive symptoms. Strategies such as mindfulness exercises (e.g., deep breathing exercises, body scans, and guided imagery), self-reflection (e.g., self-care practices, social supports, and problem-solving), and emotion-focused activities (e.g., identifying emotions, cognitive restructuring, and role-playing) can aid in emotional regulation and resiliency. It is important to involve the student as much as possible in setting personal goals related to regulating his/her emotions and to work together to establish measurable and achievable goals that can be tracked over time (Malboeuf-Hurtubise et al., 2018).

Communication Skills

Enhancing students' communication skills can facilitate the expression of emotions, needs, and concerns. Teaching assertiveness, active listening, and conflict resolution skills can support healthier interactions with peers, teachers, and family members. The student should be taught healthy listening skills, such as maintaining eye contact, nodding, and providing appropriate verbal and nonverbal cues. The student should also be taught to reflect on what the speaker is saying to ensure the student understands. Another effective communication skill is expressing emotions. The use of "I" statements (e.g., "I feel sad when…" or "I am upset because…") allows the student to be calm and use respect when communicating feelings. Other skills include empathy, conflict resolution (e.g., negotiation skills and compromising), and clarifying (McGinnis & Goldstein, 2019). It is important to note that digital communication is rising, and these skills should be extended to online environments. Digital etiquette and being mindful of tone are important skills when communicating through social media or text.

Positive Reinforcement

Recognizing and reinforcing each individual student's strengths, achievements, and progress can boost self-esteem and motivation. Whenever possible, celebrating the student's small victories and providing specific praise and encouragement to reinforce his/her strengths encourages a growth mindset, fosters a positive outlook, and promotes resiliency. Examples to keep in mind when using positive reinforcement include verbal praise, reward systems, individualized incentives, public or social recognition, certificates or rewards, special privileges, or extra time to do things the student loves (Cooper et al., 2020; Hardy & McLeod, 2020; Scott & Landrum, 2020).

Culturally Responsive Approach

Valuing students' cultural background and experiences is essential. Taking cultural factors such as beliefs, values, and traditions into account can enhance treatment relevance, engagement, and effectiveness. Being sensitive to culture ensures that interventions are appropriate and inclusive. Using tools that consider diverse family dynamics on the topic of depression can be effective. For instance, some students may come from a culture that has different beliefs on mental health. There could be a stigma surrounding poor mental health or a stigma about reaching out for help. Within the school setting, it is important to create a culture that surrounds inclusion and acceptance by celebrating diversity and promoting positive relationships and to encourage students to reach out, include others, and show kindness and support to their peers (Higgen & Mosko, 2020).

By considering these relational aspects, educators, mental health professionals, and parents/caregivers can create an environment that promotes positive relationships, emotional well-being, and effective treatment outcomes for children and adolescents within educational settings. Above all, maintaining a consistent presence in the student's life and being a reliable, dependable, and responsive model for the student will foster effective treatment outcomes.

Interviewing and Assessing for Depressive Disorders

When identifying a child or adolescent with depressive disorders, there are multiple avenues to consider. The assessment process plays a vital role in identifying depression in children and adolescents. Assessing for depression in educational settings requires a multifaceted approach that considers the unique developmental and contextual factors affecting children and adolescents. Because there are many ways to receive information, it is essential to have a systematic approach to interview and assess to effectively support individuals. This process involves gathering comprehensive information about the student's emotional well-being, behaviors, and cognitive functioning. By employing appropriate assessment techniques, educators and mental health professionals can identify potential symptoms and risk factors, determine the severity of the condition, and develop tailored interventions and support plans. The aim is to promote early detection and effective support for those experiencing depression.

Interviewing

Clinical interviewing serves as a valuable method for gathering pertinent information about children and adolescents and for gaining insight into the symptoms they may be encountering. While general inquiries directed toward parents or guardians and teachers can provide initial insights, structured clinical interviews (SCI) offer a more systematic and standardized approach to collecting this data. These SCIs enable clinicians to obtain comprehensive information about the individual's developmental and medical history, as well as his/her specific symptoms, experiences, and behaviors. By employing a structured interview approach, clinicians can ensure a thorough and consistent assessment process that aids in understanding the child or adolescent's condition. Commonly used SCIs include the *Behavior Assessment System for Children, Third Edition Structured Developmental*

History (BASC-3 SDH; Reynolds & Kamphaus, 2015) and the *Diagnostic Interview Schedule for Children, Fourth Edition* (DISC-IV; Shaffer et al., 2000).

Assessing

When considering the assessment of children and adolescents, it is crucial to prioritize empirically supported and evidence-based measures such as the BASC-3 SDH and DISC-IV. However, it is also important to consider factors like cost and efficiency. In this regard, brief rating scale screeners offer a practical and widely used option in school settings. These screeners typically involve obtaining ratings from parents, teachers, and self-reports from students themselves and then measuring how relative the scores are compared to the students' peers (National Association of School Psychologists [NASP], 2020). By using rating scales, multiple issues can be screened simultaneously, allowing for the classification of individuals who may benefit from targeted, specific interventions. It is worth noting that two common approaches for identifying children and adolescents include narrowband and broadband measures, each offering unique insights into their emotional and behavioral well-being.

Broadband Measures

Prior to identifying depressive symptoms specifically, the clinician may use broadband measures that pinpoint the areas where the child is experiencing problems. These measures use a wide range of symptoms to diagnose. These raters consider a variety of symptoms, such as anxiety, irritability, sleep disturbance, or eating disturbance, in addition to the symptoms used by narrowband raters (outlined below). Examples of broadband measures include rating scales such as the *Behavior Assessment System for Children, Third Edition* (BASC-3; Reynolds & Kamphaus, 2015); *Beck Youth Inventories, Second Edition* (BYI-2 ; Beck et al., 2005); *Behavior and Symptom Identification Scale* (BASIS-32; Eisen et al., 2019); *Mood and Feelings Questionnaire* (MFQ; Angold & Costello, 1995); *Youth Self-Report* (YSF; Achenbach & Rescorla, 2001); and *Patient Health Questionnaire for Adolescents* (PHQ-A; Johnson et al., 2002).

Narrowband Measures

Assessment tools used to identify specific criteria for depression are narrow measures. These raters use a limited set of symptoms, such as sadness, hopelessness, and loss of interest to identify cases of depression. The advantage of narrowband measures is that they are more reliable and have a higher degree of diagnostic accuracy than broad measures. Examples of narrowband measures that are used for identifying depression in children and adolescents include the *Children's Depression Inventory, Second Edition* (CDI-2, Kovacs, 2011); *Reynolds Adolescent Depression Scale* (RADS; Reynolds, 2019); *Beck Depression Inventory for Youth* (BDI-Y; Beck et al., 2005); *Child Rating Scale-Revised* (CDRS-R; Shaffer et al., 2002); and the *Diagnostic Interview Schedule for Children* (DISC-IV; Shaffer et al., 2000).

Monitoring: Assessment of Progress and Outcomes

Outcome data is pivotal for families to understand the effects of interventions as well as for professionals to make informed decisions about the need for an individual to continue receiving treatment—individually, in a group, or to discontinue. Additionally, data collected over time by a school district allows teams to make decisions regarding ongoing programming within a school-based mental health system. While the literature is helpful in informing decision makers, ultimately the local data in terms of what is working within a school is what matters when it is time to decide what interventions are working for the population. Many of the above broad-band and narrow-band instruments can be used to collect data pre-intervention, progress monitoring data, and post-intervention. Many also collect post-intervention follow-up data several weeks and months after an intervention. This data collectively helps to make individual, group, and systems-based decisions. Often professionals working in schools team-up with others to assist with the data-analysis aspect of intervention decision making due to job demands and access to resources to complete the analysis.

Case Conceptualization

Case conceptualization, or the formulation of a case, is the process in which a client and mental health professional work together to define the issues relevant to therapy. The function of this process is to guide therapy. Research has found that the more capable a mental health professional is in using case conceptualization with CBT for the treatment of depression, the more depressive symptoms in the client are reduced (Easden & Fletcher, 2018). In general, case conceptualization can be thought of as a collaborative process that incorporates the client's strengths. In CBT, case conceptualization is a process of gathering relevant history, determining maintaining factors, understanding values, and developing goals (a treatment plan).

In the treatment of depression, relevant history regarding family history of depressive disorders, duration of depressive feelings, information regarding suicidal ideations as well as attention to possible comorbid disorders are all important. In terms of maintaining behaviors, questions regarding thinking styles, structure of one's day, participation in pleasant activities, such as extra curriculars or social events, problem-solving patterns, re-occurring thoughts, and/or concerns about the future are examples of topics that are relevant to gather information about when working with a client struggling with symptoms of depression. As a part of this process, it is also important to gather an understanding for the child or adolescent's values. For example, what is working and what is not working for the child or adolescent in his/her life. If something could change, what would the child or adolescent want to change the most and why. This type of discussion during the case conceptualization process helps the client and the therapist to move on to develop meaningful, shared goals.

Some examples of CBT goals and session content for individuals or groups that are designed to target depression are provided below. When developing goals, the values of the child or adolescent as well as his/her readiness to change must be a priority during goal development. A client's readiness to change is pivotal in the case conceptualization process.

Intervention with Depressive Disorders

There are both individual and group-based interventions that are designed to prevent and intervene with children and adolescents to reduce symptoms associated with depression. While many intervention programs designed for group therapy are also used in individual therapy (and vice-versa), what is described below is what has been explored empirically in the research. Fundamentally, CBT is the approach that is used in individual therapy, which ultimately requires no manual, but rather the techniques previously reviewed in this chapter. The customization involved in individual-based CBT has produced fewer individual manuals in the literature compared to group-based manuals, which require a bit more pre-planning of materials.

Table 15.2 contains a variety of resources to consider using for individualized therapy to prevent and/or treat depression in children and adolescents. While there are many resources to use for individual therapy that address depression, there are few manuals developed for this purpose.

Table 15.2 Examples of CBT Goals and Session Content in the Treatment of Depression

Example Goals	*Example Session Content*
Find evidence for how one's thoughts impact behaviors	Fill out thought bubbles after both negative and positive events to help the child examine his/her thinking
Find evidence for how one's behaviors impact feelings	Teach the child to identify activating events and identifying a picture after that represents one's feelings (e.g., using a SUDS scale)
Identify cognitive distortions	Use direct instruction with examples and nonexamples of common cognitive distortions—playing a game using thought cards to identify these
Replace cognitive distortions	Reframe thinking by using a simple three step process—Stop, Rewind, Rethink
	Use a "Challenge that Thought" wheel that the child spins and the arrow lands on a prompt that guides he/she to re-think
Increase positive thinking patterns about self and/or the world (reduce negative thinking patterns)	Create a Gratitude journal or keep a gratitude jar Use guided practice on changing negative thoughts into positive thoughts by playing games, such as "Catch it, Check it, Change it"
Increase pleasant activities and/or coping skills	Create a menu of pleasant activities with familiar activities that have been found to be effective and ones that are new to try and track the outcome—over time the menu will grow and change
	Schedule pleasant activities (Be specific)
Improve daily routine	Develop a preferred way for the child to organize and/or plan his/her day (e.g., planner, visuals, and calendar)

Table 15.3 Individual Evidence-Based Prevention and Intervention Resources for Depression

Resource Name	*Authors*
Individual Therapy Manual for CBT of Depression	Munoz and Miranda (1996)
CBT Toolbox for Depressed, Anxious, & Suicidal Children and Adolescents	Pratt (2019)
Think Good, Feel Good Note: There is also a separate Clinician's Guide.	Stallard (2002)
The Negative Thoughts Workbook: CBT Skills to Overcome the Repetitive Worry, Shame, and Rumination That Drive Anxiety and Depression	Clarke (2020)
The Cognitive Behavioral Workbook for Depression: A Step-by-Step Program	Knaus and Ellis (2012)
CBT Toolbox for Children and Adolescents	Phifer et al. (2017)

One well-known and published individualized manual is the Individual Therapy Manual for CBT of Depression (Munoz & Miranda, 1996). The Individual Therapy Manual for CBT of Depression was originally created for adults, but later developments explored its use with adolescents and specific studies have looked at its effectiveness with diverse populations including Puerto Rican adolescents (Munoz & Miranda, 1996; Munoz et al., 2007). This intervention is a 12-session intervention designed to intervene with individuals struggling with depression. Table 15.3 includes this manual as well as other resources to consider using for the delivery of individualized work with children and adolescents in the treatment of depression.

As mentioned above, more manuals exist for group-based CBT interventions that address depression for children and adolescents. In part, this is because there is less customization with group-based work and more planning involved ahead of time to keep the group moving in the same direction and working on similar goals. A summary is provided in Table 15.4 of group-based, efficacious programs that are designed to target the prevention and intervention of depression, which vary in terms of duration and age. While these programs have been explored in the literature with mostly positive outcomes, local group-based data should be collected to determine if they are effective in specific settings.

iCBT or C-CBT

While individual and group-based online therapy is growing and presents opportunities for children and adolescents to access services outside of school, it is largely underexplored in the literature. For CBT purposes, this method of delivery is termed internet-based CBT or iCBT or computerized CBT or C-CBT (Anderson & Cuijpers, 2009; Andersson & Titov, 2014). There are both "supported" or interaction-based programs and "unsupported" or no interaction programs. The initial research on this topic has found that adolescents appear to prefer and benefit from supportive or interactive-based programs that provide feedback (Grist et al., 2018; Topooco et al., 2018). However, in adult populations, some research has found a statistically significant reduction in depressive symptoms after participation in only unsupported or no interaction programs (Leykin et al., 2014).

Applications to the School Setting

Using a CBT to intervene with depression in the school setting is ideal due to the psycho-educational nature of the content and the session structure that often involves skill development, including direct instruction and guided practice as well as review of content and homework. With 17% of adolescents aged 12–17 years old reportedly having at least one major depressive episode in their life (SAMHSA, 2021), interventions that target depression are critical to the social-emotional development of children and adolescents. As discussed earlier, children and adolescents who struggle with depression also often struggle academically in school—further emphasizing why supporting students who struggle with depression is so important. The severity of prevalence of depression in combination with the challenges in getting children and adolescents into private practices (e.g., time outside of school, cost, and transportation) underscores the value of delivering these services in a natural setting like the school.

In this chapter, information about depression including assessment and intervention methods have been shared. These methods have direct application to the school setting as they are naturally conducive to the schedule and systems already in place within these environments. Many of the assessment methods discussed can be used to collect pre-test, post-test, or progress monitoring data approaches commonly used for academic interventions. Some measures may even be used during similar times as other routine academic tasks. For example, a depression or mental health screener could be included during other school wide screeners or new depression groups might begin every quarter. In addition to these examples, many of the interventions discussed in this chapter can be adjusted to meet time/duration needs within each building in a district. For example, if there are 45 or 60-minute periods or one activity period per week, these interventions are adaptable for implementation. Finally, schools offer an opportunity for multiple observers to support children and adolescents in improving symptoms associated with depression. They are natural environments that also provide opportunity for generalization across a variety of settings (e.g., classroom, cafeteria, recess, and extra curriculars), which can be scaffolded over time to support continued development.

Table 15.4 Group Evidence-Based Prevention and Intervention Groups for Depression

Program Name	*Prevention and/or Intervention*	*Weeks or Modules*	*Ages*	*Authors*
POD-Teams	Prevention	Eight sessions (90 minutes each)	Adolescence	Garber et al. (2009)
Penn Resiliency Program	Prevention	12 sessions (90 minutes each)	9–14	Gillham et al. (2006)
Blues Program	Prevention	Six hours of sessions	15–18	Rohde et al. (2019)
Adolescent Coping with Depression Course (CWDA)	Intervention	16 sessions (two hours each)	13–19	Clarke et al. (1990)
ACTION Program	Intervention	30 sessions (one hour each)	8–13 (female)	Stark et al. (2006)
Teaching Kids to Cope	Intervention	Ten sessions (45 minutes each)	15–18 and 19–24	Puskar et al. (1997)
MATCH-ADTC	Intervention	33 modules or strategies	6–15	Chorpita and Weisz (2009)
Stressbusters	Intervention	Eight sessions (45 minutes each)	8–12	Asarnow et al. (2002)

Summary

The use of CBT to treat depression in educational settings has shown promising results. CBT equips young individuals with the tools to manage depressive symptoms and improve overall well-being. As noted within the chapter, several studies have provided empirical support for the effectiveness of CBT in this population. Research has demonstrated significant reductions in depressive symptoms, improved overall functioning, and long-term benefits, such as prevention of relapse and recurrence. CBT interventions have been successfully implemented in schools, where mental health professionals work collaboratively with educators to provide targeted support and interventions tailored to the unique needs of students.

The success of CBT can be attributed to its focus on addressing both cognitive and behavioral aspects of depression. CBT helps individuals challenge negative thoughts, reframe them in a more realistic and positive light, and develop healthier behavioral responses. CBT interventions incorporate skill-building activities, such as problem-solving, social skills training, and emotion regulation techniques. This comprehensive approach equips students with necessary tools to navigate challenges, enhance resilience, and improve overall mental health. By integrating CBT into educational settings, schools can create a supportive and empowering environment that promotes emotional and mental well-being, academic success, and positive social relationships.

Reflection Questions

1 What is one opportunity discussed in this chapter that may help you to improve your supports for students who are struggling with symptoms of depression?
2 What are one or two resources or evidence-based interventions that you want to explore to consider using with children and/or adolescents struggling with at-risk levels and/or clinic levels of depression?
3 Describe one way to utilize data to improve the way you screen or monitor students struggling with symptoms associated with depression?

References

Achenbach, T. M., & Rescorla, L. A. (2001). *Manual for the ASEBA school-age forms & profiles*. University of Vermont Research Center for Children, Youth, & Families (Vol. 80). Burlington, VT: Achenbach System of Empirically Based Assessment Research Center.

American Psychiatric Association (APA) (2022). *Diagnostic and statistical manual of mental disorders* (5th ed.). Washington DC: American Psychiatric Publishing.

Anderson, G., & Cuijpers, P. (2009). Internet-based and other computerized psychological treatments for adult depression: A meta-analysis. *Cognitive Behavioral Therapy, 38* (4), 196–205.

Andersson G., & Titov N. (2014). Advantages and limitations of internet-based interventions for common mental disorders. *World Psychiatry, 13* (1), 4–11.

Angold, A., & Costello, E. J. (1995). *Mood and feelings questionnaire (MFQ)*. Durham, NC: Duke University Medical Center.

Asarnow, J. R., Scott, C., & Mintz, J. (2002). Cognitive-behavioral treatment and family interventions for children with depression. A combined cognitive-behavioral family education intervention for depression in children: A treatment development study. *Cognitive Therapy and Research, 26*, 221–229. https://doi.org/10.1023/A:1014573803928

Barret, P. M., Farrell, L. J., Ollendick, T. H., & Dadds, M. (2006). *FRIENDS for life: Groupleaders manual for children*. Queensland, Australia: Australian Academic Press.

Beck, J. S., Beck, A. T., & Jolly, J. B. (2005). *Beck youth inventories, 2nd edition: Manual*. San Antonio, TX: Psychological Corporation.

Campbell, A. F., & Simmonds, J. G. (2011). Therapist perspectives on the therapeutic alliance with children and adolescents. *Counseling Psychology Quarterly, 24*(3), 195–209. https://doi.org/10.1080/09515070.2011.620734

Chand, S. P., Kuckel, D. P., & Huecker, M. R. (2022). *Cognitive behavior therapy*. St. Petersburg, FL: StatPearls Publishing.

Chorpita, B., & Weisz, J. R. (2009). MATCH-ADTC: *Modular approach to therapy for children with anxiety, depression, trauma, or conduct problems*. Troy, MI: Practice Wise LLC.

Clarke, A. T., Soto, G. E., Cook, J., Iloanusi, C., Akwarandu, A., & Parris, V. S. (2022). Adaptation of the coping with stress course for black adolescents in low-income communities: Examples of surface structure and deep structure cultural adaptations. *Cognitive and Behavioral Practice, 29*(4), 738–749. https://doi.org/10.1016/j.cbpra.2021.04.005

Clarke, D. (2020). *The negative thoughts workbook: CBT skills to overcome the repetitive worry, shame, and rumination that drive anxiety and depression*. Oakland, CA: New Harbinger Publications.

Clarke, G., & Lewinsohn, P. M. (1989). The Coping with Depression Course: A group psychoeducational intervention for unipolar depression. *Behaviour Change, 6*(2), 54–69.

Clarke, G., Lewinsohn, P. M., & Hops, H. (1990, August). *Adolescent coping with depression (TheCWD-A)*. Center for Health Research. Retrieved August 28, 2008, from http://www.kpchr.org/

Cook, C. R., Coco, S., Zhang, Y., Fiat, A. E., Duong, M. T., Renshaw, T. L., Long, A. C., & Frank, S. (2018). Cultivating positive teacher-student relationships: Preliminary evaluation of the establish-maintain-restore (EMR) method. *School Psychology Review, 47*(3), 226– 243. https://doi.org/10.17105/SPR-2017-0025.V47-3

Cooper, J. O., Heron, T. E., & Heward, W. L. (2020). *Applied behavior analysis* (3rd ed.). Boston, MA: Pearson Education.

Cuijpers, P., Munoz, R. F., Clarke, G. N., & Lewinsohn, P. M. (2009). Psychoeducational treatment and prevention of depression: The "coping with depression" course thirty years later. *Clinical Psychology Review, 29*(5), 449–458. https://doi.org/10.1016/j.cpr.2009.04.005

David, D., Cristea, I., & Hofmann, S. G. (2018). Why cognitive behavioral therapy is the current gold standard of psychotherapy. *Frontiers in Psychiatry, 9*(4), 1–3. https://doi.org/10.3389/fpsyt.2018.00004

Domitrovich, C. E., & Greenber, M. T. (2017). *The PATHS program for promoting social and emotional competence in children*. Champaign, IL: Research Press.

Easden, M. H., & Fletcher, R. B. (2018). Therapist competence in case conceptualization and outcome in CBT for depression. *Psychotherapy Research*. https://doi.org/10.1080/10503307.2018.1540895

Eisen, S. V., Grob, M. C., Klein, A. A., & Lefkowitz, D. S. (2019). *BASIS-32: Behavior and symptom identification scale, 5th edition: Administration and scoring manual*. Bloomington, MN: Pearson Assessments.

Fernandes, H. (2022). Therapeutic alliance in cognitive behavioural therapy in child and adolescent mental health–current trends and future challenges. *Frontiers in Psychology, 12*(610874). https://doi.org/10.3389/fpsyg.2021.610874

Flanagan, R., Allen, K., & Levine, E. (2015). *Cognitive and behavioral interventions in the schools integrating theory and research into practice*. Springer Science+Business Media. https://doi.org/1007/978-1-4939-1972-7_5

Garber, J., Clarke, G. N., Weersing, V. R., Beardslee, W. R., Brent, D. A., Gladstone, T. R., DeBar, L. L., Lynch, F. L., D'Angelo, E., Hollon, S. D., Shamseddeen, W., & Iyengar, S. (2009). Prevention of depression in at-risk adolescents: A randomized controlled trial. *JAMA, 301*(21), 215–224.

Gillham, J. E., Hamilton, J., Freres, D. R., Patton, K., & Gallop, R. (2006). Preventing depression among early adolescents in the primary care setting: A randomized controlled study of the Penn Resiliency Program. *Journal of Abnormal Child Psychology, 34*(2), 203–219. https://doi.org/10.1007/s10802-005-90147.

Gresham, F. M., & Elliot, S. N. (2017). *Social skills improvement system (SSIS) rating scales*. Bloomington, MN: Pearson.

Grist, R., Croker, A., Denne, M., & Stallard, P. (2018). Technology delivered interventions for depression and anxiety in children and adolescents: A systematic review and meta analysis. *Clinical Child and Family Psychology Review, 22*, 147–171.

Hardy, J. K., & McLeod, R. H. (2020). Using positive reinforcement with young children. *Beyond Behavior, 29*(2), 95–107. https://doi.org/10.1177/1074295620915724

Hetrick, S. E., Cox, G. R., Witt, K. G., Bir, J. J., Merry, S. N., & Turnbull, D. A. (2016). Cognitive behavioural therapy (CBT), third-wave CBT and interpersonal therapy (IPT)based interventions for preventing depression in children and adolescents. *CochraneDatabase of Systematic Reviews, 8*, CD003380. https://doi.org/10.1002/14651858.CD003380.pub4

Higgen, S., & Mosko, M. (2020). Mental health and cultural and linguistic diversity as challenges in school? An interview study on the implications for students and teachers. *PLoS One, 15*(17), e0236160. https://doi.org/10.1371/journal.pone.0236160

Individuals with Disabilities Education Act (IDEA) (2004). Individuals with disabilities education act, 20 U.S.C. § 1400.

Johnson, J. G., Harris, E. S., Spitzer, R. L., & Williams, J. W. (2002). The patient health questionnaire for adolescents: Validation of an instrument for the assessment of mental disorders among adolescent primary care patients. *Journal of Adolescent Health, 30*(3), 196–204.

Knaus, W., & Ellis, A. (2012). *The Cognitive behavioral workbook for depression: A step-by step program*. Oakland, CA: New Harbinger Publications.

Kovacs, M. (2011). *Children's depression inventory, 2nd edition: Technical manual*. Ontario, CA: Multi-Health Systems.

Krane, V., Ness, O., Holter-Sorensen, N., Karlsson, B., & Binder, P. E. (2017). 'You notice that there is something positive about going to school': How teachers; kindness can promote positive teacher-student relationships in upper secondary school. *International Journal of Adolescence and Youth, 22*(4), 377–389. https://doi.org/10.1080/02673843.2016.1202843

Lapshina, N., Crooks, C. V., & Kerry, A. (2019). Changes in depression and positive mental health among youth in a healthy relationships program. *Canadian Journal of School Psychology, 34*(4), 300–316. https://doi.org/10.1177/0829573518777154

Leykin, Y., Munoz, R., Contreras, O., & Latham, M. (2014). Results from a trail of an unsupported internet intervention for depressive symptoms. *Internet Intervention, 1*(4), 175–181.

Lind, J., Poppen, M., & Murray, C. (2017). An intervention to promote positive teacher-student relationships and self-determination among adolescents with emotional disturbance. *Career Development and Transition for Exceptional Individuals, 40*(3), 186–191. https://doi.org/10.1177/2165143416683936

Malbocuf-Hurtubise, C., Joussemet, M., Taylor, G., & Lacourse, E. (2018). Effects of a mindfulness-based intervention on the perception of basic psychological need satisfaction among special education students. *International Journal of Disability, Development, and Education, 65*(1), 33–44. https://doi.org/10.1080/1034912X.2017.1346236

March, J., Silva, S., Curry, J., Wells, K., Fairbank, J., Burns, B., & Domino, M., (2009). The treatment for adolescents with depression study (TADS): Outcomes over 1 year naturalistic follow-up. *American Journal of Psychiatry, 166*(10), 1141–1149.

March, J., Silva, S., Petrycki, S., Curry, J., Wells, K., Fairbank, J., Burns, B., Domino, M., & McNulty, S. (2004). Fluoxetine, cognitive-behavioral therapy, and their combination for adolescents with depression: Treatment for adolescents with depression study (TADS) randomized controlled trial. *JAMA, 292*(7), 807–820.

Martin, A. J., & Collie, R. J. (2019). Teacher-student relationships and students' engagement in high school: Does the number of negative and positive relationships with teacher matter? *Journal of Educational Psychology, 111*(5), 861–876. https://doi.org/10.1037/edu0000317

McGinnis, E., & Goldstein, A. P. (2019). *Skillstreaming the elementary school child: New strategies and perspectives for teaching prosocial skills*. Champaign, IL: Research Press.

Munoz, R. F., Aguilar-Gaxiola, S., & Guzman, J. (2007). *Treatment manual for cognitive behavioral therapy for depression: Adaptation for Puerto Rican adolescents*. San Fransisco, CA: San Francisco General Hospital, Depression Clinic.

Munoz, R. F., & Miranda, J. (1996). Individual therapy manual for cognitive-behavioral treatment of depression. Santa Monica, CA: RAND.

Murphy, R., & Hutton, P. (2018). Practitioner review: Therapist variability, patient-reported therapeutic alliance, and clinical outcomes in adolescents undergoing mental health treatment–a systematic review and meta-analysis. *Journal of Child Psychology and Psychiatry, 59*(1), 5–19. https://doi.org/10.1111/jcpp.12767

National Association of School Psychologists (NASP) (2020). *Providing effective social-emotional and behavioral supports after COVID-19 closures: Universal screening and Tier 1 interventions* [handout]. Author.

National Institute of Mental Health (NIMH) (2022, January). *Major Depression*. Retrieved from https://www.nimh.nih.gov/health/statistics/major-depression

Parikh, S. V., Taubman, D. S., Antoun, C., Cranford, J., Ewell Foster, C., Grambeau, M., Hunter, J., Jester, J., Konz, K., Meyer, T., Salazar, S., & Greden, J. F. (2018). The Michigan peer-to peer depression awareness program: School-based prevention to address depression among teens. *Psychiatric Services, 69*(4), 487–491. https://doi.org/10.1176/appi.ps.201700101

Phifer, L., Crowder, A., Elsenraat, T., & Hull, R. (2017). *CBT toolbox for children and adolescents*. Eau Claire, WI: PESI Publishing & Media.

Pratt, D.M. (2019). CBT toolbox for depressed, anxious, & suicidal children and adolescents. Eau Claire, WI: PESI Publishing & Media.

Puskar, K. R., Lamb, J., & Tusaie-Mumford, K. (1997). Teaching kids to cope: A preventative mental health nursing strategy for adolescents. *Journal of Child Adolescent Psychiatry Nursing, 10*(3), 18–28. https://doi.org/10.1111/j.1744-6171.1997.tb00410.x.

Reynolds, C. R., & Kamphaus, R. W. (2015). *Behavior assessment system for children* (3rd ed.). Bloomington, MN: Pearson Assessments.

Reynolds, W. M. (2019). *Reynolds adolescent depression scale, 2nd edition: Professional manual*. Lutz, FL: Psychological Assessment Resources.

Rohde, P., Stice, E., & Shaw, H. (2019). *The Blues Program: 6-session CB depressionprevention intervention group facilitator script*. Leola, PA: Oregon Research Institute.

Scott, T. M., & Landrum, T. J. (2020). An evidence-based logic for the use of positive reinforcement: Responses to typical criticisms. *Beyond Behavior, 29*(2), 69–77. https://doi.org/10.1177/1074295620917153

Shaffer, D., Fisher, P., Lucas, C. P., Dulcan, M. K., & Schwab-Stone, M. E. (2000). NIMH Diagnostic Interview Schedule for Children Version IV (NIMH DISC-IV): Description, differences from previous version, and reliability of some common diagnoses. *Journal of the American Academy of Child & Adolescent Psychiatry, 39*(1), 28–38.

Shaffer, D., Piacentini, J., & Reynolds, A. M. (2002). *Child depression rating scale-revised*. Ontario, CA: Multi-Health Systems.

Stallard, P. (2002). *Think good – feel good: A cognitive behavioral therapy workbook for children and young people*. Hoboken, NJ: Wiley.

Stark, K. D., Hargrave, J., Sander, J., Custer, G., Schnoebelen, S., Simpson, J., & Molnar, J. (2006). Treatment of childhood depression: The ACTION treatment program. In P. C. Kendall (Ed.), *Child and adolescent therapy: Cognitive-behavioral procedures* (pp. 169–216). New York: The Guilford Press.

Substance Abuse and Mental Health Services Administration (SAMHSA) (2021). *Reasons for receiving most recent mental health service in past year* (210603) [Data set]. National Survey on Drug Use and Health. Retrieved from https://www.samhsa.gov/data/sites/default/files/reports/rpt35323/NSDUHDetailedTabs2020v25/NSDUHDetailedTabs2020v25/NSDUHDetTabsSect9pe2020.htm

Topooco, N., et al. (2018). Chat- and internet-based cognitive-behavioral therapy in treatment of adolescent depression: Randomized controlled trial. *Behavioral Journal of Psychology Open*, 199–207. https://doi.org/10.1192/bjo.2018.18

United States Department of Education (2004). Individuals with Disabilities Education Improvement Act of 2004, Pub. L. No. 108-446, 118 Stat. 2647.

U.S. Department of Education (2010). *Office for Civil Rights, Free Appropriate Public Education for Students with Disabilities: Requirements under* Section 504 *of the Rehabilitation Act of 1973*. Washington, DC: Education Publications.

Weisz, J. R., Kuppens, S., Ng, M. Y., Eckshtain, D., Ugueto, A. M., Vaughn-Coaxum, R., & Fordwood, S. R. (2017). What five decades of research tells us about the effects of youth psychological therapy: A multilevel meta-analysis and implications for science and practice. *American Psychologist, 72*(2), 79–117. https://doi.org/10.1037/a0040360

Wijnhoven, L. A., Creemers, D. H., Vermulst, A. A., Scholte, R. H., & Engels, R. C. (2014). Randomized controlled Trial Testing the effectiveness of a depression prevention program ('Op Volle Kracht') among adolescent girls with elevated depressive symptoms. *Journal of Abnormal Child Psychology, 42*(1), 217–228. https://doi.org/10.1007/s10802-013-9773- 5

16
BIPOLAR DISORDER

Sally M. Weinstein and Amy E. West

Children and adolescents with bipolar spectrum disorders experience extreme and chronic mood dysregulation, including irritability, rage episodes, excessive elation or sadness, distractibility, grandiosity, a decreased need for sleep, and poor judgment. The symptoms of pediatric bipolar disorder (PBD) contribute to significant psychosocial impairment (Frías et al., 2017; Goldstein et al., 2009a, 2009b; Mendez et al., 2020) and reduced quality of life (Freeman et al., 2009). Specifically, youth with PBD demonstrate academic underperformance and disruptive school behavior, limited peer networks and poor social skills, and increased family stress (Geller et al., 2002; Mendez et al., 2020). As such, cognitive-behavioral therapy (CBT) methods for PBD have been developed as an adjunct to pharmacotherapy to address the complex constellation of symptoms and associated social, academic, and family difficulties.

Understanding Bipolar Spectrum Disorders in Youth

Bipolar spectrum disorders were rarely diagnosed in children or adolescents prior to the 1990s, and in the past 30 years, a rigorous literature has established that the spectrum of disorders (including bipolar I disorder, bipolar II disorder, cyclothymic disorder, and other specified bipolar and related disorders) occur in youth and often present differently in children with pre-pubertal onset (Goldstein et al., 2017). Youth with pre-pubertal onset may demonstrate more significant irritability, more frequent mood fluctuations within episodes, high rates of comorbid conditions, such as attention-deficit/hyperactivity disorder (ADHD) and anxiety disorders (Youngstrom et al., 2008) and a worse symptom course (Estrada-Prat et al., 2019). The different manifestation in children has contributed to PBD being underrecognized and undertreated (Khazanov et al., 2015), with potentially devastating consequences. Bipolar disorder is associated with high rates of suicidality (Hauser et al., 2013), with as many as 44% of adolescents with PBD attempting suicide before age 18 (Lewinsohn et al., 2003).

Research to date indicates that PBD represents a discrete cluster of symptoms that can be validated by reliable assessment and differentiated from other psychiatric disorders (Goldstein et al., 2017). There exists consensus that PBD can present in either "narrow" or "broad" phenotypes. Children and adolescents with the "narrow" phenotype exhibit more classic symptoms of bipolar disorder that align with DSM-5 diagnostic criteria for bipolar I or II (American Psychiatric Association, 2013). Youth meeting criteria for a diagnosis of bipolar I disorder have experienced a manic episode, defined as prominent irritability or elevated mood for one week, in addition to three accompanying symptoms

DOI: 10.4324/9781003392439-19

(or four if mood is predominantly irritable): inflated self-esteem or grandiosity, decreased need for sleep, pressured speech, racing thoughts, distractibility, increased goal-directed activity or psychomotor agitation, and impulsivity (which may manifest as hypersexuality in youth). While individuals with bipolar I often experience depressive episodes, they are not required for a diagnosis. For bipolar II disorder, youth are required to meet criteria for a past or current hypomanic episode (duration of manic symptoms occurs for four days) along with one or more past or current major depressive episodes. The "broad" phenotype in youth includes cyclothymia and other specified bipolar and related disorders. In children and adolescents, cyclothymia is defined by a period of one year or more in which the individual experiences hypomanic symptoms alternating with depressive symptoms, but symptoms do not meet full diagnostic criteria for a hypomanic or major depressive episode. Other specified bipolar and related disorders are diagnosed when symptoms do not meet criteria for a full threshold diagnosis due to reduced number, intensity, duration, or frequency. Notably, research suggests that youth with broad phenotypes experience similar levels of psychosocial impairment, suicidality, and comorbidity as youth with narrow phenotypes (Axelson et al., 2006) and, in the context of family history of bipolar disorder, are likely to convert to bipolar I or II over time (Axelson et al., 2011).

In addition, disruptive mood dysregulation disorder (DMDD) was added as a diagnostic category in DSM-5 (American Psychiatric Association, 2013). DMDD refers to marked and persistent periods of severe irritability co-occurring with emotional (e.g., explosive anger, rage) and behavioral outbursts (e.g., physical aggression, temper tantrums). The inclusion of DMDD in DSM-5 was driven by evidence suggesting that youth experiencing chronic rather than episodic irritability are more likely to develop subsequent depressive or anxiety disorders than bipolar disorder (e.g., Brotman et al., 2006; Stringaris et al., 2009). Despite ongoing discussion as to the accurate characterization of diverse presentations of mood disorders, it is widely recognized that children with both broad and narrow phenotypes of PBD (i.e., bipolar spectrum) and children with DMDD exhibit significant mood dysregulation and impairment in academic, social, and developmental domains of functioning.

A meta-analysis of international epidemiologic studies of 56,103 youth aged 7–21 years indicated that the prevalence rate of bipolar spectrum disorders in youth is 3.9% (95% confidence interval [CI] 2.6%–5.8%; Van Meter et al., 2019). Prevalence rates were lower for narrow definitions of bipolar spectrum disorders (bipolar I and II only) and higher when including the broader definition including the full spectrum of disorders. Prospective longitudinal studies of youth demonstrate high rates of recurrence of mood symptoms and episodes over time (Birmaher et al., 2009; Geller et al., 2008; Wozniak et al., 2011; Youngstrom et al., 2008); future longitudinal studies will further clarify the progression of symptoms over the course of the lifespan.

The unique symptoms of PBD are associated with adverse effects on children and families. Youth with PBD demonstrate significant disruption in normative development, manifesting in impaired functioning in social, emotional, and academic functioning (Frías et al., 2017; Goldstein et al., 2009a, 2009b; Mendez et al., 2020). Children with PBD have demonstrated academic underperformance and behavioral problems in school, social impairment, including few or no friends, frequent teasing, and poor social skills, and poor family functioning, including poor sibling relationships, and parental conflict (Frías et al., 2017; Geller et al., 2002; Wilens et al., 2003). The psychosocial impairments associated with PBD contribute to compounded risk for disruptions in social, emotional, and academic functioning throughout development. By adolescence, youth with BD exhibit low self-esteem, hopelessness, external locus of control, and poor coping (Rucklidge, 2006), high expressed emotion in family relationships, more negative life events and chronic stress (Kim et al., 2007; Rucklidge, 2006), worse school functioning (Mendez et al., 2020), poorer general neurocognitive performance (Best et al., 2017), and poorer social functioning (Best et al., 2017; Goldstein et al., 2006). The accumulation of psychosocial risk throughout childhood and adolescence makes PBD a significant public health concern, placing an enormous burden on educational and health-care systems and on the families of affected children. As adults, individuals with BD are likely to demonstrate impaired functioning, greater mental health-care utilization, and lower rates of school graduation (Lewinsohn et al., 2005). In light of these significant psychosocial risks across development, psychosocial intervention is considered an essential component of a comprehensive treatment approach for PBD.

Assessment of PBD

Appropriate treatment for bipolar spectrum disorders in children depends on a thorough and accurate diagnosis, relying on a combination of knowledge about DSM-5 criteria and an understanding of the unique symptom profiles of PBD. The diagnostic protocol for PBD involves several steps—screening for mania, establishing an actuarial estimate of the likelihood of PBD based on clinical data, evaluating diagnostic criteria with high specificity to PBD, obtaining evidence of episodes, and using a lengthy window of assessment to ensure accuracy (Washburn et al., 2011; Youngstrom et al., 2005). Screening for mania is an important 1st step in establishing the likelihood of a PBD diagnosis. The Child Mania Rating Scale (CMRS; Pavuluri et al., 2006a) developed in our program is a widely used screening tool for mania. The CMRS includes 21 developmentally specific items that correspond to DSM-IV criteria for bipolar disorder. We also developed a ten-item version, which demonstrates comparable sensitivity and specificity (Henry et al., 2008). Both versions have excellent psychometric properties and have established validity as both screening and treatment outcome measures (West et al., 2011). Once a patient has been identified through a screening process as being at risk for experiencing a manic episode (past or present), then further assessment focuses on obtaining a thorough clinical history, focusing on the assessment of bipolar-specific symptoms, such as a decreased need for sleep, grandiosity, hypersexuality, elated mood, pressured speech or racing thoughts, and increased goal directed activity. Structured diagnostic interviews, such as the Washington University Kiddie Schedule for Schizophrenia and Affective Disorders (WASH-U-KSADS, Geller et al., 1994, revised 1996) or the Kiddie Schedule for Schizophrenia and Affective Disorders, Present and Lifetime Version DSM-5 (KSADS-PL, Kaufman et al., 1997; KSADS-PL DSM-5, Kaufman et al., 2016), are useful tools to obtain a thorough understanding of mood symptoms and comorbid diagnoses. Finally, valid diagnosis requires clearly establishing an episodic nature to mood symptoms and observing the child over time if necessary in order to confirm episodicity. The use of assessment tools such as the NIMH Life Chart (Denicoff et al., 2000) can aid clinicians in assessing and measuring episodes.

CBT Conceptualization of PBD and Sequencing of CBT Sessions

PBD involves a combination of neurological underpinnings and both innate and learned patterns of emotional responses, thoughts, and behaviors. Research suggests that youth with PBD experience disturbances in the neural systems responsible for processing and modulating emotions (Pavuluri et al., 2007). As a result, these youth have difficulty regulating their emotions as they may experience a shutdown of emotional and cognitive control systems. CBT thus aims to address these impairments in affective circuitry, as well as impairments in social and family functioning, as key treatment targets through various techniques at both the child and family level. A primary component of CBT is psychoeducation to build the family's understanding of the symptoms, etiology, and chronicity of PBD, typically delivered in the initial few sessions of treatment. Therapy then incorporates a focus on the development of affect regulatory strategies to address impairments in emotion regulation, including self-monitoring of mood states, recognizing and labeling feelings, and coping skills to manage expansive, negative, and irritable moods. In addition, youth and parents may be instructed in cognitive restructuring techniques to reduce negative thought patterns (e.g., thought stopping, reframing situations positively, modifying thoughts, and use of positive self-talk/mantras during difficult situations). Parent training in behavioral management strategies that are specific to the rage episodes common in PBD can be incorporated to help families prevent and cope with these affective "storms." For example, many parents use behavioral management systems developed for children with disruptive behavior disorders, which emphasize immediate contingency enforcement, re-direction, and the implementation of consequences. Unfortunately, in the case of PBD, this method can backfire. Children whose rage is rooted in a loss of control over emotional responses (rather than a purposeful, manipulative behavior) will not respond to limit-setting in the moment; in fact, this will only exacerbate their negative emotions. Rather, parents are instructed to use calming tones and modulate their own responses so as not to model emotional reactivity and focus on defusing the situation, keeping everyone safe, and using an empathic, collaborative problem-solving approach. Consequences and limits, if necessary, can be implemented when the child is calm. This approach is far more effective than more traditional behavior management approaches in addressing affective outbursts that are common in PBD. Other strategies for regulating mood include establishing simple and predictable routines, minimizing transitions, emphasizing the timing and tone of interactions during mood episodes, and using positive reinforcement. Youth and parents are also engaged in problem-solving skills training to target interpersonal and family difficulties, as well as to enhance self-efficacy related to coping with the disorder. Similarly, social skills training focuses on role-play, listening and communication skills, and empathy to improve the interpersonal difficulties associated with PBD. Finally, parents are encouraged to engage in pleasant, relaxing activities and to utilize their support networks to help cope with the demands of caring for a child with PBD.

Together, these cognitive-behavioral interventions help address the range of cognitive, social, and interpersonal impairments that are typical of PBD and supply families with a set of tools and skills to bolster them against the negative impact of symptoms and improve their quality of life. To facilitate engagement in the treatment process, instruction in key skill areas, and internalization and uptake of skills, CBT interventions follow a structured curriculum. Each session may include a review of the week and implementation of new strategies (homework review), psychoeducation and introduction of a new skill area (CBT skill building) and assigning a task to trial during the week to promote youth and caregiver internalization and generalizability of CBT skills (homework assignment).

Empirical Support of CBT in Treatment of PBD and Role of the Family

Early intervention is essential for reducing the morbidity and mortality associated with PBD, and the importance of a multimodal treatment approach that combines pharmacotherapy and psychosocial intervention has been advocated (McClellan et al., 2007) and supported by research (see reviews by Fristad 2016; Weinstein et al., 2013). To date, three intervention protocols that comprise a class of treatments, Family Psychoeducation plus Skill Building, are collectively considered *well-established* (i.e., demonstrated efficacy through two or more randomized controlled trials [RCTs] conducted by independent research groups; Southam-Gerow & Prinstein, 2014). The interventions subsumed in this group include Child- and Family-Focused Cognitive Behavioral Therapy for pediatric bipolar disorder (CFF-CBT; West et al., 2014), Family-Focused Treatment for Adolescents (FFT-A; Miklowitz et al., 2004, 2006), and Psychoeducational Psychotherapy (PEP; Fristad, 2006; Fristad et al., 1998). Given their similar foci on family-focused psychoeducation, cognitive behavioral therapy (CBT) approaches, and communication/problem-solving skill building adjunctive to pharmacotherapy, these treatments encompass a class of interventions (Brickman & Fristad, 2022). Families are highly involved in all three interventions, although the format and nature of family involvement vary slightly as detailed below.

Interventions for PBD: Well-Established Treatments

Child- and Family-Focused Cognitive-Behavioral Therapy

CFF-CBT is an adjunctive intervention developed by our clinical research group to meet the specific developmental needs of children 7–13 with bipolar spectrum disorders and their families (Pavuluri et al., 2004; West et al., 2014, 2018). We believe that CFF-CBT comprises four innovative aspects in the treatment of PBD in that it (1) is designed to be developmentally specific to school-age children, (2) is driven by the distinct needs of these children with PBD and their families (e.g., affect regulation), (3) involves intensive work with parents parallel to the work with children in order to directly address parent's own therapeutic needs and effective parenting practices, and (4) integrates psychoeducation, CBT, mindfulness, and interpersonal therapy techniques, tailored to the unique needs of these children, to augment the effects of pharmacotherapy. Diverse therapeutic techniques are employed across multiple domains, including individual, peer, family, and school to address the impact of PBD in the child's broader psychosocial context.

The psychotherapeutic methods and core curricula used in CFF-CBT are driven by three areas of research evidence: (1) affective circuitry brain dysfunction in PBD (e.g., poor problem-solving during affective stimulation because of under activity in dorsolateral pre-frontal cortex), (2) developmentally specific symptoms of PBD, and (3) the impact of PBD on psychosocial and interpersonal functioning (e.g., poor social functioning, family stress). CFF-CBT is a 12-session protocol-driven treatment program meant to be delivered weekly over the course of three months (see Table 16.1). Each session is approximately one hour. Most sessions are for the parent and child together, but some the parent only and some the child only. Additionally, CFF-CBT has been adapted to a group format, which consists of 12 75-minute concurrent parent and child group sessions. There is established content for each session and an ideal sequence to the delivery of this content; however, the treatment protocol can be implemented in a flexible manner if the essential ingredients are included. The acronym "RAINBOW" was formed to help parents and children remember the key components of CFF-CBT. The essential components of CFF-CBT "RAINBOW" covered throughout the treatment sessions include:

R: Routine. The goal of this component is to increase affect regulation by establishing a predictable, simplified routine that will reduce emotional reactivity and difficulty with transition. Parents are also urged to integrate soothing and pleasurable activities into their own and their child's routine.

A: Affect regulation. The goal of this component is to provide psychoeducation about symptoms of PBD and the biological bases of the disorder, teach behavioral management and coping strategies, and provide affective education to the children. Children and parents are given a system to monitor their moods several times throughout each day.

I: I can do it! The goal of this component is to increase parents' and children's beliefs in their ability to cope with the disorder and to problem-solve issues that arise through skill-building activities. Parents are also encouraged to approach interactions with their children using a combination of empathy, minimal reactivity, limit setting, and a focus on positive reframing, which we believe to be most effective for children who are highly sensitive to criticism and whose negative mood states are easily triggered.

N: No negative thoughts and live in the Now! The goals of this component are two-fold. The first goal is to decrease negative and/or distorted cognitions associated with depression through cognitive restructuring (e.g., reframing unhelpful thoughts). Additionally, informed by research on the utility of mindfulness techniques in cognitive-behavioral therapy for depression (Segal

Table 16.1 Outline of Child- and Family-Focused RAINBOW Session Content and Format[a]

Session	*Participants*	*Topics Covered*
1	Child and parents together	• Orientation to treatment/goal-setting • Engagement and relationship-building with child and parents
2	Child and parents together	• Psychoeducation about PBD • Mood charting via daily mood calendar
3	Parents only	• Affect regulation skills: establishing routines and anger management • Identifying and acknowledging parents' difficult feelings
4	Child only; parent check-in	• Affect regulation skills • Labeling emotions; recognizing difficult feelings; triggers of anger and sadness
5	Child only; parent check-in	• Cognitive and behavioral ("think" and "do") coping skills • Problem-solving and positive thinking
6	Parents only	• Identifying and promoting positive qualities in child • Positive thinking and mantras; reframing negative thoughts; mindfulness strategies
7	Child only; parent check-in	• Communication skills and interpersonal problem-solving
8	Parents only	• Promoting child's social competence • Behavior management strategies • Balanced lifestyle for parents and enhancing self-care
9	Parents, child, siblings	• Psychoeducation about PBD providing to siblings • Family coping and problem-solving
10	Child and parents together	• Identifying and enhancing access of social support networks
11	Child and parents together	• Reflection on RAINBOW experience • Review of RAINBOW skills, creation of RAINBOW binder to internalize and consolidate therapy tools
12	Child and parents together	• Celebration; follow-up/maintenance plan

[a] The format of the RAINBOW Group Program is identical in length and very similar in content. Child and caregiver groups run concurrently, and session topics parallel those outlined above although extend across several sessions to allow for practice and role-play (child group) and parent discussion. Additional Child Group content areas not listed above include group rapport building through games and team-building activities (Sessions 1, 2, and 3). Psychoeducation is primarily provided in the Parent Group.

et al., 2002), the second goal is to encourage a focus on the present moment rather than dwelling on past failures or anticipating future failures. Mindfulness techniques, such as the use of positive mantras, are incorporated.

B: Be a good friend and Balanced lifestyle for parents. The first goal of this component is to improve child social functioning through skill-building activities and the identification of opportunities for practice and mastery of skills. The second goal is to increase parental well-being and coping. Parents of children with BD often suffer from physical and emotional exhaustion, frustration, guilt, and feelings of isolation (Fristad & Goldberg-Arnold, 2003). Therefore, we encourage parents to develop a more balanced lifestyle that involves findings ways to rest, replenish their energy, and enjoy life.

O: Oh, how can we solve the problem? The goal of this component is to engage parents and children in a collaborative and effective problem-solving process. Parents are encouraged to view their children as partners in the problem-solving process, to explain the pros and cons of potential solutions in an empathetic way, and to use creative approaches to problem-solving to minimize reactivity.

W: Ways to Get Support. The goal of this component is to increase social support. Isolation, shame, and lack of access may prevent families from finding support networks. Therefore, the techniques used in this component emphasize the identification and active seeking out of people who can help the child and the parents through difficult situations. School advocacy is also essential. Teachers are provided with a portfolio of information about the diagnosis, the ways in which the disorder may interfere with school functioning and recommended accommodations to promote the child's performance in school. Parents are guided in ways to further advocate for the child's needs at school.

Our group has conducted multiple studies to test the feasibility and efficacy of CFF-CBT. The preliminary open trial of CFF-CBT (Pavuluri et al., 2004) demonstrated feasibility, patient and family satisfaction, and improvement in bipolar symptoms and global functioning; these improvements were maintained over a three-year follow-up period with continued psychosocial booster sessions (West et al., 2007). In addition, an open trial of the group format of CFF-CBT indicated that the group adaptation is feasible to deliver and resulted in a significant increase in parent's report of their child's coping skills, a decrease in parenting stress, an increase in parent's knowledge and self-efficacy in coping with the disorder, and a decrease in parent-reported symptoms of mania after treatment (West et al., 2009).

An RCT compared the individual-family format of CFF-CBT with a dose-matched psychosocial treatment as usual control in children 7–13 years with bipolar spectrum disorders ($N = 69$) and their families (West et al., 2014). All youth received 12 weekly treatment sessions during the acute phase of treatment, and six monthly booster sessions were offered; all youth also received expert medication management in our specialty mood clinic. Youth and caregivers were assessed during treatment, post-treatment (12 weeks) and at a six-month follow-up. Findings demonstrated that CFF-CBT was feasible to deliver with high patient satisfaction and with greater levels of engagement among families compared to the control. Results also indicated efficacy for CFF-CBT in improving symptoms of mania and depression as well as global functioning versus the control treatment. Moreover, results suggested that CFF-CBT was relatively immune to the presence of factors that could interfere with treatment, including parent depression symptoms and higher financial stress, versus the control (Weinstein et al., 2015). Importantly, results highlighted the role of caregivers in treatment outcomes: findings indicated that improvement in symptoms and global functioning in response to CFF-CBT may be explained by changes in parenting skills and coping, family flexibility, and family positive reframing (MacPherson et al., 2016).

Psychoeducational Psychotherapy

Fristad and colleagues (Fristad et al., 1998) developed PEP as family-based adjunctive protocol for children with bipolar and depressive spectrum disorders and their parents (Fristad et al., 2002, 2009). The goals of PEP include teaching parents and children about the child's illness and its treatment, symptom management, improving problem-solving and communications skills, and providing support to parents. Important components of the treatment include direct education to parents in how to become more involved with their child's treatment and serve as an effective advocate, and the instruction of coping skills for children via the use of a "toolbox" approach that has children identify pleasant and relaxing activities in four categories (creative, physical, social, and relaxation) that can be used to combat negative emotional states. The treatment has been developed as both a multifamily group (MF-PEP) or individual-family format (IF-PEP), with similar session content but differences in session structure (eight concurrent parent and child groups or 20–24 single family sessions).

A large RCT of the multi-family format (MF-PEP) for 165 youth yielded results supporting its efficacy in reducing mood symptoms versus waitlist control plus treatment as usual (Fristad et al., 2009). The dissemination of MF-PEP to real-world settings was also; results from a small open trial revealed that MF-PEP was acceptable and feasible in community clinic settings (MacPherson et al., 2014). In addition, RCTs have examined IF-PEP (Fristad, 2006) and IF-PEP plus omega-3 fatty acids (Fristad et al., 2015) and demonstrated positive effects on youth mood symptom improvement. Moreover, IF-PEP resulted in improved family communication and expressed emotion (Fristad, 2006) with effects maintained five years post-treatment (Fristad et al., 2021).

Family-Focused Treatment for Adolescents

Miklowitz and colleagues (2004) adapted their FFT—originally developed for adults with BD—for adolescents. FFT-A aims to reduce symptoms through increased understanding about the disorder and coping skills, decreased family conflict, and improvement in family problem-solving and communication skills. FFT involves three treatment components: psychoeducation, communication enhancement training, and problem-solving skills training. The psychoeducation component involves developing an understanding of the symptoms, etiology, and course of the disorder, as well as the importance of pharmacotherapy adherence and relapse prevention. The communication enhancement training component is focused on using role-playing and rehearsal to develop skills for active listening, offering positive feedback or constructive criticism, or requesting changes in other's behavior. The problem-solving component involves helping participants to identify problems, generate solutions, and implement those solutions in everyday life. These components are delivered across 21 50-minute sessions over nine months and include the patient, parents, and available siblings. A two-year RCT of FFT-A in adolescents with bipolar spectrum disorders ($N = 58$) demonstrated that, compared to adolescents who received the control treatment (psychopharmacology plus three sessions psychoeducation), adolescents who received FFT-A had shorter times to recovery from depression, less time in depressive episodes, and lower depression severity scores for two years (Miklowitz et al., 2008). Miklowitz and colleagues (Miklowitz et al., 2014) also conducted a multi-site RCT ($N = 145$) comparing FFT-A plus pharmacotherapy to enhanced care plus pharmacotherapy. Adolescents receiving FFT-A experienced reduced severity of mania symptoms, although FFT-A was not associated with improved depression symptoms. FFT-A has been adapted for intervention with children at high risk (FFT-HR) for developing bipolar disorder by virtue of having a 1st degree relative with the illness (Miklowitz et al., 2011). Findings from the RCT of 40 high-risk youth demonstrated positive treatment effects versus control treatment (Miklowitz et al., 2013).

Interventions for PBD: Possibly Efficacious and Experimental Treatments

Dialectical Behavior Therapy for Adolescents

Goldstein and colleagues adapted dialectical behavior therapy (DBT) for adolescents with bipolar spectrum disorders with research support in an open trial (Goldstein et al., 2007) and small RCT (Goldstein et al., 2015) indicating that DBT-A is considered *possibly efficacious*. DBT (Linehan, 1993) is a psychotherapy developed for adults with borderline personality disorder, the main target of which is emotion dysregulation, including high sensitivity to emotional stimuli and extreme emotional intensity. This adapted intervention is delivered over the course of one year and is comprised of two modalities: family skills training (delivered to the family unit) and individual psychotherapy with the adolescent patient. The acute treatment period includes 24 weekly sessions that alternate between individual skill training and family therapy. Continuation treatment consists of 12 additional sessions tapering in frequency over the rest of the one year. A preliminary open trial of DBT in ten adolescents with BD found decreases in suicidality, non-suicidal self-injurious behavior, emotional dysregulation, and depression symptoms after the intervention (Goldstein et al., 2007). Further, an RCT found that youth receiving DBT-A ($N = 14$) compared to standard care ($N = 6$) demonstrated greater treatment adherence, decreased depression and mania symptoms, and decreased suicidal ideation (Goldstein et al., 2015). A larger RCT is currently underway and likely to yield additional support for DBT-A among youth with bipolar spectrum disorders.

Interpersonal and Social Rhythm Therapy for Adolescents

Hlastala and colleagues developed an adapted version of Interpersonal and Social Rhythm Therapy (IPSRT) for adolescents with BD (Hlastala et al., 2010), which can be currently classified as an *experimental treatment.* IPSRT (Frank, 2005) is a manual-based psychotherapy founded on the theory that one aspect of vulnerability for BD is instability in circadian rhythms and neurotransmitter systems involved in regulation. In this model, psychosocial stressors are hypothesized to precipitate and/or exacerbate bipolar episodes through their ability to disrupt social and sleep routines. IPSRT interventions aim to stabilize social and sleep routines and address interpersonal precipitants to dysregulation such as interpersonal disputes, role transitions, and interpersonal function deficits. IPSRT is primarily an individual treatment, but this adaptation incorporates brief family psychotherapy. A pilot study of this adapted IPSRT model indicated feasibility as well as decreased symptoms and improved functioning across treatment (Hlastala et al., 2010). A modified IPSRT-A model was also developed for adolescents at high risk for BD (i.e., with an immediate family member with BD). Although a pilot RCT yielded mixed results, findings show promise for improving sleep among high-risk youth (Goldstein et al., 2018).

Assessment of Progress and Outcomes

Monitoring treatment progress is key to maximizing therapy outcomes. Several objective assessment measures may be used throughout treatment to determine symptom response to intervention as well as objective assessment of global functioning. To monitor symptom response, the CMRS (Pavuluri et al., 2006a) can be used at regular intervals (e.g., one to three months during acute phases of treatment, every six months during maintenance phases of treatment) to collect parent-report of child mania and depression symptoms over time. Child report of depression symptoms may also be useful to collect every one to three months during acute treatment phases (e.g., Child Depression Inventory 2nd edition, CDI2; Kovacs, 2011). Measures of global functioning can quantify changes in key life domains at weekly or monthly intervals; for example, the Children's Global Assessment Scale (C-GAS, Shaffer et al., 1983) is a brief, clinician-rated measure of child functioning in family, social, and academic domains.

Application to the School Setting

Research on neurocognitive functioning in children with PBD indicates that children with PBD may be impaired in the cognitive domains of attention, working memory, executive function, verbal memory, response flexibility, reversal learning, processing speed, set shifting, and visual-spatial memory (Best et al., 2017; Dickstein et al., 2004, 2007; Frías et al., 2014; Henin et al., 2007; Pavuluri et al., 2006b) and that these deficits persist over the course of development (Pavuluri et al., 2009). Further, global neurocognitive deficits have been linked to reading difficulties in patients with PBD, and impaired vigilance has been associated with math difficulties (Henin et al., 2007; Pavuluri et al.,

2006b; Wozniak et al., 1995). Our clinical experience with PBD patients indicates significant and pervasive school difficulty, both in academic performance and social functioning. Most children with PBD require adaptations to the academic environment to help them function appropriately and many have structured educational and social interventions as part of an individualized educational plan.

The cognitive deficits associated with PBD may result in various problems with academic performance, including inattentiveness, memory and recall problems, difficulty with critical thinking, categorization, and organization, and impaired problem-solving. In addition, the symptoms and behaviors associated with PBD may manifest in problematic classroom functioning, such as peer conflict, threatening behavior, difficulty with routines and transitions, challenging of teachers, lack of follow-through with tasks and assignments, and school refusal. To help teachers better understand and address any problematic functioning, they could benefit from basic education about mood disorders (and especially how they differ from ADHD and disruptive behavior disorders), tools and techniques to use in the classroom, regular communication with mental health providers and parents, and tools for advocating for these children within the school system.

Various accommodations can be incorporated into an individualized educational plan or other structured intervention plan to help address these symptoms and behaviors. For example, students may benefit from stress-reducing accommodations to help decrease emotion dysregulation and reactivity. These could include consistent, planned breaks, decreasing stimulation and distraction in the student's environment, shortened assignments, prior notice before transitions or changes in routine, and a coping plan for outbursts, which might include permission to talk with a school counselor or go to a pre-determined "safe place" and calm down, and strategic scheduling (e.g., most difficult tasks at times of day when a child has most emotional resources). Peer conflict might be improved through interventions such as seating the student by model classmates, providing positive feedback on healthy peer interactions, and creating opportunities for successful social experiences and leadership. Finally, interventions to address academic difficulties might include reduced homework, extra tutoring, homework assignment notebooks, extended time on tests, and the use of multiple choice versus open-ended questioning. In addition to interventions to address behaviors and functional impairments, it is also important for teachers to understand the unique symptoms of PBD and implications of treatment. For example, medications used to treat PBD may cause daytime drowsiness, excessive thirst and hunger, agitation, dizziness, frequent urination, or diarrhea. Students may benefit from accommodations, such as an in-class water bottle, a permanent bathroom pass, frequent activity to combat sleepiness, and other interventions to help combat side effects from medications in addition to PBD symptoms. Although these types of accommodations can go a long way in addressing a student's difficulties in the classroom and helping teachers develop understanding, patience, and flexibility in coping with PBD in the classroom, in cases of severe illness it is not unusual for a student to need further accommodation such as a contained classroom, one-on-one classroom aides, and/or a therapeutic school placement.

Case Examples (notc: names and details have been modified to protect confidentiality)

Case Example 1: Individual/Family RAINBOW Therapy

Presenting Problem and History of Presenting Problem

Kara C.[1] was a nine-year-old female who lived at home with her biological mother, stepfather, and biological 14-year-old sister. She was referred to the RAINBOW therapy program by her child psychiatrist at the Pediatric Mood Disorders Clinic at the University of Illinois-Chicago. Initial assessment via structured interview and mood symptom rating scales (parent-, child-, and clinician-report) indicated that Kara met diagnostic criteria for Bipolar I Disorder and Generalized Anxiety Disorder.

Kara was experiencing moderate symptoms of depression and mania, including frequent irritability, mood lability, and intense periods of anger or "rage episodes." During these episodes Kara would engage in verbal and physical aggression, exhibit impaired judgment (e.g., trying to run away), and occasionally express suicidal ideation (e.g., stating *I wish I was never born* and *I want to kill myself*). Mrs. C. reported that she had difficulty containing or consoling Kara during her rage episodes. Rage only occurred at home, whereas Kara had minimal behavioral difficulties at school. Kara also had a history of periods of elated and giddy moods with increased energy, increased activity in several areas (e.g., working on several projects or playing for hours without being able to transition to other activities), motor hyperactivity, reduced sleep, and mild flight of ideas. Periods of elated moods were typically followed by an increase in irritability and depressed mood, rage, tearfulness, and feelings of worthlessness. At times, Kara would cycle between euphoric and depressed/angry states within the same day. At the evaluation, Kara's parents reported that her mood difficulties were negatively impacting all family members.

Kara attended a local public school and had a history of strong academic performance. However, she often experienced anxiety about school performance and social interactions which would manifest in somatic symptoms of distress. Despite having several friends, Kara had difficulties maintaining friendships. In addition, she experienced bullying by a peer at school.

Kara's mood difficulties began as a toddler with the onset of severe tantrums. During childhood Kara would experience weeks of stable moods, usually in the summer, punctuated by periods of cycling between elated and giddy moods to low moods and rage. Her anxiety had a gradual onset but became noticeable to parents during 2nd grade. Family history was significant for depression, substance use, and bipolar disorder. Prior mental health services included six months of unstructured play therapy which reportedly did not improve Kara's mood or behavior. At the start of therapy, Kara had recently initiated treatment with a mood stabilizer and the family had attended two medication management sessions with the child psychiatrist. She had never been hospitalized for psychiatric reasons.

Goals for Treatment

Table 16.2 outlines the goals for treatment and a sample treatment plan for Kara.

Course of Treatment

Kara's family actively participated in treatment, completing the acute treatment phase at weekly intervals and the maintenance phase at monthly intervals. Kara attended sessions with her mother, and her stepfather and older sister participated in the family session and intermittent maintenance sessions. Table 16.1 provides an outline of the content and format of the acute 12-session treatment phase; as detailed in the table, therapy sessions alternated between child-, parent-, and family-focused sessions. All child sessions included a brief family component at the conclusion of the end of session.

Treatment initially focused on *engaging the family in the treatment process, addressing expectations of and barriers to treatment, and identifying key treatment goals* (Sessions 1 and 2). Mrs. C. identified anger management, sibling discord, and transitions as key targets for treatment, and Kara added "bullies" as her goal. In addition, Kara and Mrs. C. were provided with psychoeducation regarding PBD. Bipolar disorder was described as a "brain disorder," and Kara's core symptoms were discussed in the context of documented differences in brain functioning during periods of excessive emotions to reduce blame and negative attributions surrounding Kara's rage episodes. Kara and her mother also developed a common language for her symptoms (e.g., rage episodes were named

Table 16.2 Sample Treatment Plan for Kara C

Treatment Goals	*Treatment Objectives*	*Interventions*
1 Improved mood regulation: increased positive moods, decreased sadness and irritability, increased mood stability	1 Kara/parents will increase awareness of mood patterns and improve identification and labeling of her mood states via affect education and weekly mood monitoring. 2 Family will establish simple, predictable routines. 3 Kara will learn to self-monitor the antecedents and consequences of negative feelings and will increase her ability to cope with negative affects by recognizing the triggers of such emotions. 4 Kara and her family will use cognitive and behavioral coping strategies to prevent escalation in anger and to acutely manage rage episodes. 5 Kara's parents will learn and implement behavioral management techniques to reduce Kara's anger and sadness while increasing targeted positive behaviors (e.g., establishing reward systems to increase positive behaviors; implementing consistent consequences for targeted negative behaviors).	1 Child- and Family-Focused Cognitive Behavioral Therapy for Pediatric Bipolar Disorder (manualized RAINBOW program): weekly for 60–90 minutes for 12 weeks, monthly for 60 minutes for 12 months
2 Improved understanding of pediatric bipolar disorder	Kara and her family will increase their understanding of pediatric bipolar disorder via psychoeducation regarding the symptomatology, course, neurochemical underpinnings, and challenges of the disorder.	2 Medication management: monthly for 30 minutes
3 Improved self-esteem and self-efficacy in child and family	1 Kara's family will learn and use collaborative problem-solving techniques to cope with family difficulties. 2 Kara and her family will recognize her positive qualities and engage in activities that will promote her strengths. 3 Kara and her family will identify and use positive scripts/ self-talk during times of difficulty. 4 Kara's parents' will increase their well-being and coping abilities by increasing their self-care activities and developing a balanced lifestyle.	3 Consultation with Kara's school on an as-needed basis
4 Improved interpersonal functioning with family and peers	1 Kara will engage in skill-building activities related to communication and assertiveness to improve peer relations and reduce bullying. 2 Kara's family will identify and utilize supportive networks. 3 Clinician will collaborate with Kara's school regarding the implementation of accommodations and behavioral strategies to improve peer functioning in the classroom.	

"volcanoes" and Kara's anger was described as "lava"). This process allowed Kara to distance herself from her symptoms, thereby increasing her comfort and ability to discuss these difficulties. Last, Kara's mood fluctuations were monitored on a Daily Mood Calendar: Kara used colors to indicate her mood across the day and Mrs. C. noted the triggers of mood shifts. Mornings were identified as a particularly difficult time.

Kara initially presented as anxious and guarded, manifesting in off-task behavior, silliness, and responses of "I don't know." However, she became more comfortable across early sessions, and Mrs. C. demonstrated greater understanding of the bipolar diagnosis. At the outset of treatment,

Mrs. C. expressed significant doubt about Kara's diagnosis, questioning whether this was a "phase," related to diet, or the manifestation of her anxiety. However, after Session 2, she reported increased acceptance of the diagnosis given Kara's family history and experience of the key symptoms of bipolar disorder.

The next phase of treatment (Sessions 3 through 6) focused on *affect dysregulation* and the prevention and management of Kara's rage episodes. Parent sessions dealt with the implementation of consistent, predictable routines to improve two identified areas of difficulty: mornings and abrupt transitions. Specific methods for improving Kara's morning routine were implemented at home (e.g., use of a chart for weather-appropriate clothing to minimize tense mother-daughter negotiations about getting dressed). To minimize Kara's experience of abrupt transitions, Mrs. C. began to provide ample warnings prior to transitions and posted reminders of the day's schedule. With additional problem-solving and fine-tuning across sessions, Mrs. C. reported an improvement in Kara's routine and mood in the mornings. Parent sessions also focused on helping Kara manage her anger outbursts as a family. The analogy of "putting out a fire" was used to facilitate Mrs. C.'s ability to remain neutral and calm while defusing the situation, versus engaging in the episode and exacerbating Kara's distress. Coping plans for the prevention and acute management of rage episodes were developed with Mrs. C., including ways Mrs. C. can remain calm (e.g., using a mantra, "I need to put out the fire, she is not in control"), using a code word with Kara's father and sister to enlist their support, and implementing a soothing "cool-down" area to help Kara de-escalate her anger. Coping plans also involved how and when to enforce appropriate consequences for target negative behaviors (e.g., physical or verbal aggression), such that consequences would be enforced only after Kara and others' elevated emotions had stabilized.

Additionally, parent sessions during this phase focused on Mrs. C.'s range of emotions regarding parenting a child with bipolar disorder and identifying ways to both accept and cope with the inevitable feelings of anger, helplessness, and guilt. Sessions included instruction in cognitive techniques to use during difficult situations (e.g., reframing Kara's behavior in the context of her neurocircuitry versus deliberate attempts to hurt others) as well as mindfulness techniques to help Mrs. C. focus on the present moment to manage feeling overwhelmed. Mrs. C. expressed immense relief after disclosing her difficult emotions, stating she had never admitted these feelings. She also began to recognize how her own negative emotions may contribute to Kara's escalation during rage episodes and reported greater effectiveness in helping defuse tense situations with Kara when she used coping techniques.

Child sessions with Kara focused on feelings identification, her physiological manifestations of anger ("anger clues") and increasing Kara's insight into the triggers of her negative moods, which we called her "bugs." Kara's triggers included her sister, a classroom bully, and household chores. Kara was often reluctant to describe any difficulties she experienced during the week but became very engaged in skill-building play activities on affect regulation. Games, worksheets, drawings, and role-play were used to help Kara practice cognitive and behavioral skills for coping with future "bugs" and her resulting rising anger. Yet, despite Kara's enthusiasm during session, she often resisted using her identified coping skills when triggered at home or school. Thus, it was important to normalize the experience of anger and sadness as acceptable emotions as well as the difficulty of learning new skills. Mrs. C. was encouraged to provide Kara with reassurance and support when prompting Kara's use of coping skills (e.g., "*I love you and I want to help you feel better by trying [this tool]*"). In addition, Kara felt a greater sense of self-efficacy when she created her own therapy assignments and was motivated to practice her coping skills when a reward system was employed at home. Last, Kara's experiences of anger were discussed as one small part of her identity, and family sessions focused on the promotion of Kara's strengths and competencies. Across sessions, Kara gradually increased her ability to recognize her triggers and warning signs, appropriately seek help (e.g., asking for a hug), and use positive statements to cope with her anger. Mrs. C. also became increasingly confident in her ability to soothe and redirect Kara.

As Kara's family improved in their ability to prevent and manage Kara's affect dysregulation, our focus widened to the *management of family and environmental stressors* during the 3rd phase of treatment (Sessions 7 through 10). Child sessions centered on improving Kara's communication and interpersonal problem-solving skills. For example, Kara developed various ways to respond to a peer bully and practiced these in session (e.g., direct and respectful expression of feelings, seeking help from school personnel, and use of coping songs to help Kara manage her sadness and anger in response to bullying). Parent sessions focused on promoting Kara's social competence through supervised one-on-one play activities with peers and advocating for Kara's needs in the classroom. An essential component of this phase was also our emphasis on Mrs. C.'s well-being and balance between self-care and parenting responsibilities. Mrs. C. recognized that her parenting abilities suffer when she feels "burned out." She thus identified important self-care activities to pursue, including outings with a friend, attending a church support group, and seeking help with dinner from the family. Together, Kara and Mrs. C. identified their support networks by creating a "Support Tree." Their Support Trees could then be used to seek out supportive others when feeling isolated or helpless in the future.

Last, a family session was held with Kara, her older sister, and her parents. This session was used to provide education on Kara's diagnosis and course of therapy and to improve family interactions via family problem-solving. With assistance from the therapist, family members identified their strengths as well as family-wide "bugs," practiced using feeling statements, and developed coping plans for managing their bugs as a team. Kara's family also agreed on ways to reward their positive efforts via family outings and movie nights. Kara became giddy and uncomfortable when discussing family "bugs" that involved her anger. It was important to maintain an atmosphere of acceptance and teamwork to manage the difficulties that *all* family members experience. Kara's sister also reported relief after discussing her feelings and learning about the biological underpinnings of mood symptoms.

The final sessions of the acute phase (Sessions 11 and 12) focused on preparing for the shift from weekly therapy to monthly maintenance sessions. Kara created a RAINBOW book of therapy exercises to help her remember and use these therapy tools. Mrs. C. and Kara also discussed ways to continually use therapy strategies at home, such as weekly dinner meetings to discuss family "bugs" and plan family outings. Positive family changes across treatment were reviewed and celebrated, including Kara's increased awareness of her moods and triggers and a reduction in Kara's rage episodes from near-daily outbursts to milder episodes occurring one to two times/month. Mrs. C. reported "I no longer feel like I'm walking on eggshells" and expressed confidence in her ability to manage Kara's triggers without escalation. Kara reported improved relationships with peers, her mother, and her sister.

During the maintenance phase (six monthly sessions), Kara and her mother remained engaged in treatment. Sessions included child, parent, and family components and focused on continued practice of skills and problem-solving difficulties. In addition, school consultation was provided to Kara's education team regarding bipolar disorder and strategies to enhance Kara's classroom functioning and minimize peer difficulties. An Individualized Education Plan (IEP) was developed by the school personnel to provide accommodations for her bipolar diagnosis. Accommodations included a sanctioned cool-down area outside of the classroom, greater supervision during unstructured periods to minimize bullying, and use of a private cue system between Kara and her teacher to prompt Kara's use of her coping strategies.

Outcomes

Across treatment, Kara demonstrated greater insight into her symptoms, improved self-esteem, and acceptance of her diagnosis as only "one small part of me." She improved in her ability to reframe angry thoughts (e.g., "Mom doesn't love me") and use relaxation to manage distress. An essential component of Kara's treatment success was the presentation of therapy material in a non-threatening, creative, and engaging manner, as well as helping her recognize her many positive qualities. Mrs. C.'s success in treatment was driven by her active engagement in the process, her willingness and dedication to implement novel strategies at home, and recognition of her own emotions, thoughts, and needs.

Consistent with the episodic nature of bipolar disorder, Kara's relative stability was punctuated by periods of greater difficulties (e.g., anger, aggression, feelings of worthlessness), but these had decreased in intensity, frequency, and duration across treatment. Moreover, these challenging periods were now accompanied by a mobilization of resources at the individual and family level to prevent further escalation. Kara's parents became increasingly proficient in their ability to recognize warning signs of distress and redirect Kara, and Kara was increasingly able to use coping skills independently at less intense levels of anger. Objective measures at the conclusion of the acute phase indicated significant improvement in mania and depression symptoms, family cohesion, and global functioning, and these treatment gains were maintained on objective measures at the final treatment session.

Case Example 2: RAINBOW Group Therapy

The treatment goals and concepts of CFF-CBT as outlined in Table 16.1 are also applied in a group format. The RAINBOW Group includes concurrent Parent and Child Group sessions that are reunited at the end of each session to review the child session content and therapy homework activities. The following example describes the course of one child participant's group experience.

Reason for Referral and History of the Presenting Problem

Tommy H.[2] was a 12-year-old African American male who lived with his biological mother. Tommy was referred to the RAINBOW Group from his Child Psychiatrist within the Pediatric Mood Disorders Clinic, who had provided bi-monthly family therapy services and medication management for two years. Tommy had been previously diagnosed with bipolar I disorder and ADHD, combined type. He had a history of periods of mania (elated and expansive mood, disrupted sleep, grandiosity, irritability, and psychosis) and aggression and had experienced aggressive outbursts since age two. During these outbursts, Tommy was physically aggressive toward his mother and engaged in moderate self-harm (hitting his head, scratching his arms). His aggression and psychosis had improved significantly during the past two years of treatment but he continued to experience aggressive outbursts, elated and giddy moods, distractibility, increased energy, and inattention, which resulted in difficulties at home and school. Tommy received several academic accommodations under an IEP, including reduced homework assignments and a one-on-one classroom aide. At the start of group treatment, he was experiencing frequent mood exacerbations surrounding homework. Tommy also had difficulty interacting appropriately with peers in the classroom. Thus, the RAINBOW group was recommended to improve Tommy's social functioning and mood regulation and to provide support for Ms. H.

Course of Treatment

Tommy and his mother attended all 12 RAINBOW Child and Parent Group Therapy sessions. During group treatment, the family also attended medication management sessions every one to two months. The 1st phase of the Child Group focused on rapport building and orientation to the group treatment process. Tommy was an active participant and often took a leadership role during the group sessions. He was insightful and forthcoming about his mood and attention difficulties, his experience of medication, and social challenges. However, Tommy frequently presented to the group with elevated energy, silliness, impulsivity, distractibility, and pressured and tangential speech. As a result, Tommy's participation often overshadowed and frustrated other group members. Behavioral strategies were thus implemented to promote Tommy's success and appropriate participation in the group while minimizing treatment-interfering behaviors. For example, all group members were encouraged to monitor their energy levels and to request a "chill out break" when feeling distracted or agitated: a break from group activities to lead all group members in deep breathing and stretching relaxation exercises to improve focus. Tommy and other group members were excited about the relaxation breaks and used these effectively to cope with group-interfering behaviors. In addition, a neutral cue system was developed independently with Tommy and the group leaders to signal when he was interrupting others or engaging in tangential speech. Tommy responded well to this limit setting and improved in his ability to re-direct his behavior and allow other children to participate. Given his successful response, these techniques were shared with Ms. H. to improve Tommy's behavior at home and school.

The 2nd phase of treatment focused on improving affect regulation and coping skills. Tommy showed good insight into his mood symptoms and anger triggers. He was also eager to learn and practice cognitive and behavioral skills to manage difficulties with anger, aggression, and focus during homework completion. He particularly enjoyed the therapy metaphors and frequently referred to his "bugs," "anger clues," and "cool thoughts" during the group, with his mother, and with his teachers. Tommy appeared to greatly benefit from learning relaxation strategies and reported that these were helpful in improving his mood during homework or classwork periods. However, Tommy's completion of therapy assignments (e.g., Daily Mood Calendar, coping worksheets) between sessions became problematic and was noted to lead to explosive conflicts with his mother. Thus, Ms. H. and the group leaders modified the group assignments such that Tommy received his group homework reward for verbal descriptions of his coping skills practice, rather than completing the logs or worksheets.

The final phase of group treatment emphasized social skills and self-esteem. Tommy initially could not identify his positive characteristics but was receptive to feedback from leaders and other participants, and in turn was eager to remind himself of strengths during difficult situations. He particularly benefited from in-vivo social skill-building activities with other group members. Tommy greatly improved in recognizing how his behaviors may impact others' feelings and behaviors. Ms. H. similarly reported a significant reduction in altercations with peers in the classroom setting after this phase of treatment. Although Tommy continued to struggle with aggression toward his mother when triggered, he improved in his awareness of these behaviors and motivation to improve his aggression.

Outcomes

At the conclusion of treatment, Tommy expressed pride and satisfaction with his progress but sadness about ending group. He reported improved mood, family, and peer relationships; these improvements were echoed by his mother. Ms. H. also reported receiving an immense benefit from participating in the Parent's Group, particularly in her self-efficacy and feeling supported as a parent. She reported that she enjoyed the didactic components of the group regarding PBD and parenting strategies, but most appreciated the opportunity to process her experiences with other caregivers. She hoped to create an ongoing informal support group with the other families from the program.

Summary

Research on PBD has substantially expanded since earlier versions of this book. Decades of research now support the reliability and validity of bipolar spectrum disorders in children and adolescents with evidence of continuity into adulthood. Children with PBD demonstrate significant difficulties in social, emotional, and academic functioning, underscoring the need for psychosocial treatment as an adjunctive to pharmacotherapy and with applications to the school setting. Empirically supported psychosocial interventions have been developed to address the scope of needs in youth with PBD and their families, with a class of interventions considered to be well-established in terms of research support (family psychoeducation plus skill-building interventions: CFF-CBT, PEP, and FFT-A). This class of interventions shares key elements including an adjunctive approach to pharmacotherapy, psychoeducation, development of coping skills, communication and social skills training, close involvement of family, and collaboration with the youth's educational environment to promote functioning in the school setting. Manuals are now available for clinicians to deliver each of these protocols, and treatment selection may be guided by factors such as youth age, clinical presentation, and the family environment. These interventions aim to alter the developmental trajectory of youth with PBD, thus preventing the negative consequences associated with PBD and improving overall quality of life for youth and their families. Ongoing research is examining additional interventions for adolescent and high-risk populations, as well as the predictors, moderators, and mediators of treatment to best address the question of which treatment works best for which youth, and why.

Reflection Questions

1 Why is psychosocial intervention considered an essential component of treatment best practices for youth with bipolar spectrum disorders and their families? What key treatment elements should be incorporated for treatment efficacy?
2 In what ways does PBD impact school functioning? How can school professionals implement the CBT strategies described in this chapter to create an atmosphere of acceptance and understanding within the classroom and promote functioning of youth with PBD in the school setting?
3 This chapter describes the neurobiological underpinnings of the symptoms associated with PBD. In working with a child with bipolar disorder, how can framing the child's behavior and/or difficulties within the context of their neurobiology change the way you think about and help the child within the school setting?

Evidence-Based Treatments for PBD

Intervention	*Research Support Classification*	*Resources*
Child-and Family-Focused Cognitive Behavioral Treatment for PBD (CFF-CBT/RAINBOW)	Well-established class of interventions	RCT: West et al. (2014) Manual: West et al. (2017)
Psychoeducational Psychotherapy (PEP)		Fristad et al. (1998, 2002, 2003, 2006, 2015)
Family-Focused Treatment for Adolescents with BD (FFT-A)		Miklowitz et al. (2004, 2006, 2014)
Dialectical Behavior Therapy for Adolescents with BD (DBT-A)	Possibly efficacious intervention	Goldstein et al. (2007, 2015)
Interpersonal and Social Rhythm Therapy for Adolescents (IPSRT-A)	Experimental intervention	Hlastala et al. (2010)

Notes

1 All identifying details have been changed.
2 All identifying details have been changed.

References

American Psychiatric Association (2013). *Diagnostic and statistical manual of mental disorders* (5th ed.). Washington, DC: American Psychiatric Association.

Axelson, D. A., Birmaher, B., Strober, M., Gill, M. K., Valeri, S., Chiappetta, L., Ryan, N., Leonard, H., Hunt, J., Iyengar, S., Bridge, J., & Keller, M. (2006). Phenomenology of children and adolescents with bipolar spectrum disorders. *Archives of General Psychiatry, 63*(10), 1139–1148. https://doi.org/10.1001/archpsyc.63.10.1139

Axelson, D. A., Birmaher, B., Strober, M. A., Goldstein, B. I., Ha, W., Gill, M. K., Goldstein, T. R., Yen, S., Hower, H., Hunt, J. I., Liao, F., Iyengar, S., Dickstein, D., Kim, E., Ryan, N. D., Frankel, E., & Keller, M. B. (2011). Course of subthreshold bipolar disorder in youth: Diagnostic progression from bipolar disorder not otherwise specified. *Journal of the American Academy of Child and Adolescent Psychiatry, 50*(10), 1001–16. e3. https://doi.org/10.1016/j.jaac.2011.07.005

Best, M. W., Bowie, C. R., Naiberg, M. R., Newton, D. F., & Goldstein, B. I. (2017). Neurocognition and psychosocial functioning in adolescents with bipolar disorder. *Journal of Affective Disorders, 207*, 406–412. https://doi.org/10.1016/j.jad.2016.09.063

Birmaher, B., Axelson, D., Goldstein, B., Strober, M., Gill, M. K., Hunt, J., Houck, P., Ha, W., Iyengar, S., Kim, E., Yen, S., Hower, H., Esposito-Smythers, C., Goldstein, T., Ryan, N., & Keller, M. (2009). Four-year longitudinal course of children and adolescents with bipolar spectrum disorders: The Course and Outcome of Bipolar Youth (COBY) study. *The American Journal of Psychiatry, 166*(7), 795–804. https://doi.org/10.1176/appi.ajp.2009.08101569

Brotman, M. A., Schmajuk, M., Rich, B. A., Dickstein, D. P., Guyer, A. E., Costello, E. J., Egger, H. L., Angold, A., Pine, D. S., & Leibenluft, E. (2006). Prevalence, clinical correlates, and longitudinal course of severe mood dysregulation in children. *Biological Psychiatry, 60*(9), 991–997. https://doi.org/10.1016/j.biopsych.2006.08.042

Denicoff, K. D., Leverich, G. S., Nolen, W. A., Rush, A. J., McElroy, S. L., Keck, P. E., Suppes, T., Altshuler, L. L., Kupka, R., Frye, M. A., Hatef, J., Brotman, M. A., & Post, R. M. (2000). Validation of the prospective NIMH-Life-Chart Method (NIMH-LCM-p) for longitudinal assessment of bipolar illness. *Psychological Medicine, 30*(6), 1391–1397. https://doi.org/10.1017/s0033291799002810

Dickstein, D. P., Nelson, E. E., McClure, E. B., Grimley, M. E., Knopf, L., Brotman, M. A., Rich, B. A., Pine, D. S., & Leibenluft, E. (2007). Cognitive flexibility in phenotypes of pediatric bipolar disorder. *Journal of the American Academy of Child and Adolescent Psychiatry, 46*(3), 341–355. https://doi.org/10.1097/chi.0b013e31802d0b3d

Dickstein, D. P., Treland, J. E., Snow, J., McClure, E. B., Mehta, M. S., Towbin, K. E., Pine, D. S., & Leibenluft, E. (2004). Neuropsychological performance in pediatric bipolar disorder. *Biological Psychiatry, 55*(1), 32–39. https://doi.org/10.1016/s0006-3223(03)00701-7

Estrada-Prat, X., Van Meter, A. R., Camprodon-Rosanas, E., Batlle-Vila, S., Goldstein, B. I., & Birmaher, B. (2019). Childhood factors associated with increased risk for mood episode recurrences in bipolar disorder—a systematic review. *Bipolar Disorders, 21*(6), 483–502. https://doi.org/10.1111/bdi.12785

Frank, E. (2005). *Treating bipolar disorder: A clinician's guide to interpersonal and social rhythm therapy*. New York: Guilford Press.

Freeman, A. J., Youngstrom, E. A., Michalak, E., Siegel, R., Meyers, O. I., & Findling, R. L. (2009). Quality of life in pediatric bipolar disorder. *Pediatrics, 123*(3), e446–e452. https://doi.org/10.1542/peds.2008-0841

Frías, Á., Dickstein, D. P., Merranko, J., Gill, M. K., Goldstein, T. R., Goldstein, B. I., Hower, H., Yen, S., Hafeman, D. M., Liao, F., Diler, R., Axelson, D., Strober, M., Hunt, J., Ryan, N. D., Keller, M. B., & Birmaher, B. (2017). Longitudinal cognitive trajectories and associated clinical variables in youth with bipolar disorder. *Bipolar Disorders, 19*(4), 273–284. https://doi.org/10.1111/bdi.12510

Frías, Á., Palma, C., & Farriols, N. (2014). Neurocognitive impairments among youth with pediatric bipolar disorder: A systematic review of neuropsychological research. *Journal of Affective Disorders, 166*, 297–306. https://doi.org/10.1016/j.jad.2014.05.025

Fristad, M. A. (2006). Psychoeducational treatment for school-aged children with bipolar disorder. *Development and Psychopathology, 18*, 1289–1306. https://doi:10.1017/S0954579406060627

Fristad, M. A. (2016). Evidence-based psychotherapies and nutritional interventions for children with bipolar spectrum disorders and their families. *Journal of Clinical Psychiatry, 77*, e4. https://doi.org/10.4088/JCP.15017su1c.04

Fristad, M. A., Gavazzi, S. M., & Soldano, K. W. (1998). Multi-family psychoeducation groups for childhood mood disorders: A program description and preliminary efficacy data. *Contemporary Family Therapy, 20*(3), 385–402. https://doi.org/10.1023/A:1022477215195

Fristad, M. A., Goldberg-Arnold, J. S., & Gavazzi, S. M. (2002). Multifamily psychoeducation groups (MFPG) for families of children with bipolar disorder. *Bipolar Disorders, 4*(4), 254–262. https://doi.org/10.1034/j.1399-5618.2002.09073.x

Fristad, M. A., Roley-Roberts, M. E., Black, S. R., & Arnold, L. E. (2021). Moody kids years later: Long-term outcomes of youth from the Omega-3 and therapy (OATS) studies. *Journal of Affective Disorders, 281*, 24–32. https://doi.org/10.1016/j.jad.2020.11.115

Fristad, M. A., Verducci, J. S., Walters, K., & Young, M. E. (2009). Impact of multifamily psychoeducational psychotherapy in treating children aged 8 to 12 years with mood disorders. *Archives of General Psychiatry, 66*(9), 1013–1020. https://doi.org/10.1001/archgenpsychiatry.2009.112

Fristad, M. A., Young, A. S., Vesco, A. T., Nader, E. S., Healy, K. Z., Gardner, W., Wolfson, H. L., & Arnold, L. E. (2015). A randomized controlled trial of individual family psychoeducational psychotherapy and Omega-3 fatty acids in youth with subsyndromal bipolar disorder. *Journal of Child and Adolescent Psychopharmacology, 25*(10), 764–774. https://doi.org/10.1089/cap.2015.0132

Geller, B., Craney, J. L., Bolhofner, K., Nickelsburg, M. J., Williams, M., & Zimerman, B. (2002). Two-year prospective follow-up of children with a prepubertal and early adolescent bipolar disorder phenotype. *American Journal of Psychiatry, 159*(6), 927–933. https://doi.org/10.1176/appi.ajp.159.6.927

Geller, B., Tillman, R., Bolhofner, K., & Zimerman, B. (2008). Child bipolar I disorder: Prospective continuity with adult bipolar I disorder; characteristics of second and third episodes; predictors of 8-year outcome. *Archives of General Psychiatry, 65*(10), 1125–1133. https://doi.org/10.1001/archpsyc.65.10.1125

Geller, B., Zimerman, B., Williams, M., & Frazier, J. (1994, revised 1996). *WASH-U-KSADS (Washington University at St. Louis Kiddie and Young Adult Schedule for Affective Disorders and Schizophrenia—Lifetime and present episode version-DSM-IV)*. St. Louis, MO: Washington University School of Medicine.

Goldstein, T. R., Axelson, D. A., Birmaher, B., & Brent, D. A. (2007). Dialectical behavior therapy for adolescents with bipolar disorder: A 1-year open trial. *Journal of the American Academy of Child and Adolescent Psychiatry, 46*(7), 820–830. https://doi.org/10.1097/chi.0b013e31805c1613

Goldstein, T. R., Birmaher, B., Axelson, D., Goldstein, B. I., Gill, M. K., Esposito-Smythers, C., Ryan, N. D., Strober, M. A., Hunt, J., & Keller, M. (2009a). Family environment and suicidal ideation among bipolar youth. *Archives of Suicide Research, 13*(4), 378–388. https://doi.org/10.1080/13811110903266699

Goldstein, T. R., Birmaher, B., Axelson, D., Goldstein, B. I., Gill, M. K., Esposito-Smythers, C., Ryan, N. D., Strober, M. A., Hunt, J., & Keller, M. (2009b). Psychosocial functioning among bipolar youth. *Journal of Affective Disorders, 114*(1–3), 174–183. https://doi.org/10.1016/j.jad.2008.07.001

Goldstein, B. I., Birmaher, B., Carlson, G. A., DelBello, M. P., Findling, R. L., Fristad, M., Kowatch, R. A., Miklowitz, D. J., Nery, F. G., Perez-Algorta, G., Van Meter, A., Zeni, C. P., Correll, C. U., Kim, H. W., Wozniak, J., Chang, K. D., Hillegers, M., & Youngstrom, E. A. (2017). The international society for bipolar disorders task force report on pediatric bipolar disorder: Knowledge to date and directions for future research. *Bipolar Disorders, 19*(7), 524–543. https://doi.org/10.1111/bdi.12556

Goldstein, T. R., Fersch-Podrat, R. K., Rivera, M., Axelson, D. A., Merranko, J., Yu, H., Brent, D. A., & Birmaher, B. (2015). Dialectical behavior therapy for adolescents with bipolar disorder: Results from a pilot randomized trial. *Journal of Child and Adolescent Psychopharmacology, 25*(2), 140–149. https://doi.org/10.1089/cap.2013.0145

Goldstein, T. R., Merranko, J., Krantz, M., Garcia, M., Franzen, P., Levenson, J., Axelson, D., Birmaher, B., & Frank, E. (2018). Early intervention for adolescents at-risk for bipolar disorder: A pilot randomized trial of Interpersonal and Social Rhythm Therapy (IPSRT). *Journal of Affective Disorders, 235*, 348–356. https://doi.org/10.1016/j.jad.2018.04.049

Goldstein, T. R., Miklowitz, D. J., & Mullen, K. L. (2006). Social skills knowledge and performance among adolescents with bipolar disorder. *Bipolar Disorders, 8*(4), 350–361. https://doi.org/10.1111/j.1399-5618.2006.00321.x

Hauser, M., Galling, B., & Correll, C. U. (2013). Suicidal ideation and suicide attempts in children and adolescents with bipolar disorder: A systematic review of prevalence and incidence rates, correlates, and targeted interventions. *Bipolar Disorders, 5*(5), 507–523. https://doi.org/10.1111/bdi.12094

Henin, A., Mick, E., Biederman, J., Fried, R., Wozniak, J., Faraone, S. V., Harrington, K., Davis, S., & Doyle, A. E. (2007). Can bipolar disorder-specific neuropsychological impairments in children be identified? *Journal of Consulting and Clinical Psychology, 75*(2), 210–220. https://doi.org/10.1037/0022-006X.75.2.210

Henry, D. B., Pavuluri, M. N., Youngstrom, E., & Birmaher, B. (2008). Accuracy of brief and full forms of the child mania rating scale. *Journal of Clinical Psychology, 64*(4), 368–381. https://doi.org/10.1002/jclp.20464

Hlastala, S. A., Kotler, J. S., McClellan, J. M., & McCauley, E. A. (2010). Interpersonal and social rhythm therapy for adolescents with bipolar disorder: Treatment development and results from an open trial. *Depression and Anxiety, 27*(5), 457–464. https://doi.org/10.1002/da.20668

Kaufman, J., Birmaher, B., Axelson, D., Perepletchikova, F., Brent, D., & Ryan, N. (2016). Schedule for affective disorders and schizophrenia for school-age children-present and lifetime version for DSM-5 (K-SADS-PL DSM-5). University of Pittsburgh Child and Adolescent Bipolar Spectrum Services. Retrieved from https://www.pediatricbipolar.pitt.edu/sites/default/files/KSADS_DSM_5_SCREEN_Final.pdf. (Accessed 16 February 2022).

Kaufman, J., Birmaher, B., Brent, D., & Rao, U. (1997). Schedule for affective disorders and schizophrenia for school-age children-present and lifetime version (K-SADS-PL): Initial reliability and validity data. *Journal of the American Academy of Child & Adolescent Psychiatry, 36*(7), 980–988. https://doi.org/10.1097/00004583-199707000-00021

Khazanov, G. K., Cui, L., Merikangas, K. R., & Angst, J. (2015). Treatment patterns of youth with bipolar disorder: Results from the National Comorbidity Survey—Adolescent Supplement (NCS-A). *Journal of Abnormal Child Psychology, 43*(2), 391–400. https://doi.org/10.1007/s10802-014-9885-6

Kim, E. Y., Miklowitz, D. J., Biuckians, A., & Mullen, K. (2007). Life stress and the course of early-onset bipolar disorder. *Journal of Affective Disorders, 99*(1–3), 37-44. https://doi.org/10.1016/j.jad.2006.08.022

Kovacs, M. (2011). *Children's depression inventory 2nd edition: Self-report*. North Tonawanda, NY: Multi-Health Systems.

Lewinsohn, P. M., Olino, T. M., & Klein, D. N. (2005). Psychosocial impairment in offspring of depressed parents. *Psychological Medicine: A Journal of Research in Psychiatry and the Allied Sciences, 35*(10), 1493–1503. https://doi.org/10.1017/S0033291705005350

Lewinsohn, P. M., Seeley, J. R., & Klein, D. N. (2003). Bipolar disorder in adolescents: Epidemiology and suicidal behavior. In B. Geller & M. P. DelBello (Eds.), *Bipolar disorder in childhood and early adolescence* (pp. 7–24). New York: Guilford Press.

Linehan, M. M. (1993). *Cognitive-behavioral treatment of borderline personality disorder*. New York: Guilford Press.

MacPherson, H. A., Leffler, J. M., & Fristad, M. A. (2014). Implementation of multi-family psychoeducational psychotherapy for childhood mood disorders in an outpatient community setting. *Journal of Marital and Family Therapy, 40*(2), 193–211. http://doi.org/10.1111/jmft.12013

MacPherson, H. A., Weinstein, S. M., Henry, D. B., & West, A. E. (2016). Mediators in the randomized trial of Child- and Family-Focused Cognitive-Behavioral Therapy for pediatric bipolar disorder. *Behaviour Research and Therapy, 85*, 60–71. https://doi.org/10.1016/j.brat.2016.08.014

McClellan, J., Kowatch, R., & Findling, R. L. (2007). Practice parameter for the assessment and treatment of children and adolescents with bipolar disorder. *Journal of the American Academy of Child & Adolescent Psychiatry, 46*(1), 107–125. https://doi.org/10.1097/01.chi.00002422

Mendez, I., Castro-Fornieles, J., Lera-Miguel, S., Picado, M., Borras, R., Cosi, S., Valenti, M., Santamarina, P., Font, E., & Romero, S. (2020). Functional impairment and clinical correlates in adolescents with bipolar disorder compared to healthy controls. A case-control study. *Journal of the Canadian Academy of Child and Adolescent Psychiatry = Journal de l'Academie anadienne de psychiatrie de l'enfant et de l'adolescent, 29*(3), 149–164.

Miklowitz, D. J., Axelson, D. A., Birmaher, B., George, E. L., Taylor, D. O., Schneck, C. D., Beresford, C. A., Dickinson, L. M., & Craighead, W. E. (2008). Family-focused treatment for adolescents with bipolar disorder. *Archives of General Psychiatry, 65*(9), 1053–1061. https://doi:10.1001/archpsyc.65.9.1053

Miklowitz, D. J., Chang, K. D., Taylor, D. O., George, E. L., Singh, M. K., Schneck, C. D., Dickinson, L. M., Howe, M. E., & Garber, J. (2011). Early psychosocial intervention for youth at risk for bipolar I or II disorder: A one-year treatment development trial. *Bipolar Disorders, 13*(1), 67–75. https://doi.org/10.1111/j.1399-5618.2011.00890.x

Miklowitz, D. J., George, E. L., Axelson, D. A., Kim, E. Y., Birmaher, B., Schneck, C., Beresford, C., & Craighead, W. E. (2004). Family-focused treatment for adolescents with bipolar disorder. *Journal of Affective Disorders, 82*(Suppl. 1), S113–S128. https://doi.org/10.1016/j.jad.2004.05.020

Miklowitz, D. J., Schneck, C. D., George, E. L., Taylor, D. O., Sugar, C. A., Birmaher, B., Kowatch, R. A., DelBello, M. P., & Axelson, D. A. (2014). Pharmacotherapy and family-focused treatment for adolescents with bipolar I and II disorders: A 2-year randomized trial. *The American Journal of Psychiatry, 171*(6), 658–667. https://doi.org/10.1176/appi.ajp.2014.13081130

Miklowitz, D. J., Schneck, C. D., Singh, M. K., Taylor, D. O., George, E. L., Cosgrove, V. E., Howe, M. E., Dickinson, L. M., Garber, J., & Chang, K. D. (2013). Early intervention for symptomatic youth at risk for bipolar disorder: A randomized trial of family-focused therapy. *Journal of the American Academy of Child and Adolescent Psychiatry, 52*(2), 121–131. https://doi.org/10.1016/j.jaac.2012.10.007

Pavuluri, M. N., Graczyk, P. A., Henry, D. B., Carbray, J. A., Heidenreich, J., & Miklowitz, D. J. (2004). Child- and family-focused cognitive-behavioral therapy for pediatric bipolar disorder: Development and preliminary results. *Journal of the American Academy of Child and Adolescent Psychiatry, 43*(5), 528–537. https://doi.org/10.1097/00004583-200405000-00006

Pavuluri, M. N., Henry, D. B., Devineni, B., Carbray, J. A., & Birmaher, B. (2006a). Child mania rating scale: Development, reliability, and validity. *Journal of the American Academy of Child & Adolescent Psychiatry, 45*(5), 550–560. https://doi.org/10.1097/01.chi.0000205700.40700.50

Pavuluri, M. N., O'Connor, M. M., Harral, E. M., Moss, M., & Sweeney, J. A. (2006b). Impact of neurocognitive function on academic difficulties in pediatric bipolar disorder: A clinical translation. *Biological Psychiatry. Special Issue: The Clinical and Neural Phenotype of Mood Disturbance in Children and Adults, 60*(9), 951–956. https://doi.org/10.1016/j.biopsych.2006.03.027

Pavuluri, M. N., O'Connor, M. M., Harral, E., & Sweeney, J. A. (2007). Affective neural circuitry during facial emotion processing in pediatric bipolar disorder. *Biological Psychiatry, 62*(2), 158–167. https://doi.org/10.1016/j.biopsych.2006.07.011

Pavuluri, M. N., West, A., Hill, S. K., Jindal, K., & Sweeney, J. A. (2009). Neurocognitive function in pediatric bipolar disorder: 3-year follow-up shows cognitive development lagging behind healthy youths. *Journal of the American Academy of Child & Adolescent Psychiatry, 48*(3), 299–307. https://doi.org/ 10.1097/CHI.0b013e318196b907

Rucklidge, J. (2006). Psychosocial functioning of adolescents with and without pediatric bipolar disorder. *Journal of Affective Disorders, 91*(2–3), 181–188.

Segal, Z. V., Williams, J. M. G., & Teasdale, J. D. (2002). *Mindfulness-based cognitive therapy for depression: A new approach to preventing relapse*. New York: Guilford Press.

Shaffer, D., Gould, M. S., Brasic, J., Ambrosini, P., Fisher, P., Bird, H., & Aluwahlia, S. (1983). A children's global assessment scale (CGAS). *Archives of General Psychiatry, 40*(11), 1228–1231. https://doi.org/10.1001/archpsyc.1983.01790100074010

Southam-Gerow, M. A., & Prinstein, M. J. (2014). Evidence base updates: The evolution of the evaluation of psychological treatments for children and adolescents. *Journal of Clinical Child and Adolescent Psychology, 43*(1), 1–6. https://doi.org/10.1080/15374416.2013

Van Meter, A., Moreira, A. L. R., & Youngstrom, E. (2019). Updated meta-analysis of epidemiologic studies of pediatric bipolar disorder. *The Journal of Clinical Psychiatry, 80*(3), 18r12180. https://doi.org/10.4088/JCP.18r12180

Washburn, J. J., West, A. E., & Heil, J. A. (2011). Treatment of pediatric bipolar disorder: A review. *Minerva Psichiatrica, 52*(1), 21–35.

Weinstein, S. M., Henry, D. B., Katz, A. C., Peters, A. T., & West, A. E. (2015). Treatment moderators of child- and family-focused cognitive-behavioral therapy for pediatric bipolar disorder. *Journal of the American Academy of Child and Adolescent Psychiatry, 54*(2), 116–125. https://doi.org/10.1016/j.jaac.2014.11.007

Weinstein, S. M., West, A. E., & Pavuluri, M. (2013). Psychosocial intervention for pediatric bipolar disorder: Current and future directions. *Expert Review of Neurotherapeutics, 13*(7), 843–850. https://doi.org/10.1586/14737175.2013.811

West, A. E., Celio, C. I., Henry, D. B., & Pavuluri, M. N. (2011). Child mania rating scale-parent version: A valid measure of symptom change due to pharmacotherapy. *Journal of Affective Disorders, 128*(1–2), 112–119. https://doi.org/10.1016/j.jad.2010.06.013

West, A. E., Henry, D. B., & Pavuluri, M. N. (2007). Maintenance model of integrated psychosocial treatment in pediatric bipolar disorder: A pilot feasibility study. *Journal of the American Academy of Child & Adolescent Psychiatry, 46*(2), 205–212. https://doi.org/10.1097/01.chi.0000246068.85577.d7

West, A. E., Jacobs, R. H., Westerholm, R., Lee, A., Carbray, J., Heidenreich, J., & Pavuluri, M. N. (2009). Child and family-focused cognitive-behavioral therapy for pediatric bipolar disorder: Pilot study of group treatment format. *Journal of the Canadian Academy of Child and Adolescent Psychiatry / Journal De l'Académie Canadienne De Psychiatrie De l'Enfant Et De l'Adolescent, 18*(3), 239–246.

West, A. E., Weinstein, S. M., & Pavuluri, M. N. (2017). *Child- and family-focused cognitive behavioral therapy for pediatric bipolar disorder treatment manual: Programs that work series.* New York: Oxford University Press.

West, A. E., Weinstein, S. M., Peters, A. T., Katz, A. C., Henry, D. B., Cruz, R. A., & Pavuluri, M. N. (2014). Child- and family-focused cognitive-behavioral therapy for pediatric bipolar disorder: A randomized clinical trial. *Journal of the American Academy of Child and Adolescent Psychiatry, 53*(11), 1168–1178.e1. https://doi.org/10.1016/j.jaac.2014.08.013

Wilens, T. E., Biederman, J., Forkner, P., Ditterline, J., Morris, M., Moore, H., Wozniak, J. (2003). Patterns of comorbidity and dysfunction in clinically referred preschool and school-age children with bipolar disorder. *Journal of Child and Adolescent Psychopharmacology, 13*(4), 495–505. https://doi.org/10.1089/104454603322724887

Wozniak, J., Biederman, J., Kiely, K., & Ablon, J. S. (1995). Mania-like symptoms suggestive of childhood-onset bipolar disorder in clinically referred children. *Journal of the American Academy of Child & Adolescent Psychiatry, 34*(7), 867–876. https://doi.org/10.1097/00004583-199507000-00010

Wozniak, J., Petty, C. R., Schreck, M., Moses, A., Faraone, S. V., & Biederman, J. (2011). High level of persistence of pediatric bipolar-I disorder from childhood onto adolescent years: A four year prospective longitudinal follow-up study. *Journal of Psychiatric Research, 45*(10), 1273–1282. https://doi.org/10.1016/j.jpsychires.2010.10.006

Youngstrom, E. A., Birmaher, B., & Findling, R. L. (2008). Pediatric bipolar disorder: Validity, phenomenology, and recommendations for diagnosis. *Bipolar Disorders, 10*(1 Pt 2), 194–214. https://doi.org/10.1111/j.1399-5618.2007.00563.x

Youngstrom, E. A., Findling, R. L., Youngstrom, J. K., & Calabrese, J. R. (2005). Toward an evidence-based assessment of pediatric bipolar disorder. *Journal of Clinical Child and Adolescent Psychology, 34*(3), 433–448. https://doi.org/10.1207/s15374424jccp3403_4

17
SUICIDAL BEHAVIOR

David N. Miller and James J. Mazza

Introduction and Overview of CBT for Youth Suicidal Behavior

Youth suicide is a disturbing, pervasive, and challenging public health problem in the United States (Espelage et al., 2022). Although suicide is the 10th-leading cause of death among adults, it is the 2nd-leading cause of death among young people aged 10–24. According to the CDC, in 2021 there were approximately 2,900 known suicides among youth aged 10–19, with even higher numbers among youth aged 20–24. Within the child and adolescent K-12 age range, suicide rates increase as children grow older, with elementary school-aged children at lowest risk and high school students at highest risk (Miller, 2021). Additionally, notable increases in youth suicide rates have been reported among traditionally marginalized groups, including Black youth (Bridge et al., 2018; Marraccini, Griffin, et al., 2022) and LGBTQ+ youth (Marraccini, Ingram, et al., 2022). Rates of suicidal behavior among the latter group are especially high, reflecting the high rates of bullying and discrimination LGBTQ+ youth receive.

Suicide is the most extreme form of several types of suicidal behavior, which are distinct but frequently overlapping conditions that exist on a continuum. These suicidal behaviors include suicidal ideation, making plans for suicide, suicide attempts, and suicide (Miller, 2021). Even when these suicidal behaviors do not result in death, they cause significant subjective distress among youth, their family, and their friends (Miller et al., 2009). In a national sample of US high school students conducted in 2021, 22% indicated that they seriously considered suicide, 18% reported making a suicide plan, 10% reported they attempted suicide, and 3% indicated that their suicide attempt resulted in an injury that had to be treated by a medical professional (Gaylor et al., 2023). One illustration of the complexity of youth suicidal behavior involves the sex of the individual. Specifically, although adolescent females *attempt* suicide at rate higher than adolescent males, adolescent males *die* by suicide at a rate much higher than adolescent females—a longstanding finding known as the "gender paradox" of suicide (Canetto & Sakinofsky, 1998). Clearly, an alarmingly high number of young people are at-risk for suicidal behavior, and schools have a critical role to play in youth suicide prevention efforts (Espelage et al., 2022; Mazza & Miller, 2024; Miller, 2021).

As a significant public health problem, youth suicidal behavior requires public health approaches to prevent it most effectively (Miller, 2021; Robinson et al., 2018). In schools, a public health approach to youth suicide prevention involves the implementation of a comprehensive, multi-tier system of support (MTSS) framework (Mazza & Miller, 2024; Miller, 2021). An MTSS framework

DOI: 10.4324/9781003392439-20

typically consists of three overlapping tiers that collectively represent a continuum of prevention and intervention services that increase in intensity depending on the corresponding needs of the student population (Shinn & Walker, 2010). For example, an MTSS approach to youth suicide prevention in schools would address all youth in a particular population at Tier 1 (e.g., providing all students in a high school with information about youth suicide and who and where to go to for help), youth identified as being potentially at risk for suicide at Tier 2 (e.g., group counseling for youth who exhibit depression, hopelessness, and/or substance abuse problems), and youth who were identified as engaging in suicidal behavior at Tier 3 (e.g., brief cognitive-behavior therapy [BCBT] for youth who had made a suicide attempt).

Because school personnel have such frequent contact with children and adolescents, they are uniquely positioned to prevent youth suicide. Many schools have reported significant increases in their number of students with mental health problems, such as depression, anxiety, and suicidal behavior, and this trend appears likely to continue as the US contends with the ongoing effects of the COVID-19 pandemic. Unfortunately, many school personnel, including school-based mental health professionals, report being inadequately trained to effectively prevent and respond to youth suicidal behavior (Miller & Jome, 2010; O'Neill et al., 2020). Clearly, school psychologists, school counselors, and school social workers need the knowledge and skills to provide psychotherapeutic and other interventions for students exhibiting suicidal behavior and to understand which interventions have empirical support for their effectiveness.

Research indicates that the most effective treatments for suicidal behavior are derived from cognitive-behavioral models (Bryan & Rudd, 2018; Robinson et al., 2018). Although important knowledge has been gained by researchers trained in alternative theoretical frameworks, it is widely accepted that cognitive-behavioral models may "fit" more readily with a functional approach to suicide (described in the next section). In particular, "the functional model's emphasis on understanding the contextual antecedents and consequences of suicidal thoughts and behaviors (e.g., thoughts, emotions, and behavioral responses) parallels the core conceptual principles of cognitive-behavioral theory" (Bryan & Rudd, 2018, p. 6).

In recent years, a significant evolutionary development in the advancement and refinement of cognitive-behavioral interventions for suicidal behavior has been the growth of BCBT. Although BCBT has a recent history and to date has been evaluated primarily with adults (Bryan & Rudd, 2018), it holds considerable promise as an evidence-informed intervention for youth exhibiting suicidal behavior. Given that most mental health interventions for children and adolescents are provided in schools, it is especially important for school-based mental health professionals (e.g., school psychologists, school counselors, school social workers) to become familiar with BCBT, specifically as it related to alleviating youth suicidal behavior at the Tier 3 level of support.

Understanding Youth Suicidal Behavior

Traditional approaches to treating suicidal individuals have largely been influenced by a *risk factor model* of suicide, which attempts to understand suicidal behaviors by identifying and describing their correlates (Bryan & Rudd, 2018). Treatment informed by the risk factor model "aims to reduce these risk factors under the impression that doing so will reduce the incidence and/or severity of suicidal thoughts and behaviors" (Bryan & Rudd, 2018, p. 4). A subcategory of the risk factor model is the *psychiatric syndromal model* of suicide, in which "suicidal thoughts and behaviors are described and organized according to observable characteristics and surface features of the behaviors (e.g., methods, lethality, and intent), similar to the syndromal classification schemes commonly used in the mental health and medical professions" (Bryan & Rudd, 2018, p. 4).

Although these models are intuitively appealing and have been widely applied in attempts to prevent suicide, a meta-analysis of 50 years of research found that variables that were believed to be risk factors for suicide are more accurately described as being risk factors for suicidal ideation (Franklin et al., 2017). Moreover, these risk factors are not particularly useful for prospectively predicting death by suicide, and the risk factor model has had little impact on either suicide prevention or the development of effective treatments (Franklin et al., 2017). The finding that most psychiatric disorders are correlated with suicidal thoughts but not suicidal behaviors "suggests that treatments that prioritize psychiatric disorders may not be as sufficiently specific to the mechanisms that give rise to suicidal behavior. As a result, they reduce psychiatric symptoms but not the risk for suicide attempts" (Bryan & Rudd, 2018, p. 4).

A more useful theoretical framework than either the risk factor model or the psychiatric syndromal model is the *functional model* of suicide. According to this model,

> suicidal thoughts and behaviors are conceptualized as the outcome of underlying psychopathological processes that specially precipitate and maintain suicidal thoughts and behaviors over time. From this perspective, suicidal thoughts and behaviors are not the result of any particular psychological process per se (e.g., psychiatric illness); rather, they are the result of how the psychological process is experienced by the individual within the context of his or her personal history, immediate environment, and behavioral responses. Clinically, the functional model suggests that the primary target of treatment with suicidal individuals is not the psychiatric illness itself, but rather it is the context that surrounds the emergence and maintenance of suicide risk over time.
>
> *(Bryan & Rudd, 2018, pp. 4–5)*

The utility and superiority of the functional model of suicidal behavior is now well established. For example, in a meta-analysis of 24 studies examining treatment effectiveness for suicidal ideation and suicide attempts, treatments that directly targeted suicidal thoughts and behaviors as the primary outcome (i.e., a functional approach) led to larger and statistically significant improvements in suicide risk as compared to treatments that primarily targeted psychiatric diagnosis (Tarrier et al., 2008). As noted by Bryan and Rudd (2018),

> the general consensus among suicide researchers is that the treatment of suicidal individuals should focus directly on suicide risk as opposed to psychiatric diagnosis. Unfortunately, despite the scientific evidence that supports this perspective, the majority of mental health professionals continue to be influenced heavily by the psychiatric syndromal model of treatment, a situation that is due in large part to insufficient education and training for clinicians in newer and better models of care.
>
> *(p. 6)*

Empirical Support of CBT in Treatment of Youth Suicidal Behavior

In examining the empirical literature for the treatment of suicidal behaviors generally, it should 1st be acknowledged that, to date, no interventions have been shown to prevent suicide death (Bryan, 2022). This is due primarily to the very high cost (in terms of money, resources, and time) "that would need to be incurred to conduct and implement such a study; death by suicide occurs with such infrequency that it would require a very large sample of participants to examine death as an outcome" (Bryan & Rudd, 2018, p. 6). Consequently, studies examining treatment efficacy typically use proxies for suicide that are highly associated with it, such as suicidal ideation and suicide attempts. Suicide attempt is considered the best available proxy for suicide (Bryan & Rudd, 2018), as the presence and frequency of suicide attempts is the single most powerful predictor of subsequent death by suicide (O'Connor, 2021).

Cognitive-behavioral interventions have demonstrated the most efficacy in reducing suicidal behavior, with numerous clinical trials having been conducted over several decades (e.g., Moutier et al., 2021; O'Connor, 2021; Tarrier et al., 2008). The two most investigated and promising cognitive-behavioral interventions for suicidal behavior to date are dialectical behavior therapy (DBT) and cognitive-behavior therapy (CBT). Research has demonstrated that both DBT (DeCou et al., 2019; Linehan, 1993; Linehan et al., 2006) and CBT (Brown et al., 2005; D'Anci et al., 2019; Mewton & Andrews, 2016; Tarrier et al., 2008) are evidence-based interventions for adult suicidal behavior, and there has been increasing evidence to support their efficacy with youth as well. For example, DBT has been found to be an effective intervention to decrease suicidal behavior among adolescents (McCauley et al., 2018; Miller et al., 2007). However, despite its considerable promise as an intervention for reducing suicide attempts, "wider implementation of DBT has been hindered by the fact that the treatment is very resource intensive, time-consuming, and difficult to learn" (Bryan & Rudd, 2018, p. 8). Consequently, there is a need for briefer, less complex, and more practical cognitive-behavioral treatment approaches—including those that can be used effectively with youth in schools.

One of the 1st clinical researchers to develop a BCBT for suicidal individuals were Rudd et al. (2001). Their highly structured individual therapy model included skills training in cognitive reappraisal, problem solving, and emotion regulation, as well as the development of crisis response plans for individuals experiencing a suicidal crisis. The 1st study to provide empirical support for the efficacy of a brief cognitive-behavioral intervention for preventing suicide attempts in adults was conducted by Brown and colleagues (2005), who used a ten-session, outpatient, individual cognitive-behavioral therapy that was analogous to the approach taken by Rudd et al. (2001).

In a randomized control trial comparing cognitive therapy to usual care, Brown and his colleagues (2005) found that individuals receiving cognitive therapy were 50% less likely to make a suicide attempt during the 18-month follow-up period than individuals receiving usual care (24% in cognitive therapy vs. 42% in usual care). Notably, there were minimal differences between the two groups in terms of depression, hopelessness, and suicidal ideation following treatment. The Brown et al. (2005) study demonstrated that brief, time-limited, cognitive-behavioral therapies had the potential to be as effective as more complex and extensive cognitive-behavioral therapies. In fact, meta-analytic results indicate that cognitive-behavioral therapies of longer duration are no more effective than briefer cognitive-behavioral therapies (Tarrier et al., 2008). Consequently, there has been greater attention given to BCBT for a variety of emotional and behavioral problems, including the prevention of suicidal behavior (Bryan & Rudd, 2018).

Rudd and colleagues (2015) also conducted a randomized clinical trial examining the efficacy of CBT for reducing suicidal behavior. Participants included 152 active-duty military personnel who exhibited suicidal ideation during the past week and/or made a suicide attempt within the last month. The participants were referred to the study after they were discharged from inpatient hospitalization for suicide risk, with half of the participants randomly assigned to receive BCBT and the other half randomly assigned to receive "treatment as usual," which was determined by the participants' primary mental health clinician and included individual and group psychotherapy, psychiatric medication, substance abuse treatment, and/or support groups. The participants randomly assigned to the BCBT group received 12 outpatient, individual BCBT sessions on a weekly or bi-weekly basis, with the 1st session lasting 90 minutes and all subsequent sessions lasting 60 minutes. The BCBT interventions were administered by two clinical social workers; one had recently completed her master's degree and the other was a licensed practitioner with over 20 years of experience. The results of this landmark study found that BCBT was significantly more effective than treatment as usual and "confirmed the effectiveness of BCBT as a viable alternative to longer and more time-intensive treatments like DBT" (Bryan & Rudd, 2018, p. 17). Perhaps most importantly, Rudd et al. (2015) reported a 60% reduction in risk for suicide attempts among individuals receiving BCBT, which was the largest magnitude in reduction in suicide attempt risk to date.

More recently, Sinyor and colleagues (2020) conducted a randomized control trial comparing BCBT for suicide prevention with a minimally directive supportive psychotherapy in adolescents and young adults aged 16–26. All participants in the study had been hospitalized following incidents of self-harm. Both treatment conditions included ten sessions over a 15-week period, followed by three booster sessions occurring at three-month intervals. A total of 24 individuals participated in the study (12 per condition), with one BCBT participant and two participants in the control condition dropping out prior to the 1st treatment session. Following treatment, there were significantly fewer instances of self-harm behaviors among participants in the BCBT condition (11%) as compared to those receiving treatment in the control condition (30%). Three participants in the control condition made a total of five suicide attempts during the study, whereas no participants in the BCBT condition made a suicide attempt. Although the study had a small sample size and should therefore be viewed with caution, it provides initial evidence for the promise of BCBT in reducing suicidal behavior in young people.

Relational Considerations in Treating Youth Suicidal Behavior

One of the most consistent findings in psychotherapy research has been that a strong therapeutic alliance between the therapist and the client is positively correlated with treatment outcome (Martin et al., 2000). The therapeutic alliance may be conceptualized as the mutual influence of three distinct but interrelated processes: goals, tasks, and bond. *Goals* refer to the extent to which the client and the clinician agree upon the overall objectives and purpose of the treatment. *Tasks* refer to the extent to which the client and the clinician agree upon the specific activities and techniques used in treatment to achieve mutually agreed upon goals. *Bond* refers to the extent to which the client and the clinician feel emotionally connected with each other (Bryan & Rudd, 2018).

It may be the case that

> certain cognitive-behavioral therapies such as BCBT provide a framework that supports the creation and development of an effective collaborative alliance… [which is] likely due to the fact that cognitive-behavioral therapies like BCBT are based on a collaborative model of care that explicitly invites the patient to take an active role in the development of treatment goals and the implementation of specific strategies to achieve these goals. The collaborative approach also contributes to a strong emotional bond because it helps to resolve a conflict inherent to work with suicidal patients: the patient's primary goal to reduce psychological suffering as compared to the clinician's primary goal to prevent death by suicide.
>
> *(Bryan & Rudd, 2018, p. 38)*

When assessing and treating potentially suicidal youth in schools, forming an effective therapeutic alliance is critical. Ideally, the school-based mental health clinician providing treatment will already have a strong and supportive relationship with the suicidal youth. If that is not the case (and often it is not), the clinician "should ensure that he or she behaves in a manner that makes the student feel as comfortable as possible, with the goal of establishing rapport and gaining the student's trust" (Miller, 2021, p. 120). Conducting an effective suicide risk assessment is a prerequisite to providing effective treatment and should be viewed as a critical skill set for all school-based mental health professionals, particularly those who work with adolescents. Some basic and essential elements of conducting effective school-based suicide risk assessments are discussed in the next section.

Assessing and Interviewing Potentially Suicidal Youth

King and her colleagues (2013) identified four basic principles of youth suicide risk assessment: (1) suicide risk can be understood; (2) risk for suicide is not static and therefore assessment should be ongoing; (3) risk for suicide does not always "shout out;" and (4) multiple informants facilitate a comprehensive assessment. Each of these principles will now be briefly described, followed by some important issues clinicians should be aware of when assessing potentially suicidal youth in schools.

A variety of risk factors for the increased probability of youth suicidal behavior have been identified, including (a) students with mental health problems, such as nonsuicidal self-injury, clinical depression, substance abuse problems, and/or acting out behavior problems; (b) students known to have made a previous suicide attempts; (c) minoritized populations of students, such as Native American youth; (d) LGBTQ+ students; (e) students who engage in dangerous and/or risky behavior; (f) students who have a family history of suicide; (g) students who have communicated to a desire to die by suicide; and (h) students with easy access to guns (Miller, 2021). The presence of these and other risk factors should be assessed, as well as possible warning signs for suicide.

As opposed to risk factors, which may predispose an individual to the increased probability of suicidal behavior, warning signs may indicate the more immediate possibility of a suicidal crisis (Miller, 2021). Common warning signs for the increased probability of suicidal behavior include (a) talking about wanting to die or killing oneself; (b) looking/searching for a way to end one's life; (c) increased alcohol or drug use; (d) withdrawing from others; (e) hopelessness; (f) sleeping too much or too little; (g) feeling anxious or agitated; (h) feeling trapped; and (i) anger, rage, or wanting revenge (Bryan, 2022). Unfortunately, as with risk factors, the clinical utility of warning signs in accurately predicting the probability of suicide, either individually or collectively, is limited (Miller, 2021).

Additionally, research has indicated that suicide risk is not static (King et al., 2013); it can and often does fluctuate markedly, even over brief periods of time (Bryan, 2022). Consequently, clinicians should not be fooled into believing that the results of a suicide risk assessment with a given student will be stable over time. Assessment should rather be ongoing and continue during and after treatment is provided. Guidelines for engaging in effective progress monitoring of BCBT for youth suicidal behavior are provided in a later section in this chapter.

One of the most challenging aspects of youth suicide risk assessment is that some students may not share information regarding their suicidal thoughts, intent, plans, or history with the clinician or other adults (e.g., parents). King and colleagues (2013) suggest that this reluctance on the part of youth to disclose their suicidal thoughts and/or behavior

> could be for many possible reasons: perhaps because they fear others' strong emotional or negative reactions, or because they can't find the words or courage to share their thoughts, or because they have been to the emergency department or inpatient unit before and do not want to return, or because they do not want someone to abort or interrupt their plan to die by suicide.
> *(p. 70)*

Regardless of the reason, if students demonstrate an unwillingness to disclose suicidal behavior when there is evidence it is occurring, it is especially important that clinicians make use of multiple informants. For example,

> parents can provide important information that students may not know (e.g., detailed information about previous mental health service providers; a family history of suicidal behavior or mental health problems). Even when the student is able and willing to provide information

> about his or her suicidal behavior, other adults in the student's environment can often provide supplemental information of value.
>
> *(Miller, 2021, p. 119)*

In general, the most important and useful component of an effective youth suicide risk assessment is conducting an *individual clinical interview* with the identified student. School-based clinicians should be aware that

> conducting effective suicide risk assessments is a fluid and dynamic process and not a rote and rigid one in which every student should be asked the same questions in the same sequence. Rather, the questions will vary, depending on the student's responses and developmental level and the specific issues being assessed. In other words, suicide risk assessment interviews with children and adolescents should cover pertinent areas of interest, but the way in which the process unfolds will depend to some degree on the student and his or her unique circumstances. Flexibility is required, as each case is different, even though the major issues to assess will largely remain the same.
>
> *(Miller, 2021, p. 120)*

What are the "major issues" that should be assessed in conducting youth suicide risk assessments in schools? Clearly various risk factors and warning signs should be assessed, but 1st the clinician should strive to make the student as comfortable as possible and be mentally prepared to conduct the interview. One of the biggest obstacles to mental health professionals asking clients about their suicidal thoughts is fear. Freedenthal (2018) cited four common fears about asking individuals about their suicidal thoughts: (1) the fear of putting the idea of suicide into a person's head; (2) the fear of making suicidal ideation worse by discussing it; (3) the fear of angering the person; and (4) the fear of the individual responding affirmatively when asked if they have had thoughts about killing themselves. Few if any activities will arouse more fear and anxiety in a clinician than asking someone about their suicidal behavior, and much of the basis for this fear and anxiety is the belief that talking about suicidal behavior with an individual may inadvertently and unintentionally result in an increase in suicide risk, simply by candidly discussing it. Fortunately, several studies have found this is *not* the case (e.g., Gould et al., 2005; Harris & Gough, 2017). To the contrary, research suggests that youth who openly talk about suicide with trusted adults typically have more beneficial outcomes (Miller, 2021).

More information regarding the clinical interview of suicidal youth is provided later in this chapter. As with other topics covered in it, however, a complete discussion of this important aspect of youth suicide prevention is not possible given space limitations. Readers seeking additional information on clinical interviewing with suicidal individuals are encouraged to review Bryan and Rudd (2018), Freedenthal (2018), King et al. (2013), and Miller (2021, 2022).

Case Conceptualization

The case conceptualization serves as the working model for helping the client and the clinician to understand why the client got to the point of contemplating or attempting suicide and providing a targeted treatment plan to address it. The case conceptualization flows directly from the suicide risk assessment and functions to organize the features of the client's suicidal crisis into a coherent framework known as the *suicidal mode* (Bryan & Rudd, 2018). The suicidal mode

> provides a cognitive-behavioral framework for describing the characteristics and features of suicidal episodes (which may or may not include an actual suicide attempt) and serves as the

> underlying theoretical foundation for BCBT. Structurally, the suicidal mode is comprised of four interactive and mutually influential domains: cognitive, behavioral, emotional, and physical. These four domains are conceptualized across two levels corresponding to the stable (i.e., baseline) and dynamic (i.e., acute) dimensions of risk described by the fluid vulnerability theory of suicide.
>
> *(Bryan & Rudd, 2018, p. 21)*

The suicidal mode comprises a baseline dimension of relatively stable risk factors that persist over time, as well as dynamic or state-based factors that fluctuate over time due to situational variables and triggers (Bryan & Judge, 2018). For example, possible baseline cognitive dimensions may include an individual's self-regard, cognitive flexibility, and problem solving, whereas more acute cognitive dimensions may include frequent thoughts such as "This is hopeless," "I'm trapped," or "I'm a burden" (Bryan & Rudd, 2018, p. 22). In the behavioral dimension, possible baseline behavioral dimensions may include prior suicide attempts, emotion regulation skills, and interpersonal skills, whereas more acute behavioral dimensions may include substance abuse, social withdrawal, and engaging in preparations to kill oneself (Bryan & Rudd, 2018).

Bryan and Rudd (2018), the leading researchers and clinicians in the use of BCBT for suicide prevention, suggest that the suicidal mode

> serves as the central organizing principle for the BCBT protocol; all interventions flow directly from it. The suicidal mode not only provides a simple and straightforward way for the patient to understand why he or she wants to die by suicide and/or made a suicide attempt, it also provides the patient with a rationale for each procedure and intervention used during treatment. To this end, when introducing and teaching a new intervention to the patient, the clinician should be sure to tie the concept or skill directly to the suicidal mode. Patients who clearly understand why they are being asked to use a skill and how it is supposed to work are much more likely to use the skill effectively.
>
> *(p. 25)*

Although there are no formal "prerequisites" for learning BCBT, Bryan and Rudd (2018) recommend that "clinicians who possess certain skill sets and competencies learn the treatment much faster and implement the [BCBT] protocol with greater fidelity" (p. 77). These skills and competencies include (a) training and supervision in cognitive-behavioral case conceptualization, (b) training in basic learning theory, and (c) training and supervision in motivational interviewing (Bryan & Rudd, 2018).

The suicidal mode is embedded within an important component of the *fluid vulnerability theory* of suicide. The core assumptions of fluid vulnerability theory include the following: (a) suicide risk comprises stable and dynamic properties referred to as baseline risk and acute risk. Baseline risk entails the chronic or more persistent aspect of risk whereas acute risk entails the state-based or more transient aspect of risk; (b) suicidal episodes are time-limited; (c) baseline risk varies across individuals based on one's unique constellation of historical and developmental predispositions, and these predispositions determine an individual's threshold for activation in response to triggering events; (d) acute suicidal episodes occur among sufficiently vulnerable individuals when they experience a sufficient stressful trigger; (e) individuals with high baseline risk have low thresholds for activation and therefore experience frequent and long-lasting suicidal episodes even when experiencing mild stress; (f) individuals with low baseline risk have high thresholds for activation and therefore rarely experience suicidal episodes even when experiencing extreme stress; (g) multiple suicide attempts and nonsuicidal self-injury are the clearest markers of elevated baseline risk and vulnerability to persisting risk; (h) acute suicide risk resolves when the aggravating factors that maintain the suicidal mode are deactivated or reduced; and (i) following resolution of an acute suicidal episode an individual returns to his or her baseline risk level (Bryan & Rudd, 2018).

Although the development of BCBT has been based largely on the fluid vulnerability theory and the notion of the suicidal mode, another conceptual model of suicide that is relevant to BCBT is what is known as *ideation-to-action* models of suicide. As its name indicates, ideation-to-action models "emphasize understanding how various factors contribute to suicidal ideation as well as to the transition from suicidal ideation to more serious forms of suicidal behavior, such as suicide attempts and suicide" (Miller, 2021, p. 22). Ideation-to-action models posit that it is not enough for an individual to have the *desire* to die by suicide; they must also have the *capability* to do so, such as through increased habituation over time to painful or provocative experiences, making death less daunting and fearful (Joiner, 2005). Due to space limitations, more comprehensive coverage of various ideation-to-action models cannot be provided, but interested readers are encouraged to review the interpersonal theory of suicide (Joiner et al., (2009), the three-step theory of suicide (Klonsky & May, 2015), and the integrated motivational-volitional model of suicide (O'Connor, 2021). For the implications of ideation-to-action models for youth suicide prevention in schools, see Miller (2018, 2021).

BCBT Session Structure When Working with Suicidal Youth

BCBT for suicidal behavior involves "using a phased approach that sequentially orders interventions that correspond to clinical priorities and the natural processes of suicide risk over time" (Bryan & Rudd, 2018, p. 61). Although the number of sessions need not and should not be rigid, in general BCBT has approximately 12 therapy sessions, as is consistent with the condensed timeframe of a brief intervention. These sessions are sequenced and begin with assessment, case conceptualization, and crisis response planning (Session 1), followed by the targeting of baseline behavioral risk factors (Sessions 2 through 5), transitioning to the targeting of baseline cognitive risk factors (Session 6 through 10), and concluding with relapse prevention (Sessions 11 and 12; Bryan & Rudd, 2018).

In addition to the structure BCBT has *across* sessions, there also is a structure *within* sessions. Having a consistent structure within treatment sessions is important, as it provides direction and predictability to treatment for both the clinician and the client. In general, each therapy session (after the 1st, initial section) will be structured as follows: (1) a mood check, (2) setting an agenda, (3) reviewing use of the crisis response plan, (4) reviewing skill practices since the previous session, (5) introducing a new skills and practicing the skill during the session, and (6) assigning "homework" by having the client practice newly learned skills in between sessions (Bryan & Rudd, 2018).

According to Bryan and Rudd (2018),

> BCBT is most effective when its sessions are structured and this structure is supported and followed by the clinician. The first session of BCBT is the most structured and scripted of the treatment due to the number of procedures that must be completed … [whereas] the content of BCBT's subsequent sessions are more variable due to the clinician's ability to tailor the specific sequences of interventions and procedures to the patient's unique needs….
>
> *(p. 68)*

The structure and flow of each session generally includes the following: (a) assess the individual's use of his or her crisis response plan; (b) introduce a new skill or intervention; (c) verbally describe the skill; (d) demonstrate the skill and allow the individual to practice the skill in session; (e) review the individual's experience with practicing the skill; (f) identify and problem-solve potential variables to skill use in daily life; (g) assess the individual's motivation to use the skill; (h) finalize a plan for practicing the skill between sessions; and (i) enter a lesson learned into the treatment log (Bryan & Rudd, 2018).

Components of BCBT Practice and Intervention Modules

This section provides more detailed information regarding the four phases of BCBT across the 12 sessions, with a particular focus on the 1st session, as this includes critical elements that directly affect all subsequent treatment sessions. Due to space limitations, only a general overview of these phases and the content within them can be provided. For a more detailed description of treatment phases and components in BCBT, the reader is referred to Bryan and Rudd (2018).

Session 1 (Assessment, Case Conceptualization, Crisis Response Planning)

The 1st session of BCBT has several key purposes including risk assessment, case conceptualization, and crisis response planning. Risk assessment is the 1st component of the 1st session, as the results from it determine subsequent case conceptualization and treatment planning.

Conducting an effective suicide risk assessment is critical, but unfortunately many mental health professionals are inadequately trained in this area and often lack sufficient knowledge, confidence, and skill (Schmitz et al., 2012).

As mentioned previously, the most important and critical aspect of suicide risk assessment with young people is the individual clinical interview. Due to its high stakes, however, interviewing potentially suicidal individuals can be anxiety-provoking for both clients and clinicians. For example, suicidal individuals being assessed have frequently reported that clinicians did not adequately listen to them or spend enough time with them to truly help, and they often felt unnecessarily rushed or hurried in the assessment process (Bryan & Rudd, 2018). Anxious mental health professionals may be tempted to be too controlling in clinical interviews by asking a litany of questions that may sometimes "better serve the clinician's needs for data about suicide risk than the suicidal person's needs to be heard, understood, and less alone in their pain" (Freedenthal, 2018, p. 35). The interview should not feel like an interrogation to the client (Miller, 2021).

Consequently, the 1st step in BCBT is designed to allow the individual being assessed "sufficient opportunity to explain the circumstances surrounding the suicidal crisis and to describe his or her subjective experience of it" (Bryan & Rudd, 2018, p. 63). Within the 1st few minutes of the 1st session of BCBT, the clinician conducts a narrative assessment in which the clinician invites the client to "tell the story" of their suicidal crisis, in their own words. The narrative assessment, and the 1st BCBT session generally, is critical for building rapport with potentially suicidal youth. The narrative assessment "also provides the information needed to gain an understanding of the patient's unique needs, an essential step for case conceptualization and subsequent treatment planning" (Bryan & Rudd, 2018, p. 64).

Although using this technique might not be particularly useful with younger children due to a variety of developmental issues, it can be very informative when used with adolescents. If the adolescent struggles to respond to the invitation to tell their story, or if they express confusion about where to begin, the clinician can provide an encouraging and compassionate response, such as "Feel free to start anywhere you want. There is not a right or wrong way to tell me your story" (Freedenthal, 2018, p. 35). As the adolescent tells the story of their suicidal crisis and more information regarding it is revealed, and as rapport develops and the clinician asks other questions to the adolescent about various aspects of their suicidal behavior, the clinician organizes the reported risk and protective factors into the suicidal mode framework, thus facilitating the case conceptualization process (Bryan & Rudd, 2018).

The 1st session concludes with the central intervention of BCBT: the crisis response plan. The crisis response plan

> teaches patients how to identify an impending crisis and provides a step-by-step checklist of 'what to do' when this occurs. By the end of the first session, patients have (1) discussed and

> agreed to the structure and process of BCBT, (2) gained an understanding of the factors that contributed to and sustain their suicidal crises, and (3) developed the first plan for more effectively managing their emotional distress and suicidal crises.
>
> *(Bryan & Rudd, 2018, p. 64)*

Given research suggesting that many young people contemplate suicide for a relatively brief amount of time prior to making a suicide attempt (Stanley & Brown, 2012), interventions that directly target crisis situations are critical, as they may help avert future suicide attempts. In particular, "having limited access to lethal means and effective methods of distracting from suicidal thoughts and urges play a key role in youth suicide prevention" (Monahan & Stanley, 2022, p. 79).

A crisis response or safety plan (SP) is

> individualized lists of factors that indicate the heightened risk of suicide (i.e., warning signs) and ways to prevent the person from engaging in suicidal behaviors. These plans are tailored to individuals at risk and highlight their preferred internal coping strategies, external distractors (i.e., persons and social settings), and contact information for supportive family members, friends, and mental health professionals than can assist during a crisis.
>
> *(Monahan and Stanley, 2022, p. 79)*

An important component of youth safety planning, and one that distinguishes it from adult safety planning, is the emphasis on family/parent involvement, particularly through providing psychoeducation to parents/caregivers and enhancing family communication and connection. Youth SPs should always involve a parent/caregiver,

> either during the development of the plan or after the plan has been created. In either case, caregivers should be provided with copies of their child's SP. This collaboration can increase caregiver self-efficacy in helping youth manage crises and identifying when immediate, emergency care is needed.
>
> *(Monahan & Stanley, 2022, p. 79)*

Clinicians should also coordinate with parents/caregivers in communicating with the youth's school regarding the SP and note any accommodations that may be warranted, such as unrestricted access to mental health professionals in the schools (e.g., school psychologists; school counselors) and/or having permission to leave class and practice coping skills when highly distressed (Monahan & Stanley, 2022).

Perhaps the single most critical component of an SP is lethal means counseling (LMC), which may occur during the 1st session and continue in subsequent ones. An intervention that can have a profound effect on preventing youth suicide (Monahan & Stanley, 2022), LMC involves working directly with individuals at risk for suicide, and their families, to limit access to lethal means/methods (e.g., keeping potentially lethal medications locked in a cabinet) until the risk of suicide has significantly subsided. Given that most adolescents who die by suicide make us of guns as their means/method, LMC is especially important for adolescents living in residences where firearms are present (Monahan & Stanley, 2022). Research has found that youth who live in residences with firearms have up to a five times greater risk for suicide, although this risk can diminish significantly when firearm access is limited (Barber & Miller, 2014). Limiting access to other lethal means can further help decrease the risk for suicide among young people (Barber & Miller, 2014), and parent/caregiver involvement in this process is essential.

Sessions 2–5 (Targeting of Baseline Behavioral Risk Factors)

This early phase of BCBT, which typically spans the 2nd through 5th sessions, focuses on the deactivation of the suicidal mode. As treatment begins, the youth receiving treatment has most likely recently experienced an acute suicidal crisis (e.g., made a suicide attempt) and may still be experiencing high levels of subjective distress, although they may no longer be at the peak of their acute crisis. Because this phase is when individuals in treatment are most vulnerable and most likely to make a suicide attempt, these early sessions focus on

> symptom stabilization and reduction of suicide risk, both of which are accomplished by modifying baseline behavioral risk factors for suicide. The clinician's primary tasks [for this phase] are to develop a treatment plan, elicit commitment to treatment, teach emotion regulation skills, and refine the crisis response plan.
>
> *(Bryan & Rudd, 2018, pp. 64–65)*

As such,

> interventions during this early stage of treatment are primarily comprised of safety-promoting measures and behaviorally oriented skills training activities designed to build competency in several key areas: distress tolerance, emotion regulation, and self-management. Explicit discussions about the patient's access to potentially lethal means for suicide, especially firearms, occur very early in the first phase of BCBT within the context of means safety counseling and the crisis support plan, procedures that can be used to engage family members, friends, and other supportive individuals in the treatment process…[This phase] also targets the patient's behavioral predispositions for experiencing suicidal episodes and making suicide attempts by directly targeting symptoms associated with increased risk for suicidal thoughts and behaviors.
>
> *(Bryan & Rudd, 2018, p. 65)*

Examples of possible symptoms that are directly targeted include sleep disturbance (in which youth are taught skills in the areas of sleep hygiene and stimulus control); physiological arousal associated with experiencing stress (in which youth are taught relaxation skills); and rumination, worry, and cognitive reactivity (in which youth are taught mindfulness skills) (Bryan & Rudd, 2018). Clients are also taught

> how to elicit positive emotional states and how to remember why he or she wants to continue living using the reasons for living list, which entails a handwritten list summarizing the patient's most positive life experiences, and the survival kit, which provides physical reminders of positive experiences from the patient's life.
>
> *(Bryan and Rudd, 2018, p. 65)*

The two primary goals of this early phase of BCBT treatment are to learn new behavioral skills for managing emotional distress and begin to experience some symptom relief (Bryan & Rudd, 2018).

Sessions 6–10 (Targeting of Baseline Cognitive Risk Factors)

As individuals in treatment demonstrate the ability to more effectively use the emotion regulation skills introduced in Sessions 2 through 5, symptoms of suicide often remit and/or stabilize. As this initial skill develops, BCBT transitions in Sessions 6 through 10 to a focus on undermining the suicidal belief system, thereby reducing long-term vulnerability to suicidal mode activation as well as promoting a greater sense of competency and self-efficacy (Bryan & Rudd, 2018). Interventions during this phase

> are specifically designed to develop the patient's cognitive reappraisal skills. First, the patient learns to use the ABC Worksheet to learn how one's thoughts and beliefs influence the emotions one experiences in response to triggering situations. Once this foundational skill is acquired, the patient is taught how to critically evaluate the helpfulness and usefulness of their beliefs with the Challenging Questions Worksheet and how to recognize and label different types of unhelpful beliefs with the Patterns of Problematic Thinking worksheet. In addition, the patient's sense of personal meaning in life, connectedness with others, and experience of positive emotional states is developed using activity planning and coping cards, which entails the scheduling of enjoyable activities.
>
> *(Bryan & Rudd, 2018, pp. 66–67)*

Although this phase of treatment is focused primarily on cognitive reappraisal, the practices learned in the previous phase continue to be discussed and practiced. For example, at the beginning of each session, the clinician

> continues to ask patients if they have used the crisis response plan since the previous session. If they state that they used the crisis response plan, the clinician asks them to describe the situation and circumstances that led them to use it, and the specific strategies used. If patients state that they did not use the crisis response plan, the clinician asks them how they effectively managed stressful situations such that the crisis response plan was not needed. This reinforces the effective use of emotion regulation, problem solving, and crisis management skills and bolsters the patient's sense of self-efficacy.
>
> *(Bryan & Rudd, 2018, p. 66)*

By the conclusion of this phase of BCBT, the individual receiving treatment has

> (1) learned new ways for thinking about him- or herself, the world, and others, and (2) started to acquire a new self-image and general cognitive style that reduces the likelihood of future suicidal mode activation in response to life stress.
>
> *(Bryan & Rudd, 2018, p. 67)*

The hope is that although the individual will continue to experience stress in his/her life, he or she will be better able to respond to this stress with greater adaptability and functionality (Bryan & Rudd, 2018).

Sessions 11 and 12 (Relapse Prevention)

In this final phase of BCBT (Sessions 11 and 12), the focus of treatment is on relapse prevention. The primary objective of this phase is to ensure that the individual in treatment "is sufficiently competent in using learned skills to effectively manage emotional crises without making a suicide attempt or using other maladaptive behaviors associated with the suicidal mode (e.g., substance abuse, nonsuicidal self-injury)" (Bryan & Rudd, 2018, p. 67). To help accomplish this objective, the client is presented with a relapse prevention task—an imagery exercise in which individuals visualize themselves experiencing suicidal crises and effectively resolving them. This imagery task is typically repeated several times, with each iteration becoming progressively more difficult, thereby requiring greater proficiency in demonstrating effective problem-solving skills and enhanced cognitive flexibility.

Although this final phase of BCBT typically lasts for only two sessions, additional sessions should be added if the individual is unable to adequately complete the relapse prevention task (Bryan & Rudd, 2018). After BCBT concludes, the clinician should continue to periodically monitor the individual receiving treatment and provide additional "booster sessions" if needed.

Assessment of Progress and Outcomes

Research has demonstrated that the tracking of client treatment response using standardized assessment scales has repeatedly been shown to enhance outcomes in psychotherapy when the results of these assessments are known by both the clinician and the client (e.g., Simon et al., 2013). Frequent monitoring of suicide risk and client progress is an essential component of BCBT and may be one of the factors that contributes to its effectiveness for reducing suicidal behavior (Bryan & Rudd, 2018). Although there is not currently a BCBT-specific tracking system, Bryan and Rudd (2018) suggest that the routine assessment and monitoring of the following variables is especially helpful: suicidal ideation, subjective sleep quality, suicidal beliefs, alcohol use, and general symptomatic distress.

A wide array of assessment scales and tools have been developed and can be used by clinicians to track and monitor their client's suicidal behavior. One assessment measure that may have utility with youth in schools is the Columbia Suicide Severity Rating Scale (C-SSRS), which is a brief self-report measure consisting of six questions (see cssrs.columbia.edu for more information). Regardless of which assessment measure is used, progress monitoring using a standardized, self-report measure should occur at or near the start of every treatment session. The results of that assessment should be clearly understood by the clinician and the client and should be used to evaluate treatment and modify it as necessary (Bryan & Rudd, 2018).

Applications to the School Setting

As a psychotherapeutic intervention for preventing suicide, BCBT has to date been used primarily in clinical settings with adults. Although it has a growing research base, more research on its utility for young people is clearly needed, including how to best tailor it for younger clients. Given the self-reflection and cognitive appraisal that it requires, BCBT will likely be more challenging to implement with younger children and pre-adolescents. In schools, BCBT may be particularly useful with adolescents, who are better able developmentally to engage in self-reflection and who are at much higher risk for suicide than their younger peers. Moreover, school-based mental health professionals are typically not well trained in working directly with suicidal youth, and these professionals will likely require additional training in BCBT if they wish to provide direct psychotherapeutic interventions for this challenging group of students. School mental health professionals will also want to have the support of school administrators and parents/caregivers prior to providing BCBT for suicidal youth, as without it BCBT is not likely to be successful or even implemented.

Case Study of BCBT for Youth Suicidal Behavior

To illustrate a case example of using BCBT to address youth suicidal behavior, below is a session-by-session flow of BCBT for Jamal, an adolescent male who recently made a suicide attempt. The initial treatment goals for Jamal are (1) reducing risk for future suicide attempts, (2) getting better sleep, which appeared to be affected by agitation and emotional distress, and (3) reducing his self-criticisms and core belief that he is a "failure."

Session Number	*Session Content*
1	Narrative assessment, crisis response plan, means safety plan
2	treatment planning, commitment to treatment, relaxation skills
3	Sleep stimulus control
4	Reasons for living list
5	Mindfulness skills
6	ABC (Activating Event-Beliefs-Consequences) worksheet
7	Challenging questions worksheet
8	Activity planning
9	Coping cards
10	Patterns of problematic thinking worksheet
11	Relapse prevention task
12	Relapse prevention task

An example of a treatment session for Jamal using BCBT for suicide prevention, modified from Bryan and Rudd (2018), is provided below. During BCBT with Jamal, it became apparent that one of his core beliefs is that he is a "failure" and that when he engages in thoughts about being a failure it increases his suicidal ideation. A transcript of the session between Jamal and a school-based mental health professional, which occurred in the context of targeting Jamal's baseline cognitive risk factors, is as follows:

Clinician: It sounds like there are lots of instances in which you've told yourself that you're a failure. Do you find yourself having the thought "I'm a failure" very often?

Jamal: Yeah, I guess so.

Clinician: How many times per day would you say you think about being a failure?

Jamal: I don't know. I guess at least once a day, but some days it's more.

Clinician: It sounds like you have that thought quite a bit. Given how often you have that thought, would you say it's pretty easy for you to think about how you're a failure?

Jamal: Yeah, it's pretty easy to think about that.

Clinician: Would you say it's become so easy to think about that the thought comes to you quickly, without having to give it much thought? Sort of like it just pops into your mind automatically?

Jamal: Yeah, I guess so. Yeah. It's like it's just always there when I screw up.

Clinician: Got it. So if I understand you right, this thought about being a failure comes to mind quickly, without much effort, and seems to occur over and over again, almost as though it's an automatic response. Is that right?

Jamal: Yeah, I'd say so.

Clinician: Hmmm … Well, I don't know, but that sounds a lot like a habit.

Jamal: What do you mean?

Clinician: Well, a habit is something we do over and over again without much thought, and usually we aren't even aware that we're doing it. At least that's how I think of a habit. How would you describe a habit?

Jamal: I'd probably describe it the same way.

Clinician: OK, so we're on the same page there. Based on how you just explained this thought about being a failure, it really sounds a lot like it's become a habit for you.

Jamal: Well, but it's based on facts.

Clinician: Right, you told me about all of the mistakes and errors you have made.
Jamal: Yes.
Clinician: So maybe it's both a fact and a habit?
Jamal: Yeah, maybe.
Clinician: Maybe that's it. Because you say it's based on facts, but you also talked about how it's sort of like a habit, too. What do you think?
Jamal: Yeah, I agree. That makes sense.
Clinician: OK, so what do you think we should put on the worksheet?
Jamal: I guess that I'll put that it's both.
Clinician: OK, that sounds good. Do you think it would be helpful to also jot a few words down to explain how it's a habit? It seems like that's that part of the belief that wasn't as obvious.
Jamal: Yeah, that would be good (p. 203).

The "worksheet" mentioned in the case example above refers to the Problematic Thinking Worksheet, which was introduced to Jamal during the 10th session of BCBT. At this point in his treatment, Jamal and his clinician identified several of Jamal's suicidal beliefs and were working to challenge them. Over the course of treatment, Jamal's clinician noticed that Jamal often seemed to struggle to understand how and why his maladaptive beliefs were often triggering his suicidal ideation. Consequently, Jamal's clinician asked John to complete Patterns of Problematic Thinking Worksheet (Bryan & Rudd, 2018) to assist in better understanding Jamal's maladaptive thinking patterns. Upon completing the worksheet, the clinician engaged Jamal in the following dialogue (Bryan & Rudd, 2018, pp. 211–213):

Clinician: Anything stand out to you from this worksheet?
Jamal: Well, it seems like some of my thoughts fit under different patterns.
Clinician: Yeah, that's pretty common. A lot of our unhelpful beliefs are problematic in multiple ways.
Jamal: Yeah. Another thing is that I seem to jump to conclusions and do emotional reasoning more than the others.
Clinician: What do you make of that?
Jamal: I think they're probably related to each other.
Clinician: How so?
Jamal: Well, I think that when I feel bad or upset, I assume there's a reason for it, so I'll think something about myself that matches the feeling, even if there's no evidence for it. So emotional reasoning ends up leading me to jump to conclusions.
Clinician: That's a pretty interesting observation.
Jamal: Yeah. As I look at this worksheet and we talk about it, I think that may be why I feel like things are true even though I know they aren't: the beliefs are based on my emotions.
Clinician: So it's kind of like the thoughts and beliefs are coming from your emotions?
Jamal: Yeah, that has to be it. I never thought of it that way before, but whenever I feel bad or something is when I really start to think all these things. Even if these thoughts don't make sense for the situation, I end up believing them anyway simply because I'm feeling bad.
Clinician: So what do you think we should do with this new knowledge?
Jamal: Well, one thing I can tell myself is that just because I'm feeling bad doesn't mean I've done something wrong. I think that would really help.

DBT Skills in Schools: Skills Training for Emotional Problem Solving for Adolescents

Although this chapter has focused on the use of BCBT for students exhibiting suicidal behavior (Tier 3 of a MTSS framework), a critical element of effective suicide prevention in schools is targeting *all* individuals in a population of students, such as all students in a high school (i.e., Tier 1). Consequently, school personnel who want to take a proactive approach to preventing youth suicidal behavior are strongly encouraged to consider implementing universal (Tier 1) social, emotional, and learning (SEL) programs within an MTSS model. Using a service delivery approach in schools that focuses only on those students already at risk for suicidal behavior (i.e., Tier 3),

> does little or nothing to stop the flow of youth who may experience future mental health problems. In addition, adopting this type of approach is reactionary rather than preventative and implies that students must exhibit clear and severe mental health problems (i.e., ones that are having a significant impact on their behavior at school) before they can receive mental health services.
>
> *(Miller & Mazza, 2018, p. 266)*

A frequent problem for those who experience suicidal behavior is their difficulty regulating their emotions and their frequent inability to make effective decisions and utilize adaptive coping strategies in the presence of high emotional pain. A cognitive-behavioral SEL program that directly targets these issues is *DBT in Schools: Skills Training for Emotional Problem Solving for Adolescents (DBT STEPS-A)*, developed by Mazza et al. (2016). As mentioned previously, DBT is a cognitive-behavioral, evidence-based intervention for treating suicidal behavior. In traditional DBT, the term *dialectical* is

> meant to convey both the multiple tensions that co-occur in therapy with suicidal clients as well as the emphasis in DBT on enhancing dialectical thinking patterns to replace rigid, dichotomous thinking. The fundamental dialectic in DBT is between validation and acceptance of the client as they are within the context of simultaneously helping them to change.
>
> *(Dimeff & Linehan, 2001, p. 10)*

Unlike DBT, DBT STEPS-A is not a form of individual or group psychotherapy. Instead, it is a *curriculum* intended for students and used in middle and high school settings at the universal (Tier 1) level. DBT STEPS-A was developed specifically to adapt the skills component of DBT into teacher-oriented lessons that could be implemented in general education classrooms (Mazza et al., 2016). The rationale behind this adaptation was to scale-up and expand the delivery of DBT skills so that all adolescents would have the ability to develop an effective set of skills for their own unique situations, especially during times of emotional distress.

The DBT STEPS-A curriculum comprises the four major modules that parallel the skills in DBT (Linehan, 1993, 2015): core mindfulness, distress tolerance, emotion regulation, and interpersonal effectiveness. These four modules are interrelated, with mindfulness and distress tolerance skills being on the "acceptance" side of the dialectic, whereas emotion regulation and interpersonal effectiveness skills are on the "change" side of the dialectic. Together, these skills help youth manage strong emotions (acceptance skills) and reduce the intensity of an emotion or change it (change skills).

The module of *Core Mindfulness* in DBT STEPS-A contains seven skills that are taught in three lessons. The importance of mindfulness in DBT STEPS-A cannot be understated, as it is central to all the other skills in the curriculum. Because of their importance, Core Mindfulness skills are revisited each time a module of skills is completed. The 1st skill of Core Mindfulness is "wise mind," which is a combination of *emotion mind* and *reasonable mind*. Students learn strategies to help them identify when they are in "wise mind" and when they are not. This is extremely important when students are experiencing suicidal thoughts because these thoughts most often occur in "emotion mind," when logical thinking ("reasonable mind") is impaired or not occurring, and thoughts of self-harm and suicide become more frequent and intense. Recognizing this and implementing coping strategies to reboot the logical thinking side allows "wise mind" to re-engage and make decisions that are more cognitively aligned with the client's long-term values. In other words, "wise mind" helps students recognize when they are having irrational thoughts.

How does one help students access their "reasonable mind" to help engage their "wise mind?" In DBT STEPS-A, this is accomplished by making use of what are referred to as "What" and "How" skills. There are three "What" skills: Observe, Describe, and Participate. These skills are taught and used when "emotion mind" has taken over decision-making. A unique aspect of the "What" skills is that each of them can only be done one at a time. In contrast, "How" skills refer to how an individual implements the "What" skills. There are three "How" skills: One-mindfully, Nonjudgmentally, and Effectively. Unique to the "How" skills are that all three of them can be performed at the same time. Thus, the "What" and "How" skills work together to bring the individual back to the "wise mind" of being in the present moment (i.e., not thinking about the past and not worried about the future), which helps reduce irrational thoughts.

The 2nd module on the acceptance side of the dialectic is *Distress Tolerance*. Distress Tolerance skills help students learn skills for those situations in which the intensity of their emotion becomes very strong very quickly (i.e., "emotion mind"). Distress Tolerance skills are often used in highly emotional situations to prevent them from becoming worse, given "wise mind" is likely not adequately operating. It is during these highly intense, emotional situations that students frequently engage in self-harming, self-medicating, and/or suicidal behavior. Thus, implementing Distress Tolerance skills allows sufficient time to pass during stressful/emotional situations (without making the situation worse) and for "wise mind" to reengage. There are two types of Distress Tolerance skills: "Crisis Survival" skills for short-term intense situations and "Accepting Reality" skills for long-term situations that cannot be solved immediately. Determining which type of Distress Tolerance skill to use given the situation is part of the teaching in the curriculum.

On the other side of the dialectic are the two change modules: *Emotion Regulation* and *Interpersonal Effectiveness*. Emotion Regulation skills are designed to reduce the intensity of the emotion being experienced and/or to change the emotion. To effectively reduce the intensity of the emotion or change it, the student needs to recognize that they are in "wise mind" and that Distress Tolerance skills are not needed. The Emotion Regulation skills of "check the facts" and "opposite action" align closely with CBT's emphasis on rational thinking and cognitive restructuring. In the "check the facts" skill, students examine if there are any other logical and reasonable explanations for the precipitating event that is causing their emotional reaction. If the answer is "yes" (meaning there are other logical explanations), students learn to implement the skill of "opposite action" (i.e., doing the opposite of the emotional urge the student is experiencing). For example, if the cognitive interpretation made by the student is that "no one likes me" and their subsequent behavior is to not talk with anyone and isolate themselves, the "opposite action" would be to go out and socialize with friends, which will then hopefully result in reduced emotions of sadness or shame.

The last set of skills in DBT STEPS-A is *Interpersonal Effectiveness*. This set of skills is used to develop and maintain relationships with others and to help students enhance their self-respect and confidence. Relationships with others, whether parents/caregivers, siblings, friends, and/or romantic partners, take on added importance for adolescents. Thus, learning how to interact with others to enhance getting the things students want and saying "no" to things they don't want is vital. Equally, trying to establish new relationships or maintaining ones already developed is central to establishing social support, as well as romantic and other types of relationships. Finally, helping youth learn to develop and maintain their self-respect and self-confidence underlies all their relationships. Relationship success and social support are protective factors that reduce the likelihood of youth engaging in a variety of self-destructive behaviors, including suicidal behavior.

The balanced approach of teaching youth DBT STEPS-A skills, rotating back and forth from acceptance to change, offers a unique set of skills that honors the intense emotional pain experienced by youth who are suicidal or at risk for developing suicidal behavior. Many other adolescent SEL curricula focus mainly on the "change" side of the dialectic and require youth to be in their "rational" or "wise" mind. That is not always the case, however, and in fact, it is when youth are experiencing high levels of emotional pain and irrational thinking that DBT STEPS-A provides a unique set of skills to help them endure difficult times/situations while reducing the likelihood of engaging in self-harming, self-medicating, and/or suicidal behavior. It is on the "acceptance" side of the dialectic that DBT STEPS-A provides students with unique skills not found in other universal SEL programs.

Consequently, DBT STEPS-A may be a useful Tier 1 curriculum program for preventing the development of youth suicidal behavior as well as a toolbox for mental health promotion, better empowering students to both tolerate and accept emotionally difficult events/situations and to change how students react to them. When appropriate cognitive-behavioral interventions can be used at the Tier 1 level (e.g., DBT STEPS-A) in conjunction with cognitive-behavioral interventions at Tiers 2 and/or 3 (e.g., BCBT) within an MTSS framework, the prevention of youth suicidal behavior in schools is more likely to be effective.

Summary

Youth suicidal behavior is a disturbing and significant public health problem for which effective interventions are at an early stage of development. BCBT is a promising intervention for the treatment of youth suicidal behavior. The steps for implementing BCBT were described, including the structure both within and between treatment sessions. A case example of using BCBT with an adolescent who made a recent suicide attempt was also provided. School-based mental health professionals, including school psychologists, school counselors, and school social workers, are encouraged to develop their knowledge and skills in using BCBT with suicidal youth. BCBT can be an important element within a MTSS framework in schools, one that can also include SEL programs such as DBT STEPS-A. Given the seriousness of youth suicidal behavior and the urgent need to prevent it, school personnel are ideally situated to provide effective prevention and intervention services.

Reflection Questions

1 How comfortable would you be in providing BCBT to youth in schools and what additional training do you think you would require?
2 What challenges do you see in implementing BCBT with suicidal youth in schools and how might you address them?
3 What challenges do you see in implementing DBT STEPS-A in schools and how might you address them?

References

Barber, C. W., & Miller, M. J. (2014). Reducing a suicidal person's access to lethal means of suicide: A research agenda. *American Journal of Preventive Medicine, 47*, S264–S272

Bridge, J. A., Horowitz, L. M., Fontanella, C. A., Sheftall, A. H., Greenhouse, J. B., Kellher, K. J., et al. (2018). Age-related racial disparity in suicide rates among US youth between 2001 and 2015. *JAMA Pediatrics, 172*, 697–699.

Brown, G. K., Ten Have, T., Henriques, G. R., Xie, S. X., Hollander, J. E., & Beck, A. T. (2005). Cognitive therapy for the prevention of suicide attempts: A randomized control trial. *The Journal of the American Medical Association, 294*, 563–570.

Bryan, C. J. (2022). *Rethinking suicide: Why prevention fails, and how we can do better.* New York: Oxford University Press.

Bryan, C. J., & Rudd, M. D. (2018). *Brief cognitive-behavioral therapy for suicide prevention.* New York: Guilford Press.

Canetto, S. S., & Sakinofsky, I. (1998). The gender paradox in suicide. *Suicide and Life-Threatening Behavior, 28*, 1–23

D'Anci, K. E., Uhl, S., Girardi, G., & Martin, C. (2019). Treatments for the prevention and management of suicide. *Annals of Internal Medicine, 171*, 334–342.

DeCou, C. R., Comtois, K. A., & Landes, S. J. (2019). Dialectical behavior therapy is effective for the treatment of suicidal behavior: A meta-analysis. *Behavior Therapy, 50*, 60–72.

Dimeff, L., & Linehan, M. M. (2001). Dialectical behavior therapy in a nutshell. *The California Psychologist, 34*, 10–13.

Espelage, D. L., Boyd, R. C., Renshaw, T. L., & Jimerson, S. R. (2022). Addressing youth suicide through school-based prevention and postvention: Contemporary scholarship advancing science, practice, and policy. *School Psychology Review, 51*, 257–265.

Franklin, J. C., Ribeiro, J. D., Fox, K. R., et al. (2017). Risk factors for suicidal thoughts and behaviors: A meta-analysis of 50 years of research. *Psychological Bulletin, 143*, 187–232.

Freedenthal, S. (2018). *Helping the suicidal person: Tips and techniques for professionals.* New York: Routledge Press.

Gaylor, E. M., Krause, K. H., Welder, L. E., Cooper, A. C., Ashley, C., Mack, K. A., et al. (2023, April 28). *Morbidity and Mortality Weekly Report-Supplements, 72*, 45–54.

Gould, M. S., Marrocco, F. A., Kleinman, M., Thomas, J. G., Mostkoff, K., Cote, J., et al. (2005). Evaluating iatrogenic risk of youth suicide screening programs: A randomized control trial. *Journal of the American Medical Association, 293*, 1635–1643.

Joiner, T. E. (2005). *Why people die by suicide.* Cambridge, MA: Harvard University Press.

Joiner, T. E., Van Orden, K. A., Witte, T. K., & Rudd, M. D. (2009). *The interpersonal theory of suicide Guidance for working with suicidal clients.* Washington, DC: American Psychological Association.

King, C. A., Ewell Foster, C., & Rogalski, K. M. (2013). *Teen suicide risk: A practitioner guide to screening, assessment, and management.* New York: Guilford Press.

Klonsky, E. D., & May, A. M. (2015). The three-step theory (3ST): A new theory of suicide rooted in the "ideation-to-action" framework. *International Journal of Cognitive Therapy, 8*, 114–129.

Linehan, M. M. (1993). *Cognitive-behavioral treatment of borderline personality disorder.* New York: Guilford Press.

Linehan, M. M. (2015). *DBT skills training manual* (2nd ed.). New York: Guilford Press.

Linehan, M. M., et al. (2006). Two-year randomized controlled trial and follow-up of dialectical behavior therapy vs. therapy by experts for suicidal behaviors and borderline personality disorder. *Archives of General Psychiatry, 63*, 757–766.

Marraccini, M. E., Griffin, D., O'Neill, J. C., Martinez, Jr., R. R., Chin, A. J., Toole, E. N., Grapin, S. L., & Naser, S. C. (2022). School risk and protective factors of suicide: A cultural model of suicide risk and protective factors in schools. *School Psychology Review, 51*, 266–289.

Marraccini, M. E., Ingram, K. M., Naser, S. C., Grapin, S. L., Toole, E. N., O'Neill, C., et al. (2022). The roles of school in supporting LGBTQ+ youth: A systematic review and ecological framework for understanding risk for suicide-related thoughts and behaviors. *Journal of School Psychology, 91*, 27–49.

Martin, D. J., Garske, J. P., & Davis, M. K. (2000). Relation of the therapeutic alliance with outcome and other variables: A meta-analytic review. *Journal of Consulting and Clinical Psychology, 68*, 438–450.

Mazza, J. J., Dexter-Mazza, E. T., Miller, A. L., Rathus, J. H., & Murphy, H. E. (2016). *DBT skills in schools Skills training for emotional problem solving for adolescents (DBT STEPS-A).* New York: Guilford Press.

Mazza, J. J., & Miller, D. N. (2024). Youth suicidal behavior. In L. A. Theodore, B. A. Bracken & M. A. Bray (Eds.), *Desk reference in school psychology* (pp. 377–394). New York: Oxford University Press.

McCauley, E., Berk, M. S., Asarnow, J. R., Adrian, M., Cohen, J., Korslaund, K., et al. (2018). Efficacy of dialectical behavior therapy for adolescents at high risk for suicide: A randomized clinical trial. *JAMA Psychiatry, 75*, 777–785.

Mewton, L., & Andrews, G. (2016). Cognitive-behavioral therapy for suicidal behaviors: Improving patient outcomes. *Psychology Research and Behavior Management, 9*, 21–29.

Miller, A. L., Rathus, J. H., & Linehan, M. M. (2007). *Dialectical behavior therapy with suicidal adolescents.* New York: Guilford Press.

Miller, D. N. (2018). Understanding and preventing youth suicide: Ideation-to-action theories of suicidal behavior and their implications for school-based suicide prevention. In P. Terry & R. Price (Eds.), *Understanding suicide: Perspectives, risk factors and gender differences* (pp. 165–186). Hauppauge, NY: Nova Science.

Miller, D. N. (2021). *Child and adolescent suicidal behavior: School-based prevention, assessment, and intervention* (2nd ed.). New York: Guilford Press.

Miller, D. N. (2022). Assessing risk for suicide. In S. H. McConaughy & S. A. Whitcomb, *Clinical interviews for children and adolescents: Assessment to intervention* (3rd ed.) (pp. 223–242). New York: Guilford Press.

Miller, D. N., Eckert, T. L., & Mazza, J. J. (2009). Suicide prevention programs in the schools: A review and public health perspective. *School Psychology Review, 38*, 168–188.

Miller, D. N., & Jome, L. M. (2010). School psychologists and the secret illness: Perceived knowledge, role preferences, and training needs in the prevention and treatment of internalizing disorders. *School Psychology International, 31*, 509–520.

Miller, D. N., & Mazza, J. J. (2018). School-based suicide prevention, intervention, and postvention. In A. Leschied, D. Saklofske, & G. Flett (Eds.), *The handbook of school-based mental health promotion: An evidence-informed framework for implementation* (pp. 55–66). New York: Springer Press.

Monahan, M. F., & Stanley, B. (2022). Safety planning and means safety counseling with youth. In J. P. Ackerman & L. M. Horowitz (Eds.), *Youth suicide prevention and intervention: Best practices and policy implications* (pp. 79–84). New York: Springer Press

Moutier, C. Y., Pisani, A. R., & Stahl, S. M. (2021). *Suicide prevention.* New York: Cambridge University Press.

O'Connor, R. (2021). *When it is darkest: Why people die by suicide and what we can do to prevent it.* London: Penguin Press.

O'Neill, J. C., Marraccini, M. E., Bledsoe, S. E., Knotek, S. E., & Tabori, A. V. (2020). Suicide postvention practices in schools: School psychologists' experience, training, and knowledge. *School Psychology, 35*, 61–71.

Robinson, J., Bailey, E., Witt, K., et al. (2018). What works in youth suicide prevention? A systematic review and meta-analysis. *EClinicalMedicine, 4–5*, 52–91.

Rudd, M. D., Bryan, C. J., Wertenberger, E., et al. (2015). Brief cognitive behavioral therapy effects on post-treatment suicide attempts in military sample: Results of a 2-year randomized clinical trial. *American Journal of Psychiatry, 172*, 441–449.

Rudd, M. D., Joiner, T., & Rajab, M. H. (2001). *Treating suicidal behavior: An effective, time-limited approach.* New York: Guilford Press.

Schmitz, W. M., Allen, M. H., Feldman, B. N., et al. (2012). Preventing suicide through improved training in suicide risk assessment and care: An American Association of Suicidology task force report addressing serious gaps in US mental health training. *Suicide and Life-Threatening Behavior, 42*, 292–304.

Shinn, M. R., & Walker, H. M. (Eds.) (2010). *Interventions for achievement and behavior problems in a three-tier model including RTI.* Bethesda, MD: National Association of School Psychologists.

Simon, W., Lambert, M. J., Busath, G., Vasquez, A., Berkeljon, A., Hyer, K., et al. (2013). Effects of providing patient progress feedback and clinical support tools to psychotherapists in an inpatient eating disorders treatment program: A randomized control study. *Psychotherapy Research, 23*, 287–300.

Sinyor, M., Williams, M., Mitchell, R., et al. (2020). Cognitive behavioral therapy for suicide prevention in youth admitted to hospital following an episode of self-harm: A pilot randomized controlled trial. *Journal of Affective Disorders, 266*, 686–694.

Stanley, B., Brown, G., Brent, D., Wells, K., Poling, K., Curry, J., et al. (2009). Cognitive behavior therapy for suicide prevention (CBT-SP): Treatment model, feasibility and acceptability. *Journal of the American Academy of Child and Adolescent Psychiatry, 48*, 1005–1013.

Tarrier, N., Taylor, K., & Gooding, P. (2008). Cognitive-behavioral interventions to reduce suicide behavior: A systematic review and meta-analysis. *Behavior Modification, 32*, 77–108.

18
PEDIATRIC INSOMNIA

Kristina Puzino Lenker

Pediatric Insomnia

Sleep problems are highly prevalent in children and adolescents, if left untreated, can become chronic (Kahn, 2023). Although many sleep disorders result in adverse daytime outcomes, insomnia in children and adolescents is common, affecting approximately one-third of children, and can be particularly distressing to families. Insomnia has been defined as repeated difficulty with sleep initiation, duration, consolidation, or quality that occurs despite age-appropriate time and opportunity for sleep and results in daytime functional impairment for the child and/or family (Owens & Mindell, 2011). Pediatric insomnia contributes to increased behavioral problems, difficulty with concentration, and lower test scores in cognitive tasks, and has been linked to parents' poor general health and psychological distress (Ball et al., 2019; Bruni et al., 2020; De Zambotti et al., 2018; Zhao et al., 2019).

There are multiple types of pediatric insomnia (Owens & Mindell, 2011). For the purpose of this chapter, insomnia is defined as sleep-onset delay more than 30 minutes per night, on average, or short sleep duration, less than eight hours, occurring three or more nights per week, by parent report included. Pediatric insomnia is described as behavioral insomnia of childhood (BIC) and could be classified into three separate subtypes: BIC, sleep-onset association type, limit-setting type, combined type both counterproductive sleep associations and bedtime struggles between child and parents. BIC, sleep-onset association type, is characterized by the child's dependency on specific stimulation, objects, or settings for initiating sleep or returning to sleep following an awakening, and sleep onset is prolonged without these conditions. One example is an infant who needs a pacifier to fall asleep and to return to sleep after a nighttime awakening. Another example is a child who needs his or her mother present to fall asleep or to return to sleep after a nighttime awakening. These children typically have an inability to self-soothe back to sleep in the night, due to the inability to self-soothe at bedtime (Owens & Mindell, 2011). BIC, limit-setting type, is characterized by bedtime refusal or stalling that is the result of inadequate limit-setting by a parent/caregiver. Examples include a refusal to go to bed or repeated demands at bedtime, "curtain calls," for a drink or to use the bathroom. This type of insomnia is characterized by prolonged sleep onset but not necessarily by awakenings overnight and typically occurs in children who are of preschool or school age (Owens & Mindell, 2011). BIC, combined type, is characterized by features of both sleep-onset association insomnia and bedtime resistance and represents a 3rd subtype within this diagnostic category.

 DOI: 10.4324/9781003392439-21

There is also psychophysiological insomnia, which is characterized by difficulties initiating and maintaining sleep as a result of physiologic and mental hyperarousal (i.e., racing thoughts), occurring mostly in adolescents (American Academy of Sleep Medicine, 2014). These children may excessively focus or worry about their sleep. They may have excessive cognitive and somatic arousal.

Prevalence

Researchers have reported a range of prevalence rates for pediatric insomnia, varying from 10% in Vietnam and Thailand to 25%–30% in the United States and Australia to as high as 75% in China and Taiwan (Medalie et al., 2021). Symptoms are more common in younger compared with older children and adolescents, with prevalence approximations as high as 36% in preschool children declining to roughly 11% in adolescents (Combs et al., 2016; Johnson et al., 2006). Furthermore, pediatric insomnia is more prevalent in children and adolescents diagnosed with neurologic, developmental, or psychiatric disorders (Shelton & Malow, 2021). While there does not appear to be differences in prevalence rates between young boys and girls, there are high prevalence rates of pediatric insomnia for adolescent girls (i.e., onset coinciding with puberty) (Johnson et al., 2006).

Consequences and Common Comorbidities of Pediatric Insomnia

Pediatric insomnia has broad adverse impacts on cognitive (i.e., attention, memory), motor (i.e., proneness for accidents), emotional (i.e., mood, reduced motivation), behavioral (i.e., hyperactivity, aggression), and social functioning (American Academy of Sleep Medicine, 2014). Research has demonstrated strong links between pediatric insomnia and impairments in executive functions, risk taking behaviors, poor academic performance, internalizing and externalizing symptoms, obesity, and additional poor health outcomes (Bruni et al., 2020; De Zambotti et al., 2018; Zhao et al., 2019). These links are likely complex and bidirectional, with sleep difficulties both driving and being driven by impairments in other domains. Longitudinal and experimental studies provide compelling evidence for detrimental effects and indicate that pediatric insomnia symptoms predict the onset of internalizing and externalizing disorders, substance abuse, and poor academic performance (Lovato & Gradisar, 2014; Mike et al., 2016; Zhang et al., 2022).

Empirical Support for CBT

Cognitive behavior approaches are considered the 1st-line treatment of pediatric insomnia (Kahn, 2023; Owens & Mindell, 2011). Majority of treatment modalities for pediatric insomnia are behavioral interventions, which are inherently based on learning principles that address child and parent behaviors and cognitions to improve sleep. There is strong empirical evidence for the efficacy of these behavioral interventions as shown by various comprehensive reviews of the literature. These reviews focused on behavioral treatments for bedtime problems and night wakings in young children (Kuhn & Elliott, 2003; Mindell, 1999). At the time, three interventions, unmodified extinction (ignoring all negative behaviors after lights out until a set time in the morning), graduated extinction (brief parental checks after lights out, which may decrease in frequency, again ignoring all negative behavior), and parent education/prevention, were identified as well-established and efficacious. Other interventions, including bedtime fading/positive routines (includes a positive bedtime routine, moving the child's bedtime later to match when he/she is currently falling asleep, and stimulus control techniques) and scheduled awakenings (waking and then consoling a child 15–30 minutes before the child's typical spontaneous nocturnal awakening, which is expected to assist in sleep consolidation), were identified as "probably efficacious" or as a "guideline."

Despite mounting evidence to support Cognitive Behavioral Therapy for Insomnia (CBT-I) in adults with insomnia, limited RCTs have been conducted to investigate the effectiveness of CBT-I for school-aged children (Meltzer & Mindell, 2014). In one study, Paine and Gradisar (2011) had 42 children between 7 and 13 years randomly assigned to receive either six sessions of CBT-I or a waiting list control group. Their results indicate positive effects in the CBT-I group for sleep (sleep latency, wake after sleep onset, sleep efficiency) and anxiety, which were maintained at both the one- and six-month follow-ups. However, no changes occurred in total sleep time (TST). In another RCT, school-aged children with insomnia were treated with CBT-I: Schlarb and colleagues (2018) implemented CBT-I, consisting of three sessions for children and three for parents in 112 children (age range 5–11.5 years). Results from this study show improvements in sleep problems, sleep onset latency, sleep efficiency, and nocturnal awakenings, which were maintained at 3-, 6-, and 12-month follow-up assessments. However, similar to others (Paine & Gradisar, 2011), no changes occurred in TST. This evidence is promising; however, more controlled intervention studies (focusing on collective CBT-I techniques) in school-aged children are needed to advance the field of pediatric behavioral sleep medicine.

Similar to the evidence supporting CBT-I in children, the research on the effectiveness of CBT-I in adolescents is scarce. In a recent meta-analysis, Blake and colleagues (2017) found less than ten studies that used adolescent cognitive-behavioral sleep interventions, which included only four RCTs, and only one of these RCTs included adolescents with an isolated insomnia diagnosis (de Bruin et al., 2015). The other studies that included adolescents with "insomnia symptoms"/"sleep problems" (with or without comorbid conditions) (Bei et al., 2013; Bootzin & Stevens, 2005; Blake et al., 2016; Britton et al., 2010; de Bruin et al., 2014) adolescents with insomnia and a comorbid psychiatric diagnosis (Clarke et al., 2015) adolescents with delayed sleep phase disorder (Gradisar et al., 2011) were pilot studies (Mindell et al., 2009; de Bruin et al., 2014; Clarke et al., 2015; Schlarb et al., 2010) and/or uncontrolled studies (Bei et al., 2013; Bootzin & Stevens, 2005; Britton et al., 2010; de Bruin et al., 2014; Roeser et al., 2016). Still, the results from this meta-analysis showed preliminary positive effects for CBT-I in adolescents, which can be seen in increased sleep durations, decreased sleep onset latencies, decreased wake times after sleep onset, and improved sleep efficiency. Furthermore, positive effects were found for sleep quality and daytime functioning, including daytime sleepiness and depressive and anxiety symptoms (Blake et al., 2018).

Relational Consideration in Treatment of Problem Area

The development of pediatric insomnia is influenced by a myriad of physiological (e.g., maturational, medical, and temperamental factors) and psycho-social factors (i.e., cultural influence, parental factors such as perceptions and comorbid mental health conditions, and parent–child interactions) (Sadeh & Anders, 1993; Sadeh et al., 2010). These are often significantly determined by parents or caregivers, especially during early childhood development. Research has indicated that increased parental involvement in the context of their child's sleep is an established risk factor for preschool- and younger school-aged children's behavioral sleep problems (Newton et al., 2020). Additionally, negative parenting style, comorbid mental health diagnoses of parents, and marital conflict have also been identified as caregiver-related risk factors for pediatric insomnia. In terms of adolescents with insomnia, parental divorce, adverse parenting styles, and family stress are risk factors for the development of insomnia (Sadeh et al., 2009).

Behavioral treatments for pediatric insomnia rely heavily on parents and caregivers (Meltzer & Crabtree, 2015). Common behavioral treatments promote self-regulation (or self-soothing behaviors in young children) by reducing parent involvement and allowing the child to develop the skill of self-soothing to sleep independently. If implemented consistently, the child learns that they are able to better cope with bedtime on their own, anxiety levels decline, and sleep initiation becomes easier. In contrast, the increase in independence of adolescents means that when delivering CBT-I to adolescents, we are primarily focused on the youth with insomnia (Meltzer & Crabtree, 2015). However, parents and caregivers can help to promote acceptance and reinforcement of treatment improvements, as well as keep their child enrolled in CBT-I. When developmentally appropriate, clinicians can invite parents to join the last ten minutes of the session. During this brief time, the adolescent can summarize the session and the plan moving forward. However, this decision to include parents in sessions should be driven by the adolescent and not forced.

Interviewing and Assessing Pediatric Insomnia

Similar to other pediatric sleep disorders, pediatric insomnia is often underdiagnosed (Meltzer & Mindell, 2006). A clinical history is imperative and should be collected via a semi-structured interview with parents/caregivers and the child (when age appropriate). This should include collecting information on (1) the main complaint, its duration, frequency, history, potential triggers, and previous attempts to resolve the insomnia symptoms; (2) the child's typical 24-hour sleep-wake schedule, including sleep-onset latency, sleep onset and offset times, nighttime awakenings, wake after sleep onset times, and naps (frequency, duration, and timing); (3) the consistency of their sleep-wake schedule, especially inconsistencies between weekdays and weekends or different households; (4) bedtime routines should be explored in detail to determine potential sleep promoting (i.e., bath, books, songs) or hindering behaviors (i.e., screen time, eating, rigorous physical activity); (5) the sleep environment (i.e., television in the bedroom; sleeping independently versus with a parent or sibling); (6) the use of medication, caffeine, alcohol, or other substances; (7) daytime impairment, including sleepiness, behavior, or mood being negatively affected; (8) physical and mental health comorbidities; and finally (9) the families current treatment goals, expectations, and willingness/ability to implement behavioral changes.

In many instances, a comprehensive clinical interview is adequate to diagnose pediatric insomnia (Nunes & Bruni, 2015). However, in some cases, completion of sleep diaries for about one to two weeks may be useful to further assess sleep wake patterns (i.e., if have trouble recalling sleep wake schedule, if sleep-wake schedule is variable, and most commonly if the patient is an adolescent who can complete the sleep diary independently). Objective assessment of sleep patterns may also be necessary. An actigraphy device resembles a wristwatch and samples movement at set intervals (Sung et al., 2009). This information can then be analyzed with validated algorithms. Movement indicates a wake state; a lack of movement indicates rest or sleep. Computer software calculates sleep parameters, such as TST, wake time after sleep onset, sleep latency, frequency of night awakenings, as well as timing of sleep onset and offset. A sleep diary is often used to augment the accuracy of actigraphy. Actigraphy is ideally worn for two consecutive weeks. Actigraphy can be particularly helpful in adolescents with a suspected circadian rhythm sleep-wake disorder, comorbid with pediatric insomnia.

Polysomnography can be helpful to diagnosis underlying sleep disorders that can present with symptoms of insomnia. Specifically, children and adolescents who have suspected sleep apnea, periodic limb movements of sleep, or nocturnal seizures will likely require an overnight polysomnography.

A brief tool that can assist in the screening of sleep problems in clinical and school settings is the Bedtime routines, Excessive daytime sleepiness, Awakenings during night, Regularity and duration of sleep, Sleep-disordered breathing (BEARS) algorithm. This screening tool consists of five, straight-forward questions that have demonstrated adequate reliability and validity (Mindell & Owens, 2015).

Case Conceptualization

The most consistent findings regarding the factors contributing to the development of pediatric insomnia in early childhood are related to the strong links between parental involvement in the sleep initiation process and night wakings. Research has demonstrated that infants who fall asleep while receiving significant help from their parents (i.e., while being fed, rocked, and cuddled) have a higher number of night wakings requiring parental involvement, in comparison to infants who fall asleep independently (Anuntaseree et al., 2008; Burnham et al., 2002; DeLeon & Karraker, 2007; Morrell & Cortina-Borja, 2002; Sadeh et al., 2009; Tikotzky & Sadeh, 2009; Touchette et al., 2005). From a behavioral standpoint, when parents are highly involved in their child's sleep initiation, children learn to associate falling asleep with parental presence (BIC sleep-onset association type) and fail to develop the skill of self-soothing to sleep (Meltzer & Mindell, 2006). "Self-soothers" are more likely to resume sleep by themselves when they wake up during the night, whereas "signalers" tend to cry and fuss to elicit parental assistance.

Parental behaviors during bedtime and during night awakenings seem to be influenced by the parents' cognitions (i.e., expectations, interpretations, perceptions) and emotions or mood. Therefore, an important part in CBT for pediatric insomnia focuses on changing parental thoughts regarding their child's sleep in order to initiate a behavioral change (Owens et al., 1999; Sadeh, 2005). Majority of these behavioral treatments are based on the principles of extinction: it is assumed that infant night wakings and attention-seeking behaviors are positively reinforced by parental attention and soothing behaviors such as rocking and feeding. Therefore, removal of the reinforcement (i.e., parental involvement) will lead to a decline in the night waking signaling behavior (Wade et al., 2007).

As children mature, the etiology of their insomnia becomes more complex and their treatment is more closely related to insomnia treatments for adults (i.e., CBT-I). The 3-P model of insomnia provides a framework for understanding the evolution of insomnia and the role of treatment in managing this condition (Bonnet & Arand, 2010; Riemann et al., 2010). According to this model, predisposing factors, precipitating events, and perpetuating mechanisms all contribute to the development of insomnia. The idea is that some individuals may be particularly vulnerable to sleep difficulties, because they have a "highly sensitive" biological sleep system or they may have psychological traits that predispose them to poor sleep when confronted with stressful life events. When such individuals are confronted with specific precipitating circumstances (i.e., a stressful life event such as loss of a loved one, physical or mental health conditions, onset of puberty, hospitalizations, school-work overload, or a sudden or unexpected change in their sleep schedule), they are likely to develop acute insomnia. This acute insomnia may then be perpetuated by a variety of psychological and behavioral factors that develop in reaction to sleep difficulties. For example, how people think about their sleep problem (e.g., mental or physiological arousal) and the strategies they use to cope with insomnia symptoms (e.g., staying in bed awake trying hard to sleep, engaging in behaviors incompatible with sleep such as reading, watching TV, or eating in bed), make the sleep problems persist and develop into chronic insomnia. Therefore, chronic insomnia has a self-perpetuating vicious cycle, which is maintained by these perpetuating factors, that creates a state where individuals fear sleeplessness. CBT-I is designed to target the thoughts and beliefs individuals have about sleep and the behaviors they developed that maintain insomnia.

Session Structure When Working with Problem Area

Following the assessment and diagnosis of pediatric insomnia, particularly in young children, behavioral recommendations, changes to improve sleep hygiene, bedtime routines, and changing parental responses to sleep initiation and/or maintenance difficulties would be recommended

(Meltzer & Crabtree, 2015). Typically, one to four follow-up sessions are held, which depend on progress made toward treatment goals, level of adherence, parental expectations, and troubleshooting. Generally speaking, the session structure is as follows: (1) review the sleep diary for the previous week, (2) review the extent to which the patient/parent has complied with previous recommendations, (3) engage in problem-solving issues with adherence, (4) introduce a new treatment recommendation if necessary, and (5) make referrals to medical provider if necessary. Finally, given the busy clinic visit, providing written information or handouts are ideal to optimize treatment success. When the steps for treatment are clearly and simply written out, patients and families are more likely to follow through with treatment.

For adolescents with insomnia, CBT-I sessions are typically held biweekly to ensure continuity between sessions and will last for 45–60 minutes (Edinger & Carney, 2014; Morin & Espie, 2007; Perlis et al., 2005). If scheduling issues do not permit, it is encouraged that patients are contacted by telephone or other de-identified means so that sleep diary data can be collected at least bi-weekly. Each therapy session is highly structured and will cover a different aspect of CBT-I. Although their specific content varies on the technique presented/used, most sessions are structured according to the following agenda. The very 1st item of the agenda is to review the sleep diary for the previous week. This provides a clear message to the patient that self-monitoring is expected and is an essential component of CBT-I. The next step is to check the extent to which the patient has complied with previous recommendations. After problem-solving issues with adherence, a new treatment component is introduced. Each procedure is described along with its rationale and objectives. Handouts should be provided to consolidate the new information presented during the session. The final item on the agenda is to review homework assignments for the upcoming week giving a written summary to the patient.

Accumulating evidence supports the benefits of brief behavioral treatment of insomnia (BBT-I) in typically developing adolescents and adults for improving the ability to initiate and maintain sleep and overall sleep efficiency (Germain & Buysse, 2011; Troxel et al., 2012). BBT-I, which was derived from CBT-I, consists of four sessions, two of which are phone sessions. It is shorter in duration, can be delivered in primary care and outpatient clinical settings without additional specialization in sleep medicine, and thus has the potential to increase access to such evidence-based sleep interventions. BBT-I focuses on behavioral techniques (i.e., stimulus control, sleep restriction), is based on sleep hemostasis, and utilizes a manual which facilitates its concise delivery format and ease of training a range of clinicians.

Component of Practice and Intervention Modules

Graduated Extinction

As previously mentioned, children may have developed an association between parental presence and sleep initiation, making it difficult for children to initiate independently at bedtime or resume sleep independently upon night awakenings (Meltzer & Crabtree, 2015). The key to the graduated extinction (see attachment for handout) of the sleep-onset association is slowly developing the child's ability to fall asleep independently at bedtime. An example treatment plan for a child who spends all night in his parents' bed may begin by having the child begin the night in his own bed with the parent lying with him. Once the child falls asleep, the parent leaves the child's bed. Once the child has developed the ability to fall asleep in the child's own bed for several nights, the parents move progressively further away as the child falls asleep (sitting on the child's bed, sitting on a chair by the bed, sitting or standing in the doorway). Once the child is able to fall asleep with the parent in the doorway, the parent begins leaving briefly (30–60 seconds at 1st) to complete small tasks (e.g., putting on pajamas or emptying the dishwasher). The period of absence is slowly increased until the child begins falling asleep before the parent returns. Throughout this process, the child will likely wake and return to the parents' bed at some point in the night; allowing the child to spend the rest of the night in the parents' bed is often recommended to minimize sleep disruption for everyone in the family. Once the child develops the ability to fall asleep independently at bedtime, many are able to soothe themselves back to sleep during night wakings. If this ability does not develop spontaneously, similar graduated extinction procedures can be used to teach children to soothe themselves back to sleep during night wakings.

Bedtime Pass

Even though there is insufficient evidence to classify these strategies as a guideline or standard of care, positive reinforcement is frequently recommended and successful in clinical practice (Meltzer & Crabtree, 2015). For example, with the Bedtime Pass intervention, one or more bedtime passes (e.g., notecard or token) are given to young children at bedtime, with instructions that each pass can be exchanged for a request or parental visit (e.g. drink of water, brief visit from parent). When the passes are gone, parents ignore additional requests (see attachment for handout). However, if the child still has passes left in the morning, they can be exchanged for immediate, small rewards. The number of passes allowed a child each night can be gradually reduced. As with any behavioral treatment, consistency in implementation is paramount to their success. Furthermore, allowing the child to choose their rewards (within limits) is essential for their motivation and "buy in" for this intervention.

Stimulus Control

Behavior therapy for insomnia in adolescents is aimed at achieving two goals: (1) to strengthen the association between sleep and the bed, bedtime, and the sleep environment; (2) to consolidate sleep with decreased periods of time in bed (TIB). The 1st goal is the object of stimulus control therapy, which is designed to eliminate both sleep-incompatible behaviors. The 2nd one is a function of sleep restriction, which adapts the amount of TIB.

Stimulus control (see attachment for handout) is based on the premise that insomnia is the result of maladaptive conditioning between environmental (bed/bedroom) and temporal (bedtime) stimuli and sleep-incompatible behaviors (e.g., worrying, reading, or watching television while in bed) (Edinger & Carney, 2014; Morin & Espie, 2007; Perlis et al., 2005). These stimuli have lost their discriminative properties previously associated with sleep. The main therapeutic goal is to re-establish or strengthen the associations between sleep and the stimulus conditions under which it typically occurs (bed, bedtime, and bedroom). This is accomplished by reducing the amount of time spent in bed awake, by eliminating sleep-inhibitory activities, and by keeping a consistent sleep-wake schedule. Stimulus control instructions have been developed specifically for insomnia.

Sleep Restriction

Sleep restriction consists of reducing the amount of time spent in bed so it more closely matches the actual or estimated TST (see attachment for handout) (Edinger & Carney, 2014; Morin & Espie, 2007; Perlis et al., 2005). After sleep efficiency improves, TIB is gradually increased (by 15 minute intervals) until optimal sleep duration is achieved. Sleep restriction is based on the idea that individuals with insomnia spend too much TIB, often putting effort into trying to sleep and to attempt to compensate for sleep loss. They may go to bed early hoping that this will help them to be asleep by the desired time, stay in bed late in the morning to compensate for sleep loss, or take naps during the day in order to obtain more sleep. This leads to poor sleep efficiency, more broken sleep, and inevitably perpetuates sleep difficulties. Sleep efficiency is an index of the degree of "mismatch" between TST and TIB for which the formula is sleep efficiency = (TST/TIB) × 100. A sleep efficiency that is lower than 80%–85% is usually associated with difficulties initiating/maintaining sleep, as well as with restless and unsatisfying sleep. Conversely, a sleep efficiency that is greater than 85%–90% usually means better sleep initiation/continuity and more sound and satisfying sleep. Excellent sleep efficiency does not necessarily mean adequate or satisfying sleep duration. The ideal amount of time that patients undergoing sleep restriction therapy should stay in bed is TIB = TST + 30 minutes. This ideal TIB is utilized to choose a standard wake-up time and earliest bedtime. For example, if their ideal TIB equals six hours and they decide that they want to get up each morning at 7 AM, this means that their earliest bedtime would be 1 AM. Although the recommendation for adults with insomnia is a minimum of 5.0 hours in bed, it is recommended that TIB for adolescents should never be less than 6.5 hours. In contrast, for school-aged children, a minimum TIB should not be less than 7.5 hours.

Whereas insomnia in younger children is often best targeted by behavioral strategies, cognitive strategies can be used for older youth, particularly adolescents. Cognitive restructuring, challenging negative sleep-related beliefs, or catastrophizing have been successfully used to treat insomnia in school-aged children and adolescents (Meltzer & Crabtree, 2015). CBT-I protocols for older youth may also include relaxation techniques, such as breathing exercises and progressive muscle relaxation.

Constructive Worry

Many adolescents report that stimulus control sleep restriction therapy is adequate for improving their insomnia; some continue to worry and have difficulty initiating or maintaining sleep (Edinger & Carney, 2014; Morin & Espie, 2007; Perlis et al., 2005). Some bedtime worries are a result of keeping so busy during the day that no time is available to deal with the worries. Sleep is the 1st opportunity that is quiet enough for their brain to try and complete its unfinished business. When they have problems, they tend to use their problem-solving skills to make their lives better and to relieve ourselves of anxiety. Adolescents with insomnia may use problem-solving skills at the wrong times and places, namely, bedtime. They may think about a problem, trying to solve it, but unfortunately, the anxiety caused by the problem will prolong sleep onset and maintenance. Constructive worry (see attachment for handout) is a method for managing the tendency to worry during that quiet time when sleep is supposed to be taking over. Adolescents are encouraged to complete this exercise during the early evening (at least two hours before bed), where it should only take you about 15 minutes to complete.

Assessment of Progress and Outcomes

Adequate follow-up on behavioral treatment recommendation is critical (Meltzer & Crabtree, 2015). The timing of follow-ups is important to consider, given that the clinician should give the family enough time to implement changes and see results, but not too much time that the family has neglected to begin. Commonly, follow-ups for behavioral treatment recommendations for BIC consist of inquiring with the family on progress made. However, relying on parent report only is problematic due to parent burnout and parental expectations being too high or low in terms of treatment progress. Therefore, structured and quantitative follow-up tools could greatly facilitate optimal care for children with pediatric insomnia.

Typically, the goal for improving pediatric insomnia is to achieve the following: (1) acceptable TST ranges according to the National Sleep Foundation (NSF) (Hirshkowitz et al., 2015), (2) SOL of $\leq$30 minutes, and (3) WASO $\leq$30 minutes. However, there is flexibility in these values, in that an improvement of TST and/or SOL of about 60 minutes in a child may indicate treatment effectiveness (Sadeh, 2007). Furthermore, when evaluating treatment progress, achieving parents' goals should be heavily considered in the decision-making process (Meltzer & Crabtree, 2015). Therefore, further to quantitative (TST, SOL, WASO) measures the clinician should also evaluate improvement in the child's behavior and parental satisfaction (Banaschewski et al., 2022).

In adolescents with insomnia, completing a daily sleep diary is an essential requirement in order to (1) document the nature and severity of the initial sleep problem, (2) assess night-to-night variations in sleep patterns and identify factors that contribute to improve or worsen sleep, (3) monitor treatment progress, and (4) evaluate compliance with treatment procedures (Edinger & Carney, 2014; Morin & Espie, 2007; Perlis et al., 2005). Notably, noncompliance with self-monitoring is a good predictor of noncompliance with treatment procedures; therefore, this issue needs to be addressed with motivational interviewing techniques. Sleep diary data are entered into a summary form and the clinician will have access to and use of these data during therapy sessions.

In each CBT-I visit, the clinician reviews the sleep diary to assess treatment gains and compliance and determine whether more TIB is warranted (Edinger & Carney, 2014; Morin & Espie, 2007; Perlis et al., 2005). From the sleep diary, the following data will be calculated, TST, TIB, and sleep efficiency (SE = TST/TIB) × 100. If SE is greater than 85% and they are feeling sleepy, then, their gains have met clinical expectation. This means that we will allow you 15 more minutes of TIB by either advancing your prescribed time to bed or delaying 15 minutes your prescribed wakeup time. If SE is in the 80%–85% range or greater than 85% but they are not feeling sleepy, then, their gains have been marginal in respect to clinical expectation. This means that the clinician will not change the prescribed TIB. If SE <80%, then, there have not been clinical gains. This means that the clinician will either maintain the prescribed TIB unchanged or delay the bedtime or advance the wakeup time by 15 minutes. Furthermore, collected self-report measures at each CBT-I session are ideal to track symptomology over time. For example, administering the Insomnia Severity Index (ISI), Pre-sleep Arousal Scale (PSAS), and Sleep Need Questionnaire (SNQ) will assist in guiding treatment.

Applications to the School Setting

A universal approach to improve sleep can be the implementation of sleep education programs delivered directly to students and parents, which has shown positive effects by improving both objectively and subjectively measured sleep duration in young children by around 30 minutes (Kaar et al., 2021). Rey and colleagues' intervention moved children who were having insufficient sleep (defined as less than nine hours per night of sleep for this age group) to sufficient sleep status of a mean of just over nine hours per night (Rey et al., 2020). This intervention had a total of eight lessons integrated into the schools' existing curricula which was taught over the course of one month. Teachers were trained on the program delivery and informed about sleep and health by completing a training manual on their own time. This type of training for teachers and delivery within the existing structure of the classroom may offer feasibility for other elementary schools to model in their own classroom settings. Another advantage of this program is that it can be delivered to a large number of children simultaneously and by targeting the children and parents on the importance of sleep health early has potential to negate the high prevalence of sleep disorders often diagnosed in this age group.

In general, for younger, elementary-aged children involving the parents seems the most advantageous for changing sleep duration (Kaar et al., 2021). However, merely providing parents with an informational packet or brochure is insufficient for producing substantial improvements for sleep. Researchers should consider other universal intervention methods to educate parents and families in large settings to share the program details with families and provide general knowledge on sleep health (van Rijn et al., 2020). Unfortunately, prevalence of screening and intervention for sleep disturbance is low in primary care settings, and there is a lack of specialty trained behavioral sleep medicine providers (Honaker & Meltzer, 2016). Thus, school-based delivery of sleep interventions offers a unique opportunity to reach children and families who would otherwise not receive services.

Targeted Interventions in School Setting

Intervention for sleep problems may fall outside the typical scope of practice for many school psychologists. The importance of sleep to academic functioning, as well as the ease and efficacy of brief interventions to improve sleep, suggests that expanding our role to provide support for sufficient sleep may have a significant impact on student functioning.

Many sleep problems can be treated effectively with behavioral interventions that can be implemented though brief consultation. Problematic sleep hygiene (e.g., watching TV in bed, inconsistent bed times) is the most common sleep issue experienced by children (Moore & Mindell, 2012). Several simple changes to promote effective sleep hygiene may significantly improve the quantity and quality of sleep. Consultation related to sleep hygiene often results in the establishment of a consistent sleep schedule that begins with a good bedtime routine. The routine should consist of three to four relaxing activities that move in the direction of the bedroom. A good bedtime routine might include taking a shower or bath, changing into pajamas, reading, and getting into bed. About 52% of parents report that their children's bedtime and wake time vary significantly on the weekend or during the week (Hirshkowitz et al., 2015); for these children, emphasizing consistency of bedtime and wake time may be especially important.

School psychologists' skills in behavioral interventions can be helpful in removing behaviors or associations that may interfere with sleep. One such behavior is co-sleeping, or bed sharing between students and other family members, often parents. Though co-sleeping is an accepted practice for many families and may be necessary for some families due to financial constraints, other parents want children to learn to sleep independently. Furthermore, co-sleeping may be associated with increased behavior problems at school, increased learning concerns, lower self-confidence, and increased aggressiveness with parents for some children (Pressman & Imber, 2011). In many cases, co-sleeping is difficult to reduce without a consistent behavior plan. Children may have developed a strong association between parents and sleep onset, making it difficult for children to fall asleep independently at bedtime or return to sleep independently during routine awakenings in the middle of the night. In this case, graduated extinction (as described previously) would be the behavioral recommendation to implement, which can be done by a school psychologist or counselor with training in basic behavioral principles.

When school psychologists encounter students with sleep problems that cannot be addressed in school, referral to an outside medical provider may be appropriate. Persistent daytime fatigue, behavior problems, and poor mood are all indicators that a student may suffer from insufficient sleep and need additional support beyond improvements to sleep hygiene. Some sleep disorders that may require a referral include obstructive sleep apnea, parasomnias, restless legs syndrome, and narcolepsy.

For students who may be suffering from a sleep disorder, school psychologists should partner with families and health-care professionals to make an appropriate referral. First, discussing the sleep issue with the family can develop an understanding of presenting concerns and common goals. Referral to the primary care provider for sleep assessment is often the 1st step in initiating medical treatment. School psychologists can communicate directly with outside health-care providers to provide information regarding sleep-related difficulties in school, which may help with diagnosis and treatment planning. In addition, the outside health-care professional can provide information related to the sleep problem and appropriate accommodations to support the student's success in school.

Case Study

The following case example highlights the use of CBT-I for adolescents with insomnia.

Session Protocol

The 1st session will present a conceptual cognitive-behavioral model of insomnia and the patient will receive sleep hygiene instructions (Edinger & Carney, 2014; Morin & Espie, 2007; Perlis et al., 2005). A brief presentation of Spielman's and Morin's cognitive-behavioral models (discussed earlier in this chapter) will be explained to the patients and will serve as the basis for all clinical procedures that will be used during treatment. The role of sleep-related behaviors and habits will be addressed, and a standard handout with sleep hygiene instructions will be given to the patient. Sleep restriction and stimulus control will be introduced, which have been shown to be strongly efficacious in insomnia. The goals of sleep restriction and stimulus control are (1) to reduce activities incompatible with sleep and develop positive associations of good sleep with the bedroom, (2) increase sleep-wake specificity by avoiding napping in the day and getting up if wakeful at night, (3) increase sleep efficiency by spending less TIB and build up the natural sleep drive, and (4) establish regular sleep habits and keep to a consistent pattern from night to night throughout the week. The patient will receive written instruction for homework as practice with the sleep diary is very important to achieve therapeutic goals. Because sleep restriction requires keeping to a bedtime threshold while setting a standard wakeup time and stimulus control involves getting out of bed and going to another room, all sessions should focus on addressing difficulties associated with the sleep restriction and stimulus control rules and their adherence. In some cases, stimulus control may be replaced by counterconditioning (e.g., persons with mobility problems).

In the 2nd session, we will introduce Constructive Worry which is a cognitive technique designed to decrease cognitive hyperarousal (Edinger & Carney, 2014; Morin & Espie, 2007; Perlis et al., 2005). In the context of insomnia, cognitive techniques such as constructive worry and problem solving seek to help the patient regain control over their "racing mind" or "insomnia brain." Using layman's terms, the concept of cortical hyperarousal while asleep should also be explained to the patient. This intervention requires home practice every evening before bedtime, regardless of whether the issue, worry, or concern has been addressed/solved or not. The primary goals are: (1) review data and confirm that upward titration is indicated, (2) assess treatment gains and compliance and in the case of noncompliance focus session on this issue, (3) make adjustments to the patient's sleep schedule, (a) in the case of positive clinical gains (SE >85% and sleepy), upwardly titrate total sleep opportunity by 15 minutes, (b) in the case of no or marginal gains (SE between 80% and 85%), maintain schedule and provide rationale to the patient, and (c) in the case of negative gains (SE <80%), downwardly titrate total sleep opportunity and provide rationale to the patient, (4) review sleep hygiene and provide tips to adhere to the new sleep schedule, (5) introduce Constructive Worry and its rationale and make a plan to use daily or as needed, and (6) continue to secure the patient's commitment to the program and prescribe homework and sleep opportunity.

The 3rd session will introduce Relaxation Therapy which is a method designed to decrease emotional and somatic arousal and induce sleep (Edinger & Carney, 2014; Morin & Espie, 2007; Perlis et al., 2005). In the context of insomnia, deactivation techniques such as deep breathing and progressive muscle relaxation seek to help the patient-induce sleep without putting effort onto it rather than simply reducing anxiety levels. This intervention requires home practice at least twice a day and is not expected to produce therapeutic effects within the 1st week (skill learning period). This intervention will also provide the patient with a skill to implement together stimulus control instructions. The primary goals of this session are as follows: (1) review data and confirm that upward titration is indicated, (2) assess treatment gains and compliance and in the case of noncompliance focus session on this issue, (3) make adjustments to the patient's sleep schedule (see below), (4) review sleep hygiene and provide tips to adhere to the new sleep schedule, (5) review constructive worry and cognitive restructuring and provide tips to adhere to these treatment techniques, (6) introduce relaxation therapy and its rationale, and (7) continue to secure the patient's commitment to the program and prescribe homework and sleep opportunity.

The 4th session will introduce Cognitive Restructuring which is a method designed to change a person's beliefs, expectations, appraisals, and attributions. In the context of insomnia, cognitive therapy seeks to change sleep expectations, catastrophic beliefs about the causes and consequences of insomnia, and beliefs about sleep-promoting practices (Edinger & Carney, 2014; Morin & Espie, 2007; Perlis et al., 2005). This intervention is predominantly verbal in nature and is more time consuming to implement in-session than behavioral procedures described in previous sessions. However, it is preferred that patients work at home using Thought Records and become actively involved in challenging sleep cognitions. The primary goals are as follows: (1) review data and confirm that upward titration is indicated, (2) assess treatment gains and compliance and in the case of noncompliance focus session on this issue, (3) make adjustments to the patient's sleep schedule (see below) and provide tips to adhere to the new sleep schedule, (4) review sleep hygiene, constructive worry, and relaxation therapy and provide tips to increase adherence, (5) introduce cognitive restructuring and its rationale, and (6) continue to secure the patient's commitment to the program and prescribe homework and sleep opportunity.

The 5th session will serve as a follow-up of all treatment components (Edinger & Carney, 2014; Morin & Espie, 2007; Perlis et al., 2005). The primary goals of this session are as follows: (1) review data, (2) assess treatment gains, (3) adjust the patient's sleep schedule (see below), (4) review constructive worry, relaxation therapy, and cognitive restructuring, and (5) continue to secure the patient's commitment to the program and prescribe homework and sleep opportunity.

The sixth session will also integrate all clinical procedures as to improve long-term adherence and relapse prevention (Edinger & Carney, 2014; Morin & Espie, 2007; Perlis et al., 2005). It will also include a post-treatment assessment of subjective sleep and daytime functioning scales. The same post-treatment assessment will be used at the three- and six-month follow-ups.

Case of Samantha

Samantha is a 17-year-old girl who has had difficulty falling asleep for the past five years following the onset of puberty. When she presented in clinic, her evening routine consisted of participating in extracurricular activities, dinner, and homework (which was typically completed in bed on a laptop or tablet). She would typically "try" to sleep at 11:00 PM by turning off her laptop and lying in bed on her phone. SOL was typically one hour. In contrast, on weekends and during summer months, she would attempt to fall asleep around 12:00 AM but still take an hour to initiate sleep. Samantha reported frequent night wakings, about four times per night, for which she was awake about 15 minutes per time. She would set her alarm on weekdays for 7:00 AM and often have difficulty waking up. Samantha's average sleep duration was 6.0 hours, with prolonged SOL, frequent night awakenings, and prolonged WASO. On weekends she would sleep in until 8:00 AM.

Samantha denied symptoms of any other comorbid sleep disorder (i.e., obstructive sleep apnea, restless legs syndrome, periodic limb movement disorder). In the past, Samantha has tried melatonin (of varying dosages 3–20 mg) without noticeable benefit. Samantha identified as a high achieving student who was enrolled in multiple Advanced Placement courses and heavily involved in extracurricular activities. She reported being worried that her sleep difficulties would impact her academic success, particularly "getting into college."

At the 1st session, Samantha was prescribed 6.5 hours in bed, based on her average TST of 6.0 hours. Given that she had to wake up for school at 7:00 AM, she was instructed to go to bed at 12:30 AM. She was encouraged to keep this schedule (12:30 AM–7:00 AM) across weekdays and weekends until the next session. Samantha was also instructed on how to implement stimulus control strategies, and she decided she would draw or read at her desk when unable to initiate or resume sleep within 15–20 minutes. Lastly, sleep hygiene improvements were discussed, with a focus on electronics prior to bed and while in bed, as well as developing a wind-down routine to do after homework but before bed.

At the 2nd session, Samantha reported consistently practicing stimulus control strategies for the 1st week, however by the 2nd week she didn't need to get out of bed to read. Samantha's sleep diary data indicated a SE >85% and she also reported an increased sleep need; therefore, her sleep prescription was expanded to 7.0 hours in bed (12:00 AM–7:00 AM sleep-wake schedule). Samantha's treatment adherence was reinforced and constructive worry was introduced. Samantha reported that she has many worries related to school that she often thinks about at bedtime that could be addressed with constructive worry.

At the 3rd session, Samantha's sleep diary data revealed improved adherence to treatment recommendations. However, she reported finding it difficult to "fit in" the constructive worry technique because of "the school work." Troubleshooting and motivational interviewing techniques were utilized to increase adherence to constructive worry, given her persistent cognitive arousal at bedtime. Samantha's sleep diary data indicated a SE >85% and she also reported an increased sleep need; therefore, her sleep prescription was expanded to 7.5 hours in bed (11:30 PM–7:00 AM sleep-wake schedule). Samantha's treatment adherence was reinforced and relaxation therapy was introduced.

At the 4th session, Samantha's sleep diary data revealed continued improved adherence to treatment recommendations. She reported implementing constructive worry on a nightly basis which has helped with her worries at bedtime. She also reported practicing relaxation therapy during the day and then making it a part of her wind-down routine. Samantha's sleep diary data indicated a SE >85% and she also reported an increased sleep need; therefore, her sleep prescription was expanded to 8.0 hours in bed (11:00 PM–7:00 AM sleep-wake schedule). Samantha's treatment adherence was reinforced and cognitive restructuring was introduced. One of her common negative belief about sleep was that "if I don't sleep well tonight, I won't be able to pay attention in school tomorrow." Cognitive restructuring of that negative thought was completed in session and she was encouraged to address other negative sleep-related thoughts as they arise with this technique at home.

At the 5th session, Samantha reported marginal treatment gains with her sleep dairy data indicating a SE of 82%; therefore, her sleep prescription remained the same. She attributed this to several exams that she had the previous week. Samantha denied further use of cognitive restructuring but reported continued adherence to constructive worry and relaxation techniques. Troubleshooting and motivational interviewing techniques were utilized to increase adherence to cognitive restructuring, by completing the exercise in session again with a different negative sleep-related thought.

At the 6th session, Samantha's sleep dairy data indicated a SE >85% and she also reported an increased sleep need; therefore, her sleep prescription was expanded to 8.25 hours in bed (10:45 PM–7:00 AM sleep-wake schedule). Relapse prevention was discussed in detail, with special attention to instances of high stress. It was discussed that each week if she continued to initiate sleep in less than 30 minutes and not experience night wakings, she could add 15 minutes onto her TIB each week. However, she was encouraged to not add more than 15 minutes per week, and if she was finding it difficult to initiate or maintain sleep again, to resume the previous sleep prescription for one to two weeks.

Summary

Pediatric insomnia is highly prevalent and associated with a myriad of maladaptive consequences for the child and family, yet remains largely underdiagnosed. Pediatric insomnia affects students' cognitive, academic, behavioral, emotional, and social functioning. Questions about sleep disruptions can easily be incorporated into a school psychologist's interview. Psychoeducation and brief behavioral interventions can be provided in the school setting, and referral to medical providers can lead to effective treatment of sleep disorders. Cognitive-behavioral interventions for pediatric insomnia have received strong empirical support. In addition to their positive effects on children's sleep problems, they also were found to improve the functioning and well-being of parents.

Reflection Questions

1 In what ways can you integrate screening questions about sleep into your practice?
2 What type of professional development or supervision experiences would you need to help you implement targeted, brief, behavioral strategies to improve sleep?
3 In what ways might cognitive and behavioral interventions for insomnia look different in young children and adolescents?

References

American Academy of Sleep Medicine (2014). International classification of sleep disorders (ICSD-3). American Academy of Sleep Medicine, Darien, IL.

Anuntaseree, W., Mo-Suwan, L., Vasiknanonte, P., Kuasirikul, S., & Choprapawan, C. (2008). Night waking in Thai infants at 3 months of age: Association between parental practices and infant sleep. *Sleep Medicine, 9*(5), 564–571.

Ball, H. L., Tomori, C., & McKenna, J. J. (2019). Toward an integrated anthropology of infant sleep. *American Anthropologist, 121*(3), 595–612.

Banaschewski, T., Bruni, O., Fuentes, J., Hill, C. M., Hvolby, A., Posserud, M. B., & Schroder, C. (2022). Practice tools for screening and monitoring insomnia in children and adolescents with autism spectrum disorder. *Journal of Autism and Developmental Disorders, 52*(8), 3758–3768.

Bei, B., Byrne, M. L., Ivens, C., Waloszek, J., Woods, M. J., Dudgeon, P., & Allen, N. B. (2013). Pilot study of a mindfulness-based, multi-component, in-school group sleep intervention in adolescent girls. *Early Intervention in Psychiatry, 7*(2), 213–220.

Blake, M. J., Blake, L. M., Schwartz, O., Raniti, M., Waloszek, J. M., Murray, G., & Allen, N. B. (2018). Who benefits from adolescent sleep interventions? Moderators of treatment efficacy in a randomized controlled trial of a cognitive-behavioral and mindfulness-based group sleep intervention for at-risk adolescents. *Journal of Child Psychology and Psychiatry, 59*(6), 637–649.

Blake, M. J., Sheeber, L. B., Youssef, G. J., Raniti, M. B., & Allen, N. B. (2017). Systematic review and meta-analysis of adolescent cognitive–behavioral sleep interventions. *Clinical Child and Family Psychology Review, 20*, 227–249.

Blake, M. J., Waloszek, J. M., Schwartz, O., Raniti, M., Simmons, J. G., Blake, L., & Allen, N. B. (2016). The SENSE study: Post intervention effects of a randomized controlled trial of a cognitive–behavioral and mindfulness-based group sleep improvement intervention among at-risk adolescents. *Journal of Consulting and Clinical Psychology, 84*(12), 1039.

Bonnet, M. H., & Arand, D. L. (2010). Hyperarousal and insomnia: State of the science. *Sleep Medicine Reviews, 14*(1), 9–15.

Bootzin, R. R., & Stevens, S. J. (2005). Adolescents, substance abuse, and the treatment of insomnia and daytime sleepiness. *Clinical Psychology Review, 25*(5), 629–644.

Britton, W. B., Bootzin, R. R., Cousins, J. C., Hasler, B. P., Peck, T., & Shapiro, S. L. (2010). The contribution of mindfulness practice to a multicomponent behavioral sleep intervention following substance abuse treatment in adolescents: A treatment-development study. *Substance Abuse, 31*(2), 86–97.

Bruni, O., Melegari, M. G., Esposito, A., Sette, S., Angriman, M., Apicella, M., & Ferri, R. (2020). Executive functions in preschool children with chronic insomnia. *Journal of Clinical Sleep Medicine, 16*(2), 231–241.

Burnham, M. M., Goodlin-Jones, B. L., Gaylor, E. E., & Anders, T. F. (2002). Nighttime sleep-wake patterns and self-soothing from birth to one year of age: A longitudinal intervention study. *Journal of Child Psychology and Psychiatry, 43*(6), 713–725.

Clarke, G., McGlinchey, E. L., Hein, K., Gullion, C. M., Dickerson, J. F., Leo, M. C., & Harvey, A. G. (2015). Cognitive-behavioral treatment of insomnia and depression in adolescents: A pilot randomized trial. *Behaviour Research and Therapy, 69*, 111–118.

Combs, D., Goodwin, J. L., Quan, S. F., Morgan, W. J., Shetty, S., & Parthasarathy, S. (2016). Insomnia, health-related quality of life and health outcomes in children: A seven year longitudinal cohort. *Scientific Reports, 6*(1), 27921.

de Bruin, E. J., Bögels, S. M., Oort, F. J., & Meijer, A. M. (2015). Efficacy of cognitive behavioral therapy for insomnia in adolescents: A randomized controlled trial with internet therapy, group therapy and a waiting list condition. *Sleep, 38*(12), 1913–1926.

de Bruin, E. J., Oort, F. J., Bögels, S. M., & Meijer, A. M. (2014). Efficacy of internet and group-administered cognitive behavioral therapy for insomnia in adolescents: A pilot study. *Behavioral Sleep Medicine, 12*(3), 235–254.

de Zambotti, M., Goldstone, A., Colrain, I. M., & Baker, F. C. (2018). Insomnia disorder in adolescence: Diagnosis, impact, and treatment. *Sleep Medicine Reviews, 39*, 12–24.

DeLeon, C. W., & Karraker, K. H. (2007). Intrinsic and extrinsic factors associated with night waking in 9-month-old infants. *Infant Behavior and Development, 30*(4), 596–605.

Edinger, J. D., & Carney, C. E. (2014). *Overcoming insomnia: A cognitive-behavioral therapy approach, therapist guide*. New York: Oxford University Press.

Germain, A., & Buysse, D. J. (2011). Brief behavioral treatment of insomnia. In M. Perlis, M. Aloia, & B. Kuhn (Eds.), *Behavioral treatments for sleep disorders* (pp. 143–150). London: Academic Press.

Gradisar, M., Dohnt, H., Gardner, G., Paine, S., Starkey, K., Menne, A., & Trenowden, S. (2011). A randomized controlled trial of cognitive-behavior therapy plus bright light therapy for adolescent delayed sleep phase disorder. *Sleep, 34*(12), 1671–1680.

Hirshkowitz, M., Whiton, K., Albert, S. M., Alessi, C., Bruni, O., DonCarlos, L., & Hillard, P. J. A. (2015). National Sleep Foundation's sleep time duration recommendations: Methodology and results summary. *Sleep Health, 1*(1), 40–43.

Honaker, S. M., & Meltzer, L. J. (2016). Sleep in pediatric primary care: A review of the literature. *Sleep Medicine Reviews, 25*, 31–39.

Johnson, E. O., Roth, T., Schultz, L., & Breslau, N. (2006). Epidemiology of DSM-IV insomnia in adolescence: Lifetime prevalence, chronicity, and an emergent gender difference. *Pediatrics, 117*(2), e247–e256.

Kaar, J. L., Bowen, A. E., Clark, E., Ware, M., Chandrasekhar, J. L., Gulley, L., & Simon, S. L. (2021). School-based interventions to improve sleep duration: Lessons learned and future directions. *Current Psychology, 42*, 8221–8231.

Kahn, M. (2023). Insomnia in infancy, childhood, and adolescence. *Sleep Medicine Clinics, 18*(2), 135–145.

Kuhn, B. R., & Elliott, A. J. (2003). Treatment efficacy in behavioral pediatric sleep medicine. *Journal of Psychosomatic Research, 54*(6), 587–597.

Lovato, N., & Gradisar, M. (2014). A meta-analysis and model of the relationship between sleep and depression in adolescents: Recommendations for future research and clinical practice. *Sleep Medicine Reviews, 18*(6), 521–529.

Medalie, L., Dang, T., & Casnar, C. L. (2021). Pediatric insomnia: Etiology, impact, assessment, and treatment. In D. Gozal & L. Kheirandish-Gozal (Eds.), *Pediatric Sleep Medicine: Mechanisms and Comprehensive Guide to Clinical Evaluation and Management* (pp. 333–339). Cham: Springer.

Meltzer, L. J., & McLaughlin Crabtree, V. (2015). *Pediatric sleep problems: A clinician's guide to behavioral interventions*. American Psychological Association.

Meltzer, L. J., & Mindell, J. A. (2006). Sleep and sleep disorders in children and adolescents. *Psychiatric Clinics of North America,* 29, 1059–1076.

Meltzer, L. J., & Mindell, J. A. (2014). Systematic review and meta-analysis of behavioral interventions for pediatric insomnia. *Journal of Pediatric Psychology, 39*(8), 932–948.

Mike, T. B., Shaw, D. S., Forbes, E. E., Sitnick, S. L., & Hasler, B. P. (2016). The hazards of bad sleep—Sleep duration and quality as predictors of adolescent alcohol and cannabis use. *Drug and Alcohol Dependence, 168*, 335–339.
Mindell, J. A. (1999). Empirically supported treatments in pediatric psychology: Bedtime refusal and night wakings in young children. *Journal of Pediatric Psychology, 24*(6), 465–481.
Mindell, J. A., Meltzer, L. J., Carskadon, M. A., & Chervin, R. D. (2009). Developmental aspects of sleep hygiene: Findings from the 2004 National Sleep Foundation Sleep in America Poll. *Sleep Medicine, 10*(7), 771–779.
Mindell, J. A., & Owens, J. A. (2015). *A clinical guide to pediatric sleep: Diagnosis and management of sleep problems*. Lippincott Williams & Wilkins.
Moore, M., & Mindell, J. A. (2012). Sleep-related problems in childhood. In C. A. Espie & C. M. Morin (Eds.), *The Oxford handbook of sleep and sleep disorders* (pp. 729–7450). New York: Oxford University Press.
Morin, C. M., & Espie, C. A. (2007). *Insomnia: A clinical guide to assessment and treatment*. Springer Science & Business Media.
Morrell, J., & Cortina-Borja, M. (2002). The developmental change in strategies parents employ to settle young children to sleep, and their relationship to infant sleeping problems, as assessed by a new questionnaire: the parental interactive bedtime behaviour scale. *Infant and Child Development: An International Journal of Research and Practice, 11*(1), 17–41.
Newton, A. T., Honaker, S. M., & Reid, G. J. (2020). Risk and protective factors and processes for behavioral sleep problems among preschool and early school-aged children: A systematic review. *Sleep Medicine Reviews, 52*, 101303.
Nunes, M. L., & Bruni, O. (2015). Insomnia in childhood and adolescence: Clinical aspects, diagnosis, and therapeutic approach. *Jornal de Pediatria, 91*, S26–S35.
Owens, J. A., & Mindell, J. A. (2011). Pediatric insomnia. *Pediatric Clinics, 58*(3), 555–569.
Owens, L. J., France, K. G., & Wiggs, L. (1999). Behavioural and cognitive-behavioural interventions for sleep disorders in infants and children: A review. *Sleep Medicine Reviews, 3*(4), 281–302.
Paine, S., & Gradisar, M. (2011). A randomised controlled trial of cognitive-behaviour therapy for behavioural insomnia of childhood in school-aged children. *Behaviour Research and Therapy, 49*(6–7), 379–388.
Perlis, M. L., Jungquist, C., Smith, M. T., & Posner, D. (2005). *Cognitive behavioral treatment of insomnia: A session-by-session guide* (Vol. 1). Springer Science & Business Media.
Pressman, R. M., & Imber, S. C. (2011). Relationship of children's daytime behavior problems with bedtime routines/practices: A family context and the consideration of faux-ADHD. *The American Journal of Family Therapy, 39*(5), 404–418.
Rey, A. E., Guignard-Perret, A., Imler-Weber, F., Garcia-Larrea, L., & Mazza, S. (2020). Improving sleep, cognitive functioning and academic performance with sleep education at school in children. *Learning and Instruction, 65*, 101270.
Riemann, D., Spiegelhalder, K., Feige, B., Voderholzer, U., Berger, M., Perlis, M., & Nissen, C. (2010). The hyperarousal model of insomnia: A review of the concept and its evidence. *Sleep Medicine Reviews, 14*(1), 19–31.
Roeser, K., Schwerdtle, B., Kübler, A., & Schlarb, A. A. (2016). Further evidence for the JuSt program as treatment for insomnia in adolescents: Results from a 1-year follow-up study. *Journal of Clinical Sleep Medicine, 12*(2), 257–262.
Sadeh, A. (2005). Cognitive–behavioral treatment for childhood sleep disorders. *Clinical Psychology Review, 25*(5), 612–628.
Sadeh, A. (2007). Consequences of sleep loss or sleep disruption in children. *Sleep Medicine Clinics, 2*(3), 513–520.
Sadeh, A., & Anders, T. F. (1993). Infant sleep problems: Origins, assessment, interventions. *Infant Mental Health Journal, 14*(1), 17–34.
Sadeh, A., Tikotzky, L., & Scher, A. (2010). Parenting and infant sleep. *Sleep Medicine Reviews, 14*(2), 89–96.
Sadeh, A. V. I., Mindell, J. A., Luedtke, K., & Wiegand, B. (2009). Sleep and sleep ecology in the first 3 years: A web-based study. *Journal of Sleep Research, 18*(1), 60–73.
Schlarb, A. A., Bihlmaier, I., Velten-Schurian, K., Poets, C. F., & Hautzinger, M. (2018). Short-and long-term effects of CBT-I in groups for school-age children suffering from chronic insomnia: The KiSS-program. *Behavioral Sleep Medicine, 16*(4), 380–397.
Schlarb, A. A., Liddle, C. C., & Hautzinger, M. (2010). JuSt–a multimodal program for treatment of insomnia in adolescents: A pilot study. *Nature and Science of Sleep, 3*, 13–20.

Shelton, A. R., & Malow, B. (2021). Neurodevelopmental disorders commonly presenting with sleep disturbances. *Neurotherapeutics, 18*(1), 156–169.

Sung, M., Adamson, T. M., & Horne, R. S. (2009). Validation of actigraphy for determining sleep and wake in preterm infants. *Acta Paediatrica, 98*(1), 52–57.

Tikotzky, L., & Sadeh, A. (2009). Maternal sleep-related cognitions and infant sleep: A longitudinal study from pregnancy through the 1st year. *Child Development, 80*(3), 860–874.

Touchette, É., Petit, D., Paquet, J., Boivin, M., Japel, C., Tremblay, R. E., & Montplaisir, J. Y. (2005). Factors associated with fragmented sleep at night across early childhood. *Archives of Pediatrics & Adolescent Medicine, 159*(3), 242–249.

Troxel, W. M., Germain, A., & Buysse, D. J. (2012). Clinical management of insomnia with brief behavioral treatment (BBTI). *Behavioral Sleep Medicine, 10*(4), 266–279.

van Rijn, E., Koh, S. Y., Ng, A. S., Vinogradova, K., Chee, N. I., Lee, S. M., & Chee, M. W. (2020). Evaluation of an interactive school-based sleep education program: A cluster-randomized controlled trial. *Sleep Health, 6*(2), 137–144.

Wade, C. M., Ortiz, C., & Gorman, B. S. (2007). Two-session group parent training for bedtime noncompliance in head start preschoolers. *Child & Family Behavior Therapy, 29*(3), 23–55.

Zhang, L., Yang, Y., Luo, Y., Liu, Z. Z., Jia, C. X., & Liu, X. (2022). A longitudinal study of insomnia, daytime sleepiness, and academic performance in Chinese adolescents. *Behavioral Sleep Medicine, 20*(6), 798–808.

Zhao, K., Zhang, J., Wu, Z., Shen, X., Tong, S., & Li, S. (2019). The relationship between insomnia symptoms and school performance among 4966 adolescents in Shanghai, China. *Sleep Health, 5*(3), 273–279.

19

AUTISM SPECTRUM DISORDERS

Jessica Bolton Petronis and Chuck Emig

Introduction and Overview of CBT to the Problem Area

Multiple disciplines service children and adolescents with autism spectrum disorder (ASD) in our schools through a myriad of interventions; this multidisciplinary approach is essential to address the wide variability and range of needs in the ASD population. Children and adolescents diagnosed with ASD are now more commonly treated by speech and language therapists, teachers, occupational therapists, school psychologists, and others using cognitive-behavioral therapy (CBT) programs and techniques. As our understanding of symptoms that comprise the autism spectrum has broadened, many who work with students with ASD find that traditional behaviorist approaches are not comprehensive enough to address student needs nor result in the generalization of skills to a variety of settings.

Since the 2nd edition of this book, research has continued to support the positive results of CBT with children and adolescents (Ung et al., 2014; Wang et al., 2021; Will et al., 2018). In addition, commercially available and therapist-made resources have surged in popularity. Nevertheless, more resources are needed that present ASD within a CBT framework and provide therapists with the information they need to help tailor interventions to their clients' needs using both a manualized or modular approach. This chapter aims to provide information on ASD and clinical presentations suited for CBT in school-aged children. Taken together with information provided within this book, we hope that school-based therapists can gain a broader understanding of ASD, the components of CBT practice, and how to approach CBT interventions with students with ASD.

Understanding the Specific Issue/Disorder

The estimated prevalence rates of ASD have steadily increased during the last 20 years, from 1 in 110 children in 2006 to 1 in 36 children at the time of this publication (Maenner et al., 2023). Males are still identified with ASD more frequently than females, though the ratio is not as steep as previously reported. In addition, according to the surveillance report published by the CDC, fewer differences are noted between race and ethnic groups, which may be due to better identification methods in previously underserved areas.

Diagnostic criteria for ASD in the Diagnostic and Statistical Manual of Mental Disorders (DSM) changed with the publication of the 5th edition in 2013 (American Psychiatric Association [APA],

DOI: 10.4324/9781003392439-22

2013). In the 4th edition, autistic disorder, Asperger's Disorder, and pervasive developmental disorder not otherwise specified were separate diagnoses. It was the 1st time that Asperger's disorder was recognized and was considered a positive addition by clinicians in terms of providing attention to those individuals with higher cognitive functioning and less impaired language.

The DSM-5 subsumed all previously named spectrum disorders under ASD and indicates that "individuals with well-established DSM-IV diagnosis of autistic disorder, Asperger's Disorder, or pervasive developmental disorder not otherwise specified should be given the diagnosis of autism spectrum disorder" (APA, 2013, p. 51). The diagnostic criteria are based on two core deficits: (A) persistent deficits in social communication (outlined as deficits in social-emotional reciprocity; deficits in nonverbal communicative behaviors; and deficits in developing, maintaining, and understanding relationships); and (B) restricted, repetitive patterns of behavior, interests, or activities (outlined as two or more of the following: stereotyped or repetitive motor movements, use of objects, or speech; insistence on sameness, inflexible adherence to routines, or ritualized patterns of verbal or nonverbal behavior; highly restricted, fixated interests that are abnormal in intensity or focus; hyper- or hypo reactivity to sensory input or unusual interest in sensory aspects of the environment). Specifiers for severity are included and indicate the level of support needed based on the two main symptoms, along with specifiers that indicate coexisting conditions. Symptoms must be present during the developmental period and cause impairment in functioning.

Clinicians and school personnel treating students on the autism spectrum need to understand that the diagnostic criteria include a wide range of functioning levels and may manifest with various degrees of severity. It is imperative that a solid understanding of a student's presenting strengths and needs, rather than just the diagnosis itself, be used to identify targets for treatment.

In addition to symptoms of ASD, many children and adolescents with ASD have co-occurring disorders that are the target for treatment, especially internalizing disorders. Prevalence estimates for children and adolescents with ASD and co-occurring anxiety is hard to pinpoint, with studies indicating rates ranging from 22% to 84% (Vasa & Mazurek, 2015). Increased anxiety may be a result of communication deficits, sensory sensitivities, emotional dysregulation, and social isolation. The experience of anxiety by children with Autism can further impede deficient social skills and may heighten symptoms related to perseverative or stereotyped behaviors. Much of the research conducted on the delivery of CBT with students with ASD has studied the treatment of co-occurring anxiety symptoms and disorders.

Attention-deficit/hyperactivity disorder (ADHD) is another commonly co-occurring disorder that may be a target for intervention in the school setting. In a clinical setting, CBT may be used to help treat co-occurring sleep or feeding disorders that are prevalent in children and adolescents with ASD.

To truly understand the need for more flexible and comprehensive treatments of some of the behaviors manifested by individuals with ASD, it is 1st important to look at the underlying contributor to these deficits. Current and established research has examined the role of executive functioning with ASD, as well as the idea of theory of mind (ToM) (Baron-Cohen et al., 1985) and central coherence theory (Frith, 1989). Along with these theories, research has examined some neurobiological and genetic factors that help us better understand ASD.

Executive Functions

The executive-function theory of ASD developed after difficulties with shifting, inhibition, and working memory were observed in ASD populations and theorized to be related to cognitive rigidity, perseverance in routine, and stereotyped repetitive behaviors (Landa & Goldberg, 2005; Lopez et al. 2005; McEvoy et al., 1993; Ozonoff & Jensen, 1999; Pennington & Ozonoff, 1996). Further research notes effects of executive dysfunction on mental health, adaptive behavior, and social cognition in individuals with ASD (Demetriou et al., 2018; Pugliese et al., 2016). The executive function theory of ASD suggests that, when compared to children who display normative development, the child with ASD displays deficits in executive skills that are detrimental to everyday functioning, including social skills.

Executive dysfunction has been identified in individuals across the entire autism spectrum (Landa & Goldberg, 2005; Verte et al., 2006). Specifically, several studies have established that the executive-function capacities of planning, cognitive flexibility, and emotional regulation are areas of weakness in children with Autism and may contribute to restricted, stereotyped behaviors, as well as communication difficulties and emotional dysregulation (Laurent & Rubin, 2004; Lopez et al., 2005; Ozonoff & Jensen, 1999; Verte et al., 2006). A 2019 meta-analysis concluded that because the literature supports (1) an association between executive dysfunction and ASD in the population, (2) the heritability of executive functions, and (3) higher rates of executive dysfunction within affected families than the general population, executive function meets the criteria of an endophenotype, or intermediate phenotype, of Autism (Demetriou et al., 2019). That is, executive function presents vulnerabilities in the ASD population through a link among genetics, cognitive processes, and observed behavior. Functionally, executive skills are essential in social-communicative development because individuals must coordinate language, inhibit behavioral impulses, regulate their emotions, and demonstrate cognitive flexibility while engaging in an interaction (Winner, 2008).

Theory of Mind

Based on seminal research conducted by Baron-Cohen and colleagues (1985), ToM describes how we differentiate our own thoughts and feelings from those of others, infer others' thoughts and feelings, and predict others' behaviors based on observation. In children with ASD, this is found to be a deficit. This research helped to delineate important differences between children with ASD and those with cognitive deficits, given that ToM is not an area of weakness found in individuals with intellectual deficits. This helped to establish the connection between ToM weaknesses and social-skill deficits, thus providing some specific targets for intervention to improve social functioning. One 2018 study of children and adolescents with ASD found an association between ToM weaknesses and both social communication symptoms and restricted repetitive behaviors (Jones et al., 2018); another 2018 study's findings supported a link among ToM, executive dysfunction, and ASD in children (Kouklari et al., 2018).

Central Coherence Theory

Related to the ToM and executive-functioning deficits, it has been theorized that weak central coherence plays a role in the social-skill challenges found in individuals with ASD. Central coherence explains that most people prefer to process information as a whole concept without attending to every detail. For children with ASD, processing of information happens on the level of detail. This weak central coherence prevents some children from being able to generalize ideas or activities as a whole. It has also been argued that this method of processing can be a strength during tasks requiring attention to detail and visual skills, such as when building and following visual directions (Happé & Booth, 2008; Pellicano et al., 2010). It creates social challenges for children with ASD due to the need for an understanding of socialization at the global level in order to adapt their behavior to a variety of settings and activities. Cognitive inflexibility relates to that same inability to adapt to a general understanding, as opposed to relying on narrow details. In a longitudinal study, Pellicano (2010) found that weak central coherence led to problems with ToM but did not relate to later executive-functioning deficits. This study also related weak central coherence to pragmatic language deficits, specifically when understanding figurative language.

Etiology and Neurobiology

Though these theories help explain the manifestation of symptoms and behaviors and better conceptualize Autism, they do not identify the cause of the disorder. With no one specific biological or genetic cause identified, ASD is thought to be a neurobiological disability that affects brain development during the neonatal period (McGrath & Peterson, 2020). The impact of environmental variables on brain development has also been examined, with no conclusive findings to date. A longitudinal study of 2 million people in Scandinavia, Western Australia, and Israel estimated that the direct heritability of ASD accounted for 80% of cases. It showed no evidence of maternal effects as a cause of ASD. Some environmental effects were observed, but they were generally negligible and varied by country (Bai et al., 2019). Though the exact cause is unknown to date, it does seem certain that the prevalence of this once "rare" disorder is on the rise, making ASD the most common serious developmental disorder.

Empirical Support of CBT in Treatment of the Specific Disorder

At the time of the writing of the previous edition of this book, Applied Behavior Analysis was indicated as the only efficacious treatment of ASD. The Association for Behavioral and Cognitive Therapies recognizes that, along with ABA, social skills instruction and CBT show effectiveness in teaching social skills and addressing mental health problems (Association for Behavioral and Cognitive Therapies [ABCT], 2023). Findings in the literature suggest that CBT is effective at treating co-occurring internalizing disorders in children with Autism, namely anxiety disorders, as well as improving the symptoms of ASD (Ung et al., 2015; Wang et al., 2021).

Some research suggests that children and adolescents with ASD can benefit from CBT to the same degree as their neurotypical peers despite disorder-specific deficits (Reaven et al., 2012; Schneider et al., 2011; Wood et al., 2009). Most research recognizes that some modifications to programs may need to be made to help tailor programs to the specific needs of this population (Bemmer et al., 2021; Walters et al., 2016). Research has also shown that children and adolescents with ASD are able to benefit from CBT to the same degree as their peers and, in many cases, have the prerequisite skills needed to engage in therapy (Lickel et al., 2012). Students with average cognitive ability (as measured by nonverbal IQ) were found to exhibit a capability to identify thoughts and feelings commensurate with their nondisabled peers. Students with ASD were found to have a greater weakness in feeling recognition, which should be assessed when conceptualizing the case (Lickel et al., 2012).

Relational Consideration in Treatment of Problem Area (Connecting)

By definition, students on the autism spectrum have difficulties formulating relationships. Deficits in social-emotional reciprocity and social communication skills make it difficult for the child with ASD to connect with others meaningfully. They may have one-sided peer relationships, engage in parallel play, or dominate interactions. Often, adults who interact with children on the autism spectrum need to significantly modify the situation, context, or approach to sustain an interaction. Because of these factors, formulating a therapeutic alliance with children or adolescents with ASD may be challenging in some cases.

Therapeutic alliance, or the working relationship/alliance between the therapist and child, has been found to be essential to achieving treatment goals (Bose et al., 2022; McLeod, 2011). Bordin identified the three key components of the therapeutic alliance as: agreement on goals; assignment of tasks; and development of bonds (1979). Without this relationship, a child's motivation for engaging in sessions and completing homework, as well as overall positive treatment outcomes, may be diminished.

Some barriers specific to children with ASD that may hinder the therapeutic alliance may include both child and therapist characteristics. Therapists may find it difficult to connect with children who are strongly engaged in sensory-seeking behavior during therapy or exhibit ongoing perseverative behaviors. It may be more difficult to connect with a child who exhibits weak reciprocal conversational abilities or who has difficulties picking up on nuances in language. In one study, it was found that therapeutic alliance was easier to establish with children with ASD when they were able to inhibit or regulate their emotional responses, making emotional dysregulation a factor impeding alliance (Albaum et al., 2020).

On the contrary, children on the autism spectrum may disconnect from a therapist who is rigid in their approach. They may not connect well with a therapist who relies heavily on figurative language or the use of idioms or metaphors. Research has shown that neither children nor adolescents respond well to "pushy" therapists or those they don't perceive to be genuine. The use of collaborative and informal behaviors has been found to work best with children. With adolescents, it is important that the therapist presents as an ally and works to develop trust. Some research has suggested that ethnic matching can improve therapeutic alliance with children and adolescents, though it is uncertain if this is a factor for children with ASD (Ryan et al., 2023).

To further help facilitate a positive working relationship, it is important for the therapist to have engaged in case conceptualization to understand familial, environmental, and personal factors that are relevant to the child. Understanding a child's interests (particularly any special, perseverative interests), sensory aversions or sensory interests, language abilities, and co-morbidities are crucial. More time may be needed than typical to get to know the child and build rapport. Students on the autism spectrum will likely do best with someone who can be more flexible, more patient, and who can move at a slower pace than a typical CBT session.

During sessions, therapists may converse with children while playing a game or coloring in a workbook, providing physical distance. Allowing the child to engage in an activity while talking takes pressure off the expectations for appropriate nonverbal engagement and may lower social anxiety. Additionally, providing appropriate sensory tools for use during therapy may help reduce anxiety and alleviate sensory needs. Therapists are encouraged to use a child's special interest in the therapeutic session when referencing examples or using visuals. Using visual tools and clear language can be most effective in conveying the agenda, teaching a new concept, or explaining homework (Bemmer et al., 2021). When there is a breakdown of the therapeutic alliance, it is important for the therapist to recognize it and attempt to repair it. This provides essential modeling to the student of how to problem-solve relational issues and can essentially strengthen the therapist/client bond.

A study conducted by Kalvin et al. (2021) found that telehealth for treatment of anxiety in children with ASD was advantageous for therapeutic alliance. Researchers noted that the children were able to connect with therapists by sharing aspects of their home life more easily. Children may have been more comfortable in their own physical environment, which facilitated a positive therapeutic relationship. Unless a student is educated in a virtual school setting, most school-based therapy will be conducted in person, typically in the school environment. However, a therapist can help incorporate elements from the student's home to help create comfortability in the setting, such as allowing them to bring in items or share pictures with the therapist.

Though some obvious barriers may exist that could impede the therapeutic alliance, some research has found that youth clients with ASD and co-occurring anxiety were able to formulate a relationship with their therapist to the same degree as children without ASD (Kerns et al., 2018; Klebanoff et al., 2019).

While research currently is somewhat limited, therapeutic alliance seems to be an important factor for successful therapy for youth with ASD.

Interviewing and Assessing Problem Area (Assessing)

Assessing for diagnostic purposes versus treatment planning may entail a different battery of techniques and tools. Diagnostically, clinicians may examine an individual's cognitive and academic functioning, as well as language, behaviors, and motor skills, through a variety of tools and methods. Diagnostic evaluations of ASD are typically multidisciplinary and may include a psychologist/ school psychologist, occupational therapist, speech/language clinician, developmental pediatrician, and others. For treatment, clinicians should consider any diagnostic information available, especially to help determine the extent of the child's cognitive and language functioning. This can help to tailor interventions and may further clarify targets for intervention.

For treatment purposes, the use of interviews, behavioral rating scales, and direct observations can be helpful in determining treatment goals. Interviews may be with parents, teachers, and the child to gain differing perspectives on how the child functions across environments. During the diagnostic process, the use of semi-structured interview tools, such as the Autism Diagnostic Interview–Revised (ADI-R) (Le Couteur et al., 2003), can provide developmental and functional information in the areas of communication and language skills, social interactions, and the presence of repetitive and obsessive behaviors. While interviews are helpful in developing treatment plans and conceptualizing the problem, rating scales and direct behavior observations may provide more objective data to help pinpoint specific needs and can later be used for progress monitoring purposes.

Rating Scales

Because children with ASD present with myriad difficulties that are targeted for intervention, there is not one tool that links well to intervention in terms of informing the practitioner about individual therapy needs. Most rating scales that target behaviors characteristic of ASD are diagnostic and are not specifically designed to be used in treatment planning and monitoring; therefore, practitioners must find other tools and methods to identify the area of need that may be targeted by CBT and match tools for specific areas, instead of measuring overarching symptomology. Current diagnostic rating scales may indicate to the assessment professional the degree of impairment in social skills but may not delineate what those deficits and strengths look like in a given social situation across settings. Furthermore, they may not be sensitive to changes over time. Therefore, it is important to recognize the limitations of diagnostic and broad-band rating scale measures. Social-skill, adaptive-skill, executive-functioning, or anxiety-specific scales may be more helpful in measuring need across domains that may be targeted. Some examples of social-skill rating scales include the Social Responsiveness Scale—2nd Edition (SRS-2) (Constantino & Gruber, 2012) and the Social Skill Improvement System (SSIS) (Gresham & Elliott, 2008). The SSIS provides rating-scale data as well as intervention planning guides and lessons. There are several anxiety-specific rating scales also available, both commercially and through free-share programs, that can be used in identifying anxiety symptomology. To date, The Anxiety Scale for Children-ASD (ASC-ASD©) (Rodgers et al., 2016) is the only freely available anxiety rating scale developed specifically for assessing anxiety in children with Autism.

Direct Behavior Observations

Though rating scales may elicit some important information, generally speaking, it is our opinion that rating scales are not as effective in treatment planning and progress monitoring as are direct behavior observations. Direct behavior observations, which focus on well-defined behaviors and observe the presence or absence of those behaviors, are supported within the literature as one of the most useful assessments of social skills. They allow the practitioner to observe well-defined and discrete instances of behaviors across settings to help determine the exact need of intervention, as well as environmental variables and normative peer responses (Boyd et al., 2011; Sansosti et al., 2010). One clear advantage of a school setting over a clinical setting for service delivery is the feasibility of conducting direct behavior observations.

Some standard observation forms are available to collect data. The Observation of Appropriate Social Interaction Skills (OASIS) worksheet developed by Sansosti (2003) can be utilized in an observation format. This worksheet provides 15 behaviors that can be directly observed within a set time frame to determine a percentage of appropriate skills.

The Contextual Assessment of Social Skills (CASS; Ratto et al., 2011) has been established to assess social conversational skills in children with Autism and distinguishes between social behavior and social cognition. Preliminary research identifies this as an outcome measure of social competence for adolescents participating in treatment (Simmons et al., 2021).

To help evaluate preschool social behaviors, the Autism Peer Interaction Observation Scale can be utilized. This tool was developed to differentiate between preschoolers with Autism from their peers and to provide information about preschoolers' social interactions in a natural setting. Bauminger-Zviely and Shefer (2021) reported that this tool can be used in both intervention planning and as an outcome measure.

The Playground Observation Checklist by Ingram et al. (2007) was initially developed as an assessment tool. The checklist has ten operationally defined social behaviors that can be observed during a typical 15-minute recess. Because of the concrete definitions provided that span different social behaviors, this tool could be used for both intervention planning and progress monitoring purposes, as it is deemed reliable in identifying social behaviors specific to autism-related deficits.

Additionally, we have found value in taking frequency data from well-defined behaviors specific to the intervention protocol used, as done by Crooke, Hendrix, and Rachman (2008) in their work with Think Social! (Winner, 2005). This type of observation data directly measures treatment success, and can help differentiate between successful and responsive targets of the intervention from less responsive behaviors. In turn, the data can be immediately used to modify treatment plans as needed. However, a valuable tool, careful planning and consideration must be taken into account to ensure the reliability of the instrument developed.

When collecting direct behavior observations, it is best to observe in a variety of social settings (unless the structured form demands a specific setting). In schools, this may be during lunch, recess, in-school clubs, less academically-minded courses that rely on interaction between students (cooking course, drama, etc.), or after-school activities. When looking at a variety of settings as opposed to one, observers will see the different social demands placed on students, including some settings where social behaviors can be avoided (and thus not observed) and others where social behaviors must be emitted. It is recommended that, when observing across settings, consistency is maintained in order to collect meaningful change data during treatment. Regardless of the tool used, it is advantageous for observers to conduct inter-rater reliability checks prior to data collection to determine if the definitions are well-defined enough for use by multiple raters.

Case Conceptualization (Understanding)

As addressed in this book, CBT has been established as an efficacious method for addressing many problems and difficulties for school-aged children. Deficits in ASD that CBT can address include social/cognitive deficits, perspective-taking, emotional identification and regulation, inflexible/rigid thinking patterns, and verbal/language deficits (Donoghue et al., 2011; Lopata et al., 2006). Additionally, most existing research has focused on reducing comorbid anxiety using CBT with children and adolescents with ASD.

Where ABA techniques have focused strictly on behavioral components of skill acquisition, CBT is thought to be useful in helping children and adolescents with ASD not only to acquire social skills but also to challenge their thinking and increase their emotional awareness and regulation. Because children higher on the spectrum are often more aware of their social difficulties, they may require direct instruction both in how to exhibit the behavior and to increase their understanding of why it is important. CBT interventions can provide this psychoeducation component and focus on improving the ability to organize and monitor thinking, understand cause-and-effect relationships, problem solve, exercise inhibition, and increase social cognitive abilities, such as the understanding of emotional and social situations through affective education (Anderson & Morris, 2006; Bauminger, 2002).

Treatment Planning and Intervention Strategies

When developing intervention plans for students with ASD, careful consideration must be utilized in conceptualizing individual needs. A one-size-fits-all intervention approach is not effective with this population, given the diverse manifestation of symptoms and behaviors. In CBT, case conceptualization is used to help determine individual needs to align them with the specific approach.

Case conceptualization refers not to the evaluation or diagnostic process but rather to the flexible process of data collection and hypothesis testing that guides treatment planning (Friedberg & McClure, 2015). Case conceptualization may involve evaluative procedures, such as interviews and rating scales, but may also occur throughout sessions as more hypotheses are generated and tested and new information becomes available. During case conceptualization, a student's age, cognitive and language abilities, special interests, and developmental level should be considered. Murphy and Christner (2012) suggest formulating a problem list, then gathering assessment data and developing a working hypothesis. Antecedents, activating events, impediments to change, as well as protective factors, should also be taken into account. For example, one impediment to change for a student with ASD may be a lack of affective vocabulary, which can then be addressed as a treatment goal once identified as a need.

When conceptualizing a student with ASD, further delineation and understanding of the contributing factors for "why" a student is having difficulties should be explored. Clinicians should explore and examine if the student's difficulties are due to cognitive deficiency, cognitive distortion, skill deficiency, skill dysfunction, or a combination of these. Cognitive deficiency refers to a student lacking information-processing skills, such as the executive processes described earlier. Cognitive distortion is the active, though misguided, thinking that is traditionally addressed with CBT. In Chapter 1 of this book, Mennuti and Christner discuss the role of cognitive distortions in feelings and behaviors. Skill deficiency is different from a cognitive deficiency in that a skill deficiency involves a lack of specific skills that may not have been taught to the student, though it is not necessarily due to an information-processing difficulty. For instance, this may include skills such as introduction skills, making eye contact, friendship skills, etc. Finally, there is skill dysfunction, which indicates that a student has learned the skills, yet lacks generalization to or implementation of the skills in the "real world." We have seen this many times in students with ASD, as they know the skill and can repeat it and discuss it in detail. However, despite their knowledge, they do not put the skill into action. Each of these factors requires a different type of intervention. For example, for a skill deficiency, a clinician would work to teach or increase a child's skills in certain areas, whereas, with skill dysfunction, the clinician would work to provide in vivo practice to increase generalization.

During case conceptualization, the clinician needs to consider that many differences exist in verbal and nonverbal communication norms across cultures. These cultural differences may initially manifest as skill deficits or skill dysfunction to the unfamiliar clinician. We advise clinicians to ask questions of the family or use a cultural liaison to help understand cultural communication norms. Speech and language clinicians who work with diverse populations can also be a great resource. When working with diverse populations, it is important that we, as clinicians and educators, avoid trying to "mold" majority cultural norms as a target for treatment.

Treatment Planning and Goal Setting

Taking into account information gained through case conceptualization, a treatment plan should be developed to address specific, targeted goals. While the goals are the observable and measurable anchors to determine progress, the treatment plan will address how the goals will be met based on individual strengths, needs, and personal characteristics. For example, both Corbin and Amir exhibit difficulties initiating conversations with their peers. They both wait to be spoken to before they will talk with their classmates. The therapist uncovered that Corbin experiences significant social anxiety that impedes his ability to display conversation skills, while Amir exhibits deficits in the discrete skills, and does not know how to start a conversation. Because of these important differences, their treatment plans differ.

Intervention Selection

After treatment plans and goals are developed, the next step is to select interventions that should be utilized to target each need. This is the basis of modular treatment, which refers to the selection of interventions from a variety of resources and tools, and does not follow the inflexible demands of a manualized program. While manualized programs are highly valuable and especially useful for treatment research, individuals on the autism spectrum tend to display characteristics that are not accounted for by treatment manuals designed for "typical" peers and may not fit the profile for manuals designed for individuals on the spectrum. For individuals on the autism spectrum, treatment specificity is the key to success.

One challenge that arises in utilizing a modular approach is that it requires the therapist or interventionist to have good case-conceptualization skills. Therapists must be familiar with and able to understand the literature on a variety of techniques and available manualized programs. Modular treatments should not be implemented haphazardly or "on the fly;" the use of modular interventions requires that the therapist is familiar with progress-monitoring techniques and can carefully select techniques and gather appropriate data to make treatment decisions.

Session Structure When Working with Problem Area (Guiding)

Within a CBT framework, session structure is important to the process of developing the therapeutic alliance, delivering interventions, and working toward generalizing. Beginning CBT sessions are often focused on rapport building, case conceptualization, goal setting, and treatment planning. The following sessions will focus on intervention delivery and practice. Sessions should follow a predictable structure that includes the same components, which typically include mood check-in, homework review, agenda setting, session content, homework, and feedback (Friedberg & McClure, 2015). Often, a diagnostic feature of Autism is that children greatly adhere to structures and schedules that are presented and may show distress if there is a change. The structure of CBT lends itself to the predictability that children with ASD desire. Clinicians can provide a visual outline of this schedule each week to help children see the session plan and prepare for transitions.

A CBT session will typically begin with a mood check-in to help the clinician gauge the client's current emotional status. With children and adolescents with ASD, the mood check-in itself can become a vehicle for providing affective education. The clinician should consider the use of visual aids, including feeling faces or feeling intensity thermometers, to help facilitate mood check-in. Tracking the child's ability to identify emotions over time can also provide important treatment progress.

Reviewing homework, or between-session work, is another key component of the CBT structure. This provides the therapist an opportunity to gauge (1) if a child is attempting to use skills in their naturalistic setting and (2) their success with these skills. It also helps the therapist determine if the child is prepared for new session content.

Ideally, the therapist and child would co-develop the session agenda. The therapist should have an idea of session content in order to be prepared with necessary materials but should also exhibit flexibility based on input from the child. Consider Samar, a 3rd-grade student who exhibits strong perseverative behaviors when something goes wrong. During the mood-check in, Samar recounts a playground issue to the therapist and cannot move on. In therapy, he is working on improving flexibility in his thinking but isn't open to intervention when he comes to sessions "worked up." The therapist had planned to introduce an anchoring strategy for addressing the cognitive distortion of magnifying the problem but changed the plan after gauging his mood during check-in. Though she knows he would benefit greatly from this type of cognitive intervention to quantify his problems and reactions, she understands that teaching it when he is heightened will be ill received. Instead, she works with Samar to practice relaxation strategies that were previously taught in attempts to regulate his emotionality. When Samar is able to relax, she is able to work with him on identifying his thoughts related to the situation. They record his thoughts to use for the next session.

Following the mood check-in, homework review, and agenda setting, the content of the session is delivered. This may be introducing a new intervention or engaging in practice of a previously learned strategy, depending on student need. Following the content, homework is "assigned" which should reinforce session content and provide an opportunity for the child to practice the skill in a naturalistic environment. Homework can be completed at either school or home, with the school setting often being an ideal laboratory for children to try out new skills. In a school setting, clinicians can recruit "confederates" to help the child try out new skills safely by manipulating the situation to set them up for success.

Often, children may need additional support or motivators to complete between-session work. Involving parents or guardians can serve as both oversight to ensure completion as well as a way to involve parents in intervention delivery. The same can be said for the classroom teacher. Charting completion and offering small incentives (like time to play a favorite game) can serve to increase motivation if needed. Some manualized treatment programs designed for children, like Coping Cat (Kendall & Hedtke, 2006), have homework tracking and incentives built in.

At the end of each session, it is important for the therapist to elicit feedback from the client on how they perceive the session content and delivery. This is a time when they can check for understanding and gauge if the content was well-received. Additionally, it provides a chance for the student to give therapist-related feedback. For many children, with or without ASD, providing feedback to an adult is a new and uncomfortable practice. Providing a visual may help students feel more comfortable with providing feedback. They may indicate on a Likert-type scale or through a note or drawing how helpful they think the intervention will be, their comfortability with using it or how much they understood the concepts taught. The process of providing feedback can also be an opportune time to model this skill and allow the child to practice, as it can, in turn, improve advocacy skills outside of the session.

Component of Practice and Intervention Modules (Intervening)

There are many social cognition programs currently in use for which an evidence base in the literature is emerging but not yet strong, such as the Social Thinking products (Crooke & Winner, 2022). Many of these programs adhere to CBT principles and utilize techniques to explore thoughts, challenge maladaptive beliefs, teach problem-solving skills, and provide strategies for regulation. This has been a welcome alternative to traditional, compliance-focused therapies. Although these programs have many proponents and a wealth of anecdotal data supporting their effectiveness, further research is sorely needed to validate and refine these approaches concurrent with our evolving understanding of ASD.

The following research-backed curricula are designed specifically for children on the autism spectrum and utilize a cognitive-behavioral approach.

Multimodal Anxiety and Social Skills Intervention

The Multimodal Anxiety and Social Skills Intervention (MASSI; White et al., 2013) is a CBT program designed for children ages 12–17 years old to address both core deficits and associated anxiety in children and adolescents with ASD. It utilizes both an individual and group therapy component to help teach skills and provide a naturalistic setting for practice, as well as parent coaching and homework. MASSI has shown effectiveness at improving social skills, and in some instances, decreasing anxiety (Bemmer et al., 2021; White et al., 2013).

Exploring Feelings

The Exploring Feelings programs offer direct instruction on anxiety and anger management through two books. Initial psychoeducation on emotional awareness is followed with the visual example of a toolbox to allow students to choose from strategies to help cope with these feelings. Research indicates that the Exploring Feelings: Anxiety CBT program decreases anxiety symptoms in children with ASD (McConachie et al., 2014; Wood et al., 2009)

Behavioral Interventions for Anxiety in Children with Autism

Behavioral Interventions for Anxiety in Children with Autism (BIACA; Wood et al., 2009) is an individualized, manualized/modular CBT treatment program for treating children and adolescents with ASD. The program provides flexible modules to meet individual needs to address anxiety, social skills, adaptive deficits, motivational challenges, and more. A parent component is incorporated, as well as a strong emphasis on practice and exposure. This program has been found to reduce anxiety and autism-related symptomology in children with ASD (Wood et al., 2015).

The Program for the Education and Enrichment of Relational Skills

The Program for the Education and Enrichment of Relational Skills (PEERS®) (Laugeson et al., 2014) utilizes CBT principles and has been shown to improve social functioning for adolescents with ASD (Laugeson et al., 2012, 2014). The program utilizes a small group format and provides CBT interventions such as psychoeducation, Socratic questioning, role plays, and behavioral rehearsal. Homework is incorporated as well as parent involvement. There is a specific curriculum available for implementation in school settings.

Many existing CBT techniques can address several of the deficits seen in individuals with ASD. For example, the use of behavioral rehearsal is a CBT technique designed to help clients try out new

Table 19.1 A Sample of CBT Modules for Children and Adolescents with ASD

Affect recognition	Students with ASD often have difficulty identifying their feelings and emotions, as well as those of others. Providing direct instruction and practice with these skills creates an essential foundation for introducing other higher-order concepts, like perspective-taking.
Cognitive restructuring	For individuals on the autism spectrum, cognitive distortions, such as dichotomous thinking ("all or none") or magnifying the problem, contribute to many of the challenging behaviors, including difficulties in reciprocal social interactions and emotional responses. Cognitive restructuring techniques can help individuals learn perspective-taking skills that are important in social interaction. Additionally, cognitive restructuring can help individuals with comorbid anxieties to challenge irrational thoughts and beliefs. It is recommended that a variety of techniques are used to help teach this abstract concept and are paired with visual aids.
Relaxation	Comorbid anxieties or preservative behaviors may respond to relaxation techniques, such as diaphragmatic breathing or imagery. In addition, teaching relaxation can help with somatic management for some students. Relaxation can be taught to individuals concurrently while teaching skills that may be anxiety-provoking.
Psychoeducation	There are a variety of topics that can be explored through psychoeducation with individuals with ASD, including education on their behaviors, feelings, risk factors and symptoms of internalizing difficulties, hygiene, dating, social norms, and more. Careful consideration of language skills should be given.
Behavioral rehearsal	This intervention provides an opportunity for the student to try out a new skill or behavior in a simulated situation. It is useful for students with ASD to become proficient with skills so they can be integrated into their natural repertoire. This can be used to help a student practice a newly acquired social skill in a supportive environment or can help reduce anxiety through practice exposure to a situation.

skills in naturalistic settings and report back on how others respond. For individuals with ASD, this technique is useful not only in trying out a new social skill but also in helping the individual learn how to gauge the perspectives of others as they react to the individual's exhibition of a new behavior. Table 19.1 provides examples of modules.

A clinician may determine that a manualized program does not meet a student's needs due to a specific deficit, barrier, or co-occurring challenge. In this case, the clinician may determine that a modular approach is best. If proceeding with a modular approach, clinicians will need to identify what interventions they plan to select to address specific concerns. Techniques can be utilized from a variety of sources, including manualized treatment programs. For example, a clinician may decide that they do not want to implement a manualized anxiety program but likes the way a particular program teaches cognitive distortions. During treatment planning, they may select that as a specific intervention for that child. As mentioned, therapists will need to prioritize treatment targets and determine if any one skill may be essential for the development of a different skill.

Assessment of Progress and Outcomes (Monitoring)

The process of assessing progress and monitoring treatment outcomes is important in CBT, but particularly important in the school setting when servicing children with Individualized Education Programs (IEPs). Writing observable and measurable goals, and documenting a child's progress toward these goals, is not only beneficial to the child but is required by law and protects the district from potential litigation (Individuals with Disabilities Education Act, 2004). Current case law has shown that school districts must show that services provided through an IEP have an educational benefit to the child over time (Endrew F. v. Douglas County School District RE-1, 2017). It is assumed that providers in the school-setting who provide CBT interventions to children are likely doing so through an IEP. In these situations, providers may have overlapping or differing treatment goals as well as annual IEP goals.

When monitoring progress toward treatment goals, the therapist is essentially utilizing single-case designs to determine effectiveness of the intervention for each child. The use of single-case study data is an effective and easy way for school personnel to analyze data, and is familiar for use in this setting, particularly with academic data. This is especially important in a modular approach to help determine treatment effectiveness and to ensure that the plan is "on the right track." At the onset of goal development, the clinician will need to select the behavior to monitor as well as the monitoring tool.

As mentioned earlier, behavioral rating scales are often utilized to measure social behavior and thus could be utilized to determine progress in a pre-post administration method. While the idea of this sounds good, rating scales are not always sensitive to change, especially for brief interventions, due to the diagnostic nature of most of the tools as well as the metrics used to calculate a score (raw scores are typically more change sensitive than standard or T-scores). However, rating scale data can still be of value. Gresham et al. (2010) describe the idea of "brief behavior change scales," which are more sensitive for progress monitoring. In the study, researchers took a lengthy social skills rating scale and identified a small subset of items that were used to measure change in a technically sound manner. This may help make treatment monitoring more acceptable and feasible by the raters, as well as help to identify subtle changes in behaviors. Soliciting ratings from teachers across settings using this method through electronic means can make it an easily implemented tool.

Direct Behavioral Observations, as described above, can be used in both assessing need and monitoring progress. While this is a highly useful tool, it can be time consuming to conduct at regular enough intervals needed to collect sufficient data points to monitor change. As mentioned, multi-raters can be used with careful training and reliability checks to help reduce the burden on any one person.

Data taken on behaviors elicited during the therapy session can also be utilized for progress monitoring. For example, if a student is working on feeling identification, that can easily be assessed during mood check-in within the session. Other behaviors that could be tracked within the session that may be used to monitor progress toward a goal include homework compliance, initiation of conversation, ability to sustain a back-and-forth exchange, and ability to ask questions of others. Often, a group format with other children can provide more opportunities to monitor these types of behaviors than in individual therapy.

Using data from the session, a therapist could utilize Goal Attainment Scaling, which is method that can be used to track outcome data. Goal Attainment Scaling was developed as a tool to measure progress in clinical settings due to a lack of available instruments and has since been used in school settings for both social/emotional and behaviors interventions (Coffee & Ray-Subramanian, 2009; Kiresuk & Sherman, 1968). Looking at progress in terms of percentage of change using frequency counts helps the interventionist or clinician to determine if changes made are meaningful. In addition to behaviors during the session Goal Attainment Scaling can be used to track observational, teacher, parent, or self-report, or rating scale data, as long as baseline behaviors are well defined, along with degrees of improvement or regression. For more information on Goal Attainment Scaling, we refer you to Goal Attainment Scaling: Applications, Theory and Measurement (Kiresuk et al., 2014).

Applications to the School Setting

Providers from multiple disciplines use cognitive behavioral interventions with children and adolescents with ASD in our schools. Some interventions follow manualized treatment programs, while others are implemented as an adjunct to other treatment protocols or within a modular framework. Currently, several programs exhibit effectiveness for children with ASD, including one program that follows a flexible, modular approach. Regardless of how the intervention is delivered, it is important for school-based providers to have a strong foundational knowledge of CBT. This is necessary to implement treatment with fidelity, as another potential pitfall is haphazard implementation of internet resources that are not validated.

CBT in a school setting has many advantages over a clinical setting, where clinicians have access to children in a natural environment. Direct observations and teacher input are easier to elicit. In addition, there is more opportunity for children to practice new skills in a supportive environment. Another advantage is the ease of availability to provide group-based interventions, allowing children opportunities to practice skills with other children.

For school-based providers who are new to CBT, we recommend starting small. Given the broad variety of presentations and needs of students with ASD, it may be tempting to try to "fix" everything and become overwhelmed. In order to build therapist skills and confidence, we recommend picking a target where you can make a more immediate impact.

To help make this approach applicable to the school setting, we suggest that teaming be implemented. The child with Autism will likely be working with many providers. Prioritizing problem behaviors and targets of intervention is more effective within the multidisciplinary team; otherwise, providers may be working toward similar goals using a variety of approaches, making it more difficult to track intervention progress or to identify the effective strategy. Teaming is also essential to ensure the generalizing of skills learned in the therapeutic process.

Case Study of Problem Area

Case Example: Silas

Silas is a 15-year-old boy identified with ASD. He has average intellectual functioning, but struggles significantly to engage academically and interacts with peers and teachers very little. Silas was identified in 6th grade; no concerns were raised by school staff prior to that point because Silas was always among the highest-achieving students in his grade. He interacted regularly with his grade school peers and appeared to have a few friends, though friendships were superficial. In 5th grade, concerns were raised by his math and science teachers, as he was testing below benchmark and was often not engaged in instruction (he would wear earbuds and listen to music and infrequently completed homework assignments). In addition, teachers observed that Silas would cry at times during independent seatwork or at recess; needed to visit the nurse two to three times per week for feeling sick to his stomach, despite no identified illness; and withdrew from peers at all times, but most notably during recess and lunch. It was thought that his withdrawal and disengagement from school were primarily affecting him in math and science because he had never participated in instruction enough to learn the prerequisite skills for those courses. Once he began receiving special education services through his IEP, his grades improved. Now in his 10th-grade year, Silas again displays significant social withdrawal, with specific weaknesses in reciprocal conversation and social overtures. He has started visiting the nurse frequently again for feelings of illness despite not being sick.

Silas has an intense interest in history, particularly World War II and the Battle of Britain. He states that he has tried engaging with peers about this topic, but they are not interested and have made fun of him for this interest. His 17-year-old brother also has Autism, as well as an intellectual disability, and Silas shared that he feels different from other people because he "grew up faster with taking care of my brother." Silas feels that he has no friends at school, only "acquaintances," and he even has minimal interaction with them. His social withdrawal corresponds with a renewed academic disengagement that is affecting his overall academics, but particularly Algebra, which he is currently failing despite continued special education.

Table 19.2 Treatment Goals for Silas

Goal 1: Silas will increase the number of appropriate, on-topic overtures he makes with peers during social conversations by 25%.	
Goal 2: Silas will reduce the instances in which he visits the nurse during the school day by 25%. Progress will be monitored by nurse visit data.	
Modality	With collaboration between his special education teacher and school psychologist, Silas was included in a CBT group that included six high-school students with ASD.
Frequency	The group met one time per week for 12 weeks. Sessions were 50 minutes.
Level of family involvement	Families were provided with one evening session to instruct on expectations for reviewing session homework and to help provide a common language to be used at home.
Supplemental interventions	Silas continued to receive special education during the course of this intervention; his special education teacher and the school psychologist collaborated on ways to help him generalize skills from the sessions.
Barriers to treatment	Silas's social anxiety had been causing him to withdraw; the relief and comfort he felt from withdrawal had become a powerful reinforcer, making engagement with the process difficult. A holistic approach involving all team members, particularly his case manager and his family, was essential. In addition, gradually exposing him to social situations helped ensure engagement in the therapeutic process

Table 19.2 provides goals, and a treatment plan conceptualized based on direct behavior observation data collected by his IEP team during 20-minute social situations, along with frequency data from nurse visits.

Table 19.3 offers a sample of sessions that could be done in a group with a child like Silas. Silas's presentation indicates a need for somatic management/relaxation strategies, cognitive restructuring,

Table 19.3 A Ten-Session Outline to Utilize with Silas in a Group Format

Session 1	Building Rapport/Getting to Know You
Objective	To create a therapeutic alliance and set therapy goals with group members
Activities	Utilize formats that allow for distancing while getting to know the students, such as a board game or computer game. Set goals with the use of visual aids or special interest icons
Session 2	Psychoeducation/CBT Triad
Objective	To teach students how their feelings affect thoughts and behaviors
Activities	Provide examples of scenarios in which students are participating in a group activity, specifically highlighting their thoughts and feelings during the scenario and related to an area of special interest (i.e., visiting a history museum). Provide a visual aid as students verbalize thoughts and feelings to demonstrate the relationship.
Session 3	Somatic Management—Part 1
Objective	To help students recognize somatic symptoms through body awareness and pinpointing triggers;
Activities	Provide psychoeducation on the physical experience of anxiety and our flight or fight responses. Using a body visual, have students identify where they feel symptoms of anxiety using icons to represent the feeling (i.e., butterflies, tight rope, hammer)

(*Continued*)

Table 19.3 (Continued)

Session 4	Somatic Management—Part 2
Objective	To help students utilize relaxation strategies to reduce physical symptoms of anxiety
Activities	Introduce a variety of diaphragmatic breathing techniques, such as Elevator breathing, as well as imagery and progressive muscle relaxation. Have students rate which technique is most effective for them
Session 5	Identifying Thoughts/Cognitive Restructuring
Objective	To help students identify and challenge automatic thoughts that may be maladaptive
Activities	Re-introduce the concept of automatic thoughts by utilizing thought bubbles to overlay pictures of different scenarios. Can also use *Comic Strip Conversations* (Gray, 1994) for this activity. Using a different color thought bubble, teach students how to counter their automatic thoughts with a more productive, adaptive thought
Session 6	Examining Behaviors and the Emotions of Others
Objective	To teach students what "turns off" others and how their behaviors affect their social relationships
Activities	Students will come in with an example of a social problem, which will be analyzed using a social-autopsy framework. Problem-solving skills will be taught, and alternative solutions can be role-played.
Session 7	Direct Instruction of Social Skill
Objective	To teach reciprocal conversation skills and reduce monopolization of conversation
Activities	Using a graphic organizer, Silas will create friendship webs to help identify the interests of others to use for possible conversation topics. Practice conversations through role-plays with corrective feedback from the therapist
Session 8	Direct Instruction of Social Skills
Objective	To learn awareness of conversational partners' verbal and nonverbal cues; To teach self-monitoring
Activities	When asked to engage in topics of their choosing, Silas will be provided with nonverbal picture cues of faces, and he will have to determine the degree of interest by examining the faces as the therapist presents them. After several practices with pictures, Silas will be asked to self-monitor their own conversation errors when engaged in real conversations with peers
Session 9	Generalization
Objective	To help students make connections between content learned
Activities	After engaging in behavioral rehearsal in a naturalistic setting, students will self-report on their success and failures of conversational attempts (or scenarios can be provided). Together, the group will troubleshoot their challenges and problem-solve solutions using brainstorming. Students will report on their thoughts and feelings related to their attempts in order to help make connections between successful conversations and positive feelings versus unsuccessful conversations and negative emotions and thoughts
Session 10	Feedback/Termination
Objective	To help students evaluate their progress; To gain feedback about the process and utility of therapy
Activities	Students will examine progress toward their therapy goals and discuss how they can further their own progress after termination. Students will also provide feedback about the group and its usefulness through verbal or nonverbal self-report

and social skills instruction. More than ten sessions would likely be needed to cover the content at a deeper level and ensure enough practice opportunities.

Summary

CBT has emerged in the literature as an efficacious treatment option for children and adolescents with ASD. CBT can be used to address a wide range of symptoms and problem behaviors related to ASD, as well as symptoms related to co-occurring conditions. Many school-based clinicians are familiar with some CBT programs or techniques, though they may not have a comprehensive foundational understanding of how to deliver interventions with fidelity. This chapter aimed to connect components of CBT practice to children and adolescents with ASD.

Reflection Questions

1 How has the change in diagnostic criteria for ASD contributed to the need for solid case conceptualization when treatment planning?
2 What interventions would be most helpful for a child who has deficits in social communication skills and is experiencing social anxiety?
3 What advantages does a school setting have over a clinical setting when working with children with ASD using CBT?

References

Albaum, C., Tablon, P., Roudbarani, F., & Weiss, J. A. (2020). Predictors and outcomes associated with therapeutic alliance in cognitive behaviour therapy for children with Autism. *Autism, 24*(1), 211–220.

American Psychiatric Association (APA) (2013). *Diagnostic and statistical manual of mental disorders: DSM-5.* Washington, DC: American Psychiatric Association.

Anderson, S., & Morris, J. (2006). Cognitive behaviour therapy for people with Asperger syndrome. *Behavioural and Cognitive Psychotherapy, 34*, 293–303.

Association for Behavioral and Cognitive Therapies (ABCT) (2023, June 6). Autism spectrum disorder fact sheet. *ABCT: Association for Behavioral and Cognitive Therapies*. Retrieved from https://www.abct.org/fact-sheets/autism-spectrum-disorder/

Bai, D., Yip, B. H. K., Windham, G. C., Sourander, A., Francis, R., Yoffe, R., Glasson, E., Mahjani, B., Suominen, A., Leonard, H., Gissler, M., Buxbaum, J. D., Wong, K., Schendel, D., Kodesh, A., Breshnahan, M., Levine, S. Z., Partner, E. T., Hansen, S. N., Hultman, C., Reichenberg, A., & Sandin, S. (2019). Association of genetic and environmental factors with Autism in a 5-country cohort. *JAMA Psychiatry, 76*(10), 1035–1043.

Baron-Cohen, S. Leslie, A. M., & Frith, U. (1985). Does the autistic child have a "theory of mind?" *Cognition, 21*, 37–46.

Bauminger, N. (2002). The facilitation of social-emotional understanding and social interaction in high-functioning children and autism: Intervention outcomes. *Journal of Autism and Developmental Disorders, 32*(4), 283–298.

Bauminger-Zviely, N., & Shefer, A. (2021). Naturalistic evaluation of preschoolers' spontaneous interactions: The autism peer interaction observation scale. *Autism, 25*(6), 1520–1535.

Bemmer, E. R., Boulton, K. A., Thomas, E. E. et al. (2021). Modified CBT for social anxiety and social functioning in young adults with autism spectrum disorder. *Molecular Autism, 12*, 11. https://doi.org/10.1186/s13229-021-00418-w

Bordin, E. S. (1979). The generalizablity of the psychoanalytic concept of the working alliance. *Psychotherapy: Theory, Research and Practice, 16*, 252–260.

Bose, D., Proenza, D. A., Costales, G., Viswesvaran, C., Bickman, L., & Pettit, J. W. (2022). Therapeutic alliance in psychosocial interventions for youth internalizing disorders: A systematic review and preliminary meta-analysis. *Clinical Psychology: Science and Practice, 29*(2), 124–136. https://doi.org/10.1037/cps0000052

Boyd, B. A., Conroy, M. A., Asmus, J., & McKenney, E. (2011). Direct observation of peer-related social interaction: Outcomes for young children with autism spectrum disorders. *Exceptionality, 19*(2), 94–108.

Coffee, G., & Ray-Subramanian, C. E. (2009). Goal attainment scaling: A progress-monitoring tool for behavioral interventions. *School Psychology Forum, 3*(1), 1–12.

Constantino, J. N., & Gruber, C. P. (2012). *Social responsiveness scale: SRS-2* (p. 106). Torrance, CA: Western psychological services.

Crooke, P., & Winner, M. G. (2022). Research to frameworks to practice: The social thinking methodology-layers of evidence. Retrieved from June 14, 2023. https://www.socialthinking.com/Articles?name=social-thinking-where-is-the-evidence

Crooke, P. J., Hendrix, R. E., & Rachman, J. Y. (2008). Brief report: Measuring the effectiveness of teaching social thinking to children with Asperger syndrome (AS) and high functioning Autism (HFA). *Journal of Autism and Developmental Disorders, 38*(3), 581–591.

Demetriou, E. A., DeMayo, M. M., & Guastella, A. J. (2019). Executive function in autism spectrum disorder: History, theoretical models, empirical findings, and potential as an endophenotype. *Frontiers in Psychiatry, 10*, 753. https://doi.org/10.3389/fpsyt.2019.00753

Demetriou, E. A., Song, C. Y., Park, S. H., Pepper, K. L., Naismith, S. L., Hermens, D. F., et al. (2018). Autism, early psychosis, and social anxiety disorder: A transdiagnostic examination of executive function cognitive circuitry and contribution to disability. *Translational Psychiatry, 8*(1), 200. https://doi.org/10.1038/s41398-018-0193-8

Donoghue, K., Stallard, P., & Kucia, J. (2011). The clinical practice of cognitive behavioural therapy for children and young people with a diagnosis of Asperger's syndrome. *Clinical Child Psychology, 16*(1), 89–102.

Endrew F. v. Douglas County School District RE-1, 137 S. Ct. 988 (2017).

Friedberg, R. D., & McClure, J. M. (2015). *Clinical practice of cognitive therapy with children and adolescents: The nuts and bolts* (2nd ed.). Guilford Press.

Frith, U. (1989). Autism: Explaining the enigma. *British Journal of Developmental Psychology, 3*, 465–468.

Gray, C. (1994). *Comic strip conversations: Colorful, illustrated interactions with students with autism and related disorders*. Arlington, TX: Future Horizons.

Gresham, F., & Elliott, S. N. (2008). Social skills improvement system (SSIS) rating scales. *SSIS Rating Scales*.

Gresham, F. M., Cook, C. R., Collins, T., Dart, E., Rasetshwane, K., Truelson, E., & Grant, S. (2010). Developing a change-sensitive brief behavior rating scale as a progress monitoring tool for social behavior: An example using the social skills rating system - Teacher form. *School Psychology Review, 39*(3), 364–379.

Happé, F. G. E., & Booth, R. D. L. (2008). The power of the positive: Revisiting weak coherence in ASD. *The Quarterly Journal of Experimental Psychology, 61*(1), 50–63.

Individuals With Disabilities Education Act, 20 U.S.C. § 1400 (2004).

Ingram, D. H., Mayes, S. D., Troxell, L. B., & Calhoun, S. L. (2007). Assessing children with autism, mental retardation, and typical development using the playground observation checklist. *Autism, 11*(4), 311–319. https://doi.org/10.1177/1362361307078129

Jones, C. R. G., Simonoff, E., Baird, G., Pickles, A., Marsden, A. J. S., Tregay, J., et al. (2018). The association between theory of mind, executive function, and the symptoms of autism spectrum disorder. *Autism Research, 11*(1), 95–109. https://doi.org/10.1002/aur.1873

Kalvin, C. B., Jordan, R. P., Rowley, S. N., Weis, A., Wood, K. S., Wood, J. J., Ibrahim, K., Sukhodolsky, D. G. (2021 Nov). Conducting CBT for anxiety in children with autism spectrum disorder during COVID-19 pandemic. *Journal of Autism and Developmental Disorders, 51*(11), 4239–4247. https://doi.org/10.1007/s10803-020-04845-1. Epub 2021 Jan 1. PMID: 33385281; PMCID: PMC7775616.

Kendall, P. C., & Hedtke, K. A. (2006). *Coping cat workbook* (Vol. 44). Ardmore, PA: Workbook Publishing.

Kerns, C. M., Collier, A., Lewin, A. B., & Storch, E. A. (2018). Therapeutic alliance in youth with autism spectrum disorder receiving cognitive-behavioral treatment for anxiety. *Autism, 22*(5), 636–640. https://doi.org/10.1177/1362361316685556

Kiresuk, T. J., & Sherman, R. E. (1968). Goal attainment scaling: A general method for evaluating comprehension in community mental health programs. *Community Mental Health Journal, 4*(6), 443–453.

Kiresuk, T. J., Smith, A. J., & Cardillo, J. E. (2014). Applications of goal attainment scaling. Psychology Press London, England, United Kingdom.

Klebanoff, S. M., Rosenau, K. A., & Wood, J. J. (2019). The therapeutic alliance in cognitive-behavioral therapy for school-aged children with autism and clinical anxiety. *Autism, 23*(8), 2031–2042. https://doi.org/10.1177/1362361319841197

Kouklari, E.-C., Tsermentseli, S., & Auyeung, B. (2018). Executive function predicts theory of mind but not social verbal communication in school-aged children with autism spectrum disorder. *Research in Developmental Disabilities, 76*, 12–24. https://doi.org/10.1016/j.ridd.2018.02.015

Landa, R. J., & Goldberg, M. C. (2005). Language, social, and executive functions in high functioning autism: A continuum of performance. *Journal of Autism and Developmental Disorders, 35*(5), 557–573.

Laugeson, E. A., Frankel, F., Gantman, A., Dillon, A. R., & Mogil, C. (2012). Evidence-based social skills training for adolescents with autism spectrum disorders: The UCLA PEERS program. *Journal of Autism and Developmental Disorders, 42*, 1025–1036.

Laugeson, E. A., Park, M. N. (2014). Using a CBT approach to teach social skills to adolescents with autism spectrum disorder and other social challenges: The PEERS® method. *Journal of Rational-Emotive and Cognitive Behavior Therapy, 32*, 84–97. https://doi.org/10.1007/s10942-014-0181-8

Laurent, A. C., & Rubin, E. (2004). Challenges in emotional regulation in asperger syndrome and high-functioning autism. *Topics in Language Disorders, 24*(4), 286–297.

Le Couteur, A., Lord, C., & Rutter, M. (2003). *Autism diagnostic interview-revised*. Los Angeles, CA: Western Psychological Services.

Lickel, A., MacLean, W. E., Blakeley-Smith, A. et al. (2012). Assessment of the prerequisite skills for cognitive behavioral therapy in children with and without ASD. *Journal of Autism and Developmental Disorders, 42*, 992–1000. https://doi.org/10.1007/s10803-011-1330-x

Lopata, C., Thomeer, M. L., Volker, M. A., & Nida, R. E. (2006). Effectiveness of a cognitive-behavioral treatment on the social behaviors of children with Asperger disorder. *Focus on Autism and Other Developmental Disabilities, 21*(4), 237–244.

Lopez, B. R., Lincoln, A. J., Ozonoff, S., & Lai, Z. (2005). Examining the relationship between executive functions and restricted, repetitive symptoms of autistic disorder. *Journal of Autism and Developmental Disorders, 35*(4), 445–461.

Maenner, M. J., Warren, Z., Williams, A. R., Amoakohene, E., Bakian, A. V., Bilder, D. A., ... & Shaw, K. A. (2023). Prevalence and characteristics of autism spectrum disorder among children aged 8 years—Autism and developmental disabilities monitoring network, 11 sites, United States, 2020. *MMWR Surveillance Summaries, 72*(2), 1.

McConachie, H., McLaughlin, E., Grahame, V., Taylor, H., Honey, E., Tavernor, L., ... & Le Couteur, A. (2014). Group therapy for anxiety in children with autism spectrum disorder. *Autism, 18*(6), 723–732.

McEvoy, R. E., Rogers, S. J., & Pennington, B. F. (1993). Executive function and social communication deficits in young autistic children. *Journal of Child Psychology and Psychiatry and Allied Disciplines, 34*(4), 563–578.

McGrath, L. M., & Peterson, R. L. (2020). Autism spectrum disorder. In B. F. Pennington (Ed.), *Diagnosing learning disorders: A neuropsychological framework* (3rd ed., pp. 258–311). New York: Guilford Press.

McLeod, B. D. (2011). Relation of the alliance with outcomes in youth psychotherapy: A meta-analysis. *Clinical Psychology Review, 31*, 603–616. https://doi.org/10.1016/j.cpr.2011.02.001

Murphy, V. B., & Christner, R. W. (2012). A cognitive-behavioral case conceptualization for children and adolescents. In R. B. Mennuti, R. W. Christner, & A. Freeman (Eds.), *Cognitive-behavioral interventions in educational settings: A handbook for practice* (pp. 81–114). Routledge/Taylor & Francis Group.

Ozonoff, S., & Jensen, J. (1999). Brief report: Specific executive function profiles in three neurodevelopmental disorders. *Journal of Autism and Developmental Disorders, 29*(2), 171–177.

Pellicano, E. (2010). Individual differences in executive function and central coherence predict developmental changes in theory of mind in autism. *Developmental Psychology*, *46*, 530–544. https://doi.org/10.1037/a0018287

Pellicano, E., Smith, A. D., Ledger-Hardy, L., Briscoe, J., Hood, B., & Gilchrist, I. D. (2010). Children with autism are neither systematic nor optimal foragers. *Proceedings of the National Academy of Sciences, 108*(1), 421–426.

Pennington, B. F., & Ozonoff, S. (1996). Executive functions and developmental psychopathology. *Journal of Child Psychology and Psychiatry, 37*, 51–87.

Pugliese, C. E., Anthony, L. G., Strang, J. F., Dudley, K., Wallace, G. L., Naiman, D. Q., et al. (2016). Longitudinal examination of adaptive behavior in ASD: Influence of executive function. *Journal of Autism and Developmental Disorders, 46*(2), 467–477. https://doi.org/10.1007/s10803-015-2584-5

Ratto, A. B., Turner-Brown, L., Rupp, B. M., Mesibov, G. B., & Penn, D. L. (2011). Development of the contextual assessment of social skills (CASS): A role play measure of social skill for individuals with high-functioning Autism. *Journal of Autism and Developmental Disorders, 41*, 1277–1286.

Reaven, J., Blakeley-Smith, A., Culhane-Shelburne, K., & Hepburn, S. (2012). Group cognitive behavior therapy for children with high-functioning ASD and anxiety: A randomized trial. *Journal of Child Psychology and Psychiatry, 53*(4), 410–419.

Rodgers, J., Wigham, S., McConachie, H., Freeston, M., Honey, E., & Parr, J. R. (2016). Development of the anxiety scale for children with autism spectrum disorder (ASC-ASD). *Autism Research, 9*(11), 1205–1215.

Ryan, R., Berry, K., & Hartley, S. (2023 May). Review: Therapist factors and their impact on therapeutic alliance and outcomes in child and adolescent mental health – A systematic review. *Child and Adolescent Mental Health, 28*(2), 195–211. https://doi.org/10.1111/camh.12518. Epub 2021 Nov 11. PMID: 34763371.

Sansosti, F. J. (2003). Effectiveness of social story interventions for children with asperger's syndrome. *USF Tampa Graduate Theses and Dissertations.* Retrieved from https://digitalcommons.usf.edu/etd/1464

Sansosti, F. J., Powell-Smith, K. A., & Cowan, R. J. (2010). *High-functioning autism/asperger syndrome in schools: Assessment and intervention.* New York: Guilford Press.

Schneider, S., Blatter-Meunier, J., Herren, C., Adornetto, C., In-Albon, T., & Lavallee, K. (2011). Disorder-specific cognitive-behavioral therapy for separation anxiety disorder in young children: A randomized waiting-list-controlled trial. *Psychotherapy and Psychosomatics, 80*(4), 206–215.

Simmons, G. L., Ioannou, S., Smith, J. V., Corbett, B. A., Lerner, M. D., & White, S. W. (2021). Utility of an observational social skill assessment as a measure of social cognition in autism. *Autism Research, 14*(4), 709–719.

Ung, D., Small, B. J., Selles, R. R., & Storch, E. A. (2014 Sept). A systematic review and meta-analysis of cognitive behavioral therapy for anxiety in youth with high-functioning ASD. *Child Psychiatry & Human Development.*

Vasa, R. A., & Mazurek, M. O. (2015 Mar). An update on anxiety in youth with ASD. *Current Opinion in Psychiatry, 28*(2), 83–90. https://doi.org/10.1097/YCO.0000000000000133. PMID: 25602249; PMCID: PMC5764108.

Verte, S., Geurts, H. M., Roeyers, H., Oosterlaan, J., & Sergeant, J. A. (2006). Executive functioning in children with an autism spectrum disorder: Can we differentiate within the spectrum? *Journal of Autism and Developmental Disorders, 36*(3), 351–372.

Walters, S., Loades, M., & Russell, A. (2016). A systematic review of effective modifications to cognitive behavioural therapy for young people with ASD. *Journal of Autism and Developmental Disorders, 3*, 137–153. https://doi.org/10.1007/s40489-016-0072-2

Wang, X., Zhao, J., Huang, S., Chen, S., Zhou, T., Li, Q., Luo, X., & Hao, Y. (2021 May). Cognitive behavioral therapy for ASD: A systematic review. *Pediatrics, 147*(5), e2020049880. https://doi.org/10.1542/peds.2020-049880. PMID: 33888566

White, S., Ollendick, T., Albano, A., Oswald, D., Johnson, C., Southam-Gerow, M. A., Kim, I., & Scahill, L. (2013). Randomized controlled trial: Multimodal anxiety and social skill intervention for adolescents with autism spectrum disorder. *Journal of Autism & Developmental Disorders, 43*(2), 382–394.

Will, M. N., Currans, K., Smith, J., Weber, S., Duncan, A., Burton, J., Kroeger-Geoppinger, K., Miller, V., Stone, M., Mays, L., Luebrecht, A., Heeman, A., Erickson, C., & Anixt, J. (2018). Evidenced-based interventions for children with autism spectrum disorder. *Current Problems in Pediatric and Adolescent Health Care, 48*(10), 234–249.

Winner, M. (2005). *Think social!* San Jose, CA: Think Social Publishing.

Winner, M. G. (2008). *A politically incorrect look at evidence-based practices and teaching social skills: A literature review and discussion.* San Jose, CA: Think Social Publishing.

Wood, J. J., Drahota, A., Sze, K., Har, K., Chiu, A., & Langer, D. A. (2009). Cognitive behavioral therapy for anxiety in children with ASD: A randomized, controlled trial. *Journal of Child Psychology and Psychiatry, 50*(3), 224–234.

Wood, J. J., Ehrenreich-May, J., Alessandri, M., Fujii, C., Renno, P., Laugeson, E., Piacentini, J. C., De Nadai, A. S., Arnold, E., Lewin, A. B., Murphy, T. K., & Storch, E. A. (2015). Cognitive behavioral therapy for early adolescents with ASD and clinical anxiety: A randomized, controlled trial. *Behavior Therapy, 46*(1), 7–19.

20
EXECUTIVE FUNCTIONING DEFICITS

Laura W. Monahon and Kathryn Arcari

Introduction and Overview of CBT to the Problem Area

Executive function is a term used to refer to a set of cognitive processes and skills that are carried out by the prefrontal regions of the brain (Goldstein et al., 2014). Executive functions include processes such as initiating and monitoring tasks, sustaining and switching attention, and self-regulation, all of which support a person's ability to successfully develop and execute a plan to meet a goal, follow multi-step directions, ignore distractions, and manage their emotions. As such, these capacities must be appropriately developed to ensure that an individual functions and feels well in their environment. Conversely, individuals who experience deficits in executive functioning can be negatively impacted in a number of functional domains. For children and adolescents with executive functioning difficulties, the impact is most commonly felt in school, where they can experience academic, behavioral, and social frustration and failure. In short, schools are places that consistently demand a high degree of executive functioning skills, and when these skills are lacking, students can suffer.

Interventions to support children and adolescents with executive functioning deficits can take many forms. Teachers can help in myriad ways, including setting up the physical space to reduce distractions, developing consistent routines and clear rules, and reinforcing positive, prosocial behaviors. Implementing these supports will likely benefit all students and will provide a boost to those students with executive functioning deficits. However, there will be times when more is needed. In addition to school-wide and classroom-wide supports, some students will benefit from individualized therapeutic interventions to treat the negative emotional correlates that result from executive functioning deficits. Cognitive-behavioral therapy (CBT) has been shown to be widely effective in teaching and strengthening executive functioning skills while improving mood and emotional regulation skills in children and adolescents (Derella, 2019).

This chapter will explore the connection between CBT and improved executive functioning, school performance, and mood in children and adolescents. Foundational CBT principles including collaborative empiricism, psychoeducation, agenda setting, problem solving, and cognitive restructuring will be reviewed and applied to the treatment of executive functioning deficits. Conceptualization of executive functioning and the impact on core beliefs, automatic thoughts, feelings, and behaviors will also be considered and applied within a case study format.

DOI: 10.4324/9781003392439-23

Understanding the Specific Issue/Disorder

For most students, middle school is a time of increased executive functioning load, with the need for interacting with multiple teachers and classroom rules and routines over the course of a single school day. Boyer and colleagues (2015) further delineate environmental changes that occur in adolescence that tax students' executive functioning, including diminished help provided by parents and teachers, increased expectation for independent planning of long-term projects, studying for tests, and turning in assignments, and a general increase in the number of homework assignments for which students need to be responsible. Perhaps most importantly, the middle school and high school years typically represent an increase in tasks that inherently have delayed reinforcement and reward, including paying attention in class (to do well on an assignment or test that may be weeks away) and completing longer-term homework assignments and projects (Zeman et al., 2002).

Imagine that you are a student who struggles to sustain attention in school. Consider what the functional impact would be during a typical day in middle school. Will you remember your materials for each of your classes? When is the best time to visit your locker to gather what you need and drop off what you don't need? What happens when your math teacher has a different daily routine than your science teacher, and, more importantly, how quickly are you expected to remember the various routines once reminders are faded? These demands represent only a small sampling of what most middle schoolers are expected to manage on a daily basis. How do we imagine those students with executive functioning deficits might be feeling at the end of a week? Now, what if we compound those negative feelings across 13 weeks of a marking period? Week by week, many of these students are building a history of failure and underachievement. Is it any wonder that they begin to develop negative core beliefs regarding their ability to be effective; beliefs that then generate dysfunctional cognitions which lead to disturbances of mood, including depression, anxiety, anger, and even guilt (Golombek et al., 2020; Safren et al., 2004; Young et al., 2019)? And, as indicated previously, we must also consider how these mood disturbances further prevent the application of appropriate compensatory strategies, thereby compounding the difficulties yet again (Warren et al., 2021).

To be certain, the difficulties experienced by students with executive functioning deficits are not limited to academic frustration and failure. Impairments in social functioning are also well documented in individuals who struggle with executive functioning. Numerous studies have concluded that students with executive functioning deficits may be as capable as their typical peers at initiating social relationships; however, these individuals tend to have significantly more trouble maintaining these relationships (Grenell et al., 1987; Landau & Milich, 1988; Renshaw & Asher, 1983). Generally speaking, individuals who experience EF deficits tend to have a decreased ability to adjust their thoughts and actions to manage the dynamic demands of the social world. Specific deficits in flexible social communication, conflict resolution, and self-regulation often create barriers to the give-and-take that is necessary to maintain social relationships, be they peer-to-peer or child/adolescent-to-adult.

Several diagnosable conditions are associated with executive functioning disorders such as attention-deficit/hyperactivity disorder (ADHD), autism spectrum disorder (ASD), and post concussive syndrome (PCS) or mild traumatic brain injury (mTBI). Perhaps the most well-associated disorder with executive dysfunction in school is ADHD. Students with ADHD often present with disorganization, difficulty with planning, struggles with shifting and mental flexibility, trouble initiating tasks, difficulties with emotional regulation, and many other management needs of daily life (Barkley, 1990, 2006). Although medication has been shown to have a positive effect on executive functioning in the treatment of ADHD, several compensatory techniques can also be taught that will aid in long-term learning of management and produce better outcomes. Allowing students to learn, practice, adjust, and self-monitor what works for them can be a rewarding experience that allows for students to learn to predict when they require new or adjusted techniques both now and in the future.

Another disorder in which the individual can present with executive functioning struggles is ASD. Children with ASD present with difficulties regulating emotional responses, initiating, and appropriate inhibition in social scenarios, among other struggles (Otterman et al., 2019). Teaching explicit exercises that will change the manner in which students with ASD approach situations and providing practice of these techniques both in session and in vivo can often empower children with ASD to not only improve skills but also improve locus of control and self-reliance.

Individuals who have suffered a concussion with longer lasting effects, such as those with PCS or mTBI, often begin to demonstrate executive functioning difficulties (Ransom et al., 2016) that perhaps they have never experienced previous to their concussion. This can present an additional frustration when working with this student. Falling back on traditional executive functioning training, while also paying close attention to how the student is feeling and reacting to these difficulties, is an important component when working with this population.

Empirical Support of CBT in Treatment of Specific Disorder

As with many developmental capacities, some children and adolescents seem to develop and apply effective executive skills naturally while others struggle and can lag behind their peers (Dawson, Guare). These functional impairments, or lags, have diverse negative impacts, not the least of which is academic underachievement. Specifically, successful application of effective executive function strategies leads to increased efficiency, which supports learning and academic achievement. Not surprisingly, these successes often result in boosts in students' sense of self-efficacy and self-confidence, which then motivates them to continue to target their efforts to achieve specific academic goals (Meltzer et al., 2004). This connection between motivation, academic self-concept, and self-efficacy is well established, not only with students for whom learning is relatively easy but also for students who have been identified as having learning and/or attentional deficits (Meltzer et al., 2004).

So what happens when the positive cycle of successful application of executive functioning skills and the resulting boost in self-confidence and self-efficacy does not occur? Dawson and Guare (2014) note that teachers and parents, both important stakeholders in students' academic and emotional development and success, can sometimes assume that these students are "simply being oppositional by refusing to do something that is well within [their] capacity" (p. 24). This often results in a power struggle that leaves parents and teachers feeling frustrated and students feeling misunderstood and defeated. Even in cases such as these, all parties share a goal of increasing students' capacity to function independently. This is often accomplished through a combination of environmental modifications to support weaker executive functioning, as well as the direct teaching of skills and motivating children to practice (Dawson and Guare).

Safren and colleagues (2004) developed a conceptual model of an approach to treating the functional impairments associated with chronic executive functioning deficits. This model first identifies core neuropsychiatric impairments, such as difficulties with attention, working memory, inhibition, self-regulation, and set shifting that contribute to functional impairments in individuals with poor executive functioning (Miyake et al., 2000; Safren et al., 2004). Additionally, individuals who experience these impairments also frequently have significant difficulty conceptualizing and implementing appropriate compensatory strategies that could serve to offset the impairment. These compensatory strategies include activities that support organization of materials, task planning, and time management (Safren et al., 2004). Put simply, this is a sort of compounding problem: deficits in executive functioning not only *create* the problem(s) but are also instrumental in blocking the pathway to *solving* the problem(s).

Let's apply the Safren model to a typical middle school student with executive functioning difficulties. When Alex, a 5th grade student, first presented to the counselor due to angry outbursts in class during independent work time, he described a "build up" of feelings that he could not control sometimes. After several weeks of data collection, including a classroom observation, in which the counselor was able to watch one of Alex's outbursts in real time, the issue became clear. The initial difficulty observed was that Alex struggled to initiate tasks during independent study and work time. The classroom teacher, having had many years of experience with students with executive functioning deficits, had set up several compensatory techniques for Alex during these periods of time including timers, picture schedules, and clear, written out schedules of work to be completed with each time period. However, she would then leave him to his work. Despite all of these techniques, Alex would fidget, become distracted with other stimuli in the classroom, and disrupt the other students attempting to complete the assigned work. When the teacher would cue him back to the work, he would become agitated with the eventual angry outburst, sending him out of the classroom for disciplinary action. It was clear to the counselor that in addition to setting up these techniques, Alex required the additional support of learning or re-learning how to effectively utilize these instruments. Despite the good intentions of the teacher, Alex required more explicit learning due to his inability to not only initiate the classroom work but also initiate the use of the tools given to him and monitor if and when these tools worked for him.

CBT has a rich history of effectively treating many of the negative emotional correlates that result from executive functioning deficits. Countless studies have supported using a CBT approach to address mood disturbances across the lifespan, including treating symptoms of anxiety, depression, and anger in children and adolescents. Not surprisingly, children and adolescents who have difficulty regulating their emotions secondary to executive functioning deficits tend to show it in the form of emotional and/or behavioral symptoms (Aldao et al., 2016). Fortunately, just as the relationship between effective compensatory strategies and mood regulation is bidirectional, so is the relationship between executive functions and effective CBT interventions, particularly in regard to internalizing disorders. Specifically, CBT has been shown to be effective in increasing emotional regulation skills in children and adolescents (which, in turn, can result in improved mood and functioning in school) (Derella, 2019; Suveg et al., 2009). As such, implementing a CBT approach to support mood and functioning via increasing emotional regulation skills provides a double benefit.

Further, Pruessner and colleagues (2020) found that executive functions such as cognitive flexibility and cognitive control are critical for emotional regulation, not only from a neurobiological perspective but also in terms of selecting effective strategies and developing a plan for their implementation. From a therapeutic perspective, using CBT to teach individuals (via psychoeducation and other CBT-informed strategies) about their strengths and limitations in the areas of cognitive control, flexibility, and emotional regulation sets the stage for not only improved executive functioning but also more meaningful interpersonal interactions and more social success.

Additional CBT techniques also have promising implications for treating executive functioning deficits in and of themselves as well as the negative thoughts and emotions that often accompany them (Safren et al., 2005; Vidal-Estrada et al., 2012). Asnaani and colleagues (2020) and others have made a case that application of and practice using foundational CBT principles and strategies such as cognitive restructuring, problem solving, and, more recently, mindfulness lead to improved executive functioning as well as reduced difficulties with emotional regulation (Emerson et al., 2005; Huang et al., 2019; Mohlman, 2008).

While psychopharmacological interventions are hallmark in the treatment of many executive functioning difficulties, they are not without limitations, including high rates of dropout, potential for dependency, and limited treatment response with persistent residual symptoms (Pan et al., 2019; Toren et al., 2000). One diagnosis that is often associated with executive functioning deficits is ADHD

(Holmes et al., 2010). ADHD is a diagnosis based not only on the criteria of deficits in attention and central nervous system hyperactivity (American Psychiatric Association [APA], 2022) but also an inability to manage typical external demands that can be at best overwhelming and at worst debilitating, also referred to as deficits in executive functioning. These deficits include struggles with inhibition, impulsivity, set shifting and cognitive flexibility, organization, planning, higher order thinking and problem solving, working memory, and self-monitoring (Groves et al., 2022; Monteiro, 2022).

When working with children and adolescents with ADHD, it is often helpful and necessary to address their executive functioning struggles first and foremost as these are frequently the most disruptive yet actionable behaviors that they present. However, due to the neurobiology involved in the diagnosis of ADHD, it is oftentimes challenging to have the child or adolescent fully engage in the process of therapy itself and follow through with required practice and reinforcement to ensure skill acquisition and thought modification (Tripp, 2009). The group of medications commonly referred to as the stimulant group of medications can help many students with ADHD improve executive functioning (Miklós et al., 2019; Tripp, 2009), such as directing attention in session, which in turn allows the therapist and student to achieve the work they set out to do within the time they are given as well as helps the student to achieve the goals set forth throughout the week, such as homework or data collection, for example. For a complete review of psychopharmacological stimulants and non-stimulants utilized with the ADHD population, see Groom and Cortese (2022). In brief, one example of the stimulant class of medications, methylphenidates may work to compensate for some of the dopamine cell firing that is sought after in reinforcing events, or preferred activities, which in turn is associated with an increase in symptoms in individuals with ADHD (Tripp, 2009). These preferred activities become replacement behaviors for non-preferred activities, such as homework or chores, and lead to executive dysfunction such as lack of initiation and procrastination. Balancing the proven effectiveness of psychopharmacological interventions with these potential limitations supports utilizing CBT as a primary or adjunctive treatment intervention.

Relational Consideration in Treatment of Problem Area (Connecting)

As indicated in previous sections, executive functioning deficits impact multiple areas of functioning across multiple settings. When developing a treatment plan to address the impact of executive functioning deficits, consideration must be given to aspects such as assessing a client's capacity for self-awareness, selecting appropriate and engaging interventions, and determining pacing to best manage the cognitive load of treatment. While these are certainly necessary steps in ensuring that a treatment plan yields maximum positive results, practitioners must also consider them in the context of connecting with and relating to the client. Hallmarks of CBT such as establishing rapport, building and maintaining a therapeutic alliance through use of collaborative empiricism, and providing a rationale for treatment are critical components to any effective CBT-based intervention. Additionally, the practitioner will also use psychoeducation not only to decatastrophize and normalize the problem(s) but also to empower clients with an understanding of the treatment framework (i.e., the cognitive model).

Meta-analytic studies have consistently demonstrated that establishing an effective rapport at the outset of treatment is important in any therapeutic milieu (Bose et al., 2022; McLeod, 2011). Specifically, Marker and colleagues (2013) found a positive correlation between effective therapeutic alliance and symptom reduction in their sample of children being treated for anxiety. This is especially important in CBT, as successful rapport-building is the cornerstone of building and maintaining a strong therapeutic alliance. Importantly, findings also suggest that the role of establishing rapport and building a therapeutic alliance is most effective at the outset of treatment. Put simply, there is ample research that suggests that "starting strong" with children and adolescents in therapy can be predictive of positive outcomes (Kendall et al., 2023).

What does "starting strong" look like when using a cognitive-behavioral approach to treating children and adolescents with executive functioning deficits and resulting emotional dysregulation and distress? The answer is both complex and simple: while there is no single activity or strategy that is guaranteed to allow the practitioner to connect with their client, the goal of connecting and engaging with the child or adolescent (or adult!) is quite straightforward. As Kendall and colleagues (2023) explain, a primary goal of initial therapy session(s) is centered on the client developing a sense of positive connection with both the therapist and the process. Not only can this initial positive connection pave the way for a strong therapeutic alliance, but it can also serve to reinforce engagement with the process of therapy for the child or adolescent, which is likely to pay dividends over the course of treatment.

In terms of specific rapport-building activities, most practitioners will find themselves building a library of options throughout the tenure of their practice. These "getting to know you" activities can range from structured games (which can be effective in engaging and learning about young children) to informal conversations (commonly preferred by older children and adolescents). One activity that is sufficiently flexible to use with a variety of ages is a "This or That" list. This is an easy-to-play word game in which the participants (e.g., the client and the therapist) choose between two items, indicating a preference for one over the other. The list can be presented in a variety of formats, including simply listing the items or providing pictures as reference, and can easily be adapted for non-readers. As the participants select and respond to list items, they are sharing their own preferences while getting to know the likes and dislikes of their game partner. On the part of the client, this back-and-forth exchange will frequently prompt further discussion about the reasons for and possibly some personal experiences related to their preferred choices. For the therapist, it provides an appropriate means of using limited and highly structured self-disclosure to connect with their client. Finally, this type of activity can be extended into future therapy sessions by reserving a few minutes at the beginning or end of a session to try out a new list.

As Dobson (2022) notes, since the establishment of CBT as an effective treatment modality, there are "critical features of both the therapist and the relationship between the therapist and client that optimize the likelihood of therapeutic success." Key among these features is the concept of collaborative empiricism. This term is frequently interpreted and expressed as the therapist and client as functioning as "co-scientists" in the therapeutic process, a term that effectively conveys the meaning of collaborative empiricism in a manner that is easier for young clients to access. Specifically, collaborative empiricism involves the therapist and client working together as a team (i.e., as collaborators) to 1st understand and then address problems through therapeutic interventions and activities (Dobson, 2022). As with any scientific endeavor, data from the therapeutic tasks (conducted both in and out of session) are then reviewed to determine the effectiveness of the intervention. In CBT, the therapist and the client are both maintained as stakeholders in the data-analysis process; after all, the therapist has advanced training in the theory and practice of CBT, but the client is the expert of their own experience.

Finally, within the context of providing school-based therapeutic services, it is not uncommon that students are referred for treatment based on someone else's assessment of that student's need (e.g., a parent or caregiver, a teacher, a school administrator). As such, it is often necessary for the therapist to determine their client's perception of and motivation for treatment. In-session interviewing can be utilized to gather this data and can also be utilized to understand and validate any ambivalence that the child or adolescent may have toward working with the therapist and/or participating in treatment (Kendall et al., 2023).

This process can also be facilitated and supported by the use of psychoeducation. Along with collaborative empiricism, psychoeducation has long been identified as a crucial component of CBT, both broadly and specifically when working with children and adolescents (Chiappini et al., 2020; Compton et al., 2004). In the context of CBT, psychoeducation is typically utilized to increase a client's knowledge about the difficulties they are experiencing and also about the method of treatment that the therapist believes will help with problem resolution and improved functioning and mood (e.g., CBT). This technique has extensive empirical support. Numerous studies have shown how the use of psychoeducation in the context of individual CBT with students promotes more positive automatic thoughts and increases their sense of self-efficacy, while simultaneously reducing thoughts of stress and confusion (Freire et al., 2020; Kaplan et al., 2023; Nakao et al., 2021). Similarly, a study conducted by Kürümlüoğlugil and Tanrıverdi (2022) found that clients who participate in CBT-based psychoeducation have fewer cognitive distortions related to interpersonal interactions, decreased dysfunctional attitudes, and lower rates of negative automatic thoughts.

Engaging in psychoeducation with children and adolescents with executive functioning deficits and resulting social and emotional difficulties focuses on increasing their understanding about what these difficulties feel/look like, where they come from, and how they can be supported, treated, and remediated. Psychoeducation can also be used to dispel any myths about what the client is experiencing (Kendall et al., 2023). Specifically, in the case of executive dysfunction, children and adolescents may believe that they are the only student in their classroom who experience struggles related to capacities such as attention, shifting, or self-monitoring. Inaccurate perceptions such as these increase the client's negative thoughts and perceptions of themselves and can lead to depressed or anxious mood, inaccurate processing of environmental and/or social cues, and a diminished sense of social competency. In cases such as these, the therapist can first use rapport building/interviewing techniques (as described above) to uncover the misperceptions. Then, psychoeducation can be used to correct inaccuracies while also normalizing and validating the client's experience. This discussion provides the therapist with an opportunity to begin to set expectations for treatment. Specifically, the goal of therapy in this case would be twofold: teach strategies to improve executive functioning and/or to reduce the impact of executive dysfunction *and* develop skills to help the client cope with the emotional discomfort they experience. By focusing on coping, rather than eliminating, negative emotions, the therapist will empower the client to be aware of and better manage their feelings when they do arise (as they will while the client is actively in treatment and if/when treatment is discontinued). In other words, the therapist will teach the client how to cope with executive dysfunction and anxious, depressive, or angry thoughts without letting them disrupt what the client wants or needs to do in life.

Interviewing and Assessing Problem Area (Assessing)

Assessing the existence of executive functioning struggles in school-aged children involves several factors, including self-monitoring and appraisal, reports, and observations from others in the child's life, including caretakers and educators, and direct observation if available (Mares et al., 2007). In gathering information from several different reporters, including the therapist, the breadth of the problem, given its many different presentations, can truly be measured and the extent of the student's difficulties and how they adversely affect his or her functioning can be observed and understood.

Self-monitoring is important for gaining insight into the student's experience of their struggles. Self-awareness, or lack thereof, can often be a part of executive dysfunction. Utilizing Socratic questioning, a technique that uses questions instead of statements to assess the problem and draw conclusions (Toolin, 2016), will allow the student to gain insight and independent discovery into their problem areas. Below is an example of Socratic questioning used to assess how much a student's procrastination has affected his poor homework performance.

Therapist: Tell me about your approach to homework?
Student: So I usually do it the night before it's due, since I work best under pressure.
Therapist: So what you are telling me is that you do your best work when you feel the pressure of a due date bearing down on you? What information do you have to support this?
Student: I don't know, it's just how I always did it and how my mind works. It's just the way I am.
Therapist: Ok, so I hear that you believe that you perform best when you feel that pressure, however, is it safe to say that you have missed several homework assignments over the course of this marking period?
Student: Well yea but sometimes I forget, or I have stuff to do, like sports, and don't I have time.
Therapist: How could you structure homework time a little differently to account for things like sports or needing more time for longer assignments?
Student: I guess starting things earlier might help....

In this example, the student presents the problem independently without the therapist directly questioning the obvious (to the therapist) breakdown in his thought process. Even with insight, however, the process of questioning and helping the student come to these conclusions may require repetition over several sessions. In addition to interviews, charting behaviors to further build evidence may be helpful to aid the student in gaining additional insight into cognitive distortions or beliefs about how he does his "best work." Lastly, there are many empirically supported self-report measures of executive functioning for older children, starting around the age of 12 years. These measures provide standardized scores of specific clinical scales, such as initiation, shifting, and planning/organization, while some also offer index scores, such as externalizing/internalizing problems. Some specific measures include the Behavior Rating Inventory of Executive Functioning-2nd Edition published by Psychological Assessment Resources and the Comprehensive Executive Function Inventory (CEFI) published by Western Psychological Services.

Gaining information from others is integral in assessing executive dysfunction in children and adolescents. As mentioned, it is likely that children and adolescent students with executive functioning difficulties will have less self-awareness or insight into their own executive dysfunction (Steward et al., 2017). Therefore, teachers' and parents' or caregivers' perspectives are important in identifying and truly understanding areas of concern. When available, a thorough history of the behavior is also useful. Additionally, parent- and teacher-report versions of the self-reports given to the students can determine where the caregiver and teacher perceive the problem(s) to be and can also help the therapist to understand the differences in perceptions of each individual involved in the case. This multi-source data will help to inform treatment and will also help to determine each person's role in the development and implementation of the treatment plan.

Direct observation of the problem behaviors can be invaluable for the practitioner. For example, imagine that you are working with Sara, a middle-school student with executive functioning deficits who is having difficulties maintaining friendships in school. In session, Sara explains that, while her peers are friendly toward her, she believes that "everyone else is better friends with each other" which leaves her feeling isolated and lonely. Between sessions, you have the opportunity to observe Sara in her Math class. You note that she chats briefly with students who are seated near her at the beginning and end of class; however, socialization opportunities are limited in that setting. In an effort to gather additional data about Sara's social functioning, you decide to observe her in the most social of middle school settings: the lunchroom. You observe Sara enter the lunchroom with a group of peers and walk toward a table where some students who you recognize from her Math class are seated. Next, you observe Sara turn around and walk quickly toward the exit. Several minutes later, she returns with her lunchbox (which she had forgotten to retrieve from her locker on the way to lunch). She walks back to the table and takes the only seat available at the far end of the table. You observe Sara attempt to join in the conversation at the table, but, in the noise of the lunchroom, it appears that her friends cannot hear her. She is observably frustrated by this and turns in her seat so that her back is facing the group. When one of her tablemates leans over to talk to Sara, you observe her shrugging her shoulders and resisting eye contact. When the end-of-the-period bell rings, Sara stands up immediately and turns to look at the students at her table. When no one looks her way, she slams her lunchbox closed and stomps toward the exit. Later, in session, when you ask Sara about lunch, she states, "Everyone was ignoring me the whole time. They aren't my friends. I am going to just sit by myself from now on."

By observing Sara in her natural environment, the therapist is provided first-hand knowledge of not only Sara's behavior but also the behavior of her peers. Armed with this data, the therapist can then form hypotheses about what may be reinforcing (directly or indirectly) the problem behavior(s). In the case of Sara, the therapist observed that forgetting her lunchbox caused Sara to miss the first several minutes of the lunch period. Upon returning to the lunchroom, not only had Sara missed social time, but she was also left with a seat that acted as a barrier to further socialization. When faced with these situational variables, it appears that Sara made the assumptions that, "Nobody is talking to me. They are ignoring me and aren't my friends." These negative thoughts caused Sara to feel isolated, which, given her difficulties with self-awareness and emotional regulation, soon developed into frustration and anger. Sara then expressed these feelings with behaviors such as turning away and ignoring her peers, which inadvertently exacerbated the problem. All in all, the situation likely confirmed Sara's belief that she is unable to form meaningful friendships. Because the therapist was able to directly observe this situation and not rely only on Sara's perception of it, they can help to guide treatment planning to include strategies that address elements that Sara has not considered. These might include helping Sara to improve her organization and planning skills so that she remembers to bring her lunchbox to the cafeteria, as well as improving her self-awareness and emotional regulation skills through the use of cognitive restructuring, perspective taking, and decatastrophizing.

Functional behavior analysis is often the first assessment that occurs in a school setting where a student's behavior is being called into question for treatment. A functional analysis of the behaviors will help to determine the factors contributing to the behaviors and those that are reinforcing to the behaviors. The observer will determine the antecedents and consequences of the behaviors displayed as well as any additional stimuli that elicit conditional responses (CRs), be they cognitive, emotional, and/or behavioral (Young et al., 2019). The environmental context in which the behaviors occur may also be important and contributing to the behaviors; for example, is this happening during recess, class time, transitions, etc.? With first hand knowledge and observation of the behaviors, the clinician is then able to engage with the student in a collaborative way when discussing the behaviors and perhaps help the student to begin to understand the maladaptive thought processes that are attached to those behaviors more expeditiously in session.

With the input from all sources, the therapist is now ready to help the student identify target behaviors and the maladaptive beliefs that perpetuate those behaviors. Behavioral change begins by labeling cognitive distortions, presenting evidence that challenges set behaviors, and beginning to develop new strategies and techniques to improve problem behaviors and associated thoughts and feelings.

Case Conceptualization (Understanding)

Effective executive functioning capacities are necessary to navigate the demands of daily living across multiple environments successfully. With children and adolescents, their primary workplace is often school, which comes with a host of dynamic academic and social demands. When executive functioning skills are working well, students have an increased capacity to thrive, both academically and socially. These opportunities for success breed additional opportunities for success, creating a cycle of optimized functioning, which paves the way for increased positive mood, as well as increased self-efficacy and self-confidence. Conversely, when executive functioning capacities are not adequate or are ineffective, a cycle of failure and self-doubt is likely to occur. For some students, this begins at an early age. For others, the cycle begins with the executive functioning demands of school outpace their executive functioning abilities, which commonly happens toward the middle school years. Regardless of when the gap between demands and skills occurs, a child or adolescent faced with daily "failures" in areas that require application of executive functioning skills quickly learns that they just do not measure up. These failures can impair functioning in multiple ways and tend to impact academic and social functioning (the two primary "jobs" of school) quickly and repeatedly.

When this occurs, it is not difficult to imagine that these students are likely to develop negative core beliefs that are centered around inadequacy and incompetence. These core beliefs could include fixed and global statements such as "I am dumb," "I am not as smart as I thought that I was," "I am a failure," and/or "I am not likable." When faced with a situation that requires the application of a level of executive functioning that these students are not able to meet, these core beliefs give rise to negative automatic thoughts, such as "I will never be able to do this," "Even when I try hard (at school, with peers), I still fail," "Everyone else is more successful at these tasks than I am," and "Everyone thinks I'm dumb." Additionally, these settings often promote repeated comparison to higher-achieving peers, both on the part of the individual (i.e., comparing themselves to others who are experiencing more success) and by adults (i.e., teachers and parents). Even when this comparison by others is well intended, it has the potential to do harm as it further perpetuates the individual's negative perception of self. Finally, those students whose executive functioning deficits impact them later in their academic career (i.e., when the demands of middle school or high school outpace their executive functioning skills) might also bear the additional burden of "knowing that they used to be smart/capable/socially adept," which can exacerbate the frequency and/or intensity of their thoughts and feelings of inadequacy.

As described above, treating individuals with executive functioning deficits utilizing cognitive-behavioral techniques can not only result in improved understanding and application of effective executive functioning skills but can also reduce negative cognitions and improve mood and emotional regulation (Emerson et al., 2005; Huang et al., 2019; Mohlman, 2008; Safren et al., 2005; Vidal-Estrada et al., 2012). As such, when planning treatment, CBT techniques such as psychoeducation (including a focus on metacognition), cognitive restructuring, and problem solving should be at the forefront of the plan. Additionally, collaborative goal-setting tasks will be critical and, generally speaking, should be implemented at the outset of treatment.

When implemented in the context of a CBT treatment plan, effective goal-setting exercises serve the critical dual purpose of affirming the need for treatment while assuring that treatment goals remain relevant to the client. When we consider this in the context of working with children and adolescents with executive functioning deficits in a school setting, the need for skilled goal setting becomes even more important. Specifically, it will often be the case that students with executive functioning deficits will be referred for treatment by someone who has identified that there is a need for intervention and is invested in helping improve the functioning and mood of the student (i.e., a stakeholder). Typically, these initial observations and analyses are made with input from multiple stakeholders, including parents, teachers, guidance counselors, and coaches. Notice the absence of an important stakeholder here—the student. While this is not always the case, oftentimes decisions about what a student needs and how best to meet those needs are made without input from the student, at least initially. This is even more likely to happen with individuals who struggle with their executive functions, as self-awareness is a form of metacognition, which falls under the umbrella of executive functioning. Put plainly, students with poor executive functioning often lack the self-awareness to know what isn't working and how to go about fixing it. As such, utilizing goal-setting strategies and activities that allow the therapist and the student to work collaboratively to determine what areas need to be addressed can serve as powerful tools for improving the efficacy of treatment.

Additionally, setting goals collaboratively within the context of a CBT session helps to maintain structure and focus both within and across sessions. This is a foundation for all effective CBT treatment and is perhaps even more critical when working with clients who struggle with internal mechanisms that support focus and attention (i.e., executive functions). By providing an explicit external structure that outlines agreed-upon goals and the roadmap by which those goals will be addressed (in the form of a treatment plan), the therapist helps to reduce the client's cognitive load. When this occurs, not only is treatment more productive, but it demonstrates to the client that incremental and effective change is possible, even when their struggles might seem overwhelming.

Session Structure When Working with Problem Area (Guiding)

Most CBT interventions use a combination of guided discovery, didactic exploration of the skill(s) being addressed, and appropriate reinforcement to accomplish therapeutic goals. Additionally, foundational components of CBT, such as agenda setting, pacing, and session structure, become especially critical when working with children and adolescents with executive dysfunction (Roscoe et al., 2022). When developing an effective treatment plan, practitioners must not only consider the areas to be targeted, but they must also conduct a careful and thoughtful analysis of *how* the interventions will proceed. For example, consider the process of agenda setting with a child or adolescent who has executive functioning deficits. Defined broadly, agenda setting within the context of CBT is an opportunity for the therapist and client to work together to determine the focus of the session. For their part, the therapist is trained to use the agenda-setting process to maintain a sense of collaboration and connection with the client, while ensuring that specific problem(s) will be addressed during the session. When applied effectively, agenda-setting empowers the client to partner with the therapist and develop the skills needed to influence their own treatment, thus supporting an ongoing dynamic of collaborative empiricism. When working with children and adolescents with executive functioning deficits, therapists must be aware that the very nature of their deficits often make it difficult for these clients to participate in agenda setting. Put simply, individuals who experience real-world difficulties with task initiation, planning, prioritizing, time management, and self-awareness/metacognition (all component skills of agenda setting) will bring these difficulties into therapy with them. Does this mean that the therapist should forgo trying to set an agenda (or, perhaps even worse, simply set the agenda on behalf of the client)? Certainly not. As indicated above, skipping or co-opting the agenda-setting component of a CBT session would undermine the collaborative problem-solving approach that is a hallmark of CBT. Instead, when working with children and adolescents with executive functioning deficits, the therapist must remain aware that clients may need explicit instruction and support in order to develop the skills needed to participate in the process of agenda setting. By bearing this in mind, an effective CBT practitioner can use agenda-setting as a therapeutic intervention that not only will facilitate increased participation in therapy but will simultaneously support the development of critical skills that will improve their client's functioning outside of therapy.

As with agenda setting, there are other components of CBT that will necessarily be impacted by client deficits. Just as intervention strategies are selected based on the tasks that need to be accomplished (e.g., homework completion, organization of time and materials, managing social demands) and the requisite skills needed to accomplish the tasks (e.g., initiation, sustained attention, emotional regulation), CBT session structure must also be tailored to meet the specific needs of the client. To this end, Dawson and Guare (2014) differentiate between two types of tasks: those that we are not entirely capable of accomplishing and those that, while we are capable of accomplishing, we simply do not want to do or "just don't like doing" (p. 431). In a practical sense, the results can look the same (i.e., the task does not get accomplished); however, the distinction can be important in the context of structuring CBT for children and adolescents who are struggling to complete necessary tasks, as is often the case with executive dysfunction. Analysis of the type of task in conjunction with consideration of the type of deficit (e.g., "can't do it" or "don't like/want to do it") allows the therapist to structure the CBT session that increases positive outcomes while addressing deficits that would otherwise hinder progress early on in the treatment process. Specifically, when a students is struggling with a task or area of functioning because they "can't do it," interventions should first include psychoeducation focused on building awareness of what is needed to successfully complete the task, as well as self-awareness regarding the skills and capacities the students currently has and does not have to be successful. Next, tasks can be broken down into small steps, which are then explained and practiced until the child or adolescent becomes fluent. In session, this process often involves didactic instruction (i.e., teaching the client what to do), guided practice with feedback, and role play. The therapist and client then determine naturalized settings in which the skill(s) are needed and, finally, the client commits to practicing the skills outside of therapy, with the understanding that more practice and rehearsal will be available as needed.

When it is determined that the child or adolescent possesses a requisite skill to be successful, yet does not demonstrate the ability or willingness to apply the skill successfully, interventions typically take on a different focus. In this case, the therapist's primarily goal is to help the child or adolescent learn to ignore or override the desire to quit (i.e., simply not perform the task or not perform it consistently) and/or the desire to engage in more enjoyable preferred tasks instead (Dawson & Guare, 2014). Interestingly, this can be accomplished in somewhat the same manner as the "can't do it" tasks described above. The therapist can effectively use psychoeducation to help the child or adolescent understand the connection between executive functioning difficulties and successful task completion (even when we know how to complete the task). Next, the therapist and client can work together to break down the task into small steps in order to determine how to create a first step that feels easy enough for the client to do without feeling the urge to quit or to do something more fun. Finally, both approaches described above involve scaffolding of a task, which Dawson and Guare (2014) aptly explain as, "The key is to determine how far the child can get on her own and then intervene – not by doing the task for her but by offering enough support…to get her over the hump and moving on to success" (p. 432).

Component of Practice and Intervention Modules (Intervening)

Problem Area: Forgetting Materials at Home Such as Lunch Box, Water Bottle, Reading Book, Instrument, and Tablet

This is a common difficulty observed in students with executive functioning challenges and involves a few executive functioning struggles. The child may have difficulty *organizing* herself in the morning and her materials may consistently be scattered throughout the house instead of gathered together the night before in one place to conveniently grab when she is ready to walk out. She may attempt to gather her materials ahead of time but her *working memory* deficits may cause her to forget one or two items consistently. She may begin to gather her materials for school and then may be *distracted* by something else and not *complete the task.* Below are a few suggestions on how to intervene with a student who consistently forgets materials at home, collaborating with the student and her parents or caregivers at home as well as her teacher at school.

1 (Home) Begin with a checklist in an area where she will gather the materials each night before she goes to bed, i.e. the area where she keeps her bookbag. On this checklist should be each item she will need when she walks out the door for the bus in the morning. The checklist should be clear and bulleted with simple, short language:

   - Flute
   - Water bottle
   - Lunch box
   - Reading book
   - Tablet

2 (Home) Utilize a smart device, such as Alexa, Siri, or Google, to set a reminder both in the evening to remind her to gather her items and in the morning to check her list before leaving. Many times, lists are developed for students, but they are not effective if the student does not remember to check the list.
3 (School) If she arrives at school and all items have arrived with her, reinforce with a basic behavior chart, following the rules of reinforcement, i.e. begin with rewarding her for three days of items arriving then up the stakes once consistently achieved.
4 (Both) Natural consequences can be very important in this particular situation. When the student did not remember an item before intervention began, her mother would run the forgotten item to her, resulting in no consequence for her forgetting. In getting her mother to agree not to do this, the student now understands that she will have to do without if she does not remember. In contrast, remembering her items, being reinforced with her chart, feeling responsible and accomplished for achieving this, and thinking "I can do this myself; I don't need my mom to bring me my stuff after all" will also be a reinforcing natural consequence.
5 (School) Lastly, teaming her up with a peer buddy, perhaps someone who also needs assistance in this area, so they can look at their in-school checklists together and pack their bookbags together will be reinforcing as she will now have a partner in her goal. This will also allow her to understand that she is not the only student "in the world" who experiences these struggles or "falls short" in these areas. If a peer is not available for this purpose, then it will be helpful for her to meet with a teacher, paraprofessional, or even check in with her guidance counselor at the end of the day to review her checklist of items to go home.

Assessment of Progress and Outcomes (Monitoring)

For the case above, several monitoring measures can be employed to help determine if this particular intervention is working, if adjustments should be made, or when it is time to adjust the schedule of reinforcement. In addition, other executive functioning difficulties may present during these times due to external demands changing academically, socially, and recreationally. For example, in the above example, if the student begins a sports season, she may begin to forget her mouth guard for field hockey resulting in missed practices and subsequently missed game time as a consequence for not practicing. This will likely, in turn, leave her with a sense of poor self-adequacy and failure. Simple measures can be put into place to help determine what is and is not working and additional areas that should be addressed in her plan.

1 Using an EF inventory—Utilizing statistically driven measures (such as the BRIEF-2) or having the student collaborate with the therapist to create his or her own data keeping measure will allow the student to track and "see" progress or areas of need from a data driven perspective.

2 Diary keeping is an effective tool for students in self-monitoring and self-assessing progress in CBT interventions (Evans-Jones, 2011). Having the student record their own experience of their progress and areas that they see success and needs for growth can be both useful in intervention as well as building self-awareness and feelings of self-efficacy (Evans-Jones, 2011).
3 Charting behaviors can be visually effective, especially for younger children. This will not only allow the child to see when their target behavior is improving but also helps to track when there will be a reinforcer or reward.

Applications to the School Setting

Although we have access to decades' worth of data affirming the efficacy of using CBT to treat children and adolescents, studies suggest that there is still a dilemma of accessibility (Dobson, 2022; Kendall et al., 2023). In other words, there is an increasingly unmet need for mental health services for children and adolescents (National Association of School Psychologists [NASP], 2021; Thompson et al., 2008). Specifically, data provided by the US Department of Health and Human Services reveal that approximately 20% of children and adolescents experience a problem with their mental health during their school-aged years (NASP, 2021). Sadly, most of these children and adolescents do not receive the necessary therapeutic interventions that prevent the persistence and exacerbation of their difficulties. While the barriers to accessing appropriate and effective mental health care are myriad for a variety of children (and well beyond the scope of this discussion), disparities in access to care are particularly prevalent among minority students and within low-income communities (NASP, 2021). In fact, according to data reported by the Substance Abuse and Mental Health Services Administration (2019), among the 3.8 million adolescents aged 12–17 who report a major depressive episode, nearly 60% do not receive any treatment. Similarly, the majority of adolescents who exhibit symptoms of anxiety also do not receive treatment, and among those who do, there are frequently lengthy delays between onset of symptoms and access to treatment (Chavira et al., 2004; Heiervang et al., 2007). It is statistics such as these that underscore the mental health crises facing many of our children and adolescents.

What about the youth who do not have access to effective mental health treatment? We have the data to support the need for and importance of this, but how do these children and adolescents access services? According to the National Association of School Psychologists (NASP), the answer is short: in school. Recall the 2019 data provided by the Substance Abuse and Mental Health Services Administration referenced above. Of the roughly 40% of adolescents who received mental health treatment, approximately two-thirds of them did so in school (NASP, 2021). Per NASP (2021), schools are an optimal place to provide mental health services to children and adolescents. In some instances, including in rural regions, schools represent the *only* access to therapeutic services. Finally, studies show that students are more likely to seek help when services are available in their schools (NASP, 2021). From a more prosaic perspective, providing evidence-based mental health interventions, including CBT, in schools makes sense because that is where children and adolescents spend the majority of their time (Mychailyszyn et al., 2011; NASP, 2021).

Achieving a more widespread application of effective and empirically supported interventions is paramount to treating the critical mental health needs of children and adolescents. Choosing CBT as a driver of these interventions in schools is also a clear choice. It has already been established that CBT is widely empirically validated for use with children and adolescents. Additionally, utilizing CBT to remediate executive functioning deficits and the resulting negative automatic thoughts and emotions that further impact an individual's mood and functioning is also a data-driven decision. Thus, applying data-based interventions in the place where children and adolescents spend several hours a day, often facing the very demands and stressors that result from executive functioning deficit is certainly best practice.

Case Study of Problem Area

JM is a 7th-grade student at Lincoln Middle School. During the fall of his 7th-grade school year, he starts out strong, both academically and socially. However, as the first marking period continues and the workload increases, his grades gradually begin to trend downward. JM's teachers are concerned about his falling grades and make a referral to Dr. Smith, the school psychologist. When Dr. Smith reviews JM's academic and behavioral data after Winter break, she notes that, not only are JM's grades lower than at any prior time in his academic history (i.e., predominantly Cs in core classes with the exception of History, which has traditionally been his favorite class), but he has also begun to demonstrate mild behavioral problems in the classroom. Specifically, his teachers are reporting that JM is frequently speaking out of turn (although not disrespectfully), walking in late for class continually, speaking to his buddies when he should be working on independent work, and frequently asking to go to the bathroom. In an effort to create a full picture of JM's functioning across settings, Dr. Smith reaches out to JM's mother to gather data about any changes in functioning outside of school. Through this conversation, Dr. Smith learns that JM's mother is also concerned about his declining grades. Ms. M. also reports changes in JM's behavior at home that are worrisome to her. She has observed that JM has become increasingly moody, has been isolating in his room more than he ever has, and has been talking back more frequently. She also notes that while JM has always been a bit disorganized, his room is messier than it has ever been. Ms. M. sums up the interview by stating, "I just don't know what's been going on with him. He's always been my easy kid; now I'm starting to get worried."

Next, Dr. Smith schedules a time to meet JM. At first, JM reacts as a typical adolescent student, reporting that he is "fine" and that "seventh grade is just hard." Dr. Smith probes this topic by asking pointed questions about JM's reported difficulties, such as "Are you handing in your homework on time?", "How is your performance on tests?", and "Do you realize when you do not do well, or are you surprised by your grades?" JM becomes teary in the office and begins to report that he is struggling both academically and socially. He describes himself as "very disorganized" and explains that, even though he typically does his homework, he frequently forgets to hand it in or to submit it. JM also reports that sometimes he "just completely forgets" that he has an assignment to complete at all.

Table 20.1 Initial Treatment Goals

Initial Treatment Goals for JM
1 Organization/Planning: Getting JM to not only write down assignments ahead of time, remember to check his planner for the assignments and complete them, but also have him hand in all completed assignments
2 Completing tasks (e.g., handing in homework): Establishing a plan with the teachers to cue JM if he has not handed in his assignments by the end of the class period. Working on also establishing a reinforcer for JM when he remembers to hand in all assignments independently without cueing
3 Task monitoring/Self-monitoring: Having JM note briefly in his planner whether or not he completed these assignments and required cueing. Tracking this information on a self-report inventory created by JM and his therapist each week at the beginning of the session to determine progress
4 Regulating emotions and coping with frustration: When JM requires "alone time" in his room, having a note on his door that indicates this. However, also encouraging him open up to his mother for 15 minutes (or more) each evening to summarize how his day went, including his social day
5 Social demands and navigating different personalities: Encouraging JM to reach out to one of his "old buddies" and one new friend each week in an attempt to begin to meld the two groups together. When a topic becomes too uncomfortable for him in one group, he will then actively seek out another group where he knows someone and is comfortable interacting with that person. He will attempt to jot down these interactions in a diary each night or every other night and will share his progress in session with the therapist

He states that he does not want to do badly in school and has never forgotten to do homework "on purpose." JM feels badly, not only because of his poor grades but also for disappointing his teachers and his mother when he fails to do an assignment.

When asked about his social functioning in 7th grade, JM reports that he is unable to navigate the social demands of middle school as well as he had when he was in elementary school. JM has always been a student who was well liked by his peers and adults in school; however, when the middle school melded with two other elementary schools, JM felt pressured to maintain his "popular" status but was unsure of how to interact with all of the new kids. He explains that he had grown up with many of his closest friends since they were in daycare together. JM describes having to manage new social interactions and establish new friends as "confusing and sometimes scary." He also reports that many of his friends are "into girls" and he really isn't yet, so this was another area where he felt lost and confused. When asked about how he handles these emotions, JM states that he often listens to music in his room and tries to forget about his day. He also reports that he feels that he "shouldn't cry in front of other kids," so he will also isolate himself when he feels upset or avoids situations where he may get upset (Tables 20.1 and 20.2).

Table 20.2 Sample Session Outline

Week/Session	*Information Covered Within Session*
I	Introduction of the principles of CBT, psychoeducation about executive functioning/dysfunction, and related social/emotional problems that arise with these difficulties
II	Identify areas of concern and prioritize what is most distressing for the student, question current behaviors/ways of doing things, thoughts behind current behavior/actions, challenge evidence that supports or does not support current behavior/actions
III	Begin to generate alternatives to current thoughts and behaviors, assess how he/she feels about these alternatives, i.e. avoiding work that must be done versus scheduling out time to tackle work in smaller more manageable chunks with a feeling of accomplishment for each time these goals are achieved
IV	Identify possible consequences to alternative actions • How could these consequences lead to different thoughts, feelings, and overall outcomes? (feelings of frustration and stress over accomplishment and control) • What are potential long-term outcomes of these new actions/consequences/thoughts? (academic successes, free time for socialization, less stress in the family dynamic, etc.)
V	Brainstorm potential obstacles or barriers that may get in the way of these alternative ways of doing and thinking (additional projects, new social "threats," a bad grade). Develop a plan for how to identify an obstacle and then to respond by attempting another action: What is your Plan B? Can the student shift and is this a new way of functioning for the student as this too is an executive function?
VI	Putting the plan into action: collaboratively crafting a behavioral experiment to test the new plan. How will we evaluate outcomes? Standard measures, self-measures, diary keeping, charting?
VII	Evaluating effectiveness of the experiment: • Did it work? • What were the consequences or outcomes of the new behavior? • Was Plan B needed? If so, why was it needed? Was Plan B successful? • Next steps?
VIII	Begin again with new set of thoughts/behaviors until the student begins to effectively implement these steps into their own ability to problem solve through executive functioning challenges

Summary

Executive functioning struggles are a common difficulty for students and cause significant disturbances in academic, behavioral, emotional, and social functioning. When experiencing executive dysfunction, students can have difficulty with initiation, self-monitoring, planning, inhibition, flexibility of thought, directing attention, task monitoring, organization of materials and time, and emotional regulation, to name a few. These struggles affect school performance and social performance, and can have adverse behavioral manifestations. Students' thoughts can be disrupted with self-deprecating statements such as "I am dumb," "I am less than," and "I can't." As these thoughts and behaviors are perpetuated due to the students' poor executive functioning and inability to fix the problem, beliefs surrounding poor self-reliance, poor self-efficacy, and poor self-esteem increase, resulting in dysfunctional cognitions. These negative core beliefs and dysfunctional cognitions eventually cause mood disturbance such as anxiety and depression. With effective CBT, the therapist and the student are able to collaborate through well-established and empirically driven techniques to turn this cycle of self-defeating behaviors, thoughts, and feelings into a positive cycle of behavior change, increased academic self-efficacy, increased confidence, improved motivation, and ability to achieve goals.

Reflection Questions

1 Executive functions permeate most aspects of a person's life. Consider how a student with executive functioning deficits is impacted as they move throughout their school day. What implications does this have for their learning, behavioral functioning, and social-emotional well-being?
2 Providing CBT on an individual basis to students with executive functioning deficits is an example of an intensive school-based intervention. What are some adjunctive interventions/supports that could be implemented at the universal and targeted level to address these deficits?
3 What are potential barriers to treatment (both intrinsic and external) that a child or adolescent might face that are specifically related to their executive functioning difficulties? How would you troubleshoot these?

References

Aldao, A., Gee, D. G., De Los Reyes, A., & Seager, I. (2016). Emotion regulation as a transdiagnostic factor in the development of internalizing and externalizing psychopathology: Current and future directions. *Development and Psychopathology, 28*(4), 927–946. https://doi.org/10.1017/S0954579416000638

American Psychiatric Association (APA) (2022). Neurodevelopmental disorder. In G. Baird (Ed.), *Diagnostic and statistical manual of mental disorders* (5th ed., text rev., pp. 35–99). Published by Author, Washington, DC.

Asnaani, A., Tyler, J., McCann, J., Brown, L., & Zang, Y. (2020). Anxiety sensitivity and emotion regulation as mechanisms of successful CBT outcome for anxiety-related disorders in a naturalistic treatment setting. *Journal of Affective Disorders, 267*, 86–95. https://doi.org/10.1016/j.jad.2020.01.160

Barkley, R. (1990). *Attention deficit hyperactivity disorder: A handbook for diagnosis and treatment*. New York: Guilford Press.

Barkley, R. A. (2006). *Attention deficit hyperactivity disorder: A handbook for diagnosis and treatment*. New York: Guilford.

Bose, D., Proenza, D. A., Costales, G., Viswesvaran, C., Bickman, L., & Pettit, J. W. (2022). Therapeutic alliance in psychosocial interventions for youth internalizing disorders: A systematic review and preliminary meta-analysis. *Clinical Psychology: Science and Practice, 29*(2), 124–136. https://doi.org/10.1037/cps0000052

Boyer, B. E., Geurts, H. M., Prins, P. J., & Van der Oord, S. (2015). Two novel CBTs for adolescents with ADHD: The value of planning skills. *European Child & Adolescent Psychiatry, 24*(9), 1075–1090. https://doi.org/10.1007/s00787-014-0661-5

Chavira, D. A., Stein, M. B., Bailey, K., & Stein, M. T. (2004). Child anxiety in primary care: Prevalent but untreated. *Depression and Anxiety, 20*(4), 155–164. https://doi.org/10.1002/da.20039

Chiappini, E. A., Gosch, E. A., Compton, S. N., Olino, T. M., Birmaher, B. B., Sakolsky, D., Peris, T. S., Piacentini, J., Albano, A. M., Keeton, C. P., Walkup, J. T., Ginsburg, G. S., & Kendall, P. C. (2020). In-session involvement in anxious youth receiving CBT with/without medication. *Journal of Psychopathology and Behavioral Assessment, 42*(6), 1–12.

Compton, S. N., March, J. S., Brent, D., Albano, A. M., 5th, Weersing, R., & Curry, J. (2004). Cognitive-behavioral psychotherapy for anxiety and depressive disorders in children and adolescents: An evidence-based medicine review. *Journal of the American Academy of Child and Adolescent Psychiatry, 43*(8), 930–959. https://doi.org/10.1097/01.chi.0000127589.57468.bf

Dawson, P., & Guare, R. (2014). Interventions to promote executive development in children and adolescents. In S. Goldstein & J. A. Naglieri (Eds.), *Handbook of executive functioning* (pp. 427–444). Springer. https://doi.org/10.1007/978-1-4614-8106-5

Derella, O. J., Johnston, O. G., Loeber, R., & Burke, J. D. (2019). CBT-enhanced emotion regulation as a mechanism of improvement for childhood irritability. *Journal of Clinical Child and Adolescent Psychology: The Official Journal for the Society of Clinical Child and Adolescent Psychology, American Psychological Association, Division 53, 48*(sup1), S146–S154. https://doi.org/10.1080/15374416.2016.1270832

Dobson, K. S. (2022). Therapeutic relationship. *Cognitive and Behavioral Practice, 29*(3), 541–544. https://doi.org/10.1016/j.cbpra.2022.02.006

Emerson, C. S., Mollet, G. A., & Harrison, D. W. (2005). Anxious-depression in boys: An evaluation of executive functioning. *Archives of Clinical NNeuropsychology: The Official Journal of the National Academy of Neuropsychologists, 20*(4), 539–546. https://doi.org/10.1016/j.acn.2004.10.003

Evans-Jones, C. (2011). *The CBT handbook: Cognitive behavioural therapy* (1st ed.). Routledge. https://doi.org/10.4324/9781315174082

Freire, C., Ferradás, M. D. M., Regueiro, B., Rodríguez, S., Valle, A., & Núñez, J. C. (2020). Coping strategies and self-efficacy in university students: A person-centered approach. *Frontiers in Psychology, 11*, 841. https://doi.org/10.3389/fpsyg.2020.00841

Goldstein, S., Naglieri, J. A., Princiotta, D., & Otero, T. M. (2014). Introduction: A history of executive functioning as a theoretical and clinical construct. In S. Goldstein & J. A. Naglieri (Eds.), *Handbook of executive functioning* (pp. 427–444). Springer. https://doi.org/10.1007/978-1-4614-8106-5

Golombek, K., Lidle, L., Tuschen-Caffier, B., Schmitz, J., & Vierrath, V. (2020). The role of emotion regulation in socially anxious children and adolescents: A systematic review. *European Child & Adolescent Psychiatry, 29*(11), 1479–1501. https://doi.org/10.1007/s00787-019-01359-9

Grenell, M. M., Glass, C. R., & Katz, K. S. (1987). Hyperactive children and peer interaction: Knowledge and performance of social skills. *Journal of Abnormal Child Psychology, 15*(1), 1–13. https://doi.org/10.1007/BF00916462

Groom, M. J., & Cortese, S. (2022). Current pharmacological treatments for ADHD. *Current Topics in Behavioral Neurosciences, 57*, 19–50. https://doi.org/10.1007/7854_2022_330.

Groves, N. B., Wells, E. L., Soto, E. F., Marsh, C. L., Jaisle, E. M., Harvey, T. K., & Kofler, M. J. (2022 Jun). Executive functioning and emotion regulation in children with and without ADHD. *Research on Child and Adolescent Psychopathology, 50*(6), 721–735. https://doi.org/10.1007/s10802-021-00883-0. Epub 2021 Nov11.

Heiervang, E., Stormark, K. M., Lundervold, A. J., Heimann, M., Goodman, R., Posserud, M. B., Ullebø, A. K., Plessen, K. J., Bjelland, I., Lie, S. A., & Gillberg, C. (2007). Psychiatric disorders in Norwegian 8- to 10-year-olds: An epidemiological survey of prevalence, risk factors, and service use. *Journal of the American Academy of Child and Adolescent Psychiatry, 46*(4), 438–447. https://doi.org/10.1097/chi.0b013e31803062bf

Holmes, J., Gathercole, S. E., Place, M., Alloway, T. P., Elliot, J. G., & Hilton, K. A. (2010). The diagnostic utility of executive function assessments in the identification of ADHD in children. *Child and Adolescent Mental Health, 15*(1), 37–43. http://doi.org/10.1111/j.1475-3588.2009.00536.x

Huang, F. Y., Hsu, A. L., Hsu, L. M., Tsai, J. S., Huang, C. M., Chao, Y. P., Hwang, T. J., & Wu, C. W. (2019). Mindfulness improves emotion regulation and executive control on bereaved individuals: An fMRI study. *Frontiers in Human Neuroscience, 12*, 541. https://doi.org/10.3389/fnhum.2018.00541

Kaplan, V., Düken, M. E., Kaya, R., & Almazan, J. (2023). Investigating the effects of a cognitive- behavioral-therapy-based psychoeducation program on university students' automatic thoughts, perceived stress, and self-efficacy levels. *Journal of Research & Health, 13*(2), 87–98. http://dx.doi.org/10.32598/JRH.13.2.2125.1

Kendall, P. C., Ney, J. S., Maxwell, C. A., Lehrbach, K. R., Jakubovic, R. J., McKnight, D. S., & Friedman, A. L. (2023). Adapting CBT for youth anxiety: Flexibility, within fidelity, in different settings. *Frontiers in Psychiatry, 14*, 1067047. https://doi.org/10.3389/fpsyt.2023.1067047

Kürümlüoğlugil, R., & Tanrıverdi, D. (2022). The effects of psychoeducation on cognitive distortions, negative automatic thoughts and dysfunctional attitudes of patients diagnosed with depression. *Psychology, Health & Medicine, 27*(10), 2085–2095. http://doi.org/10.1080/13548506.2021.1944654

Landau, S., & Milich, R. (1988). Social communication patterns of attention deficit disordered boys. *Journal of Abnormal Child Psychology, 16*, 69–86.

Mares, D., McLuckie, A., Schwartz, M., & Saini, M. (2007 Aug). Executive function impairments in children with attention deficit hyperactivity disorder: Do they differ between school and home environments? *Canadian Journal of Psychiatry, 52*(8), 527–534. https://doi.org/10.1177?070674370705200811

Marker, C. D., Comer, J. S., Abramova, V., & Kendall, P. C. (2013). The reciprocal relationship between alliance and symptom improvement across the treatment of childhood anxiety. *Journal of Clinical Child and Adolescent Psychology: The Official Journal for the Society of Clinical Child and Adolescent Psychology, American Psychological Association, Division 53, 42*(1), 22–33. https://doi.org/10.1080/15374416.2012.723261

McLeod, B. D. (2011). Relation of the alliance with outcomes in youth psychotherapy: A meta-analysis. *Clinical Psychology Review, 31*(4), 603–616. https://doi.org/10.1016/j.cpr.2011.02.001

Meltzer, L J., Reddy, R., Sales, L., Roditi, B., Sayer, J., & Theokas, C. (2004). Positive and negative self-perceptions: Is there a cyclical relationship between teachers' and students' perceptions of effort, strategy use, and academic performance? *Learning Disabilities Research & Practice, 19*(1), 33–44.

Miklós, M., Futó, J., Komáromy, D., & Balázs, J. (2019 Oct 10). Executive function and attention performance in children with ADHD: Effects of medication and comparison with typically developing children. *International Journal of Environmental Research and Public Health, 16*(20), 3822. https://doi.org/10.3390/ijerph16203822

Miyake, A., Friedman, N. P., Emerson, M. J., Witzki, A. H., Howerter, A., & Wager, T. D. (2000). The unity and diversity of executive functions and their contributions to complex "frontal lobe" tasks: A latent variable analysis. *Cognitive Psychology, 41*(1), 49–100. https://doi.org/10.1006/cogp.1999.0734

Mohlman, J. (2008). More power to the executive? A preliminary test of CBT plus executive skills training for treatment of late-life GAD. *Cognitive and Behavioral Practice, 15*(3), 306–316. https://doi.org/10.1016/j.cbpra.2007.07.002

Monteiro, E. M. (2022). An ecologically valid understanding of executive functioning. *Psychology in Schools, 59*(7), 1390–1401. https./doi.org/10.1002/pits.22627

Mychailyszyn, M. P., Beidas, R. S., Benjamin, C. L., Edmunds, J. M., Podell, J. L., Cohen, J. S., & Kendall, P. C. (2011). Assessing and treating child anxiety in schools. *Psychology in the Schools, 48*(3), 223–232. https://doi.org/10.1002/pits.20548

Nakao, M., Shirotsuki, K., & Sugaya, N. (2021). Cognitive-behavioral therapy for management of mental health and stress-related disorders: Recent advances in techniques and technologies. *BioPsychoSocial Medicine, 15*(1), 16. https://doi.org/10.1186/s13030-021-00219-w

National Association of School Psychologists (NASP) (2021). *Comprehensive school-based mental and behavioral health services and school psychologists* [handout]. Author. Retrieved from https://www.nasponline.org/resources-and-publications/resources-and-podcasts/mental-and-behavioral-health/additional-resources/comprehensive-school-based-mental-and-behavioral-health-services-and-school-psychologists

Otterman, D. L., Koopman-Verhoeff, M. E., White, T. J., Tiemeier, H., Bolhuis, K., & Jansen, K. W. (2019 Oct 22). Executive functioning and neurodevelopmental disorders in early childhood: A prospective population-based study. *Child Adolesc Psychiatry Ment Health,* 13–38. https://doi.org/10.1186/s13034-019-0299-7

Pan, M. R., Huang, F., Zhao, M. J., Wang, Y. F., Wang, Y. F., & Qian, Q. J. (2019). A comparison of efficacy between cognitive behavioral therapy (CBT) and CBT combined with medication in adults with attention-deficit/hyperactivity disorder (ADHD). *Psychiatry Research, 279*, 23–33. https://doi.org/10.1016/j.psychres.2019.06.040

Pruessner, L., Barnow, S., Holt, D. V., Joormann, J., & Schulze, K. (2020). A cognitive control framework for understanding emotion regulation flexibility. *Emotion (Washington, DC), 20*(1), 21–29. https://doi.org/10.1037/emo0000658

Ransom, D. M., Burns, A. R., Youngstrom, E. A., Vaughan, C. G., Sady, M. D., & Gioia, G. A. (2016 Nov). Applying an evidence-based assessment model to identify students at risk for perceived academic problems following concussion. *Journal of the International Neuropsychological Society, 22*(10), 1038–1049. https://doi.org/10.1017/S1355617716000916

Renshaw, P. D., & Asher, S. R. (1983). Social knowledge and sociometric status: Children's goals and strategies for social interaction. *Journal of Learning Disabilities, 17*, 560–567

Roscoe, J., Bates, E., & Blackley, R. (2022). 'It was like the unicorn of the therapeutic world': CBT trainee experiences of acquiring skills in guided discovery. *The Cognitive Behaviour Therapist, 15*, E32. https://doi.org/10.1017/S1754470X22000277

Safren, S. A., Otto, M. W., Sprich, S., Winett, C. L., Wilens, T. E., & Biederman, J. (2005). Cognitive-behavioral therapy for ADHD in medication-treated adults with continued symptoms. *Behaviour Research and Therapy, 43*(7), 831–842. https://doi.org/10.1016/j.brat.2004.07.001

Safren, S. A., Sprich, S., Chulvick, S., & Otto, M. W. (2004). Psychosocial treatments for adults with attention-deficit/hyperactivity disorder. *The Psychiatric Clinics of North America, 27*(2), 349–360. https://doi.org/10.1016/S0193-953X(03)00089-3

Steward, K. A., Tan, A., Delgaty, L., Gonzales, M. M., & Bunner, M. (2017). Self-awareness of executive functioning deficits in adolescents with ADHD. *Journal of Attention Disorders, 21*(4), 316–322. https://doi.org/10.1177/1087054714530782. Epub 2016 Jul 28

Suveg, C., Sood, E., Comer, J. S., & Kendall, P. C. (2009). Changes in emotion regulation following cognitive-behavioral therapy for anxious youth. *Journal of Clinical Child and Adolescent Psychology: The Official Journal for the Society of Clinical Child and Adolescent Psychology, American Psychological Association, Division 53, 38*(3), 390–401. https://doi.org/10.1080/15374410902851721

Thompson, A., Issakidis, C., & Hunt, C. (2008). Delay to seek treatment for anxiety and mood disorders in an Australian clinical sample. *Behaviour Change, 25*(2), 71–84. https://doi.org/10.1375/bech.25.2.71

Toolin, D. (2016). *Doing CBT: A comprehensive guide to working with behaviors, thoughts, and emotions*. New York: The Guilford Press.

Toren, P., Sadeh, M., Wolmer, L., Eldar, S., Koren, S., Weizman, R., & Laor, N. (2000). Neurocognitive correlates of anxiety disorders in children: A preliminary report. *Journal of Anxiety Disorders, 14*(3), 239–247. https://doi.org/10.1016/s0887-6185(99)00036-5

Tripp, G., & Wickens, J. R. (2009 Dec). Neurobiology of ADHD. *Neuropharmacology, 57*(7–8), 579–589. https://doi.org/10.1016/j.neuropharm.2009.07.026. Epub 2009 Jul 21.

Vidal-Estrada, R., Bosch-Munso, R., Nogueira-Morais, M., Casas-Brugue, M., & Ramos-Quiroga, J. A. (2012). Psychological treatment of attention deficit hyperactivity disorder in adults: A systematic review. *Actas Españolas de Psiquiatria, 40*(3), 147–154.

Warren, S. L., Heller, W., & Miller, G. A. (2021). The structure of executive dysfunction in depression and anxiety. *Journal of Affective Disorders, 279*, 208–216. https://doi.org/10.1016/j.jad.2020.09.132

Young, K. S., Sandman, C. F., & Craske, M. G. (2019). Positive and negative emotion regulation in adolescence: Links to anxiety and depression. *Brain Sciences, 9*(4), 76. https://doi.org/10.3390/brainsci9040076

Zeman, J., Shipman, K., & Suveg, C. (2002). Anger and sadness regulation: Predictions to internalizing and externalizing symptoms in children. *Journal of Clinical Child and Adolescent Psychology, 31*(3), 393–398. https://doi.org/10.1207/153744202760082658

21

SCROLL LESS, LIVE MORE

CBT Strategies for Balanced Media and Device Use

Jessica L. Stewart and Ray W. Christner

In the past decade, significantly more people have owned smartphones (30%–85% between the years 2011 and 2012; Laricchia, 2022), including children and adolescents, and devices are an integral part of the lives of not only working adults but also youth in educational settings. Thus, media and device use (MDU) has rapidly increased. Constructive MDU practices have become intrinsic to modern education, from elementary levels to advanced degrees, including accessing classroom lessons and curriculum content, using digital platforms and online resources to complete assignments and for learning, studying, sharing resources, viewing educational content, creating e-flashcards, completing group projects, etc. In many schools, students engage with the curriculum via individual devices (e.g., one-to-one iPad programs, personal district-provided chromebooks) from the start of homeroom through the final bell and to complete homework at night. Feasibly, students may spend anywhere from 6 to 12 hours "in front of a screen" to keep up with academic expectations.

For both children and adults, MDU is likely a combination of necessary time (e.g., for schoolwork, connecting to one's social network and family, finding resources to support productivity, gaining knowledge relevant to one's health and well-being) and also pleasurable recreational time (e.g., gaming, scrolling social media, watching videos, accessing pornography, or online browsing). While there are, of course, immense positives of technology in exposing individuals to new concepts, ideas, information, perspectives, and social support, there are detrimental consequences of excessive and unhealthy MDU. Those who do not balance their use are negatively impacted by excessive and unhealthy MDU, contrasting starkly with those who harness media and devices in healthy ways (Stockings et al., 2016).

While experts offer considerations for MDU at different developmental levels (American Academy of Child and Adolescent Psychiatry, 2020; the American Academy of Pediatrics, 2021), these guidelines have moved away from simple "screen time" and instead now stress understanding the *functional impact* MDU has on the child's or adolescent's physical, mental, emotional, and social health, and ability to absorb information, learn, and meet life goals. Uncontrolled device use can lead to issues like disrupted sleep patterns, weight problems, reduced academic performance, poor self-image and body image issues, reduced physical activity, heightened stress, increased risk for anxiety and depression, and social concerns (American Academy of Child and Adolescent Psychiatry, 2020) including isolation, especially when digital interactions minimize the need for face-to-face socialization and connection. For students with learning difficulties, including ADHD, these issues (e.g., sleep or appetite disturbance, emotional challenges) exacerbate difficulties. In addition, when

DOI: 10.4324/9781003392439-24

used as a tool for coping with unwanted emotions, MDU limits one's ability to develop healthier ways to relax, cope, or find enjoyment off-screen. The key to determining what constitutes "unhealthy" MDU lies in understanding the extent to which such usage negatively impacts an individual's overall well-being and functioning, such as interpersonal relationships, health and well-being, and one's ability to meet their goals (including performing as a student). In these ways, unhealthy MDU mirrors addictive behaviors, such as gambling and substance abuse. Thus, we propose that the ideal intervention for problematic MDU would include components of treatment approaches that have been proven effective for addressing addictions, namely, *cognitive-behavior therapy that incorporates a harm reduction approach.*

Typically associated with substance abuse treatments, harm reduction strategies focus not on outright cessation but on mitigating the adverse effects of addictive behavior. While we are not talking solely about "addiction" when we are referring to unhealthy MDU, we believe utilizing a harm reduction approach can offer significant advantages when addressing the negative implications of excessive or problematic screen, media, and device use on youth well-being and functioning because it encourages more conscious awareness of the factors contributing to problematic aspects of this behavior *and* stresses the importance of empowering youth to build a healthier, more balanced relationship with that behavior—rather than seeing it as all "good" or "bad." The goal is to facilitate minimal negative impact of one's unavoidable relationship with technology. In a world increasingly dependent on screens, this is especially important for youth who will need to be empowered with the tools necessary to build a sustainable relationship with their MDU. A harm reduction approach provides insights into the implications of unhealthy use and expands intervention to facilitate a healthy relationship with technology (Tatarsky, 2003). However, the success of harm reduction methods depends heavily on participants' desire and voluntary commitment to change (McMahon et al., 2019). In the context of MDU, we believe that both increasing one's explicit understanding of the negative consequences of their device use *and* empowering their ability to choose alternative ways to address factors that contribute to their MDU (e.g., emotional coping, social needs, neurochemical reinforcement) will be instrumental in facilitating a greater commitment to moderate device use, thus reducing "dependency."

Harm reduction therapy was first incorporated as a component of formal treatment for internet addiction in adults by Young in 1995, who included this framework as the 3rd phase of her model known as CBT-IA (Cognitive Behavioral Therapy—Internet Addiction). While behavior therapy focused on reducing time on the internet, and cognitive restructuring addressed maladaptive thought patterns (including denial) that perpetuated the addictive and compulsive behavior, harm reduction strategies aimed to identify and treat coexisting issues such as psychiatric, vocational, and social/interpersonal (relationship) problems resulting from (although also contributing to) one's excessive internet use. In this chapter, we present our model of intervention that includes not only behavioral modification (including goal setting) and cognitive interventions (e.g., restructuring distortions and fear-based thinking, building self-esteem and competency) but also addresses emotional coping (including mindfulness-based practices), social dynamics and problem-solving, and physiological/neurobiological factors (e.g., mechanisms related to self-regulation and executive functioning) and does so through intervention modules that facilitate skill acquisition and application in each of these interrelated domains.

These modules are designed for application in both individual therapy and group-format interventions including prevention-focused, universal intervention in the school setting. Addressing these concerns within a group setting provides a number of benefits, from modeling and social comparison to accountability and a "natural laboratory" for building skills practice (Stewart & Christner, 2024). Greer and colleagues (2016) highlighted the benefits of peer involvement in harm reduction approaches, emphasizing its role in enhancing group therapy outcomes and fostering the acquisition and implementation of effective decision-making skills. Denning (2010) similarly stressed the important role that loved ones' support can play in the long-term success of harm reduction methods for substance abuse. We believe the involvement of positive peer and family member influence is also important within a harm reduction approach to modifying unhealthy MDU. This is especially true given that guardians can structure a youth's environment and access to screens and devices. They also can reinforce therapeutic principles and skills at home if they are involved in the intervention. We propose that strong familial support and constructive peer relationships can act as a protective factor, potentially reducing an individual's vulnerability to detrimental MDU habits (Stewart et al., 2024).

CBT Conceptualization of MDU

Within a growing field of research and treatment, many articles and books are singularly devoted to problematic MDU. An in-depth review of the expanding literature on factors contributing to the development of unhealthy MDU is beyond the scope of this chapter. In summary, theories attempt to differentiate between functional internet, media, gaming, and device use—that affords the user benefits for productivity, connectivity, simple leisure activity, and other aspects of wellness—and pathological use, which can be generalized in nature or of a more specific, function-based problem (e.g., internet gambling or pornography). Theories also attempt to explain the mechanisms contributing to unhealthy MDU, including neurobiological predispositions (e.g., neural structures and dopamine receptors), behavioral conditioning (e.g., classical conditioning, reinforcement principles), social factors (e.g., connectivity and finding a sense of belonging), cognitive aspects (e.g., cognitive biases and distortions, reduced sense of self-worth), and emotional coping (e.g., depression, escapism, numbing). The work of Brand and colleagues (2016), for example, presents a model that emphasizes the interplay between predisposing factors (e.g., neurobiological or psychological traits), moderators (e.g., coping styles and cognitive biases), and mediators (e.g., affective and cognitive responses to situational prompts and internet-related cognitive biases), along with reduced executive function skills, as together driving the onset and maintenance of addictive behavior. Our conceptualization of unhealthy MDU is most closely aligned with this work. However, we also stress the importance of behavioral aspects (certainly executive function skills, as well as conditioning principles) and social factors when conceptualizing not only the problem but also skills-focused interventions. The goal of CBT to address problematic MDU within a harm-reduction framework is to improve students' cognitive, emotional, and behavioral competencies so they will (1) be less likely to use MDU to address these needs and (2) more effectively manage life demands to minimize consequences related to their use of devices.

Clinicians must have a basic understanding of each of these factors and how they interact with (and potentially reinforce) each other in order to fully appreciate the function the MDU serves—especially when it persists despite the negative consequences the person experiences. Functional impact is determined by considering one's effective engagement in daily life activities, relationships, physical health, and psychological well-being. It is important to think about the mechanisms underlying an individual's drive to engage in MDU and determine which may be contributing most to that use being problematic, as well as which may be best targeted for intervention (e.g., neurobiological factors may not be changeable). We offer the following thoughts on each of the factors we feel contribute to unhealthy MDU.

Physiological and Neurobiological Processes

Research has definitively established the concept of neuroplasticity: that brains can structurally and functionally change and are adaptable. Specific to MDU, increasing research has also established that, especially for children during critical developmental periods, extensive screen use (and especially gaming) is leading to changes in neural tissue and function (Sigman, 2017). In particular, the development of problematic MDU is increasingly understood as being associated with maladaptive changes to regions associated with addiction: the frontal lobe (which is primarily responsible for executive function skills, such as inhibitory control) and the limbic system (which is largely responsible for emotion). These structures are thought to be responsible for components of addictive behavior, such as pleasure, reward, craving, emotional management, learning, memory, impaired executive functioning, and decision-making (Brand et al., 2016). Increasingly, these maladaptive interactions are seen as bidirectional in that gaming and unhealthy MDU, for example, may change brain structures and processes, which then contribute to continued seeking and engaging in stimulating behaviors.

Structural abnormalities in dopamine-rich areas of the brain have been observed for those with unhealthy MDU. There is also evidence for predisposing risk factors that may make someone more susceptible *to engage* in compulsive behavior or addiction. For example, prenatal exposure to higher levels of androgens has been associated with problematic video game addiction (Kornhuber et al., 2013). Also, variation in specific genes coding for the dopamine D2 receptor and dopamine degradation enzyme was associated with excessive internet gaming and "higher reward dependency" (Han et al., 2007). Differences in a cholinergic receptor that plays a role in nicotine addiction were found to be present for those with problematic social media use (Montag et al., 2012). These are just a few examples of the growing research substantiating neurochemical and neurostructural differences that may be associated with unhealthy MDU. The good news is that there is increasing evidence that positive changes also occur in functional connectivity in the brain in response to appropriate treatment (Zhang et al., 2016).

Most clinicians will not know their clients' genetic makeup or what structural abnormalities may be present in critical brain regions. However, we *can* (and should) be mindful when conceptualizing an individual's situation and, subsequently, any approach to intervention that neurological dysfunction contributes in part to unhealthy MDU—from predisposing neuroanatomical differences and imbalances in neurotransmitters governing emotion, behavior, and regulation, to neuroadaptive changes (changes in the structure and function of the brain *because* of excessive screen activities). We recommend getting a sense of a student's executive function skills prior to intervening to reshape or restructure behavior or belief systems around MDU, as this is an important way to assess the manifestation of unseen neurobiological factors. This will help clinicians avoid imposing behavior change goals that are beyond a student's capacity to achieve successfully or autonomously. Reduced executive functioning (e.g., inhibition, planning, time management) detracts from conscious decision-making even when the will is there to modify behavior. Because of these complex interactions between brain chemistry and connections that regulate and motivate behavior, children and adolescents may not be able to *choose* to stop engaging in a behavior, even when explicitly told to or when negative results will occur (e.g., grounding, removal of privileges). This is especially true for younger children.

Further, engagement in MDU results in positive chemical changes that are reinforcing, such as a "high" or lift in mood, the warmth of a connection to peers or social support, a sense of reward or achievement, and the feeling of pleasure. Thus, these benefits may limit one's motivation to reduce the behavior. The individual would need to have strong inhibitory capacities, mental flexibility, planning skills, and positive problem-solving skills to proactively and intentionally structure their efforts to forego the gains of MDU. We believe that executive functioning skills are one of the most critical areas of intrapersonal growth that can be directly targeted as part of any harm reduction approach to intervention (discussed in more detail below).

Behavioral Principles of Reinforcement

In order to improve problematic behavior, clinicians must include principles of behavior modification and reinforcement, likely learned in an introductory psychology class, in their conceptualization and approach. Concepts such as reward, positive reinforcement, negative reinforcement, negative punishment, and positive punishment can be confusing (especially the last one!). Yet, each of these is an important contributor to unhealthy MDU. Remember that, essentially, reinforcement is about increasing a behavior, while punishment is about decreasing that behavior. "Positive" refers to adding something to accomplish that increase or decrease, while "negative" refers to the removal of something undesirable. Those who are not familiar with these concepts (like most of the youth attending therapy and their family members) may assume, for example, that "negative reinforcement" might be the same as punishment. However, it actually refers to the idea that a behavior will be repeated (reinforced) if it *removes* something undesirable. For example, those who engage in excessive MDU are often motivated to do so, at least partially, by a desire to reduce a negative emotion (e.g., feelings of isolation or loneliness, the discomfort of anhedonia associated with depression, excessive worry) or increase a positive emotion (e.g., sense of belonging and connection) (Brand et al., 2016). As such, intervention must include (in developmentally appropriate ways) educating students about and incorporating principles of both positive and negative reinforcement and punishment to help them identify what their MDU brings into their lives (whether desired or not) and what they may be able to remove or add into their lives by reducing their MDU. This will empower students to appreciate the importance of cause and effect and intentional choice in changing behavior.

Clinicians should also understand schedules of reinforcement, such as intermittent rewards, that may also play a role in unhealthy MDU. You may remember Skinner's work (1953) that identified the power of an intermittent reinforcement schedule. When behavior is reinforced unpredictably, it will strengthen and be more difficult to extinguish. Being rewarded at unexpected intervals is more powerful than being rewarded consistently and predictably for behavior. As an award-winning game designer noted, aspects of games must be uncertain (e.g., the outcome, the game's path, perception, complexity), or it will not hold our interest (Costikyan, 2013). Does the child have a hard time limiting gameplay (e.g., "Just one more round so I can see if I can make it to the end of the level!") or are they unable to stop scrolling or monitoring posting on social media because they are awaiting the feedback of others as the "reward" (e.g., "I need to see how many likes I can get for this post")? These are examples of intermittent reinforcement prolonging one's MDU.

Social Factors

Aspects of social psychology principles also contribute to MDU, such as social thinking (how we perceive the world and ourselves within it), social influence (e.g., issues of stereotypes and biases, why we conform, how to persuade others), and social behavior (e.g., aggression, helping behaviors, attraction and relationships) (Sage Publications, 2019). Social psychologists have long studied—and proven—that the feelings and beliefs about the self (self-esteem) are impacted by the way others treat us and show they value us. The sociometer model posits that self-esteem is a gauge of perceived social value, whereby self-esteem is higher to the extent we feel accepted and appreciated (think: "liked" on social media) but lower to the extent we feel rejected or not liked by others (Leary & Baumeister, 2000; Leary & Downs, 1995).

Additionally, students may remain excessively engaged with MDU to avoid falling behind a shared social experience among their peers (e.g., friends moving ahead in online gaming, things being shared online about what is happening within a friend group, online auctions/shopping, news about something happening in the community or larger world that is important to the person). This includes the concept known as FOMO or for fear of missing out. Youth typically want to stay connected and be a part of their social group so as not to miss what "everyone else" gets to be a part of and to avoid loneliness, jealousy, a sense of rejection, etc. Maintaining an active presence within online activity is meant to deter these negative feelings (think: negative reinforcement) and provide a sense of connection and belonging (think: positive reinforcement). This sense of belonging is especially important if a student feels isolated, rejected, or neglected in their home, school, or community environments, such as if they identify with a marginalized group (e.g., the LGBTQ+ community).

MDU affords us an opportunity to connect for social support to others who share our identities, experiences, struggles, and interests, allowing for the development of meaningful, connected relationships and a sense of belonging that has long been identified as a factor in both physical and mental health and resiliency (Weziak-Bialowolska et al., 2022). Once this connectedness is established, reducing engagement in one's online activity or community may be experienced as withdrawal—chemically and emotionally—and as a sense of loss. In addition to FOMO and the drive to reduce this negative emotional state, youth may perceive that not being involved in something would change *others*' perceptions about them or their place in their social group. Thus, reducing the frequency or duration of MDU would be seen as threatening to the person's social status or happiness, potentially triggering defensive reactivity (think: resistance to treatment) and further solidifying their investment in the activity (to avoid the perceived loss). We often hear from adolescents who may have come to realize their MDU is unhealthy that they "can't stop, or else…(this thing) will happen." Students may avoid treatment recommendations or interventions meant to lessen MDU so as to avoid perceived social consequences.

These social psychology principles typically contribute to a drive to seek the approval of others and to avoid criticism, to stay connected and to avoid rejection and isolation. These are great examples of positive reinforcement: receiving praise leads me to continue to post similar things. This also provides a chemical response, such as a "high" (think: the dopamine hit from accomplishment, especially for a desirable skill that sets me apart from my peers). Collectively, this is an example of the interconnectedness of social, cognitive, emotional, behavioral, and neurobiological factors. In addition, social psychology tells us that behavior is a function of the interaction between personality and environment (Sage Publications, 2019). These factors need to be taken into account when conceptualizing a student's MDU. For example, certain personality characteristics are associated with using online communication applications or sites excessively, such as extraversion and openness to experience, narcissism, impulsivity and attention deficits, low self-esteem, social anxiety, and coping style (Brand et al., 2016).

Cognitive and Emotional (Psychological) Processes

A cognitive-behavioral conceptualization would, of course, include aspects of an individual's core belief system (especially of the self, others, and how the world works), automatic thoughts, emotional experiences that result from one's interpretations of events, and behavioral reactivity meant to cope with or regulate those emotions. We suggest clinicians specifically consider students' beliefs related to empowerment, accomplishments, and competencies, as they may be connected to any special talent or persona supported by their MDU. For example, a youth who may struggle in school or to meet expectations in their home environment may feel inadequate in real life. But if online they are seen as socially desirable (e.g., they are a trusted confidant of others, funny and provide others with entertainment), offer something valued by others, or talented in game play, then MDU provides them a way to feel "special" and more competent. Similarly, those with negative mood states (such as anxiety and depression) would be more likely to engage in excessive MDU as an escape from (or numbing of) those negative mood states. They may believe that engaging in their activities of choice is the only way they can be happy. Again, readers are directed to the summaries by Brand and colleagues (2016) and Kuss and Pontes (2019) for factors contributing to various MDU addictions, including gaming addiction in children, which highlights that escapism (the desire to avoid difficulties in their real lives) is the "strongest motivational factor predicting video game addiction." Unfortunately, escapism also leads to increased psychiatric distress.

The need to achieve and perform are additional factors in gaming addiction, as is the desire for fun, catharsis or autonomy, and boredom. In terms of social networking addiction, "the most popular motives include relationship maintenance, passing time, entertainment, and companionship" (Kuss & Pontes, 2019). These authors also point out that internet use expectancies play a role in motivating behavior because they involve anticipation of how the internet or gaming behavior may help to distract and improve mood, whether by reducing a negative mood state or introducing or enhancing a positive one. When considering how to support a student's efforts to reduce the frequency of MDU, clinicians need to think about how the individual views the MDU and the ***meaning*** *they* give to it: as a tool, escape, source of pleasure, sense of identity, or other motivation that draws their investment. What function does this behavior serve, whether consciously or unconsciously motivated?

As discussed above, harm reduction approaches to therapy are integrated, biopsychosocial approaches rather than sequential models of treatment. Students will simultaneously be addressing each of these contributing factors (cognitive, emotional, social, behavioral, and physiological responses) to their MDU. They must understand the interrelated aspects of each component and how these factors impact their short- and long-term goals in order to commit to making changes. When intervention is provided within a group therapy format, individuals receive the benefits of peer support, accountability, creative problem-solving, modeling, and so on to help facilitate advancement through stages of change and success in modifying behavior (Stewart & Christner, 2024). Within the group format, members can see these interactions in the examples of others and work to recognize, in themselves, the relationships between and among each of these factors in order to understand how best to interrupt unhealthy patterns of MDU and limit the harm their current choices cause in their lives in the future, ultimately finding a healthier balance in their MDU.

Cultural Considerations

Clinicians should remain aware of how students' unique identities and backgrounds shape their nonverbal communication, openness, and engagement in therapy, affecting their disclosure of personal and psychological experiences. Understanding cultural nuances is vital throughout the therapeutic process, from assessment to intervention to outcome. This involves recognizing diverse beliefs on mental health, authority, family privacy, and spirituality, as highlighted by Stewart and Christner (2024). Yet, broad knowledge of cultural tendencies is insufficient; clinicians must collaborate with each individual to understand personal and familial contexts to grasp the complexity of these interactions.

Pedersen and Pope (2016) stress the need for inclusive cultural empathy in therapy, particularly with youth from marginalized or traumatized backgrounds. This approach helps avoid assumptions, enhances understanding, and ensures appropriate actions, aiding effective engagement and therapeutic outcomes. The conversations around modifying unhealthy media use (MDU) must account for cultural perspectives on technology, recognizing varying views on what constitutes excessive use and its impact on functionality. For example, the DSM-5 identifies Internet Gaming Disorder, with prevalence differing globally, indicating cultural disparities in viewing and managing MDU (American Psychiatric Association [APA], 2022; Lin et al., 2014; Rumpf et al., 2014).

Cultural differences extend to perceptions of MDU's impact on academic performance and self-image, with, for example, Eastern cultures often seeing excessive use as a loss of parental control and a source of shame (Rao, 2019), contrasting with Western views that attribute it to the youth's individual shortcomings. Religious and socioeconomic factors also influence MDU perceptions and practices. For example, social media can provide a sense of community for marginalized religious groups, while excessive use may conflict with religious norms or highlight socioeconomic disparities that affect youth's well-being and sense of inclusion (Alvstad, 2010; Lim & Sng, 2020; Livingood et al., 2022; Manning et al., 2019; Marizan, 2016; Neumaier, 2020). Understanding the functional impact of one's MDU through a cultural lens can be complex, requiring clinicians to take time to understand the identity-related contexts of youth, including generational differences within families (which often underlie how families may see MDU as "problematic"). This awareness helps tailor interventions, by appreciating contextual factors that motivate behavior and perceptions of technology use, in order to reduce harm while maintaining benefits.

Protective Factors

Following the US Surgeon General's advisory on May 23, 2023, highlighting the risks of young people's social media use, it is critical to understand and address these dangers. Preliminary studies suggest significant impacts on youth mental health, prompting calls for action from tech companies, policymakers, researchers, and caregivers to safeguard young users. Many are wondering what factors determine which youth are most at-risk and what safeguards can protect vulnerable users. The alarming statistic from Crittenden (2019) that 95% of adolescents have access to smartphones, with half reporting near constant use, underscores the importance of parental vigilance and strategies like limited screen time and device-free periods to foster self-discipline and ensure healthier balance.

The Surgeon General's 2023 Advisory advocates for a Family Media Plan to encourage open discussions about safe device use, including privacy settings and avoiding harmful content. This approach, coupled with adults modeling responsible media use (consistent with Social Learning Theory), can guide children toward balanced MDU. Encouraging participation in extracurricular activities offers alternative forms of entertainment, connection, purpose, and self-esteem, potentially reducing device dependency and enhancing life skills.

Despite efforts to counteract excessive MDU, the societal push toward digital engagement is strong, with research indicating links between unrestricted social media use and mental health issues like depression and anxiety. Therefore, bolstering protective strategies is crucial for youth well-being. This chapter discusses employing CBT within a harm reduction framework to manage unhealthy MDU and offers a preventative strategy that could be integrated into school health curricula to enhance children and adolescents' media literacy and healthy use habits.

Assessment

Once clinicians understand how to conceptualize contributing factors of unhealthy MDU and the various aspects that need to be taken into account (including cultural factors unique to the individual and the interaction between individual and environment), they must define what constitutes "unhealthy" MDU. As mentioned, this needs to move beyond simply the hours one is engaged with a screen or device (although this is also telling and should not be ignored!). For starters, we suggest considering the following key principles

1 **Quality Over Quantity**: The impact of MDU largely depends on the content consumed and the activities engaged in while using these devices. Spending several hours on educational, creative, or productive tasks may have different consequences than an equal amount of time spent on

"mindless" scrolling or passive consumption, viewing violence or pornographic material, cyber-bullying, or consuming emotional or distressing stories and news.

2 **Individual Variability**: Individuals have varying thresholds for the amount of screen time and the nature of the content they consume without experiencing negative effects on their mental, physical, social, and emotional well-being. What might be excessive for one person could be manageable for another, depending on individual characteristics, experiences, cultural considerations, and risk versus protective factors. We must understand that individual impact to identify "harm."
3 **Purpose and Balance**: The key is to have harmony that aligns with one's individual needs and goals. Unhealthy MDU often occurs when screen time begins to interfere with essential aspects of life, such as sleep, relationships, work or school performance, emotional well-being, and physical health, or when one is engaged excessively in one particular kind of activity to the detriment of developing other hobbies, connections, opportunities, and even simply experiencing unstructured time that is important for the mental health of children and adolescents.
4 **Context Matters**: The context in which screen time occurs is also crucial. For example, screens used for education may have different implications than those used for leisure or entertainment or for avoiding or coping with emotional matters (e.g., social anxiety and depression). Likewise, the presence of social interaction during screen time can significantly influence its impact (e.g., a group of adolescents sitting in the same room but operating independently on their screens versus teens engaging in cooperative gameplay).

Understanding the functional impact of MDU is key, particularly when it interferes with essential activities such as homework, exercise, socializing, and sleep. Problematic MDU often results in behavioral changes, including irritability, rule-breaking, anxiety, and withdrawal. The significance of MDU as a factor in the functioning and well-being challenges of today's youth is undeniable, evident across clinical settings. A thorough initial assessment is crucial before starting intervention, encompassing emotional health, executive functions, learning profiles, substance use, mood, social skills, family and cultural contexts, and protective factors. This assessment aims to evaluate MDU's extent and its effect on daily life, determine treatment readiness, and set intervention goals. It also helps identify co-occurring conditions and potential barriers to progress, to guide treatment planning and ongoing progress monitoring, especially in CBT for MDU harm reduction.

For group interventions, clinicians must judiciously consider the nature and effects of members' MDU when deciding group composition, acknowledging that achieving an "ideal" group may be challenging due to diverse motivations for and impacts of MDU among members (see Stewart & Christner, 2024). Ensuring a safe and productive group dynamic is paramount, including screening out individuals whose online activities might harm other group members (e.g., sexual or racially harmful behavior). In some cases, individual therapy may be more suitable than group settings.

Given that the basics of assessment are covered elsewhere in this book (see Chapters 1 and 2), we forego a detailed review of specific tools and approaches related to interviewing and collecting data, focusing instead on clinically relevant concepts, tools, and considerations for evaluating and treating unhealthy MDU in children and adolescents, with an emphasis on formulating effective treatment approaches. However, in Table 21.1, we do offer suggested questions specific to MDU.

In addition to asking questions regarding MDU, there are specific rating scales that can be used in assessing MDU. This does not replace broadband measures we might use to rule out anxiety, depression, executive functions, or other emotional or behavioral difficulties. Instead, the narrowband measures focus more specifically on behaviors related to the MDU concerns. Several instruments have been adapted from previously validated tools to provide a broad view of media and device abuse (Király et al., 2015). For example, *Young's Internet Addiction Diagnostic Questionnaire* (IADQ) and *Internet Addiction Test* (IAT) were partially developed based on the original diagnostic criteria for

Table 21.1 Questions about MDU

- How much time do you spend playing on a device (phone, tablet, computer, or game console) each day after school and on the weekend?
- Can you tell me what you usually do with your devices every day, like where and when you use them the most?
- Are there any apps, games, or websites that you find really hard to stop using once you start?
- Have you ever missed out on sleep, homework, or hanging out with friends because you were using your devices?
- How do you feel if you can't use your device for a long time? Do you feel worried, lonely, or grumpy?
- What's it like for you when you stop using your devices, whether because you want to or someone asks you to?
- Do you ever use your phone or computer to take a break from feeling bored, stressed, or sad?
- Have you and your family or friends ever argued about how much you use your devices?
- After using your devices a lot, have you ever felt things like your eyes hurting, getting headaches, or finding it hard to sleep?
- Do you think using your devices a lot makes it harder for you to pay attention or do well in school or other fun activities?
- Have you ever tried to use your devices less? How did that go?
- How often do you do stuff that doesn't involve screens, like sports or other hobbies?
- Are there things you wish you could do more of but feel like you can't because you're spending too much time on devices?
- What rules does your family have about using devices and what do you think about them?
- What does social media mean to you and do you ever feel like you have to act a certain way online?

Table 21.2 Examples of Narrowband Rating Scales for MDU

Bergen Social Media Addiction Scale (BSMAS; Andreassen et al., 2012)	Assesses the degree of addiction to social media (originally for Facebook but now expanded)
Internet Gaming Disorder 20 (IGD-20) Pontes et al., 2014)	Measures the nine Internet Gaming Disorder criteria suggested in DSM-5
Problematic Internet Use Questionnaire (PIUQ) (Demetrovics et al., 2008)	Measure problematic or addictive internet use
Problematic Online Gaming Questionnaire (POGQ) (Pápay et al., 2013)	Measures problematic or addictive online gaming behavior
Social Media Disorder Scale (SMD) (van den Eijnden et al., 2016)	Assesses the severity of social media disorder based on the nine DSM-5 criteria for internet gaming disorder, adapting them to a social media context
Social Media Use Integration Scale (SMUIS) (Jenkins-Guarnieri et al., 2013)	Evaluates the degree to which social media use is integrated into daily activities and social practices
Social Networking Activity Intensity Scale (SNAIS) (Li et al., 2016)	Measures the intensity and the nature of individuals' use of social networking sites
The Adolescent Compulsive Internet Use Scale (ACIUS) (Lopez-Ferandez et al., 2019)	Assesses the severity of compulsive internet use with adolescents
The Internet Addiction Test (IAT) (Young, 2017)	Assesses excessive device use, including prolonged internet or app usage on smartphones and other devices
The Media and Technology Usage and Attitudes Scale (MTUAS) (Rosen et al., 2013)	Measures the frequency and duration of media and technology use across different devices
The Problematic Media Use Measure (PMUM) (Domoff et al., 2019)	Assesses problematic media use across various devices and screens, including smartphones, tablets, and computers
The Screen Time Questionnaire (Vizcaino et al., 2019)	Assesses daily screen time across different devices and activities
The Smartphone Addiction Scale (SAS) (Kwon et al., 2013)	Assesses smartphone addiction and its severity through device usage patterns and behaviors

gambling disorder (Young, 1998, 2017). With the increased awareness of unhealthy MDU, additional instruments have been specifically developed for use with this population. It is beyond this chapter to discuss these in great detail. In Table 21.2, we offer several examples that clinicians might consider when assessing MDU.

Modular-Based Intervention

Stewart et al. (2024) advocate for a CBT-based harm-reduction approach tailored for MDU within group settings. This semi-structured, adaptable intervention model emphasizes a modular format, allowing for customization according to individual needs and personal goals, while ensuring a structured framework facilitating the acquisition of knowledge and skills necessary for behavior change, competent coping, and effective self-regulation. The flexibility within each module accommodates the unique needs of individual students based on assessment results, case conceptualization, and desired change. Of note, some students will require interventions beyond what is appropriate or feasible within an educational setting (e.g., to address issues such as severe emotional problems, acute trauma, developmental social disorders, and sexually addictive behaviors). Clinicians should have determined the need for additional or supplemental services during the initial assessment process and collaborated with other professionals to meet those needs.

Below, we offer a brief description of the intervention modules that serves as a guide for progressing in a structured, sequential manner through educational and targeted skill-building components we have found to be most effective with youth engaging in unhealthy device use. The modules are grounded in cognitive-behavioral theory and harm-reduction principles, informed by research and our clinical experience, designed to mitigate problematic MDU. Below, we discuss each module, and in Table 21.3, we offer examples of language and interventions to support each component.

Paving the Way with Successful Goal-Setting

Setting goals is an important part of CBT, offering substantial benefits within the collaborative therapeutic processes. This helps establish the connection between the clinician and the individual and offers a way for the student to share their perspectives to help determine the support needed. Clear goals provide individuals a path toward behavioral changes, guiding their focus during therapy sessions toward achieving these objectives. Effective goal setting serves a dual purpose: *reducing maladaptive behaviors* and *promoting overall well-being*. For instance, a student might aim to "charge my phone outside my bedroom nightly" or "reduce daily gaming by one hour." Yet, since such goals may initially seem unappealing, integrating them with personal, rewarding objectives can boost motivation. Students are encouraged to envision the positive shifts in their lives post-MDU adjustment, like using newfound time for beneficial activities, such as extra academic support, doing artwork, playing sports, learning a musical instrument, or hanging out with friends.

Incorporating "mini-goals" within each session is essential for building accountability, enhancing engagement, and tracking progress toward broader objectives. These could involve tasks like mastering educational content, participating actively during sessions, or completing "homework" between sessions. For example, a student committed to lessening daily screen time by 15 minutes might show a significant drop in their weekly average, something celebrated within the session. A student struggling to limit video gaming to 60 minutes on school nights might find encouragement in discussing what worked on the days they met their goal. Clinicians using this approach not only acknowledge the individual's efforts but also facilitate a problem-solving dialogue to overcome any encountered obstacles.

Developing Self-Understanding through Psychoeducation

Prior to starting specific behavioral and cognitive strategies, it's essential for individuals to grasp the underlying factors contributing to the behavior or negative emotions they want to improve and understand the reasons for the interventions. Psychoeducation serves as a foundation from which individuals can understand the role their MDU plays in promoting risk and impacting well-being, and appreciate the dynamics driving their use (that were previously outlined during case conceptualization) so that interventions make sense within the context of their goals, increasing compliance and follow-through. Topics such as how their brain influences mood and motivation, how social connections impact well-being, and the theoretical model of CBT (the connection between thoughts-feelings-behaviors) facilitate a sense of self-awareness rooted in evidence and logical reasoning.

Building Self-Awareness for Competent Coping

After having a foundational knowledge of how neurobiological, social, emotional, behavioral, and cognitive factors influence behavior, we move students toward improving emotional regulation. This process involves accurately identifying emotions, understanding their intensity, building tolerance, and learning to manage and express them constructively, including seeking social support. It's vital to acknowledge that difficult emotions manifest not only as feelings but also as physical discomfort and mental distress, such as anxiety, self-doubt, or confusion. Acknowledging that positive emotions are also felt physically supports awareness of how our choices (like MDU) may be motivated by desire to avoid discomfort, which limits development of more effective coping strategies.

Improved emotional awareness and regulation enable individuals to handle adverse feelings better and diminish the need to resort to MDU for escape or gratification. By understanding the factors that drive both negative and positive emotions, individuals can expand coping skills to include alternatives to MDU, to support distress tolerance and foster fulfilling and healthy emotional states. This module will likely extend over multiple sessions, as it aims to equip students with the skills to navigate their emotional landscape more effectively and incorporates opportunities for repeated practice (in and between sessions).

Changing the Narrative: Flipping Your Inner Script

This module, potentially extending over several sessions, focuses on refining students' awareness and management of their thought processes. It emphasizes the critical skill of using thought records to identify and modify maladaptive thoughts that cause distress. The aim is to provide students with the skills to recognize and reframe distorted, inaccurate, or exaggerated interpretations of events ("thinking traps") to mitigate the severity of the negative emotions they produce.

The process involves challenging and changing negative self-perceptions, doubts about personal abilities, misconceptions about social interactions, and any misbeliefs related to their MDU. By addressing, for example, one's thoughts about *only* feeling comfortable in online interactions or fearing rejection in face-to-face encounters, this module helps individuals realize the limitations of dichotomous or "black-and-white thinking." Maladaptive thoughts cause distress, exaggerate the importance of MDU, and limit one's confidence (and, then, often willingness) to make changes.

Addressing maladaptive thoughts and beliefs directly is beneficial not only for reducing distress and altering detrimental behaviors like excessive MDU but also for correcting skewed perceptions about one's capabilities and the perceived risks of changing those behaviors. The goal here is to foster a more balanced perspective, rooted in facts rather than fears or assumptions, enhancing one's competence and overall well-being. By teaching students to identify the thoughts that may lead to irrational or exaggerated responses and guiding them to reframe these thoughts, the module aims to empower students with the ability to "flip the script" on their cognitive distortions, paving the way for healthier, more intentional decision-making and lifestyle choices.

Moving from Chaos to Control: Building Your Brain's Command Center

The role of executive function in regulating MDU is highlighted, as it significantly influences an individual's capacity for intentional decision making. For children who understand the negative impact of their MDU but find it challenging to make in-the-moment decisions, issues with executive functions like inhibition or planning can hinder their ability to consider consequences before acting. This is particularly evident in scenarios where immediate gratification (e.g., watching a highly anticipated video) overshadows responsibilities, causing distraction from important tasks.

Furthermore, deficiencies in executive functions related to time management and planning can lead to stress within family dynamics or affect participation in extracurricular activities due to poor punctuality or preparedness. Recognizing executive functioning as a pivotal element in excessive MDU underscores the necessity for targeted interventions that enhance these cognitive processes. By focusing on strengthening executive functions, interventions can more effectively support individuals in making healthier decisions regarding their MDU, thereby mitigating its adverse effects on their daily lives, relationships, and overall well-being.

Solving Problems for Success

After improving emotional regulation, establishing decision-making skills, setting personal objectives for managing MDU, and finding balance with other aspects of life, we shift to viewing challenges as manageable through a systematic process that aligns actions with personal goals while minimizing consequences. This approach enhances executive functions like inhibition, adaptability, and self-regulation, further strengthening one's overall competence. This module teaches a structured problem-solving process long recognized for facilitating purposeful goal-based decision-making while taking responsibility for the repercussions of one's choices. Students are taught to define MDU-related problems clearly and brainstorm various solutions before then weighing the advantages and disadvantages of each option. This exercise in deliberate decision-making helps them appreciate and accept the trade-offs involved in their choices, encouraging more balanced and intentional MDU.

For instance, reducing social media use can feel threatening if there is concern about losing online friends and social connection. Problem-solving will help students learn to balance their online presence with in-person activities (also important for social health) that provide the connection and belonging they seek. For those accessing digital entertainment to excess (e.g., through the personalized content of TikTok and YouTube), problem-solving helps youth understand how time spent in unproductive, purely entertaining activity reduces time and energy available for other areas of healthy life functioning (e.g., school, work, physical activity, sleep, in-person socializing), so they can make informed choices that allow for balanced use and fewer negative consequences.

Discussing the potential outcomes of all solutions first helps students make informed decisions that reflect their priorities and willingness to accommodate certain downsides, while balancing what they want. This comprehensive approach not only aids in developing practical solutions but also in enhancing self-regulation capabilities. By evaluating the outcomes of their choices and adjusting decisions based on practice in the "real-world," students refine their problem-solving skills, leading to increased self-efficacy and a more balanced relationship with MDU.

Sustaining Healthy Digital Habits

The concluding module, occurring over two or three sessions, aims to solidify the understanding and application of knowledge and skills for managing MDU more intentionally: from proactive emotional regulation and effective coping, to purposeful goal setting, planning, and problem-solving of potential consequences. This reinforcement occurs through interactive methods tailored to each student's developmental stage, including role-playing exercises where students teach back learned concepts, potentially in group settings or through digital presentations. These activities are designed not only to enhance comprehension but also to improve retention and effective implementation.

A key component involves formal and informal progress monitoring to assess skill mastery and the readiness to apply these strategies outside the therapeutic setting. Methods range from rating scales or paper-pencil "tests" (e.g., of vocabulary and concepts), to innovative digital quiz platforms that engage students in a familiar, enjoyable format. Activities, such as creating and performing before-and-after skits in sessions that depict skills application offer a dynamic way to review and reinforce learning. These exercises encourage active participation, critical reflection, and the practical application of coping mechanisms, cognitive reframing, and decision-making processes.

Furthermore, we encourage having individuals compile a "portfolio" of their journey, reflecting on their growth, challenges, and plans for maintaining a balanced relationship with MDU. This not only serves as a tangible reminder of concepts, skills, their goals, and their progress, but also aids in identifying future support needs and potential obstacles. Engaging family members in the final session can provide additional insights, preparing students for real-world application and long-term success. Ultimately, this module supports sustained behavioral change, preparing students with the tools for a healthier, more balanced engagement with digital media.

Application within School Setting: Case Study

To highlight using CBT and harm-reduction with youth in schools, we want to introduce you to Sophie, a 14-year-old girl experiencing declining academic performance and increasing anxiety levels over the past year. Her parents and teachers have described Sophie's situation as an "obsession with her phone." In addition to her recreational use, Sophie also is on a device throughout her school day. Sophie spends approximately 10–12 hours daily in front of screens, including for academic work, social media, gaming, and streaming videos. Unfortunately, this excessive screen time has led to disrupted sleep patterns, weight gain, and social isolation, exacerbating her preexisting anxiety and contributing to academic decline. She already receives school-based mental health services for anxiety and worry. As part of her session with the school psychologist, Sophie discussed how she feels her MDU is "making everything worse," though she has struggled to better manage it on her own. They decide to focus more on MDU within her sessions.

Through the interview and assessment, Sophie and the psychologist determined her "triggers" include fearing she will miss out on something shared on social media (e.g., FOMO), and that if she is not "in the know," others might think she doesn't care and begin excluding her. Sophie easily set a primary goal: "I want to be able to have at least two hours every night that are tech-free." She worries this might be "too stressful" to tackle all at once, so they decide to start with 30 minutes a night of non-screen time when her phone is placed in a different room. While there are emotional and social factors, most of the in session time with Sophie initially was to "flip the script" and work on challenging and reframing the fear-based thoughts that drove her unhealthy use. Although addressed, less time was devoted to the development of emotional regulation skills given that assessment confirmed previous counseling had effectively built her toolbox of coping skills she could articulate and use well. Executive functioning was less of a concern for Sophie, though planning skills were reinforced

Table 21.3 Sample Activities for MDU Treatment Modules

1 Paving the way for successful goal setting

- o Introduce the concept of setting and prioritizing goals as a way to make positive changes. Have students brainstorm a list of possible goals they could work on, then write on a whiteboard and discuss the feasibility of each. Have them pick two goals they feel they would benefit from (or they can come up with one on their own). Help them turn each goal into SMART goals (specific, measurable, achievable, relevant, and time-bound). For between-session work, have them break each SMART goal into smaller, manageable steps and create a "plan of action."
- o Introduce students to the importance of visualizing success and using self-affirmations to boost self-belief. Use a visualization activity and ask students to close their eyes and imagine themselves achieving their goals with MDU. Have them picture what they feel, see, and hear. Play video on "positive thinking" (we like using https://www.youtube.com/watch?v=kO1kgl0p-Hw&t=4s). Have students create their positive thoughts or affirmations related to their goals.

2 Developing insight/psychoeducation

- o Show a short video about the fight or flight response (we like using https://youtu.be/rpolpKTWrp4?si=ko3yM3i_QO5zgbxc). Ask students to list two or three situations that cause them to feel strong negative emotions, including where and how these are felt in the body. And then list two or three situations that cause positive emotions, including bodily sensations.
- o Teach the T-F-B connection using an example relevant to the student. For example, with middle schoolers, share about a teen who receives a grade of 62 back on their math test: what did that student think, feel, and do in response to that "trigger"? Then, model how the person's thoughts and feelings would be different if the context changed (e.g., that student had been receiving 45s on previous tests) to exemplify how perspective and resulting emotional responses can change based on our interpretation of the trigger
- o Give students a blank "thought record," read a scripted scenario of a child (similar age) experiencing a difficult moment, and ask them to list the resulting T-F-B

3 Empowering self-awareness for competent coping

- o Mindful awareness and observing one's experiences (thoughts, feelings, and bodily sensations):
  - • Introduce students to mindful meditation to learn to attend to their senses and perceptions (including emotion) without necessarily working to change them
  - • Use muscle tension/relaxation activities that help students recognize the difference between physical states (e.g., progressive muscle relaxation, how difficult it is to hold a tight fist while deep breathing)
- o Differentiating emotions:
  - • Share or create collaboratively with the student examples of anger as a masking emotion for something else, usually more vulnerable feelings (e.g., hurt, embarrassment, guilt)
  - • Use scenarios that exemplify the difference between emotions, such as anxiety versus discomfort, anger/irritation versus boredom and restlessness, happiness, and contentment versus simply the absence of loneliness.
- o Learning to gauge emotions on a range and not as "all or nothing states":
  - • Have students build a "feeling thermometer" of any negative emotion (e.g., anger, anxiety, sadness) relevant to them as well as a positive emotion (e.g., safe, happy, loved), with some experience that produces that emotion at all points from 0 to 10 (similar to creating a SUDS scale for anxiety treatment)

4 Changing the narrative: Flipping your inner script

- o A free association activity that requires students to complete a series of sentence starters that all begin with My use of (media/device)…, such as: brings me, makes me feel, makes others feel, makes others think, means I can, means I don't, etc. Then have members fill in a 2nd group of sentences based on the starter, "If I didn't (media/device use)…," such as: "I would feel," "I would spend my time," "I could," "my family would," "in school I could," "my friends would," etc.

(*Continued*)

Table 21.3 (Continued)

- o Introduce the common cognitive distortions (see Stewart & Christner, 2024) often referred to as "Thinking Traps," "Junk Thoughts," or "Perceptual Prisons," discuss examples relevant to the student, and then ask students to create an example of each distorted thought specifically related to MDU (e.g., generate a few traps within small groups, assign one or two traps to each group member). Send a copy home for between-session work for students to identify within another column of their thought records (thinking trap).

5 Going from chaos to control: Building your brain's command center

- o To foster *mental flexibility* (which promotes more effective problem-solving, discussed more below), engage in collaborative brainstorming with the student:
  - For example, students could identify as many uses as possible for a brick. Or generate a list of food options for a picnic, which will also ask students to begin thinking of the possible "consequences" to solutions (e.g., why ice cream may not be the best choice if the picnic is far away, there are no ice packs, etc.)
  - Having students ask others for help brainstorming supports flexibility because they will likely receive differing perspectives on a given prompt. Another activity could require students to have to explain or defend the rationale of the perspective (once given) of another "hypothetical" student or someone else in their life
- o *Self-monitoring* is an important skill that precedes self-regulation and can be improved through structured practice
  - First, students discuss and make a list of what they would like to manage better in their lives and start with something fairly trivial, such as decreasing the amount of time they say "like" before other words (e.g., "like, I already told you," or "like, I know)
  - In the case of MDU, we might have students identify what area of MDU is most problematic for them (e.g., do they watch TikTok or YouTube for hours prior to bedtime, do they neglect to nourish their bodies by skipping lunch and dinner because they are so engrossed in gaming). This can begin as an in-session assignment to determine what type of MDU is most problematic for the individual and transition to homework to monitor how much time the MDU that they identified occurs. The students will keep track throughout the week, recording the start time and end time they engage in the MDU they identified as most problematic
  - However, this can also be used to self-monitor other MDU activities that the individual did not identify. For example, a student may have identified online gaming as the most problematic, but after tracking the use of all MDU, they realize they actually spend more time on social media
  - This activity will highlight a truth that one cannot achieve through estimation and which produces dissonance between beliefs and behavior that is necessary to promote lasting behavior change

6 Solving problems for success

- o Have students brainstorm in-person social interactions to try when changing MDU. Have them list the anticipated pros (e.g., getting to know someone better, including mannerisms, real-time back-and-forth reciprocal interaction, chemical changes that occur during bonding) and potential cons (e.g., anxiety about looking "stupid" or not making a good impression, worries it will be "boring" or not a good time). They then use cognitive skills to balance their "thinking traps" about the replacement activity by creating more positive, empowering self-talk before implementing their choice: "Even if I don't love it, it could still be something I enjoy (like a 6 if it's not a 10)" or "I'm trying something different which maybe I didn't even know I could like"
- o Have students list "barriers" or "roadblocks" to changing MDU. Using a metaphor of a GPS rerouting someone who is trying to get to a certain place when there is construction and detours, have the student come up with options to "reroute" around the MDU roadblocks. Once a list of options is created, have students rank them in a hierarchy of options they believe would help them best

(*Continued*)

Table 21.3 (Continued)

7 Final module: Maintenance assurance o Have students write down their "long-term" goal for MDU in moderation. Have them write it in specific terms and write it on a 3 × 5 card. Underneath the goal, have them write the strategies that will be the most useful for them. On the back, have them list the barriers they might face and, next to it, what they will do to "reroute" from barriers. As an alternative, this can be done on a computer and printed. We encourage students to make a couple of copies and place one in the phone case or on their gaming system or computer as a reminder

Source: Copyright ©2024 Ray W. Christner and Jessica L. Stewart.

when behavioral experiments she engaged in to monitor if the thoughts around FOMO were accurate. After a few days successfully having 30 minutes of screen-free time, Sophie, on her own, began increasing the time.

After about three weeks of desired "off" time and Sophie sleeping better and feeling less anxious, a setback occurred. During her non-screen time one night, her friend made a post but Sophie did not respond. She was confronted next day by her friend and accused of not caring. This real-life setback was important in treatment, as it allowed her to consider genuine drawbacks of her goal-based choices, recognize and directly cope with the emotions of a challenging social situation, and develop a thoughtful plan for how to address it. This offered an opportunity for problem solving process to consider various responses to her friend while not compromising her self-care and progress. Assertiveness was practiced via role play. While Sophie continues to be on devices throughout school and at times recreationally, her use has decreased by her own choice and the functional difficulties have improved. She is sleeping better and her grades are now typical for her. Most importantly, she is more aware of socially driven thoughts and emotions, and more comfortable making balanced choices in line with her goals.

Summary

In the era of omnipresent technology, the rise in MDU in both adults' and children's lives is unprecedented. This proliferation has facilitated significant educational advancements and accessibility, embedding devices deeply into the fabric of academic settings. However, this integration comes with nuanced challenges, particularly for youth. Excessive and unbalanced MDU can lead to detrimental outcomes, including disrupted sleep patterns, diminished academic performance, and heightened anxiety and depression, highlighting the necessity for discerning and managing MDU effectively. CBT incorporating harm reduction strategies emerges as a promising approach that aims to mitigate the adverse effects of excessive MDU while promoting a healthier, more balanced relationship with technology.

We proposed an intervention model emphasizing a modular-based, adaptable framework tailored to individual needs, reinforcing the notion that intervention must be multifaceted to address the complex interplay of behavioral, cognitive, emotional, social, and neurobiological factors contributing to unhealthy MDU. Through a modular-based approach, we seek to equip students with the necessary tools to navigate their digital engagements more mindfully and effectively. The inclusion of harm reduction principles further enriches this approach by fostering an understanding of MDU's functional impact, encouraging individuals to recognize and adjust their usage patterns voluntarily. Our goal is not to stop MDU but to help individuals be good consumers of technology so they can maintain a healthy balance between meeting one's responsibilities (including to the self) and engaging in enjoyable activities (which is perfectly reasonable in moderation) while safeguarding their physical, mental, and social health. Schools are the perfect place to incorporate this kind of intervention, as MDU has an important role in education, yet as educators, our goal remains to pair academic progress with overall wellness.

Reflection Questions

1 How might you use information about MDU and harm-reduction to create school-wide or population-based interventions as part of a school's wellness program?
2 How do the five main factors of CBT conceptualization for MDU interact with the students you work with?
3 How might you use the modular approach presented to develop group programming within your school?

References

Alvstad, E. (2010). Encounters between believers and non-believers in a symbolic universe: Religious dialogue and controversy on the Internet. *Nordic Journal of Religion and Society, 23*(1), 71–86. https://doi.org/10.18261/ISSN1890-7008-2010-01-05

American Academy of Child and Adolescent Psychiatry (2020). *Screen time and children. No.54.* Retrieved from https://www.aacap.org/AACAP/Families_and_Youth/Facts_for_Families/FFF-Guide/Children-And-Watching-TV-054.aspx#:~:text=For%20children%202%2D5%2C%20limit,about%20and%20use%20parental%20controls

American Academy of Pediatrics (2021). *Beyond screen time: A parent guide to media use*. Washington, DC: Author. https://doi.org/10.1542/peo_document099

American Psychiatric Association (2022). Diagnostic and statistical manual of mental disorders (5th ed., text rev.). https://doi.org/10.1176/appi.books.9780890425787

Andreassen, C. S., Torsheim, T., Brunborg, G. S., & Pallesen, S. (2012). Development of a Facebook addiction scale. *Psychological Reports, 110*(2), 501–517.

Brand, M., Young, K. S., Laier, C., & Wölfling, K. (2016). Integrating psychological and neurobiological considerations regarding the development and maintenance of specific Internet-use disorders: An Interaction of Person-Affect-Cognition-Execution (I-PACE) model. *Neuroscience and Biobehavioral Reviews, 71*, 252–266.

Costikyan, G. (2013). *Uncertainty in games*. Cambridge: MIT Press

Crittenden, C. (2019). The kids are online—and alright. *Issues in Science and Technology, 36*(1), 43–47.

Demetrovics, Z., Szeredi, B., & Rózsa, S. (2008). The three-factor model of Internet addiction: The development of the Problematic Internet Use Questionnaire. *Behavior Research Methods, 40*, 563–574.

Denning, P. (2010). Harm reduction therapy with families and friends of people with drug problems. *Journal of Clinical Psychology, 66*(2), 164–174. https://doi.org/10.1002/jclp.20671

Domoff, S. E., Harrison, K., Gearhardt, A. N., Gentile, D. A., Lumeng, J. C., & Miller, A. L. (2019). Development and validation of the problematic media use measure: A parent report measure of screen media "addiction" in children. *Psychology of Popular Media Culture, 8*(1), 2–11. https://doi.org/10.1037/ppm0000163

Greer, A. M., Luchenski, S. A., Amlani, A. A., Lacroix, K., Burmeister, C., & Buxton, J. A. (2016). Peer engagement in harm reduction strategies and services: A critical case study and evaluation framework from British Columbia, Canada. *BMC Public Health, 16*(1), 1–9. https://doi.org/10.1186/s12889-016-3136-4

Han, D. H., Lee, Y. S., Yang, K. C., Kim, E. Y., Lyoo, I. K., & Renshaw, P. F. (2007). Dopamine genes and reward dependence in adolescents with excessive Internet video game play. *Journal of Addiction Medicine, 1*, 133–138.

Jenkins-Guarnieri, M. A., Wright, S. L., & Johnson, B. (2013). *Social Media Use Integration Scale (SMUIS)* [Database record]. APA PsycTests.

Király, O., Urbán, R., Griffiths, M. D., Ágoston, C., Nagygyörgy, K., Kökönyei, G., & Demetrovics, Z. (2015). The mediating effect of gaming motivation between psychiatric symptoms and problematic online gaming: An online survey. *Journal of Medical Internet Research, 17*(4), e88. https://doi.org/10.2196/jmir.3515

Kornhuber, J., Zenses, E. M., Lenz, B., Stoessel, C., Bouna-Pyrrou, P., Rehbein, F., Lkiem, S., & MöBle. (2013). Low 2D:4D Values are associated with video game addiction. *PLoS One, 8*(11), e79539. Retrieved from https://www.ncbi.nlm.nih.gov/pmc/articles/PMC3827365/

Kuss, D. J., & Pontes, H. M. (2019). *Internet addiction.* Boston, MA: Hogrefe Publishing.
Kwon, M., Kim, D.-J., Cho, H., & Yang, S. (2013) The smartphone addiction scale: Development and validation of a short version for adolescents. *PLoS One, 8*(12). https://doi.org/10.1371/journal.pone.0083558
Laricchia, F. (2022, December 6). *US smartphone ownership 2011 to 2021*. Statista. Retrieved from https://www.statista.com/statistics/219865/percentage-of-us-adults-who-own-a-smartphone/
Leary, M. R., & Baumeister, R. F. (2000). The nature and function of self-esteem: Sociometer theory. In M. P. Zanna (Ed.), *Advances in experimental social psychology* (pp. 1–16). San Diego, CA: Academic Press.
Leary, M. R., & Downs, D. L. (1995). Interpersonal functions of the self-esteem motive: The self-esteem system as a sociometer. In M. Kernis (Ed.), *Efficacy, agency, and self-esteem* (pp. 123–144). New York: Plenum.
Li, J., Lau, J. T. F., Mo, P. K. H., Su, X., Wu, A. M. S., Tang, J., & Qin, Z. (2016). *Social Networking Activity Intensity Scale (SNAIS)* [Database record]. APA PsycTests.
Lim, F. K., & Sng, B. B. (2020). Social media, religion and shifting boundaries in globalizing China. *Global Media and China, 5*(3), 261–274. https://doi.org/10.1177/2059436420923169
Lin, I. H., Ko, C. H., Chang, Y. P., Liu, T. L., Wang, P. W., Lin, H. C., … & Yen, C. F. (2014). The association between suicidality and Internet addiction and activities in Taiwanese adolescents. *Comprehensive Psychiatry, 55*(3), 504–510. http://doi.org/10.1016/j.
Livingood, W. C., Bautista, M. A. B., Smotherman, C., Azueta, D., Coleman, J., Grewal, R., Stewart, E., Orlando, L. A., & Scuderi, C. (2022). Comparative study of different SES neighborhood clinics for health literacy and internet access. *Digital Health, 8*. https://doi.org/10.1177/20552076221123715
Lopez-Ferandez, O., Griffiths, M. D., Kuss, D. J., Dawes, C., Pontes, H. M., Justice, L., Rumpf, J., Bischof, A., et al. (2019). Cross-cultural validation of the Compulsive Internet Use Scale in four forms and eight languages. *Cyberpsychology, Behavior, and Social Networking,* 451–464. http://doi.org/10.1089/cyber.2018.0731
Manning, L., Ferris, M., Narvaez Rosario, C., Prues, M., & Bouchard, L. (2019). Spiritual resilience: Understanding the protection and promotion of well-being in the later life. *Journal of Religion, Spirituality & Aging, 31*(2), 168–186.
Marizan, P. (2016). *American muslims tackle terrorism with teens' best tool: The internet.* Washington, DC: NPR, Retrieved from https://www.npr.org/2016/01/27/464593565/american-muslims-tackle-terrorism-with-teens-best-tool-the-internet.
McMahon, N., Thomson, K., Kaner, E., & Bambra, C. (2019). Effects of prevention and harm reduction interventions on gambling behaviours and gambling related harm: An umbrella review. *Addictive Behaviors, 90*, 380–388. https://doi.org/10.1016/j.addbeh.2018.11.048
Montag, C., Kirsch, P., Sauer, C., Markett, S., & Reuter, M. (2012). The role of the CHRNA4 gene in internet addiction: A case-control study. *Journal of Addiction Medicine, 6*, 191–195.
Neumaier, A. (2020). The big friendly counter-space? Interreligious encounter within social media. *Religion, 50*(3), 392–413. https://doi.org/10.1080/0048721X.2020.1754605
Pápay, O., Urbán, R., Griffiths, M. D., Nagygyörgy, K., Farkas, J., Kökönyei, G., Felvinczi, K., Oláh, A., Elekes, Z., & Demetrovics, Z. (2013). Psychometric properties of the problematic online gaming questionnaire short-form and prevalence of problematic online gaming in a national sample of adolescents. *Cyberpsychology, Behavior and Social Networking, 16*(5), 340–348. https://doi.org/10.1089/cyber.2012.0484
Pedersen, P. B., & Pope, M. (2016). Toward effectiveness through empathy. In P. B. Pedersen, W. J. Lonner, J. G. Draguns, J. E. Trimble, & M. R. Scharron-del Rio (Eds.), *Counseling across cultures* (7th ed.) (pp. 13–30). Thousand Oaks, CA: SAGE Publications.
Pontes, H. M., Király, O., Demetrovics, Z., & Griffiths, M. D. (2014) The conceptualisation and measurement of DSM-5 internet gaming disorder: The development of the IGD-20 test. *PLoS One, 9*(10), e110137. https://doi.org/10.1371/journal.pone.0110137
Rao, Y. (2019). From confucianism to psychology: Rebooting internet addicts in China. *History of Psychology, 22*(4), 328–350.
Rosen, L. D., Whaling, K., Carrier, L. M., Cheever, N. A., & Rokkum, J. (2013). The media and technology usage and attitudes scale: An empirical investigation. *Computers in Human Behavior, 29*(6), 2501–2511. https://doi.org/10.1016/j.chb.2013.06.006
Rumpf, H. J., Vermulst, A. A., Bischof, A., Kastirke, N., Gürtler, D., Bischof, G., et al. (2014). Occurrence [sic] of Internet addiction in a general population sample: A latent class analysis. *European Addiction Research, 20*(4), 159–166. http://doi.org/10.1159/000354321
Sage Publications (2019). *Introduction to social psychology.* Retrieved from https://us.sagepub.com/sites/default/files/upm-assets/90582_book_item_90582.pdf
Sigman, A. (2017). Screen dependency disorders: A new challenge for child neurology. *Journal of the International Child Neurology Association, 17*(119), 1–13.

Skinner, B. F. (1953). *Science and human behavior.* New York: Macmillan.

Stewart, J. L., & Christner, R. W. (2024). Finding strength in numbers: An introduction to Cognitive Behavior Group Therapy (CBGT) with youth. *The handbook of cognitive behavior group therapy for children and adolescents* (2nd ed.). Routledge.

Stewart, J. L., Christner, R. W., Mulligan, C., & Fox, E. (2024). Building healthy media and device habits: A CBT-based roadmap. In *The handbook of cognitive behavior group therapy for children and adolescents* (2nd ed.). Routledge.

Stockings, E., Hall, W. D., Lynskey, M., Morley, K. I., Reavley, N., Strang, J., Patton, G., & Degenhardt, L. (2016). Prevention, early intervention, harm reduction, and treatment of substance use in young people. *The Lancet Psychiatry, 3*(3), 280–296. https://doi.org/10.1016/s22150366(16)00002-x

Tatarsky, A. (2003). Harm reduction psychotherapy: Extending the reach of traditional substance use treatment. *Journal of Substance Abuse Treatment, 25*(4), 249–256. https://doi.org/10.1016/s0740-5472(03)00085-0

van den Eijnden, R. J. J. M., Lemmens, J., & Valkenburg, P. M. (2016). The social media disorder scale. *Computers in Human Behavior, 61*, 478–487. https://doi.org/10.1016/j.chb.2016.03.038

Vizcaino, M., Buman, M., DesRoches, C., et al. (2019). Reliability of a new measure to assess modern screen time in adults. *BMC Public Health, 19*, 1386. https://doi.org/10.1186/s12889-019-7745-6

Weziak-Bialowolska, D., Bialowolski, P., Lee, M. T., Chen, Y., VanderWeele, T. J., & McNeely, E. (2022) Prospective associations between social connectedness and mental health. Evidence from a longitudinal survey and health insurance claims data. *International Journal of Public Health, 67*, 1604710. https://doi.org/10.3389/ijph.2022.1604710

Young, K. S. (2017). *The Internet Addiction Test (IAT).* Woodale, IL: Stoelting.

Young, K. S., & Rogers, R. C. (1998). The relationship between depression and internet addiction, *Cyberpsychology, Behavior, & Social Networking, 1*(1), 25–28.

Zhang, J. T., Ma, S. S., Li, C. S. R., Liu, L., Xia, C. C., Lan, J., Wang, L. J., Liu, B., Yao, Y. W., & Fang, X. Y. (2016). Craving behavioral intervention for internet gaming disorder: Remediation of functional connectivity of the ventral striatum. *Addiction Biology, 23*(1), 337–346. https://doi.org/10.1111/adb.12474

22

SEXUALIZED BEHAVIORS AND SOCIAL MEDIA

Christy A. Mulligan, Justin Ayoub and Sarah Liberti

Introduction to the Problem

In a recent Pew Research Study, half of all teens aged 13–17 report using the Internet almost constantly. Ninety percent of these youth are on at least one social media platform, the most popular being YouTube (Pew Research Study, 2022), and 71% of young people use more than one social media option (Lenhart et al., 2015). This data alone is both startling and troubling, especially in recent light of the scores on the National Assessment of Educational Progress (NAEP), often referred to as the Nation's Report Card, which showed a decline of four points in reading and nine points in mathematics for 13-year-olds during the 2022–2023 school year (https://www.nationsreportcard.gov/highlights/ltt/2023/). Although there may be competing reasons for this decline, such as the COVID-19 pandemic, the ubiquitous use of social media and the Internet, in general, suggests different priorities for youth today. These priorities include online socialization, viewing influencer reels, or other media content, while reading for pleasure has fallen in popularity among all age groups but most dramatically (18%) in the 13-year-old demographic. This is likely a very common age for youth to engage in social media, replacing reading and other academic endeavors.

In Western society, youth's sexual curiosity, expression, and experimentation are all typical and considered normative aspects of development (Tolman & McClelland, 2011). Most teens view online social networks as one of the most important platforms for socializing, connecting, communicating, and building one's identity, e.g., self-expression (Pew Research Study, 2022). Youth often use social media in positive ways that are developmentally appropriate, such as exploring their identity, promoting their independence, and trying to gain support and strengthen their relationships with their peers (Radovic et al., 2017). Developing this online identity may help adolescents increase their self-esteem by showing individualism through their profiles (Gonzales & Hancock, 2011) or gaining positive reactions to their posts or photos (Moreno & Kolb, 2012; Valkenburg et al., 2006; Williams & Merten, 2008). Therefore, we have a delicate balance between allowing youth to maintain their level of connection with their peers and keeping them safe from online bullying, predators, or misusing social media.

Portrayals of casual sex are prevalent in the media and can be easily accessed through the Internet (Bridges et al., 2010; Brosius et al., 1993) and mainstream media (Wright, 2009). Previous findings on the association between sexually explicit media content and young people's permissive attitudes toward sex (Brown & L'Engle, 2009; Omori et al., 2011; Peter & Valkenburg, 2010) suggest that

DOI: 10.4324/9781003392439-25

youths' willingness to engage in casual sex may increase as their viewing of sexually explicit depictions increases. A typical mainstream media that ranks among the genres with the highest sexual content is reality TV (Fisher et al., 2004; Kunkel et al., 2007). Sexual situations in reality TV often revolve around casual sex. There has been an explosion of this type of reality television in recent years, and exposure to such content has been related to youths' permissive attitudes toward sex (Bond & Drogos, 2014) and their beliefs about having sex on the 1st date or with multiple partners (Riddle & De Simone, 2013). In addition, these shows are discussed among youth on social media and "in real life" (IRL), which may exacerbate the permissive behavior because these youth find the reality TV figures attractive, cool, or desirable.

When youth create and share sexual content of themselves, e.g., sexy "selfies" on social network sites (Hall et al., 2012; Hinduja & Patchin, 2008; Moreno et al., 2009; Peluchette & Karl, 2009), these images may be interpreted as the youth being sexually open or accessible (Peluchette & Karl, 2009; Ringrose & Eriksson Barajas, 2011) welcoming others to the potential of their willingness to engage in casual sex. This perception is promoted by initial evidence that online sexually nuanced photos are associated with having experience with casual sex (Bobkowski et al., 2012). Youth who post these risqué photos or create posts with sexual undertones are at greater risk for engaging in casual sexual relations outside of a committed relationship, which is viewed as risky sexual behavior (Kotchick et al., 2001). Moreover, these youth frequently do not have their social media settings marked as private, and those who are not "friends" or screened "followers" gain access to these photos. These consequences may extend further than their inappropriate online social media use and impact school functioning, family relationships, and IRL friendships.

The wide use of technology also comes with risks, such as cyberbullying or harassment, sexting, depression (O'Keefe & Clarke-Pearson, 2011), and involuntary exposure to unwanted sexual content (Smith et al., 2016). Youths' exposure to sexualized images, or even pornographic or violent sexual content, has been linked to a desensitization to sexually violent stimuli and a more permissive attitude toward high-risk sexual behaviors (Yao et al., 2010). Youth who use social media or the Internet are typically in the safety of their home; this distance provided by their remote environment could increase the desensitization process. Youth may find chatting with an adult or another peer in a sexual manner exciting and sending explicit photos of themselves as a low-risk behavior. These youth's lack of awareness regarding their safety, coupled with the risk that the recipient may share their messages or explicit photos, exposes them to vulnerability. If their content gets distributed, it can lead to significant stress, anxiety, and depression.

Overview of CBT to Sexualized Behavior and Social Media

Unhealthy media device use (MDU) was recently reviewed and conceptualized from a cognitive-behavioral perspective (Stewart et al., 2024). Sexualized behaviors in relation to social media are certainly of a similar ilk. There is likely no argument that for some youth, their use of social media is problematic and maladaptive (Shensa et al., 2017), which could be identified from symptoms such as a fixation with social media, an inability to control social media use, and continued social media use even though they have suffered negative consequences (Worsley et al., 2018). Problematic social media (PSM) use has been found to have many adverse effects, such as stress (Hawk et al., 2019), reduced well-being (Kross et al., 2013; Lin et al., 2016; van Rooij et al., 2017), distractedness (van Zoonen et al., 2017), poor school performance (Turel & Qahri-Saremi, 2016), and many other negative emotions (Pontes et al., 2018). This may be exacerbated when the youth is posting sexualized images of themselves and getting "likes" or multiple requests to "follow." Receiving this type of reinforcement can validate and promote the likelihood of continued posting of sexualized content.

Although the research on the use of cognitive-behavioral therapy (CBT) to address sexualized behaviors in the use of social media is scant, it has been helpful as an effective treatment in the prevention of Internet addiction and other compulsive behaviors (Andreassen, 2015; Kuss & Griffiths, 2011). Some researchers believe that the problematic use of social media is a new and rising type of behavioral addiction (Andreassen, 2015; Kuss & Griffiths, 2011; Ryan et al., 2014). Although the Diagnostic and Statistical Manual of Mental Disorders (DSM) does not recognize social media as an addiction, it does share similar symptoms with other addictions (Ryan et al., 2014; Van den Eijnden et al., 2016), such as withdrawal (Stieger & Lewetz, 2018) relapse (Baumer et al., 2013) and time distortion (Turel et al., 2018a, 2018b). Comparable to other types of addictions, social media use can be described by the reward-based learning process (Brewer, 2019), meaning that because social media use is typically a distinct high-reward behavior, it is more likely to be performed again versus a low-reward behavior (Hofmann & Van Dillen, 2012). This behavioral phenomenon is commonly considered the cause of both substance and behavioral addictions (Grant et al., 2010). Therefore, we must also address which replacement behaviors will be healthier and allow similar peer validation regarding positive comments, likes, or follow requests.

When conceptualizing sexualized behavior alongside unhealthy social media, it is crucial to understand the maladaptive cognitions (Wang et al., 2015) that support its use. The cognitive-affective-behavioral paradigm purports that behavior is guided by emotion, and emotion is determined by cognition (Breckler, 1984). Youth who engage in unhealthy social media use are at risk for low self-esteem, narcissism, and loneliness (Andreassen et al., 2017; Błachnio et al., 2016; Hormes et al., 2014). There is evidence that youth who have dysfunctional cognitions about social media may be more inclined to engage in social media addictive behaviors (Davis, 2001; Caplan, 2010; Mai et al., 2012; Pontes et al., 2018). A recent study investigating the key cognitive factors contributing to unhealthy social media use supports this theory, revealing that maladaptive cognitions significantly predict excessive social media use (Pontes et al., 2018). Therefore, a possibly effective way to treat unhealthy social media use is by using cognitive restructuring techniques to promote change in youths' maladaptive cognitions.

Empirical Support of CBT in the Treatment of Sexualized Behavior and Social Media

CBT is a form of psychotherapy based on the premise that irrational beliefs and maladaptive thoughts lead to emotional and behavioral disturbances. CBT posits that thoughts, feelings, and behaviors are interactional, and the primary goal is to assist the client in identifying and restructuring irrational thoughts and beliefs. It is an active and directive form of therapy in which the therapist and client set the agenda for the course of treatment and each session (Tolin, 2016). CBT is an effective treatment for several disorders, including anxiety, depression, schizophrenia, and insomnia (David et al., 2018; Fordham et al., 2021; Hofmann et al., 2012).

Both social media use and sexual behavior can be maladaptive and problematic. Bearing this in mind, practitioners must identify targets of intervention as well as treatment goals, as PSM use and problematic sexual behavior may require different treatment modalities. The literature on interventions for PSM use is scarce. PSM use can involve a preoccupation with social media, difficulty moderating social media use, and continued use even after experiencing adverse consequences (Worsley et al., 2018; Zhou et al., 2021). In a more recent meta-analysis, psychotherapeutic interventions (i.e., counseling, CBT) were more effective than abstinence-based interventions for reducing social media use and improving overall well-being (Plackett et al., 2023).

There is body of research examining the effectiveness of group CBT for internet addiction. In a sample that included 50 adults aged 18–30, Alavi and colleagues (2021) found that those in the

CBT group showed significant reductions in internet addiction and an increase in quality of life compared to participants in the control group. Another study of 50 adolescents aged 12–17 indicated that group CBT improved emotional, cognitive, and behavioral symptoms (Du et al., 2010). Unfortunately, these studies had small samples and did not compare CBT to other psychotherapies. There is also uncertainty about how these treatments fare across various cultural groups. A meta-analysis that included 13 studies on CBT (both individual and group) for internet addiction found that CBT had a significant effect on reducing internet addiction. However, all these studies were conducted in China (Liu et al., 2017), which could limit generalizability to a Westernized population.

The primary treatment for sexually harmful behavior is multisystemic therapy (MST) (Henggeler et al., 2009). MST is an intensive family and community-based treatment targeted at youth with serious social, emotional, and behavioral problems who are at risk for out-of-home placement (Letourneau et al., 2013; Littell et al., 2021). MST practitioners apply interventions and target the individual, family, peer, and school communities that may be contributing to problem behavior; caregivers are seen as essential to program success. Therapists integrate evidence-based treatments, such as behavioral parent training, pragmatic family therapy, CBT, and MST, to address clinical issues at different levels. MST is effective in reducing youth delinquency, substance use, externalizing symptoms, and deviant sexual interest/risk behaviors (Henggeler et al., 2009; Letourneau et al., 2009, 2013); however, a more recent meta-analysis achieved mixed results (Littell et al., 2021). Nonetheless, this research on MST is encouraging as a treatment option, as some youths are engaging in high-risk sexual behavior that can be detrimental to their mental and physical health. Furthermore, practitioners can glean strategies from MST, such as collaborating with parents or increasing supervision, when working with youth exhibiting sexually problematic behavior.

Empirical support for CBT as a standalone treatment for problematic sexual behavior is not promising, as a recent literature review indicated that CBT did not improve outcomes in comparison with no treatment, treatment as usual, or alternative interventions (Sneddon et al., 2020). Nonetheless, CBT can help youths with problematic sexual behavior by addressing denial, enhancing accountability, restructuring cognitive distortions, and preventing relapse. Goals also include building problem-solving skills, improving social skills, fostering empathy for victims, and increasing self-awareness (Letourneau et al., 2013; Sneddon et al., 2020). Thus, while CBT may not be the main component of the treatment for problematic sexual behavior, it should be incorporated into the larger framework of treating youth who are engaging in risky sexual behavior online and IRL.

Factors of the Therapeutic Connection

It is well-known by practicing clinicians that the therapeutic relationship plays a critical role in both adult and youth psychological treatment (Labouliere et al., 2017). Specifically, when treating youth within a CBT framework, the therapeutic relationship is considered especially critical in encouraging active participation, collaboration, and the discussion of emotions (Shirk et al., 2008). Therefore, having a strong therapeutic relationship may enhance trust and openness between the youth and their therapist and be a principal component for progress.

The youth's presenting problem is important for conceptualizing and determining which initial CBT techniques and behavioral experiments should be attempted (Brown et al., 2014). When youth have a strong therapeutic relationship during their sessions, this can help in building the dialogue in unpacking potentially embarrassing or difficult topics such as sexualized posts on social media. A majority of the empirical research surrounding the therapeutic relationship has concentrated on the collaboration of tasks and goals, with a heavy focus on the bond between therapist and youth (Bordin, 1979). There is a moderate association (r = .26) between the therapeutic relationship and positive outcomes in CBT in depressed youth (Shirk et al., 2008).

Some variables are significant for the youth and their parent(s), such as their willingness to participate in treatment, their feelings around the acceptability of treatment, and their commitment/motivation to therapy; parent and youth willingness to participate in treatment were all moderately related to treatment outcome (Karver et al., 2005). These are important findings because, unlike adults who are likely to seek out treatment independently of others and do not need permission, youth need their parent's consent to engage in the treatment, which may add a complex layer to the therapeutic connection. For example, youth may be powerless to schedule sessions consistently, may have transportation issues, or may only be eligible for a maximum number of sessions based on their parent's insurance. Therefore, we cannot underscore the importance of parents' onboarding and buy-in in the youth's therapeutic process.

Interestingly, with the rise in problems with the overuse or misuse of technology, some younger clients are turning to text-based treatments. Therefore, there have been questions surrounding whether a therapeutic alliance is as important when clients are not treated face to face. There is evidence to indicate that alliance levels in Internet-based CBT (ICBT) are comparable to those in face-to-face therapy (Berger, 2017). However, there have been mixed results when investigating the outcomes of the therapeutic alliance, with some studies finding a positive relationship between the therapeutic alliance and outcome (Bergman et al., 2013) and some that do not (Andersson et al., 2012; Preschl et al., 2011; Sauer-Zavala et al., 2012). Research on youth is sparse, but one study (Andersson et al., 2012) suggests a positive and significant relationship between alliance and outcomes in ICBT for adolescents.

Interviewing and Assessing Problem Area

A critical part of assessing social media use is determining when it becomes problematic or maladaptive. A clear indicator is when social media use precludes participation in other important life activities, such as completing homework, socializing with others outside of the digital context, participating in extracurricular activities, engaging in physical activity, maintaining personal hygiene, and getting adequate sleep. The amount of time spent on social media is another indicator, although the purpose of social media use should be considered. Engaging in productive and creative activities is different from scrolling through platforms in search of entertainment. Individuals may differ in their tolerance for social media use, with some being able to manage longer amounts of time than others without experiencing negative consequences (Stewart et al., 2024).

When social media use is determined to be problematic, it is essential to understand the function that it is serving. Healthier functions of social media use include connecting with friends, gaining emotional support, gaining information, increasing diverse experiences, and finding people with similar identities and interests (Anderson & Jiang, 2018). Social media use can also benefit vulnerable populations, as they may lack local access to support networks (Berger et al., 2022; Craig et al., 2021). Additionally, practitioners should assess at a broader level, looking for comorbid symptoms of anxiety, depression, withdrawal, and other emotional problems, which may need to be concurrently addressed.

Interviewing youth regarding sexual behavior can seem to be a daunting task. Interviews for less sensitive clinical issues can be challenging, and the youth may feel uncomfortable disclosing certain information in these situations. Considering the sensitive nature of the content to be discussed, practitioners should place a greater emphasis on confidentiality and the limits thereof, explaining what information will be shared and with whom may put the youth at ease. Informing the youth that questions regarding sexual practices are asked to everyone may also be helpful; practitioners will want to ensure that questions are developmentally appropriate, given the youth's age and level of functioning. Furthermore, allowing the youth the opportunity to ask questions/discuss concerns may assist them in feeling validated (Pfeffer et al., 2017). Practitioners should strive to create a safe, nonjudgmental space and present themselves as a resource for clients. As with any clinical interview, practitioners should make a concerted effort to establish rapport before delving into more sensitive issues.

The clinical interview should include the evaluation of how often the youth engages in social media, as well as the duration and type of activities they are interested in. Practitioners will want to collect information about their mood when engaging in social media and when told to stop; their cognitions and thinking patterns about social media can then be evaluated. The Centers for Disease Control and Prevention (2022) has offered guidance for practitioners discussing sexual issues with clients, and these can be adapted to children and adolescents. They endorse posing questions about sexting and the consumption of highly sexualized media, as well as if they engage in high-risk sexual behaviors, e.g., unprotected sex or a high number of sexual partners. We also recommend gathering information from the youth about how social media has affected their daily functioning, e.g., missed school assignments or other social activities due to their use, as well as lack of sleep or conflicts with family and friends. Finally, the practitioner should understand whether the youth client sees their social media use as a problem and evaluate their readiness to change (Stewart et al., 2024).

In addition to a clinical interview, practitioners can use rating scales to gain information about the various symptoms the child may be experiencing. Broad-band scales will assist in getting a general sense of the youth's emotional functioning. One such measure is the *Behavior Assessment System for Children, Third Edition* (BASC-3™; Reynolds & Kamphaus, 2015), which examines the emotional and behavioral symptoms of the youth. The BASC-3™ can be used for youth aged 2–21 and has various reporting methods (i.e., self, parent, teacher). Another instrument is the *Child Behavior Checklist* (CBCL; Achenbach & Rescorla, 2001), which is appropriate for youth aged 6–18. Similar to the BASC-3™, the CBCL has multiple reporting methods (self, caregiver, and teacher). Both the BASC-3™ and CBCL have general and clinical samples that allow practitioners to compare and assess the severity of symptoms.

Assessment of executive functions may also be warranted, as emergent literature indicates an association between executive functioning deficits and PSM use (Aydin et al., 2020; Pichardo et al., 2021). Two noteworthy instruments are the *Behavior Rating Inventory of Executive Function®, Second Edition* (BRIEF®2; Gioia et al., 2015) and the *Comprehensive Executive Function Inventory®* (CEFI®; Naglieri & Goldstein, 2013). These rating scales assess various aspects of executive functioning, are appropriate for children and adolescents aged 5–18, and allow for multiple informants (self, parent, teacher). Results from these scales can be helpful for treatment planning and implementing interventions specifically targeting executive functions or aspects thereof.

There has been a growing interest in the psychological effects of social media over the past 15 years; this interest has given rise to the development of narrow-band scales to assess social media use. One option is the *Social Media Disorder Scale* (SMDS; van den Eijnden et al. 2016), adapted from the *DSM-5* (American Psychiatric Association, 2013) criteria for internet gaming disorder. It is a nine-item yes/no scale intended for adolescents that assesses problematic uses of social media. The SMDS has acceptable psychometric properties on various aspects of reliability and validity (Boer et al., 2022; van den Eijnden et al., 2016). The nine-item SMDS has recently been adapted for parent use (SDMS-P; Austermann et al., 2021) to allow practitioners to get parents' perspectives on the youth's social media use.

Measuring specific sexual behaviors and practices more objectively is an integral part of the assessment process, and there are a few options specifically for sexual behavior. The *Adolescent Sexual Behavior Inventory-Self-Report* (ACSBI-S; Friedrich et al., 2004) is an option for practitioners. It is a 45-item self-report scale normed on a clinical population that assesses sexual knowledge, sexual risk, divergent sexual interests, concerns about appearance, and fear. A parent report version can also be used to get caregivers' perspective. Currently, there is a need for an instrument validated on youth that includes other types of risky sexual behaviors that are prevalent among teenagers, such as sexting or exchanging sexual content on social media.

Case Conceptualization

Internal experiences and states are important in conceptualizing youth and their Internet use. According to Gerwin et al. (2018), youths' interest in digital media is developmentally appropriate because it is a space to connect with peers outside of the home and family. Gerwin and colleagues purport that it is developmentally natural for youth between the ages of eight and 12 to be influenced by their peers rather than their families. Hence, if peers are regularly using digital media to socialize and communicate, it can be expected that youth will also use this outlet. Digital outlets also provide a space for adolescents to connect with others who share their interests and struggles (Gerwin et al., 2018). Such opportunities are critical to development, especially if in-person opportunities to socialize and relate to others are limited.

Evidence indicates that certain risk factors may increase the likelihood of adolescents engaging in risky internet behavior. According to Noll and colleagues (2013), adolescents who have experienced maltreatment, defined as abuse and neglect, show a connection between participating in risky online activities and exhibiting general behavioral issues. More specifically, the researchers highlighted that adolescent girls who have been victims of maltreatment exhibit elevated levels of depressive symptoms, engage in high-risk nonsexual behaviors, experience inadequate parenting, encounter online sexual solicitations, and are unintentionally exposed to online sexual content.

There is evidence that youth who have sexually offended have been abused themselves (Krause et al., 2022). However, if there is a relationship between childhood sexual abuse and youth who engage in sexually harmful behavior, available research suggests that this may impact the onset of the behavior but not the maintenance of it (Seto & Lalumière, 2010). It is also important to note that although some studies report high rates of previous sexual abuse in sexually harmful youth, only a small number of sexually abused youths become abusers, and not all sexually harmful youth have been sexually victimized (Burton et al., 2002).

In working with youth whose lives have been impacted by their internet usage, it is critical to perceive the underlying contexts in which the client exists. Brand et al. (2016) articulated the theoretical model of Interaction of Person-Affect-Cognition-Execution (I-PACE), which explicitly addresses factors that contribute to the "development and maintenance of addictive behaviors" for Internet usage (p. 253). I-PACE addresses three components: predisposing variables, affective and cognitive responses to external or internal stimuli, executive functions, inhibitory control, and the decision to use certain Internet applications (Brand et al., 2016). Finally, I-PACE recognizes that youths' executive functioning skills, inhibitory control, and the process of deciding to use certain applications decrease in individuals experiencing Internet addiction. Overall, the I-PACE model grants clinicians space to conceptualize youth comprehensively facing Internet addiction by contextualizing the individual's internal and external experiences.

Most of the literature on case conceptualization for youth engaging with sexualized behaviors on social media references CBT-based models. It is critical to remember that cognitive therapy case conceptualizations must be parsimonious, coherent, meaningful, and justifiable to be considered high quality (Kuyken et al., 2005). There has been criticism about the absence of sociocultural and biological mechanisms and elements of the therapeutic relationship that can impact the holistic view of the youth client (Haarhoff et al., 2011); therefore, these elements must be addressed. We endorse identifying patterns and connections between thoughts, behaviors, and emotions so clinicians can formulate a comprehensive understanding of the causes and effects of the youth's inappropriate social media use; therefore, a plan can be developed, and goals can be established to lead them on a path to improved relationships and mental health.

Session Structure

Clinicians working with youth presenting with either sexual deviancy or appropriate sexual behaviors must determine if social media use is associated with such behaviors. Bettmann et al. (2020) encouraged therapists to use their clinical judgment to determine if a youth's social media use is "problematic or merely [a way to] help the client meet needs in an adaptive and convenient way" (p. 376). They further explained that social media uniquely influences every youth's life. Therefore, it is critical to determine if social media influences any of the youth's harmful behaviors and emotions.

In structuring sessions, the clinician must explore multiple associations social media may have on the client's behaviors and emotions. As mentioned above, Bettmann and colleagues (2020) advocated for applying clinical judgment in perceiving if social media adversely impacts their clients. They also noted that social media use is linked with intentional emotional suppression; frequently, youths will turn to social media as an outlet to avoid experiencing their strongest and potentially most painful feelings. Thus, across sessions, therapists should "utilize interventions that help clients to label, express, and explore emotions while moderating emotional arousal" (p. 376).

In constructing sessions, clinicians should also consider the role of the youth's family. Among a sample of individuals addicted to social media, Mousa (2023) found a positive relationship with family as well as isolation and boredom. When structuring sessions, Mousa advocated for family members to become familiar with the applications associated with the youth's behaviors. Thus, therapists working with individuals who use social media excessively will want to incorporate the youth's family in their sessions for both psychoeducational and therapeutic purposes. Families can be educated about the function(s) of their loved one's behaviors and be involved in the therapeutic process of addressing underlying feelings of isolation and boredom.

Hou and colleagues (2019) also studied young adults with social media addiction and found this use to be associated with poor academic performance. Hou and colleagues also found that reduced levels of self-esteem accounted for social media addiction and an overall poor quality of mental health. In structuring sessions with young clients who engage with social media in an addictive manner, clinicians should incorporate practices that address youths' peer relationships in school and outside of school, as well as their overall self-esteem.

Moreover, sessions with young people who use social media to extreme or inappropriate degrees may also want to be galvanized to address online dating and online sexual behaviors in general. Harren et al. (2021) found that PSM use, problematic online dating (POD), and problematic online sexual behaviors (POSB) are all associated with one another, were "negatively correlated to body esteem, and were positively related to cognitive distortions, sexual depression, sexual preoccupation, and sexual desire" (p. 2281). Additionally, Harren and colleagues revealed PSM, in particular, had a negative relationship with one's sexual esteem. Meaning that the more frequently a youth is engaged in PSM use, the less confidence they hold in their sexuality. When structuring sessions with those utilizing social media in risky ways, clinicians should be prepared to address the client's self-image, sexuality, thoughts of sex, as well as blocks or distortions among their thought processes.

For youths involved in sexting with others, either via smartphone or social media app, e.g., Snapchat, Facebook Messenger, or WhatsApp, sessions must recognize the youth's social environment. Gregg et al. (2018) noted that adolescents were more likely to participate in the sending of explicit messages "if they thought their peers would approve, felt pressured by their peers, or had observed their peers sexting" (p. 430). Therefore, in session, the concepts of peer pressure and boundary-setting should be explored. Additionally, youth were less likely to acknowledge potential long-term consequences of their engagement in sexting if they experienced higher levels of sensation-seeking and impulsive decision-making (Gregg et al., 2018). In terms of structuring sessions with youth who frequently sext, coping skills and behavior changes for both sensation-seeking and impulsive decision-making may be practical.

Component of Practice and Intervention Modules

Throughout this chapter, we have explored youth's overuse and inappropriate use of social media. For many youths, social media can be an opportunity to avoid experiencing and recognizing difficult emotions (Bettman et al., 2020). When intervening with youth who use social media in problematic manners, clinicians must use practices that provide them with the space to explore, name, and experience the complex emotions they desire to avoid.

Similarly, Stewart et al. (2024) pushed for youth to accurately perceive their emotions by naming them as well as determining the degree to which they feel the emotion(s). The clinician must validate the experience of painful emotions internally and externally, working with the youth to understand that emotions are experienced as physical sensations (Stewart et al., 2024). The therapist and client should explore underlying influences that contribute to their need to use social media in risky ways.

Mousa (2023) stated that the objectives of CBT in working with university students with social media addiction include identifying reasons that contribute to their addiction (*why* does one turn to social media?), addressing how their addiction has adversely impacted their lives, naming emotions that are connected to the addiction, as well as "guiding the addict to think correctly, enhance [their] awareness, and adopt correct beliefs, which will make [them] behave moderately in life, away from the social media addiction" (p. 188).

Once objectives have been identified and clarified, Mousa (2023) applied the CBT framework presented in Table 22.1 in his study with university students experiencing social media addiction.

Mousa's (2023) CBT intervention can be modified when working with youth who engage in inappropriate sexualized behavior influenced by excessive social media use. In the 2nd phase of treatment, the assessment of potential contributing factors should also include motivating forces behind their sexually inappropriate behavior. Also, during the 2nd phase, the clinician can assess for irrational

Table 22.1 Objectives of CBT

First phase	Establish rapport for clients to accept the intervention and participate effectively
Second phase	• Assess the clients' social media addiction by determining potential contributing factors that sparked the social media addiction • This assessment should include any irrational thoughts the client holds and measure the severity of the addiction • Explain the dangers associated with social media addiction to potentially decrease the client's drive to turn to social media
Third phase	• Work with the client to replace unhealthy thoughts with "right thoughts" to ease negative emotions (p. 188). Such emotions may include despair, frustration, anger, anxiety, and fear
Fourth phase	• Inform clients of "new behavioral skills that guide them to logical thinking, correct perception, and sound beliefs that would help them adopt positive behaviors in life" (p. 188)
Fifth phase	• Closely monitor the client's behavior associated with social media addiction
Sixth phase	• End the CBT intervention by engaging in regular follow-ups with the client at an appropriate time

Source: Mousa (2023, p. 188).

thoughts the client holds, specifically about sexual behaviors. The 2nd phase may also be altered by having the clinician explain the dangers of inappropriate sexual behaviors alongside the dangers of social media addiction. Lastly, in the 5th phase, sexualized behavior must also be closely monitored.

Overall, cognitive-based treatments encourage those excessively using the Internet and social media to address their thoughts and behaviors connected to their usage directly. They acknowledge that this disordered behavior has been triggered by unacknowledged emotions and maintained through unhealthy thought processes. Whichever counseling technique applies to youths who misuse social media or engage in sexually risky behaviors, Laundry et al. (2017) advised that parental monitoring most likely serves as a protective factor in youths who frequently use social media and engage in risky sexual behaviors. The more involved parents are in youths' lives, the less likely youths are to carry out sexually risky behaviors. This suggests parents must take steps to monitor and supervise youth struggling with sexualized behaviors on social media, which will create safe avenues for meeting their developmental needs.

There are many treatment options available. However, the research on typical youth engaging in sexualized behaviors within the confines of social media and how to address these behaviors from a CBT or other psychological treatment modality is scant. Therefore, adapting treatments from peripheral areas within the literature, e.g., gaming, internet abuse, and juvenile sex offending, to offer evidence-based solutions to address youth who engage in inappropriate sexualized behavior on social media may be warranted. We believe this research is forthcoming, as youth are continually bombarded with sexual images online, and this content is often shared among their peer groups. It is an important topic to address so we can combat unhealthy stereotypes and unrealistic body images, which can impact self-esteem. It is also critical for the adults in youths' lives to demystify sex and unpack what leads to a mutual connection and healthy sexual relationships.

Assessment of Progress and Outcomes: Monitoring

Several formal measurements were mentioned earlier in the Interviewing and Assessing the Problem Area section of this chapter. Therefore, we will not review each one again, but we endorse the use of both narrow and broad-band scales to monitor improvements in youth's risky sexual behavior on social media.

In addition to formalized tools, practitioners can use their clinical judgment to observe changes in particular symptomology. Regarding sexually risky behaviors, Doornwaard et al. (2014) found that youth who frequently engage in sex-related online behaviors "are at increased risk for developing negative body and sexual self-perceptions" (p. 1109). These researchers also noted that youth with higher levels of sexually explicit Internet material use predicted decreased satisfaction with sexual experiences (Doornwaard et al., 2014). Thus, it infers that youth who decrease their sexually explicit Internet material use report a decrease in negative self-perceptions of the body and sexuality as well as higher levels of sexual satisfaction. Doornwaard and colleagues also concluded from their research that youths' use of social networking sites, in general, may elicit the youth to self-evaluate critically. Therefore, if excessive or inappropriate engagement with social networking sites decreases, the clinician may observe the youth possessing a more positive self-image.

Among a sample of university students, Hou et al. (2019) noted that social media addiction was negatively associated with general mental health and academic performance. It assumes that if a youth's social media addiction weakens, the youth and clinician may observe an overall strengthening of their mental health as well as better academic productivity. This may produce other positive consequences, such as involvement in social activities and stronger connections with family and friends.

Furthermore, youths' progress may also be monitored by regularly assessing how they continue to use social media. Gerwin et al. (2018) noted that adolescents can utilize social networks for positive engagements that are developmentally and socially appropriate. For instance, they wrote, "Social networks and communication via various electronic means allow teens to identify and connect with communities that share their interests and struggles, even if they are physically or socially isolated offline" (p. 352). Through treatment, the youth may change their engagement with Internet platforms from mostly inappropriate and disruptive to valuable and productive; youths may then distinguish between healthy and unhealthy ways of using Internet platforms for communication and socialization.

Similarly, the continuous involvement of the youths' parents in monitoring their child's Internet engagement to prevent sexually risky behaviors is critical (Laundry et al., 2017). Therefore, if the clinician understands that the youth's parent(s) are involved in what the youth is using online, there is a possibility that the youth is engaging in fewer sexually risky behaviors. We advocate that this is critical in decreasing youths' problematic Internet/social media use. Although treatment with a skilled clinician is important, the parents who live with the youth must provide supervision to monitor inappropriate versus appropriate online usage. Therefore, parent training and collateral sessions are essential to help the clinician understand progress.

School Applications

School practitioners are in a unique position to treat PSM use, as they often have consistent access to the youth, their teachers, and their parents. School practitioners interact with students daily and can use this to their advantage in terms of tracking social media use and working through issues relating to social media use in real time. They can take a proactive and preventative approach to educating the students they serve on healthy versus problematic uses of social media (Savina et al., 2017). This may include school-wide presentations addressing the risks of social media use, such as cyberbullying, content that encourages harmful or dangerous behavior (e.g., disordered eating or self-harm), facing racism or hate speech, confronting misleading or inaccurate information, and involuntary exposure to unwanted sexual content (Smith et al., 2016; Weir, 2023). School practitioners may also discuss the potential risks and emotional consequences of acting impulsively on social media, oversharing, posting inappropriate content, or sharing sexually risqué or explicit photos/videos of themselves or others. Finally, school practitioners can inform students about the legal ramifications of sharing content that is considered child pornography (Savina et al., 2017).

As youth spend much of their time in school, school practitioners can work with youth in individual or group settings. Cognitive-behavioral techniques discussed earlier in this chapter may be easily integrated into counseling sessions. School practitioners can work with youth to identify harmful and PSM habits. Further, these practitioners can assist youth in identifying maladaptive thinking patterns related to social media and modifying and restructuring these thoughts.

Youth typically have access to their phones during the school day; school practitioners, with permission from parents, may work with the youth on their social media habits and adverse consequences resulting from inappropriate social media use in real time. In conjunction with parents, school practitioners can assist in abstinence efforts by creating a system in which the student turns their phone in to school staff at the beginning of the day and retrieves it at the conclusion of the day, thereby reducing the temptation of social media/device use.

On a broad level, school practitioners should conduct parent training workshops on social media use. School practitioners should seek to inform parents of the benefits and risks of social media, and parents should be encouraged to engage their children in discussions about the risks and negative consequences of social media. Teaching parents to be mindful of unhealthy social media habits, such as preoccupation and continued use, even after experiencing adverse consequences, can place parents in the best position to keep their children safe.

The school's role in treatment for sexually harmful behavior is complex. It must be clearly delineated, as most school practitioners have not had training or supervision in treating sexually harmful youth (Mulligan et al., 2016) and behaviors. In these instances, treatment specifically for sexually harmful behavior is usually not appropriate for school practitioners, and a referral to more specialized treatment (e.g., MST) should be made (Mulligan et al., 2016). Nonetheless, school practitioners can have a role in treatment. They should coordinate with outside providers to obtain strategies or support that may be helpful for the student (Mulligan et al., 2016). School practitioners may play a key role in competency development (Schladale, 2010). This may include building pro-social, moral reasoning, academic, workforce development, and independent living skills (Torbet & Thomas, 2005). Building these competencies can aid significantly in building self-esteem and self-efficacy and decrease the likelihood of continued engagement in sexually harmful behavior.

Case Study of Problem Area

When working with youth who are struggling with sexualized behavior and social media overuse, we need to educate and help them see the impact these behaviors are having on the quality of their lives. Therefore, investigating school life, peer life, family life, and extracurricular activities is essential. Similar to Stewart et al. (2024) in their approach to addressing unhealthy MDU, we endorse a reduction approach for social media and an abstinence approach to address posting sexualized images/posts on their social media. Although we do not want to cut youth off entirely from social media, as this is a large part of their social connections with others, we do encourage safety 1st and moderation 2nd. Therefore, helping youth see the benefits of abstaining from posting sexualized images reduces the likelihood that they will be targeted, bullied, or treated inappropriately by others.

Although this is not an exhaustive set of treatment goals, it is a starting point where clinicians can work with youth within a CBT framework to reduce the unhealthy ways they use social media. In Table 22.2, we offer sample sessions and activities that may be useful when working with youth who engage in sexualized behaviors on social media.

Introduction to CBT/Rapport Building

For many youths, this may be their 1st time in treatment, so it is crucial to prioritize establishing rapport with the youth. One way to do this is by demystifying the CBT process. Providing psychoeducation about CBT, what it is and what it is not, can go a long way in helping the youth feel comfortable. We would like to understand what the youth thinks is the presenting problem to determine their readiness to change or their level of engagement in the therapeutic process. For example, does the youth view their behavior as "costing" them, e.g., grades, stress with family/friends, unwanted attention? Once the therapist establishes this understanding, they can begin conceptualizing the youth client.

Understanding the Problem

Many youths may not view their sexualized behaviors on social media as problematic. Therefore, they may fail to see the danger of loose privacy settings, which may allow adult predators access to their personal social media pages. Helping youth understand the presenting problem and healthy versus unhealthy social media use through Socratic Questioning can have many beneficial effects in therapy (Clark & Egan, 2018). The benefits of this process include developing critical thinking skills that will allow the clinician to guide the youth into understanding maladaptive cognitions and unhelpful processes (Padesky, 1993; Padesky & Beck, 2003). Once youth concede that their sexualized

Table 22.2 Sample Sessions

Session/Goal	*Activities*
1 Introduction to CBT/rapport building	• Introductions • Setting the agenda • Psychoeducation on the CBT approach and techniques • Exploring the presenting problem • What has the problem "cost" the youth?
2 Understanding the problem	• Setting the agenda • Understanding healthy vs. unhealthy Internet/social media use • Identifying their readiness to change
3 Goal setting	• Setting the agenda • Check-in and rapport-building • Collaboratively working on setting goals • Identifying risky online sexual behavior
4 Brainstorming replacement behaviors	• Setting the agenda • Determining satisfactory replacement behaviors • Connecting how the replacement behaviors are reinforcing
5 Understanding how thoughts affect feelings	• Setting the agenda • Discriminate between what is a thought and what is a feeling • Learning how thoughts can affect feelings • Introduce the ABC model • Determining motivation to change—pros/cons
6 Learning how thoughts can change feelings	• Setting the agenda • Asking the youth to provide examples in relation to their thoughts when they post sexualized images on social media and how they feel afterward • Changing negative thoughts to positive or neutral thoughts—check in on how that feels
7 Understanding how replacement behaviors can affect feelings	• Setting the agenda • Discussing feelings about the replacement behavior • Unpacking how needs are being met through the replacement behavior • Self-esteem check-in
8 Planning for maintenance and relapse prevention	• Setting the agenda • Identifying positive supports • Identifying relapse strategies • Identifying a long-term plan for success

behaviors on social media are negatively impacting different areas of their lives, they can then begin to work on the next step, which is finding healthy replacement behaviors.

Goal Setting

In a cognitive behavioral framework, goal setting is a collaborative process between the youth client and the therapist. As mentioned in the section on factors of therapeutic connection, the therapeutic relationship is an important factor in the collaboration of goal setting, which can lead to better outcomes. Reviewing and teaching the youth what is risky online behavior can help shift their behaviors. Collaborating on goals the youth chooses to tackle is the 1st step to uncovering the cognitive triangle of thought, feelings, and behaviors and how this relates to the presenting problem.

Brainstorming Replacement Behaviors

This process may be trickier than anticipated, as "likes" and "followers" are especially reinforcing for youth. Despite the long-term potential costs, they can achieve temporary gains to their self-esteem and self-worth surrounding their popularity in this modality. Beginning with an interest inventory or determining what was reinforcing to the youth before joining social media sites is important. Regardless, finding a replacement for posting sexualized images of themselves would be ideal, albeit understanding the motivation other than the immediate gratification of positive attention is worthy of exploration.

Understanding How Thoughts Affect Feelings

It is important to teach the youth client the thought-feeling connection. Discuss with them the concept of automatic thoughts and how these thoughts spontaneously come to mind. Introduce the ABC Model (Activating event, Beliefs, Consequences) to them (Ellis, 1991). Using examples with the ABC model for their presenting problem can be helpful for them to make connections about how changing their beliefs can lead to positive emotional outcomes. It is here that we challenge negative thoughts that may arise and provide strategies to combat their negative thoughts.

Learning How Thoughts Can Change Feelings

Our thoughts significantly impact our feelings; with the help of cognitive restructuring, we can help the youth identify and change irrational or negative thought patterns, which may be holding them back from treatment gains. Through cognitive restructuring, youth will learn to replace irrational or distorted thoughts with more realistic or balanced ones, positively affecting their emotional responses (Ciharova et al., 2021). This shift in thinking allows youths to gain better control over their feelings and reactions to various situations and will hopefully delay the posting of a sexualized image of themselves.

Understanding How Replacement Behaviors Can Affect Feelings

Replacement behaviors are critical in the treatment of social media misuse. Social media is especially reinforcing, so finding an activity or behavior that will decrease use to moderation and curb any sexualized activity online is critical. When youth can identify and replace harmful behaviors with positive alternatives, they will often experience a shift in their emotional states. For example, if they impulsively post a sexual image of themselves, this may create stress about how others might perceive this image or how many likes they will get, which can lead to stress or anxiety. However, if they go for a run instead of engaging in social media, this can lead to both physical and brain benefits (Hashimoto et al., 2021). Unpacking how this new behavior has impacted their feelings is a critical component of long-lasting change.

Planning for Maintenance and Relapse Prevention

When planning for maintenance and relapse prevention, the youth must know they can always return to treatment. There should be a schedule or a way to check in after one month and then again in three months. It is important to identify the support in the youth's life and provide strategies to prevent relapse, such as identifying triggers, developing coping strategies, and engaging in mindfulness or preferred hobbies. We also encourage a longer-term plan for success, including regular self-reflection to monitor their emotional and mental well-being. It is also important to recognize early signs of distress so they can ask for the support they may need and prevent any escalation in behaviors. Lastly, developing and maintaining healthy routines, such as exercise, good nutrition, and sleep hygiene, may contribute to their overall stability and reduce the likelihood of relapse.

The above are sample sessions and CBT techniques that may help to enable the youth to abstain from sexualized behavior on social media and use it for authentic connections with peers. These sessions may go beyond eight weeks, with sessions on building self-esteem and treating any comorbid symptoms they may experience.

Summary and Conclusion

This chapter discusses the impact of social media on the sexual behaviors of youth. While social media can be a positive outlet for self-expression and connecting with peers, it can also lead to negative consequences, such as exposure to inappropriate content and an increased risk of engaging in risky sexual behavior. The goal is to provide practitioners with the tools to conceptualize this problem, monitor improvements or declines, and provide treatment strategies to address these youths' needs. Although there are few studies on this specific population of youth and how they respond to CBT, there is enough literature on the treatment of associated and comorbid symptoms, e.g., anxiety, depression, impulsivity, and so on, that respond well to cognitive and behavioral strategies. We hope this chapter adds to the awareness of treatment providers that social media is a serious issue, regardless if the youth is engaging in sexualized behaviors; the time it steals from our youth creates risk for declines in their academics, social skills, and overall emotional wellness.

Reflection Questions

1 In what ways do you think social media platforms influence adolescents' understanding and expression of sexuality? Consider the balance between positive aspects of identity exploration and the potential for risky sexual behaviors.
2 Reflect on the role of CBT in addressing PSM use and sexualized behavior among youth. How might these strategies be applied within your own practice, school, or home to support healthier digital engagement?
3 Considering the challenges and risks associated with adolescent social media use, what steps can parents, educators, and mental health professionals take to create a safer and more supportive digital environment for youth? Reflect on specific actions that could be implemented in your community or institution.

References

Achenbach, T. M., Rescorla, L. A. (2001). *Manual for the ASEBA school-age forms & profiles*. Burlington: Research Centre for Children, Youth and Families, University of Vermont.

Alavi, S. S., Ghanizadeh, M., Mohammadi, M. R., Jannatifard, F., Esmaili Alamuti, S., & Farahani, M. (2021). The effects of cognitive-behavioral group therapy for reducing symptoms of internet addiction disorder and promoting quality of life and mental health. *Trends in Psychiatry and Psychotherapy*, *43*, 47–56.

American Psychiatric Association (2013). Diagnostic and statistical manual of mental disorders (DSM-5) (5th ed.). Washington, DC: American Psychiatric Association.

Anderson, M., & Jiang, J. (2018). Teens, social media & technology 2018. Pew Research Center, 31(2018), 1673–1689.

Andersson, G., Paxling, B., Wiwe, M., Vernmark, K., Felix, C. B., Lund- borg, L., Furmark, T., Cuijpers, P., & Carlbring, P. (2012). Therapeutic alliance in guided internet-delivered cognitive behavioural treatment of depression, generalized anxiety disorder and social anxiety disorder. *Behaviour Research and Therapy, 50*(9), 544–550. https://doi.org/10.1016/j.brat.2012.05.003

Andreassen, C. S. (2015). Online social network site addiction: A comprehensive review. *Current Addiction Reports, 2*(2), 175–184.

Andreassen, C. S., Pallesen, S., & Griffiths, M. D. (2017). The relationship between addictive use of social media, narcissism, and self-esteem: Findings from a large national survey. *Addictive Behaviors, 64*, 287–293.

Andersson, G., Paxling, B., Wiwe, M., Vernmark, K., Felix, C. B., Lund- borg, L., Furmark, T., Cuijpers, P., & Carlbring, P. (2012). Therapeutic alliance in guided internet-delivered cognitive behavioural treatment of depression, generalized anxiety disorder and social anxiety disorder. *Behaviour Research and Therapy, 50*(9), 544–550. https://doi.org/10.1016/j.brat.2012.05.003

Austermann, M. I., Thomasius, R., & Paschke, K. (2021). Assessing problematic social media use in adolescents by parental ratings: Development and validation of the social media disorder scale for parents (SMDS-P). *Journal of Clinical Medicine, 10*(4), 617.

Aydın, O., Obuća, F., Boz, C., & Ünal-Aydın, P. (2020). Associations between executive functions and problematic social networking sites use. *Journal Of Clinical and Experimental Neuropsychology, 42*(6), 634–645.

Baumer, E. P. S., P. Adams, V. D. Khovanskaya, T. C. Liao, M. E. Smith, V. S. Sosik, and K. Williams. 2013. "Limiting, Leaving, and (re)Lapsing: An Exploration of Facebook non-use Practices and Experiences." Conference on Human Factors in Computing Systems - Proceedings, 3257–3266. doi:10.1145/2470654.2466446

Berger, T. (2017). The therapeutic alliance in internet interventions: A narrative review and suggestions for future research. Psychotherapy Research, 27(5), 511–524. https://doi.org/10.1080/10503307.2015 .1119908

Berger, M. N., Taba, M., Marino, J. L., Lim, M. S., & Skinner, S. R. (2022). Social media use and health and well-being of lesbian, gay, bisexual, transgender, and queer youth: Systematic review. *Journal of Medical Internet Research, 24*(9), e38449.

Bergman Nordgren, L., Carlbring, P., Linna, E., & Andersson, G. (2013). Role of the working alliance on treatment outcome in tailored internet- based cognitive behavioural therapy for anxiety disorders: Randomized controlled pilot trial. *JMIR Research Protocols, 2*(1), e4. https:// doi.org/10.2196/resprot.2292

Błachnio, A., Przepiorka, A., & Pantic, I. (2016). Association between Facebook addiction, self-esteem and life satisfaction: A cross-sectional study. *Computers in Human Behavior, 55*, 701–705.

Bobkowski, P. S., Brown, J. D., & Neffa, D. R. (2012). "Hit Me Up and We Can Get Down" US youths' risk behaviors and sexual self-disclosure in MySpace profiles. *Journal of Children and Media, 6*(1), 119–134.

Boer, M., Stevens, G. W., Finkenauer, C., Koning, I. M., & van den Eijnden, R. J. (2022). Validation of the social media disorder scale in adolescents: findings from a large-scale nationally representative sample. *Assessment, 29*(8), 1658–1675.

Bond, B. J., & Drogos, K. L. (2014). Sex on the shore: Wishful identification and parasocial relationships as mediators in the relationship between Jersey Shore exposure and emerging adults' sexual attitudes and behaviors. *Media Psychology, 17*(1), 102–126.

Bordin, E. S. (1979). The generalizability of the psychoanalytic concept of the working alliance. *Psychotherapy: Theory, Research & Practice, 16*(3), 252.

Brand, M., Young, K. S., Laier, C., Wölfling, K., & Potenza, M. N. (2016). Integrating psychological and neurobiological considerations regarding the development and maintenance of specific Internet-use disorders: An Interaction of Person-Affect-Cognition-Execution (I-PACE) model. *Neuroscience & Biobehavioral Reviews, 71*, 252–266.

Breckler, S. J. (1984). Empirical validation of affect, behavior, and cognition as distinct components of attitude. *Journal of Personality and Social Psychology, 47*(6), 1191.

Brewer, J. (2019). Mindfulness training for addictions: Has neuroscience revealed a brain hack by which awareness subverts the addictive process? *Current Opinion in Psychology, 28*, 198–203. https://doi.org/10.1016/j.copsyc.2019.01.014

Bridges, A. J., Wosnitzer, R., Scharrer, E., Sun, C., & Liberman, R. (2010). Aggression and sexual behavior in best-selling pornography videos: A content analysis update. *Violence Against Women, 16*, 1065–1085. https://doi.org/10.1177/1077801210382866

Brosius, H. B., Weaver III, J. B., & Staab, J. F. (1993). Exploring the social and sexual "reality" of contemporary pornography. *Journal of Sex Research, 30*(2), 161–170.

Brown, J. D., & L'Engle, K. L. (2009). X-rated: Sexual attitudes and behaviors associated with US early adolescents' exposure to sexually explicit media. *Communication Research, 36*(1), 129–151.

Brown, R. C., Parker, K. M., McLeod, B. D., & Southam-Gerow, M. (2014). Building a positive therapeutic relationship with the child or adolescent and parent. In E. S. Sburlati, H. J. Lyneham, C. A. Schniering, & R. M.

Rapee (Eds.), *Evidence-based CBT for anxiety and depression in children and adolescents: A competencies-based approach* (pp. 63–78). Oxford: John Wiley & Sons. https://doi.org/10.1002/9781118500576
Burton, D. L., Miller, D. L., & Shill, C. T. (2002). A social learning theory comparison of the sexual victimization of adolescent sexual offenders and nonsexual offending male delinquents. *Child Abuse & Neglect, 26*(9), 893–907.
Caplan, S. E. (2010). Theory and measurement of generalized problematic Internet use: A two-step approach. *Computers in Human Behavior, 26*(5), 1089–1097.
Centers for Disease Control and Prevention (2022). Retrieved from https://www.cdc.gov/healthyyouth/sexualbehaviors/index.htm
Ciharova, M., Furukawa, T. A., Efthimiou, O., Karyotaki, E., Miguel, C., Noma, H., ... & Cuijpers, P. (2021). Cognitive restructuring, behavioral activation and cognitive-behavioral therapy in the treatment of adult depression: A network meta-analysis. *Journal of Consulting and Clinical Psychology, 89*(6), 563.
Clark, G. I., & Egan, S. J. (2018). Clarifying the role of the Socratic method in CBT: A survey of expert opinion. *International Journal of Cognitive Therapy, 11*, 184–199.
Craig, S. L., Eaton, A. D., McInroy, L. B., Leung, V. W., & Krishnan, S. (2021). Can social media participation enhance LGBTQ+ youth well-being? Development of the social media benefits scale. *Social Media+ Society, 7*(1), 2056305121988931.
David, D., Cristea, I., & Hofmann, S. G. (2018). Why cognitive behavioral therapy is the current gold standard of psychotherapy. *Frontiers in Psychiatry, 9*, 4.
Davis, R. A. (2001). A cognitive-behavioral model of pathological Internet use. *Computers in Human Behavior, 17*(2), 187–195.
Doornwaard, S. M., Bickham, D. S., Rich, M., Vanwesenbeeck, I., van den Eijnden, R. J., & Ter Bogt, T. F. (2014). Sex-related online behaviors and adolescents' body and sexual self-perceptions. *Pediatrics, 134*(6), 1103–1110.
Du, Y. S., Jiang, W., & Vance, A. (2010). Longer term effect of randomized, controlled group cognitive behavioural therapy for Internet addiction in adolescent students in Shanghai. *The Australian and New Zealand Journal of Psychiatry, 44*(2), 129–134. https://doi.org/10.3109/00048670903282725
Ellis, A. (1991). The revised ABC's of rational-emotive therapy (RET). *Journal of Rational-Emotive & Cognitive-Behavior Therapy, 9*(3), 139–172. https://doi.org/10.1007/BF01061227
Fisher, D. A., Hill, D. L., Grube, J. W., Bersamin, M. M., Walker, S., & Gruber, E. L. (2004). Sex on American television: An analysis across program genres and network types. *Journal of Broadcasting & Electronic Media, 48*, 529–553.
Fordham, B., Sugavanam, T., Edwards, K., Stallard, P., Howard, R., Das Nair, R., ... & Lamb, S. E. (2021). The evidence for cognitive behavioural therapy in any condition, population or context: A meta review of systematic reviews and panoramic meta-analysis. *Psychological Medicine, 51*(1), 21–29.
Friedrich, W. N., Lysne, M., Sim, L., & Shamos, S. (2004). Assessing sexual behavior in high-risk adolescents with the Adolescent Clinical Sexual Behavior Inventory (ACSBI). *Child Maltreatment, 9*(3), 239–250.
Gerwin, R. L., Kaliebe, K., & Daigle, M. (2018). The interplay between digital media use and development. *Child and Adolescent Psychiatric Clinics, 27*(2), 345–355.
Gioia G. A., Isquith P. K., Guy S. C., Kenworthy L. (2015). *Behavior rating inventory of executive function® (BRIEF®2)* (2nd ed.). Lutz, FL: PAR Inc.
Gonzales, A. L., & Hancock, J. T. (2011). Mirror, mirror on my Facebook wall: Effects of exposure to Facebook on self-esteem. *Cyberpsychology, Behavior, And Social Networking, 14*(1–2), 79–83.
Grant, J. E., Potenza, M. N., Weinstein, A., & Gorelick, D. A. (2010). Introduction to behavioral addictions. *The American Journal of Drug and Alcohol Abuse, 36*(5), 233–241.
Gregg, D., Somers, C. L., Pernice, F. M., Hillman, S. B., & Kernsmith, P. (2018). Sexting rates and predictors from an urban midwest high school. *Journal of School Health, 88*(6), 423–433.
Haarhoff, B., Gibson, K., & Flett, R. (2011). Improving the quality of cognitive behaviour therapy case conceptualization: The role of self-practice/self-reflection. *Behavioural and Cognitive Psychotherapy, 39*(3), 323–339.
Hall, P. C., West, J. H., & McIntyre, E. (2012). Female self-sexualization in MySpace. com personal profile photographs. *Sexuality & Culture, 16*, 1–16.
Harren, N., Walburg, V., & Chabrol, H. (2021). Studying social media burnout and problematic social media use: The implication of perfectionism and metacognitions. *Computers in Human Behavior Reports, 4*, 100117.
Hashimoto, T., Shepard, D. L., Kuboyama, T., Shin, K., Kobayashi, R., & Uno, T. (2021). Analyzing temporal patterns of topic diversity using graph clustering. *The Journal of Supercomputing, 77*, 4375–4388.

Hawk, S. T., van den Eijnden, R. J., van Lissa, C. J., & ter Bogt, T. F. (2019). Narcissistic adolescents' attention-seeking following social rejection: Links with social media disclosure, problematic social media use, and smartphone stress. *Computers in Human Behavior*, *92*, 65–75.

Henggeler, S. W., Schoenwald, S. K., Borduin, C. M., Rowland, M. D., & Cunningham, P. B. (2009). *Multisystemic therapy for antisocial behavior in children and adolescents*. New York: Guilford Press.

Hinduja, S., & Patchin, J. W. (2008). Cyberbullying: An exploratory analysis of factors related to offending and victimization. *Deviant Behavior*, *29*(2), 129–156.

Hofmann, S. G., Asnaani, A., Vonk, I. J., Sawyer, A. T., & Fang, A. (2012). The efficacy of cognitive behavioral therapy: A review of meta-analyses. *Cognitive Therapy and Research*, *36*, 427–440.

Hofmann, W., & Van Dillen, L. (2012). Desire: The new hot spot in self-control research. *Current Directions in Psychological Science*, *21*(5), 317–322.

Hormes, J. M., Kearns, B., & Timko, C. A. (2014). Craving Facebook? Behavioral addiction to online social networking and its association with emotion regulation deficits. *Addiction*, *109*(12), 2079–2088.

Hou, Y., Xiong, D., Jiang, T., Song, L., & Wang, Q. (2019). Social media addiction: Its impact, mediation, and intervention. *Cyberpsychology: Journal of Psychosocial Research on Cyberspace*, *13*(1), Article 4. https://doi.org/10.5817/CP2019-1-4

Karver, M. S., Handelsman, J. B., Fields, S., & Bickman, L. (2005). A theoretical model of common process factors in youth and family therapy. *Mental Health Services Research*, *7*(1), 35–52.

Kotchick, B. A., Shaffer, A., Miller, K. S., & Forehand, R. (2001). Adolescent sexual risk behavior: A multi-system perspective. *Clinical psychology review*, *21*(4), 493–519.

Krause, C., Barra, S., Landolt, M. A., Bessler, C., & Aebi, M. (2022). Sexualized behavior among adolescents who sexually offended. *Archives of Sexual Behavior*, *51*(8), 4047–4061.

Kross, E., Verduyn, P., Demiralp, E., Park, J., Lee, D. S., Lin, N., ... & Ybarra, O. (2013). Facebook use predicts declines in subjective well-being in young adults. *PloS one*, *8*(8), e69841.

Kunkel, D., Farrar, K. M., Eyal, K., Biely, E., Donnerstein, E., & Rideout, V. (2007). Sexual socialization messages on entertainment television: Comparing content trends 1997–2002. *Media Psychology*, *9*(3), 595–622.

Kuss, D. J., & Griffiths, M. D. (2011). Online social networking and addiction—a review of the psychological literature. *International Journal of Environmental Research and Public Health*, *8*(9), 3528–3552.

Kuyken, W., Fothergill, C. D., Musa, M., & Chadwick, P. (2005). The reliability and quality of cognitive case formulation. *Behaviour Research and Therapy*, *43*(9), 1187–1201.

Labouliere, C. D., Reyes, J. P., Shirk, S., & Karver, M. (2017). Therapeutic alliance with depressed adolescents: Predictor or outcome? Disentangling temporal confounds to understand early improvement. *Journal of Clinical Child & Adolescent Psychology*, *46*(4), 600–610.

Lenhart, A., Duggan, M., Perrin, A., Stepler, R., Rainie, H., & Parker, K. (2015). Teens, social media & technology overview 2015.

Letourneau, E. J., Henggeler, S. W., Borduin, C. M., Schewe, P. A., McCart, M. R., Chapman, J. E., & Saldana, L. (2009). Multisystemic therapy for juvenile sexual offenders: 1-year results from a randomized effectiveness trial. *Journal of Family Psychology*, *23*(1), 89.

Letourneau, E. J., Henggeler, S. W., McCart, M. R., Borduin, C. M., Schewe, P. A., & Armstrong, K. S. (2013). Two-year follow-up of a randomized effectiveness trial evaluating MST for juveniles who sexually offend. *Journal of Family Psychology*, *27*(6), 978.

Lin, L. Y., Sidani, J. E., Shensa, A., Radovic, A., Miller, E., Colditz, J. B., ... & Primack, B. A. (2016). Association between social media use and depression among US young adults. *Depression and Anxiety*, *33*(4), 323–331.

Littell, J. H., Pigott, T. D., Nilsen, K. H., Green, S. J., & Montgomery, O. L. (2021). Multisystemic Therapy® for social, emotional, and behavioural problems in youth age 10 to 17: An updated systematic review and meta-analysis. *Campbell Systematic Reviews*, *17*(4), e1158.

Liu, J., Nie., J., & Wang, Y. (2017). Effects of group counseling programs, cognitive behavioral therapy and sports intervention on internet addiction in East Asia: A systematic review and meta analysis. *International Journal of Environmental Research and Public Health, 14*(12), 1–17.

Mai, Y., Hu, J., Yan, Z., Zhen, S., Wang, S., & Zhang, W. (2012). Structure and function of maladaptive cognitions in Pathological Internet Use among Chinese adolescents. *Computers in Human Behavior*, *28*(6), 2376–2386.

Moreno, M. A., & Kolb, J. (2012). Social networking sites and adolescent health. *Pediatric Clinics of North America, 59*(3), 601–612. http://dx.doi.org/10.1016/j.pcl.2012.03.023

Moreno, M. A., Parks, M. R., Zimmerman, F. J., Brito, T. E., & Christakis, D. A. (2009). Display of health risk behaviors on MySpace by adolescents: prevalence and associations. *Archives of Pediatrics & Adolescent Medicine*, *163*(1), 27–34.

Mousa, S. E. A. (2023). The effectiveness of cognitive-behavioral therapy in alleviating social media addiction among university youth groups. *Egyptian Journal of Social Work, 15*, 175–200. Retrieved from http://ejsw.journals.ekb.eg/

Mulligan, C. A., Ayoub, J., & Kostelnik, C. E. (2016). *Sexually harmful youth: Successful reintegration to school*. Springer Science + Business Media. https://doi.org/10.1007/9783-319-47397-0

Naglieri, J. A., & Goldstein, S. (2013). *Comprehensive executive functioning inventory*. Toronto: MultiHealth Systems.

Noll, J. G., Shenk, C. E., Barnes, J. E., & Haralson, K. J. (2013). Association of maltreatment with high-risk Internet behaviors and offline encounters. *Pediatrics, 132*(2), 510–517. https://doi.org/10.1542/peds.2012-1281

O'Keefe, G. S., & Clarke-Pearson, K. (2011). Clinical report: The impact of social media on children, adolescents, and families. *Pediatrics, 127*(4), 800–804. https://doi.org/10.1442/peds.20110054

Omori, K., Zhang, Y. B., Allen, M., Ota, H., & Imamura, M. (2011). Japanese college students' media exposure to sexually explicit materials, perceptions of women, and sexually permissive attitudes. *Journal of Intercultural Communication Research, 40*, 93–110. https://doi.org/10.1080/17475759.2011.581031

Padesky, C. A. (1993). *Socratic questioning: Changing minds or guiding discovery*. London: Paper presented at the A keynote address delivered at the European Congress of Behavioural and Cognitive Therapies.

Padesky, C. A., & Beck, A. T. (2003). Science and philosophy: Comparison of cognitive therapy and rational emotive behavior therapy. *Journal of Cognitive Psychotherapy, 17*(3), 211–224.

Peluchette, J., & Karl, K. (2009). Examining students' intended image on Facebook: "What were they thinking?!". *Journal of Education for Business, 85*, 30–37. https://doi.org/10.1080/08832320903217606

Peter, J., & Valkenburg, P. M. (2010). Processes underlying the effects of adolescents' use of sexually explicit Internet material: The role of perceived realism. *Communication Research, 37*, 375–399. https://doi.org/10.1177/0093650210362464

Pew Research Study (2022). Internet, smartphone and social media use. Retrieved from https://www.pewresearch.org/global/2022/12/06/internet-smartphone-and-social-mediause-in-advanced-economies-2022/

Pfeffer, B., Ellsworth, T. R., & Gold, M. A. (2017). Interviewing adolescents about sexual matters. *Pediatric Clinics of North America, 64*(2), 291–304. https://doi.org/10.1016/j.pcl.2016.11.001

Pichardo, C., Romero-López, M., Ruiz-Durán, A., & García-Berbén, T. (2021). Executive functions and problematic internet use among university students: The mediator role of self esteem. *Sustainability, 13*(19), 11003. MDPI AG. http://dx.doi.org/10.3390/su131911003

Plackett, R., Blyth, A., & Schartau, P. (2023). The impact of social media use interventions on mental well-being: Systematic review. *Journal of Medical Internet Research, 25*, e44922. https://doi.org/10.2196/44922

Pontes, H. M., Taylor, M., & Stavropoulos, V. (2018). Beyond "Facebook addiction": The role of cognitive-related factors and psychiatric distress in social networking site addiction. *Cyberpsychology, Behavior, and Social Networking, 21*(4), 240–247.

Preschl, B., Maercker, A., & Wagner, B. (2011). The working alliance in a randomized controlled trial comparing online with face-to-face cognitive-behavioral therapy for depression. *BMC Psychiatry, 11*(1), Article e189. https://doi.org/10.1186/1471-244X-11189

Radovic, A., Gmelin, T., Stein, B. D., & Miller, E. (2017). Depressed adolescents' positive and negative use of social media. *Journal of Adolescence, 55*, 5–15.

Reynolds, C. R., & Kamphaus, R. W. (2015). *Behavior assessment system for children* (3rd ed.). Bloomington, MN: Pearson.

Riddle, K., & De Simone, J. J. (2013). A Snooki effect? An exploration of the surveillance subgenre of reality T.V. and viewers' beliefs about the "real" real world. *Psychology of Popular Media Culture, 2*, 237–250. https://doi.org/10.1037/ppm0000005

Ringrose, J., & Eriksson Barajas, K. (2011). Gendered risks and opportunities? Exploring teen girls' digitised sexual identities in postfeminist media contexts. *International Journal of Media and Cultural Politics, 7*, 121–138. https://doi.org/10.1386/macp.7.2.121_1

Ryan, T., Chester, A., Reece, J., & Xenos, S. (2014). The uses and abuses of Facebook: A review of Facebook addiction. *Journal of Behavioral Addictions, 3*(3), 133–148.

Sauer-Zavala, S., Boswell, J. F., Gallagher, M. W., Bentley, K. H., Ametaj, A., & Barlow, D. H. (2012). The role of negative affectivity and negative reactivity to emotions in predicting outcomes in the unified protocol for the transdiagnostic treatment of emotional disorders. *Behaviour Research and Therapy, 50*, 551–557. https://doi.org/10.1016/j.brat.2012.05.005

Savina, E., Mills, J. L., Atwood, K., & Cha, J. (2017). Digital media and youth: A primer for school psychologists. *Contemporary School Psychology, 21*(1), 80–91. https://doi.org/10.1007/s40688-017-0119-0

Schladale, J. (2010). Enhancing community collaboration to stop sexual harm by youth. In K. Harrison (Ed.), *Managing high risk sex offenders in the community: Risk management, treatment and social responsibility* (pp. 172–184). London: Willan Publishing.

Seto, M. C., & Lalumière, M. L. (2010). What is so special about male adolescent sexual offending? A review and test of explanations through meta-analysis. *Psychological Bulletin, 136*(4), 526–575. https://doi.org/10.1037/a0019700

Shensa, A., Escobar-Viera, C. G., Sidani, J. E., Bowman, N. D., Marshal, M. P., & Primack, B. A. (2017). Problematic social media use and depressive symptoms among U.S. young adults: A nationally-representative study. *Social Science & Medicine (1982), 182*, 150–157. https://doi.org/10.1016/j.socscimed.2017.03.061

Shirk, S. R., Gudmundsen, G., Kaplinski, H. C., & McMakin, D. L. (2008). Alliance and outcome in cognitive-behavioral therapy for adolescent depression. *Journal of Clinical Child and Adolescent Psychology, 37*, 631–663. https://doi.org/10.1080/15374410802148061

Smith, L. W., Liu, B., Degenhardt, L., Richters, J., Patton, G., Wand, H., Cross, D., Hocking, J. S., Skinner, S. R., Cooper, S., Lumby, C., Kaldor, J. M., & Guy, R. (2016). Is sexual content in new media linked to sexual risk behaviour in young people? A systematic review and meta-analysis. *Sexual Health, 13*, 501–515. https://doi.org/10.1071/SH16037

Sneddon, H., Grimshaw, D., Livingstone, N., & Macdonald, G. (2020). Cognitive-behavioural therapy (CBT) interventions for young people aged 10 to 18 with harmful sexual behaviour. *Cochrane Database of Systematic Reviews, 6*, CD009829. https://doi.org/10.1002/14651858.CD009829.pub2

Stewart, J., Christner, R. W., Mulligan, C. A., & Fox, E. (2024). Harm reduction: An alternate approach to compulsive and addictive behaviors. In R. W. Christner, J. Stewart & C. A. Mulligan (Ed.), *Handbook of cognitive behavior group therapy for children and adolescents.* New York: Routledge.

Stieger, S., & Lewetz, D. (2018). A week without using social media: Results from an ecological momentary intervention study using smartphones. *Cyberpsychology, Behavior, and Social Networking, 21*(10), 618–624.

Tolin, D. F. (2016). *Doing CBT: A comprehensive guide to working with behaviors, thoughts, and emotions*. New York: Guilford.

Tolman, D. L., & McClelland, S. I. (2011). Normative sexuality development in adolescence: A decade in review, 2000–2009. *Journal of Research on Adolescence, 21*, 242–255. https://doi.org/10.1111/j.1532-7795.2010.00726.x

Torbet, P., & Thomas, D. (2005). *Advancing competency development: A white paper for Pennsylvania.* Pittsburgh, PA: National Center for Juvenile Justice. Retrieved from https://www.ncjj.org/pdf/whitepaperfinal.pdf

Turel, O., Brevers, D., & Bechara, A. (2018a). Time distortion when users at-risk for social media addiction engage in non-social media tasks. *Journal of Psychiatric Research, 97*, 84–88.

Turel, O., Cavagnaro, D. R., & Meshi, D. (2018b). Short abstinence from online social networking sites reduces perceived stress, especially in excessive users. *Psychiatry Research, 270*, 947–953.

Turel, O., & Qahri-Saremi, H. (2016). Problematic use of social networking sites: Antecedents and consequence from a dual-system theory perspective. *Journal of Management Information Systems, 33*(4), 1087–1116.

Valkenburg, P. M., Peter, J., & Schouten, A. P. (2006). Friend networking sites and their relationship to adolescents' well-being and social self-esteem. *CyberPsychology & Behavior, 9*(5), 584–590.

Van den Eijnden, R. J., Lemmens, J. S., & Valkenburg, P. M. (2016). The social media disorder scale. *Computers in Human Behavior, 61*, 478–487.

Van Rooij, A. J., Ferguson, C. J., Van de Mheen, D., & Schoenmakers, T. M. (2017). Time to abandon internet addiction? Predicting problematic internet, game, and social media use from psychosocial well-being and application use. *Clinical Neuropsychiatry, 14*(1), 113–121.

Van Zoonen, W., Verhoeven, J. W., & Vliegenthart, R. (2017). Understanding the consequences of public social media use for work. *European Management Journal, 35*(5), 595–605.

Wang, C., Lee, M. K., & Hua, Z. (2015). A theory of social media dependence: Evidence from microblog users. *Decision Support Systems, 69*, 40–49.

Weir, K. (2023, September). Social media brings benefits and risks to teens. Here's how psychology can help identify a path forward. *Monitor on Psychology, 54*(6), 46–53.

Williams, A. L., & Merten, M. J. (2008). A review of online social networking profiles by adolescents: Implications for future research and intervention. *Adolescence, 43*, 253–274.

Worsley, J. D., Mansfield, R., & Corcoran, R. (2018). Attachment anxiety and problematic social media use: The mediating role of well-being. *Cyberpsychology, Behavior, and Social Networking, 21*(9), 563–568.

Wright, P. (2009). Sexual socialization messages in mainstream entertainment mass media: A review and synthesis. *Sexuality & Culture, 13*, 181–200. https://doi.org/10.1007/s12119-009-90505

Yao, M. Z., Mahood, C., & Linz, D. (2010). Sexual priming, gender stereotyping, and likelihood to sexually harass: Examining the cognitive effects of playing a sexually-explicit video game. *Sex Roles, 62*, 77–88. https://doi.org/10.1007/s11199-009-9695-4

Zhou, X., Rau, P.-L. P., Yang, C.-L., & Zhou, X. (2021). Cognitive behavioral therapy-based short-term abstinence intervention for problematic social media use: Improved well-being and underlying mechanisms. *Psychiatric Quarterly, 92*(2), 761–779. https://doi.org/10.1007/s11126-020-09852-0

PART IV

Closing Reflections

23

CBT CHICKEN SOUP

Collective Wisdom to Bring It All Together

Ray W. Christner and Rosemary B. Mennuti

Throughout this book, we have engaged in a comprehensive exploration of cognitive-behavioral therapy (CBT) and its strong interplay with relational theory. In the front matter, we dedicated this book to Dr. Arthur Freeman. It was through each of our relationships with Art that resulted in us working together and, ultimately, developing a prosperous professional relationship and enduring friendship. It seems only fitting that we conclude this book with a metaphor shared with both of us and many other students whom Art mentored about imagining CBT as the process of making chicken soup.

Art would share a story about his grandmother making chicken soup without a recipe but making it based on how she wanted it to look like, taste like, and smell like (aka, the outcome). At its core, most recipes for chicken soup involve essential ingredients—chicken, water, vegetables, and spices. Yet, the beauty of chicken soup lies in its versatility; each cook brings their unique touch to the recipe, adjusting ingredients, cooking times, and seasonings until they reach the desired outcome, suiting their taste and the preferences of those for whom they cook. Art would highlight the similarity to CBT, which provides a foundational framework—its techniques, principles, and methodologies—but it is the clinician's role to tailor this framework to the individual needs of their clients, much like adjusting a recipe. The relational aspects of CBT are akin to the spices in our soup; they can transform the basic into the sublime, enriching the therapy's effectiveness and enhancing its flavor.

Throughout each chapter of this book, the authors have delved into the intricacies of CBT for children and adolescents with specific concerns, emphasizing the importance of customizing the therapeutic experience to address the unique personality of each student. To varying degrees, they skillfully explored integrating relational dynamics into the fabric of CBT. The relational factors are evident in every chapter, supporting its value in our work with children. However, even more important is the approach at which authors used relationship with specific areas of concerns and the child's relational abilities. It is the personalization and the deep understanding connection that help merge CBT and relational theories. Our aim in using the Integrative-Relational Model of CBT is to recognize that the therapeutic relationship is not just a backdrop but a central thread that runs throughout each interaction and intervention. The integration is not merely an addition but a seamless weaving of relational considerations throughout all components of CBT, ensuring that the therapy is not only effective but also deeply meaningful to the individual's experiences, preferences, needs, and goals.

Tailoring evidence-based theoretical model and application of CBT to the individual involves an acute understanding of the person sitting across from us—their history, story, struggles, strengths, and relational landscape. Intervention requires a dynamic and flexible approach, where the clinician is a

DOI: 10.4324/9781003392439-27

guide, coach, collaborator, and support, navigating the therapeutic process with sensitivity, creativity, and connection. This process is not linear but an interactive practice of exploration, understanding, intervention, and reflection. Just as a cook tastes and adjusts the soup throughout the cooking process, so too must the clinician be attuned to the individual's responses, ready to modify strategies and techniques to meet the individual's evolving needs best. We achieved our goal of highlighting this by providing evidence-based CBT programs and case examples, illustrating how they can be used in a personalized and relational manner with youth.

As we draw the curtain to conclude this book, it is clear that CBT, much like the process of making chicken soup, is both a science and an art. It combines the solid foundation of evidence-based practices with the nuanced art of relational engagement, offering a rich and flexible framework for addressing a wide range of concerns presented by children and adolescents. Our goal for this book was to provide chapters that not only provide evidence-based programs and interventions but did so while embracing the relational aspects throughout all components of CBT. With this, we hope to impart that relational CBT is not just a method of treatment but a process of transformation and healing—one that is as unique and varied as the individuals we have the privilege to work with.

Our challenge and opportunity as CBT practitioners lie in continuously refining our skills, deepening our understanding, and expanding our capacity for empathy and connection. In doing so, we not only honor the complexity and dignity of those we engage with but also contribute to the ongoing evolution of theory and practice of CBT. We hope that our thoughts encourage you to move forward with curiosity, compassion, and a commitment to the craft of therapy, ever mindful of the profound impact we can have on the lives of those children, adolescents, parents, and school staff who seek our guidance and support. We both thank Dr. Arthur Freeman for starting us on our journey in CBT and encouraging us to push the boundaries. Now, it is time to enjoy a nice bowl of chicken soup.

APPENDIX: REPRODUCIBLE HANDOUTS FROM EACH CHAPTER

Form 1: Clinical Psychological Evaluation Interview Guide

Clinical Psychological Evaluation Interview Guide

Developed by Ray W. Christner, Psy.D., NCSP, ABPP

Identifying Information

Name: ______________________________

Preferred Name/Nickname: ____________ **Date of Birth:** ____________ **Age:** ______

Assigned Sex at Birth: ☐ Male ☐ Female **Gender Identity:** ☐ Male ☐ Female ☐ Transgender ☐ Other: ____________

Educational Level: ____________ **Ethnoracial Identity:** ____________

Preferred Pronouns: ☐ He/Him/His ☐ She/Her/Hers ☐ They/Them/Their ☐ Other: ____________

Reason for Referral

Get to Know the Person (Tell me about you. What are your interests, likes, and dislikes?)

Details About Presenting Areas of Concerns/Differences/Symptoms

Functional Strengths/Impairment (How do these things affect everyday life? When do things go better?)

Why are you looking for support with this now?

What supports, interventions, or accommodations are you aware of?

What is the outcome you are

Clinical Psychological Evaluation Interview Guide
Page 1 of 4

Individual History (This should clarify information provided by the individual/caregiver comprehensive history form.)

Strengths

Family History

Social History

Developmental History

Gross motor difficulties: crawl, walk, bicycle, gym, sports	☐ Yes ☐ No	**Details:**
Fine motor difficulties: tracing, shoe laces, writing	☐ Yes ☐ No	
Language difficulties: words, sentences, pragmatics	☐ Yes ☐ No	
Odd behaviors: rocking, flapping, odd play, self-harm	☐ Yes ☐ No	

Medical and Mental Health History

Because of the relationship between physical and mental health concerns, the evaluating clinician should question and document the following to rule out possible medical causes of symptoms and common sequelae of mental health concerns.

Possible Medical Causes of Symptoms

1. Hearing and vision assessment
2. Thyroid disease
3. Neurofibromatosis (café au lait spots)
4. Potential cases of anoxia (asthma, CF, cardiovascular disease)
5. Genetic syndromes and facial or dysmorphic characteristics
6. Fetal alcohol spectrum disorder: growth retardation, small head circumference, smaller eye openings, indistinct philtrum
7. Physical abuse: fractures, burn marks, unexplained injuries
8. Sleep disorders: enlarged tonsils/adenoids, difficulty breathing, sleep apnea
9. Growth delay or failure to thrive
10. PKU, cardiovascular issues, epilepsy, and unstable diabetes
11. Traumatic brain injury

Sequelae of Some Mental Health Disorders

1. Abuse
2. High pain threshold
3. Irregular sleep, delayed sleep phase, short sleep cycle
4. Comorbid developmental coordination disorder or difficulties with motor skills
5. Eating difficulties: picky eater, not able to sit to eat
6. Evidence of injury from coordination difficulties
7. Sensory issues: visual, auditory, tactile/texture, olfactory, gustation
8. Impulsive actions: spending, sex, driving infractions

Functioning and Lifestyle Issues

Exercise: ______

Nutrition: ______

Self-care, personal hygiene: ______

Sleep routine and quality: Bedtime: ______ Time Asleep: ______ Wake up time: ______ # Sleep hours: ______

Sleep problems (BEARS): Bedtime resistance: ☐ Yes ☐ No Regularity: ☐ Yes ☐ No
Excessive daytime sleepiness: ☐ Yes ☐ No Snoring: ☐ Yes ☐ No
Awakenings: ☐ Yes ☐ No

Adverse Childhood Experiences/Trauma History

Alcohol/Substance Use History

Clinical Psychological Evaluation Interview Guide
Page 2 of 4

Legal History

School/Educational History

Learning Disorders identified: ☐ No ☐ Dyslexia ☐ Dyscalculia ☐ Dysorthographia ☐ Dysgraphia ☐ Dysphasia ☐ Other

Work/Vocational History

Current and Previous Treatments/Interventions/Supports

(Include medical, medication, psychosocial, etc. for the presenting problem)

Current Treatment/Interventions/Support	Dose/Frequency	Duration of Tx	Outcome/Side Effects

Previous Treatment/Interventions/Support	Dose/Frequency	Duration of Tx	Outcome/Side Effects

Important Risk Factors to Identify

Risk Factor	Yes or No	Details and Attitude Toward Changes
Excessive screen time	☐ Yes ☐ No	
Accident-prone	☐ Yes ☐ No	
Extreme sports	☐ Yes ☐ No	
Smoking	☐ Yes ☐ No	
Alcohol	☐ Yes ☐ No	
Drugs	☐ Yes ☐ No	
Financial	☐ Yes ☐ No	
Relationships	☐ Yes ☐ No	
Parenting	☐ Yes ☐ No	
Family conflict	☐ Yes ☐ No	
Discipline issues	☐ Yes ☐ No	
Witness to violence	☐ Yes ☐ No	
Trauma	☐ Yes ☐ No	
Physical abuse	☐ Yes ☐ No	
Emotional abuse	☐ Yes ☐ No	
Sexual abuse	☐ Yes ☐ No	
Foster placements	☐ Yes ☐ No	
Significant losses	☐ Yes ☐ No	
Illnesses	☐ Yes ☐ No	
Other:	☐ Yes ☐ No	
Other:	☐ Yes ☐ No	

Treatment Adherence/Attitudes

Is the individual/caregiver open to medication management? ☐ Yes ☐ No
Can the individual swallow pills? ☐ Yes ☐ No
Is the individual/caregiver open to psychosocial treatments (e.g., behavior management, psychotherapy, etc.? ☐ Yes ☐ No
Is the individual/caregiver open to accommodations/support for home/school/work? ☐ Yes ☐ No
Is the individual/caregiver open to pursuing other medical therapies (e.g., OT, PT, etc.)? ☐ Yes ☐ No
Is the individual/caregiver open to the completion of further psychological/neuropsychological testing? ☐ Yes ☐ No

General Notes & Observations:

Clinical Psychological Evaluation Interview Guide

Page 4 of 4

Form 2: Cognitive-Behavior Case Conceptualization Worksheet

Cognitive-Behavior Case Conceptualization Worksheet

Ray W. Christner, Psy.D., NCSP, ABPP & Rosemary B. Mennuti, Ed.D.

Name: ______________________________

Preferred Name/Nickname: ______________ **Date of Birth:** ____________ **Age:** ______

Assigned Sex at Birth: ☐ Male ☐ Female **Gender Identity:** ☐ Male ☐ Female ☐ Transgender ☐ Other: ____________

Educational Level: ____________ **Ethnoracial Identity:** ____________

Preferred Pronouns: ☐ He/Him/His ☐ She/Her/Hers ☐ They/Them/Their ☐ Other: ____________

Self-View (How do they describe themselves and their interests)
Relational View (How do they see themselves in relationships)
Reported Concerns
Antecedents/Triggers
Developmental Considerations
Ethnoracial/Cultural Considerations
Wellness and Resiliency Factors
Individual – Family – Peer – Education – Employment – Community –
Roadblocks and Barriers to Progress
Individual – Family – Systemic – Teacher/Classroom – Employment –
Readiness to Change
☐ Noncomtemplation ☐ Anticomtemplation ☐ Precomtemplation ☐ Contemplation ☐ Action Planning ☐ Action ☐ Prelapse ☐ Lapse ☐ Relapse ☐ Maintenance

Relevant Assessment Data (as needed)
(e.g., cognitive, academic, broadband & narrow band ratings)

Working Hypothesis(es)

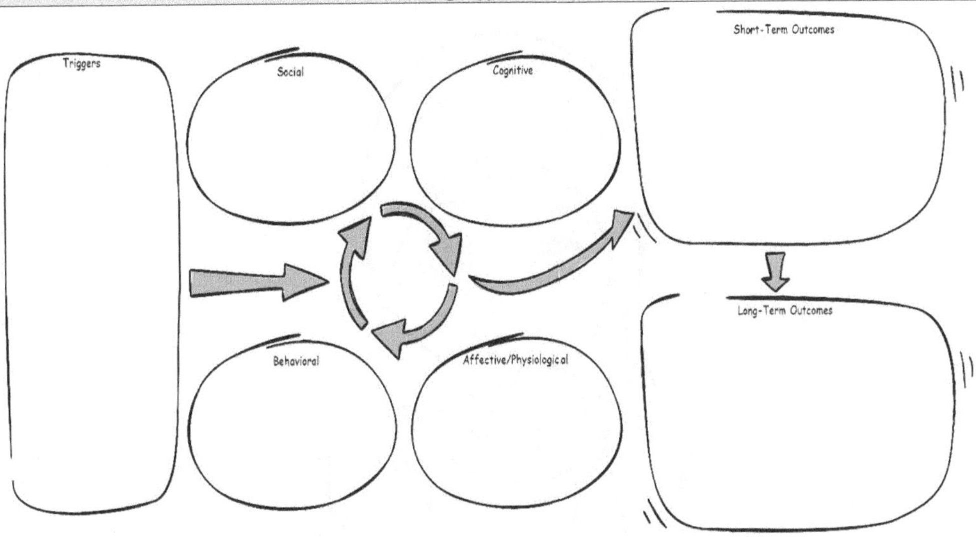

Summary Statement(s):

Diagnostic Impressions/Educational Classification

Goals Setting

1.
2.
3.
4.

Levels of Care

☐ Supportive Care	☐ Group Intervention
☐ Ultra Brief Care	☐ Teacher Consultation
☐ Brief Care	☐ Parent Consultation
☐ Standard Care	☐ Systemic Consultation
☐ Extended Care	☐ Referral to: ________
☐ Other: ________	☐ Other: ________

Frequency of Recommended Services

Initial Frequency: ☐ Weekly ☐ Twice a Month ☐ Monthly ☐ Quarterly ☐ As Needed

Anticipated Number of Sessions:

Form 3: How Does Your Body Feel Today

How Does Your Body Feel Today?

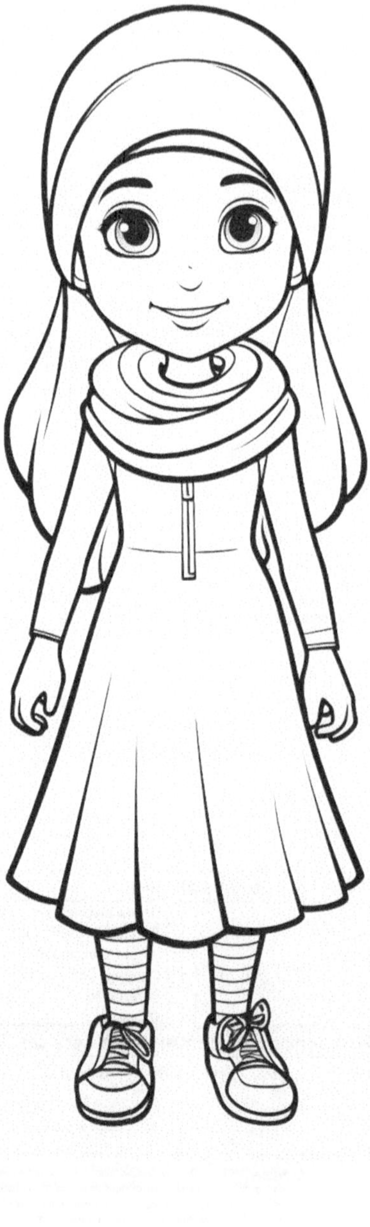

How Does Your Body Feel Today?

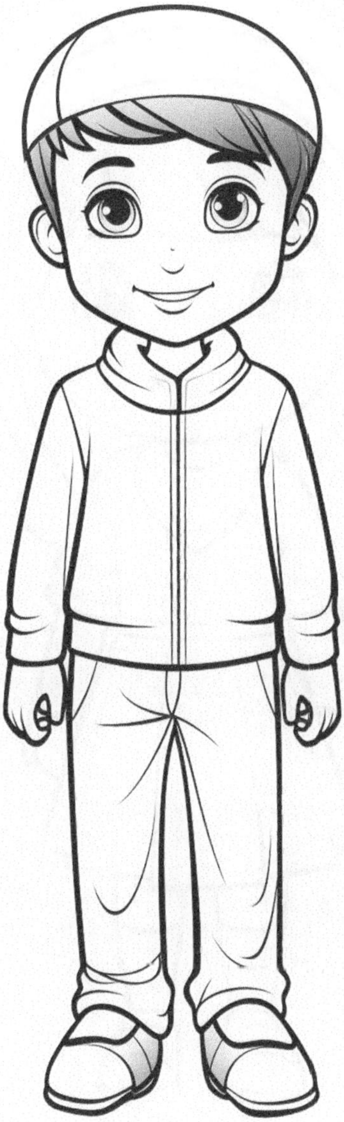

How Does Your Body Feel Today?

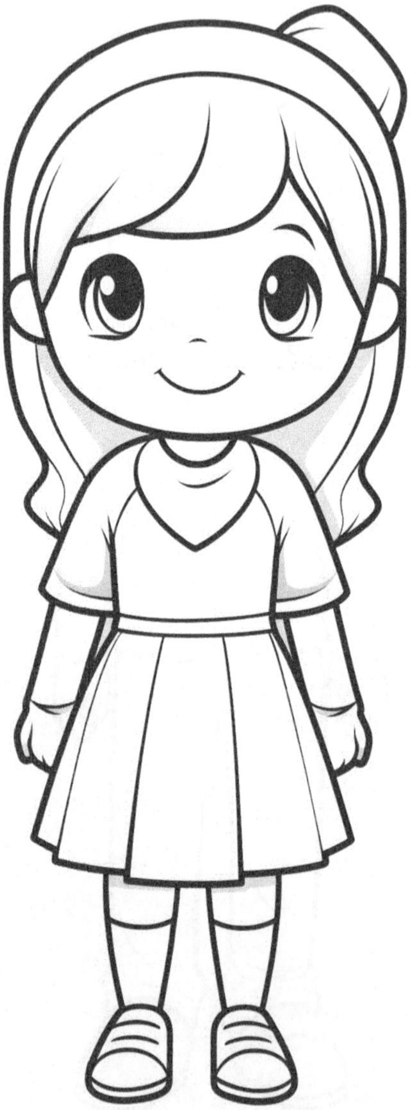

How Does Your Body Feel Today?

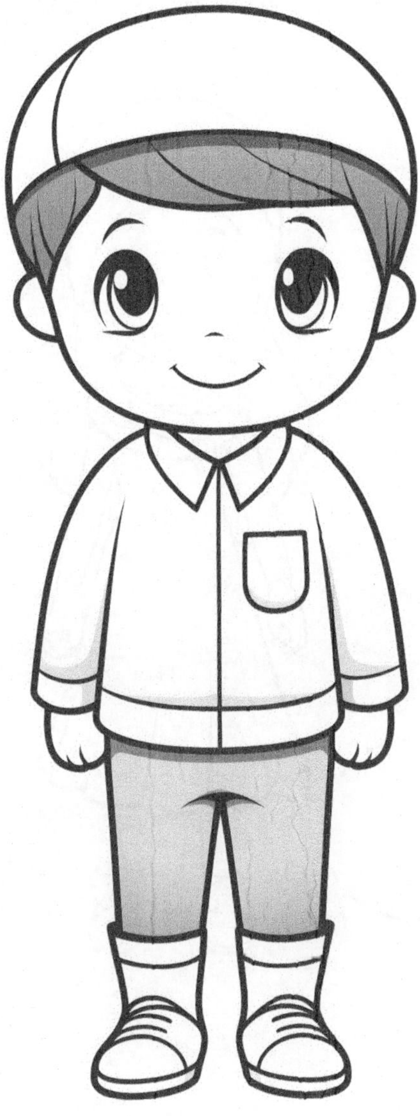

How Does Your Body Feel Today?

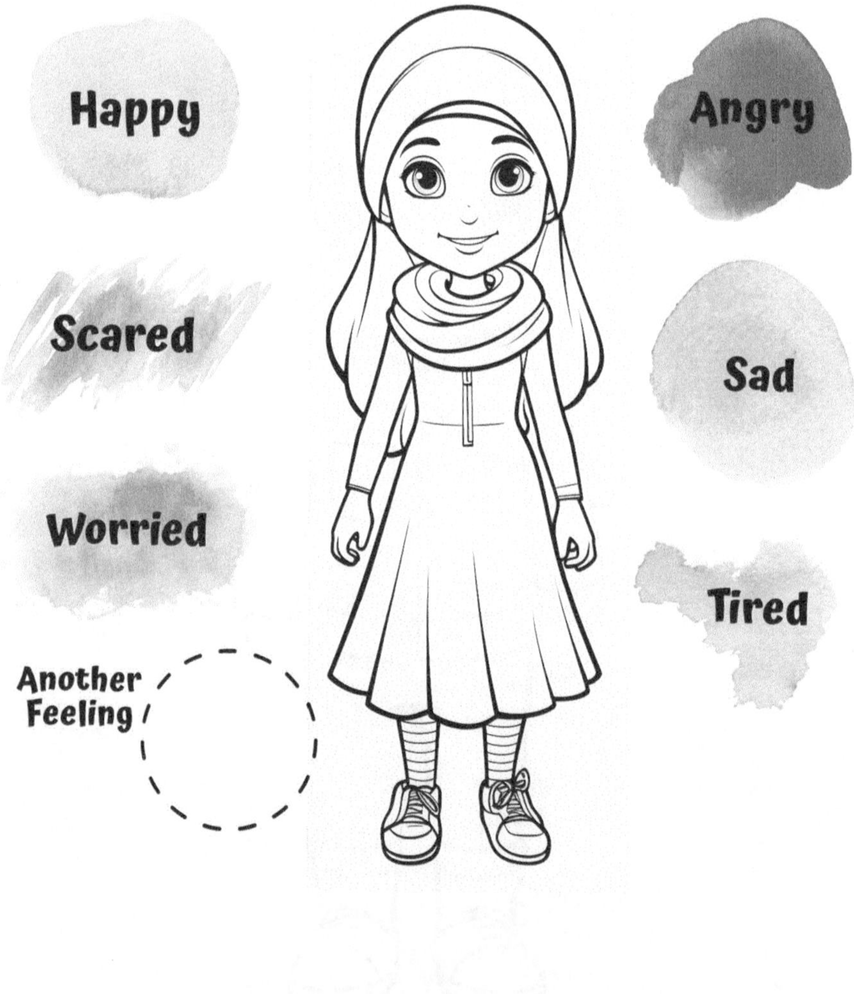

How Does Your Body Feel Today?

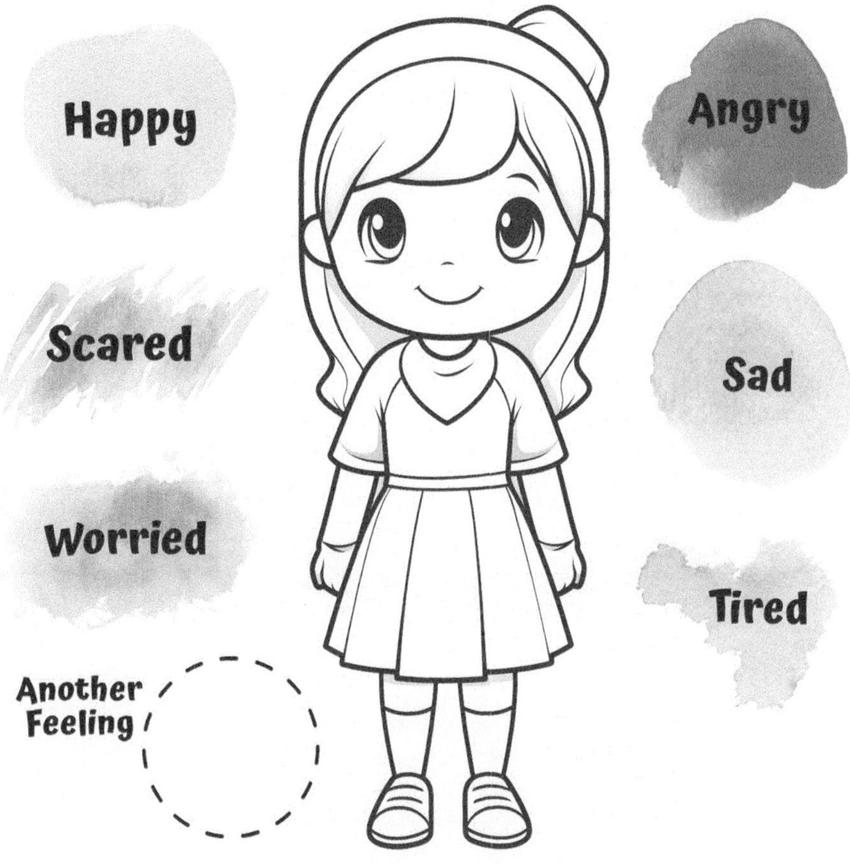

INDEX

Note: **Bold** page numbers refer to tables; *italic* page numbers refer to figures and page numbers followed by "n" denote endnotes.